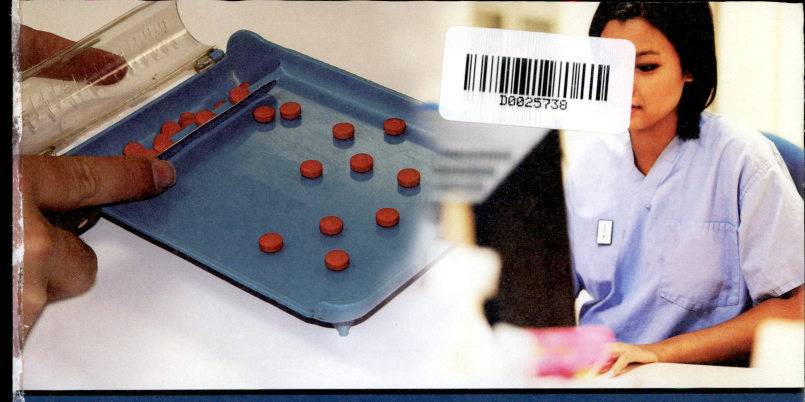

The Pharmacy Technician
FOUNDATIONS AND PRACTICES

MIKE JOHNSTON, CPhT

Karen Davis, CPhT • Jeff Gricar, CPhT, Med

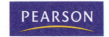

PEARSON

Upper Saddle River, NJ 07458

Library of Congress Cataloging-in-Publication Data

Johnston, Mike, CPhT.
  The pharmacy technician: foundations and
practices/Mike Johnston; contributing authors,
Karen Davis, Jeff Gricar.
    p. ; cm.
  Includes bibliographical references and index.
  ISBN-13: 978-0-13-228309-0
  ISBN-10: 0-13-228309-3
  1. Pharmacy technicians. 2. Pharmacy.
I. Davis, Karen, CPhT. II. Gricar, Jeff. III. Title.
  [DNLM: 1. Pharmacy. 2. Pharmaceutical Preparations.
3. Pharmacists' Aides. 4. Technology, Pharmaceutical.
QV 704 J73p 2009]
  RS122.95.J63 2009
  615'.1023dc22   2008013594

Notice: Care has been taken to confirm the accuracy of information presented in this book. The authors, editors, and the publisher, however, cannot accept any responsibility for errors or omissions or for consequences from application of the information in this book and make no warranty, express or implied, with respect to its contents.

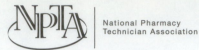

National Pharmacy
Technician Association

The NPTA logo is a trademark of the
National Pharmacy Technician Association

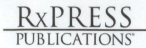

RxPRESS
PUBLICATIONS

The Straden-Schaden and RxPress logos are
both trademarks of Straden-Schaden, Inc.

Publisher and Editor-in-Chief: Julie Levin Alexander
Assistant to Publisher: Regina Bruno
Executive Editor: Joan Gill
Development Editor: Jill Rembetski, Triple SSS Press Media Development, Inc.
Associate Editor: Bronwen Glowacki
Editorial Assistant: Mary Ellen Ruitenberg
Director of Marketing: Karen Allman
Senior Marketing Manager: Harper Coles
Marketing Specialist: Michael Sirinides
Marketing Assistant: Lauren Castellano
Managing Editor, Production: Patrick Walsh
Production Liaison: Julie Li
Production Editor: Trish Finley, GGS Book Services PMG
Media Project Manager: Stephen Hartner
Manufacturing Manager: Ilene Sanford
Manufacturing Buyer: Pat Brown
Composition: GGS Book Services PMG
Director, Image Resource Center: Melinda Patelli
Manager, Rights and Permissions: Zina Arabia
Manager, Visual Research: Beth Brenzel
Manager, Cover Visual Research & Permissions: Karen Sanatar
Image Permission Coordinator: Fran Toepfer
Printer/Binder: Quebecor World Color/Versailles
Senior Design Coordinator: Maria Guglielmo-Walsh
Creative Design Director: Christy Mahon
Cover Designer: Mary Siener
Cover Photos: (top left) iStock; (top right, bottom left and right) photos.com
Cover Printer: Phoenix Color Corporation

Pearson Education Ltd., London
Pearson Education Singapore, Pte. Ltd
Pearson Education Canada, Inc.
Pearson Education–Japan
Pearson Education Australia PTY, Limited
Pearson Education North Asia, Ltd., Hong Kong
Pearson Educación de Mexico, S.A. de C.V.
Pearson Education Malaysia, Pte. Ltd.
Pearson Education, Upper Saddle River, New Jersey

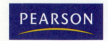

10 9 8 7 6 5 4 3 2 1
ISBN-13: 978-0-13-228309-0
ISBN-10: 0-13-228309-3

This textbook is dedicated to the memory of

Emily Jerry

Emily passed away, at the age of 2,
as a result of a medication error made by a
pharmacy technician. I hope that this textbook,
along with more stringent regulations, will help
prevent such tragedies in the future.

Contents

chapter **4**

Pharmacy Law and Ethics   42

chapter 8

Technology in the Pharmacy 150

chapter 9

Inventory Management and Health Insurance Billing 162

V. Special Topics   681

chapter 32
Pediatric and Neonatal Patients   682

chapter 33
Geriatric Patients   695

chapter 34
Biopharmaceuticals   703

APPENDICES

Preface

Introduction

The Pharmacy Technician: Foundations and Practices addresses today's comprehensive educational needs for one of the fastest growing jobs in the United States: that of the pharmacy technician. The pharmacy technician career is ranked number 60 among the 100 fastest-growing jobs in the United States and 19th among the 500 best jobs for people with a conventional personality type. According to the U.S. Bureau of Labor Statistics, the pharmacy technician career is growing at approximately 30 percent, a much higher rate than other jobs in the health professions. This equates to more than 39,000 pharmacy technician job openings available every year.

In addition to the tremendous workforce demand for pharmacy technicians, professional regulations and requirements are being established for pharmacy technicians across the United States. With many state boards of pharmacy either considering, or having already enacted, requirements for mandatory registration, certification, and/or formal education, the need for a comprehensive and up-to-date pharmacy technician textbook like *The Pharmacy Technician: Foundations and Practices* has never been greater.

Learning Made Easy

The core chapter features include:

- Clearly defined chapter learning objectives inform students of the expected educational outcomes and provide instructors with tools to measure their students' mastery of the material presented.
- Chapter introductions and summaries provide students with a clearer understanding of the scope and rationale for the content being covered.
- Key terms listed at the beginning of each chapter familiarize students with new terminology; key terms are then bolded and defined within the text to reinforce students' learning.
- Numerous full-color illustrations and photographs allow students to visualize content.
- Step-by-step procedures in relevant chapters provide students with clear directions on how to perform the numerous tasks required of pharmacy technicians.
- "Workplace Wisdom" boxes feature tips, comments and advice from a seasoned pharmacy technician.
- "Profiles in Practice" boxes offer practical exercises that simulate real-world pharmacy problems,

giving students the opportunity to apply their learning.

- Chapter review exercises at the end of every chapter assess student comprehension. Exercises include multiple-choice questions, Internet-based assignments, and critical thinking questions.

Organization of the Text

The Pharmacy Technician: Foundations and Practices contains 5 sections and 34 chapters. The following is a brief description of each section and its chapters.

Section I—Introduction to Pharmacy

The first section of the book (Chapters 1–5) provides students with an introduction to pharmacy practice and establishes a framework for the student to build upon. This section includes a comprehensive account of the history of medicine and pharmacy (Chapter 1); an examination of the characteristics, traits, and attributes of a professional pharmacy technician (Chapter 2); a discourse on effective communication, customer service, and patient care (Chapter 3); a detailed explanation of pharmacy law and ethics matters (Chapter 4); and an exhaustive review of medical terminology and abbreviations used in pharmacy practice (Chapter 5).

Section II—Pharmacy Practice

The second section of the book (Chapters 6–11) provides students with an understanding of contemporary pharmacy practice. This section includes a detailed explanation of community-based pharmacy operations (Chapter 6); a thorough explanation of health-system-based pharmacy operations (Chapter 7); an overview of the use of technology in the pharmacy (Chapter 8); an overview of inventory management and insurance billing (Chapter 9); an introduction to nonsterile, or extemporaneous, compounding (Chapter 10), and an introduction to aseptic technique and preparation of sterile products (Chapter 11).

Section III—Pharmacy Calculations

The third section of the book (Chapters 12–17) provides students with systematic understanding of how to properly perform pharmacy and dosage calculations. This section includes a review of basic math skills necessary to perform advanced pharmacy calculations (Chapter 12); an overview of the various systems of measurement used in pharmacy practice (Chapter 13); a detailed explanation of how to do various dosage calculations (Chapter 14);

an introduction on how to perform concentration and dilution calculations (Chapter 15); an overview of how to solve alligations (Chapter 16); and an overview of how to do parenteral-based calculations (Chapter 17).

Section IV—Pharmacology

The fourth section of the book (Chapters 18–31) provides students with a thorough comprehension of pharmacology, including anatomy and physiology. This section includes an introduction to the subject of pharmacology (Chapter 18), an explanation of biopharmaceutics (Chapter 19), and an overview of the various drug classification systems (Chapter 20). It also contains a thorough review of anatomy, physiology, and pharmacology by body system, related to the skin (Chapter 21), the eyes and ears (Chapter 22), the gastrointestinal system (Chapter 23), the musculoskeletal system (Chapter 24), the respiratory system (Chapter 25), the cardiovascular system (Chapter 26), the immune system (Chapter 27), the renal system (Chapter 28), the endocrine system (Chapter 29), the reproductive system (Chapter 30), and the nervous system (Chapter 31).

Section V—Special Topics

The fifth section of the book (Chapters 32–34) gives students an introduction to special considerations in pharmacy practice. This section includes a review of special practice considerations related to pediatric and neonatal patients (Chapter 32), a review of special practice considerations related to geriatric patients (Chapter 33), and an introduction to the use of biopharmaceuticals (Chapter 34).

Appendices

- *Appendix A: Top 200 Drugs* is a current listing of the most-prescribed medications in the United States, in the order of popularity. The drugs are listed by trade name, with generic names and class/indications included.
- *Appendix B: OTC Product Guide* is a comprehensive listing of the over-the-counter medications, devices, and products most often recommended and sold in pharmacies. The products are categorized by use/indication.
- *Appendix C: Advanced Career Path Options* offers students a closer look at various advanced practice settings, including long-term care, home infusion service, mail-order pharmacy, nuclear pharmacy, and federal pharmacy.
- *Appendix D: Professional Resources* provides students with detailed information on certification,

accreditation, regulations, professional organizations, and government agencies.
- *Appendix E: References* offers students a review of the reference and resource books most commonly used in pharmacy practice.
- *Appendix F: Practice Certification Exams* offers students three unique exams that simulate the national certification exam in both content coverage and question format. Each exam contains 100 questions developed using the content outline of the Pharmacy Technician Certification Board (PTCB) national certification exam. Answers to the exams appear in the Instructor's Resource Manual.

The Learning Package

The Student Package
- *Textbook*
- *Student Workbook & Laboratory Manual*: The Student Workbook contains key terms, chapter objectives, chapter outlines, critical thinking questions, practice exercises, review questions, and end-of-workbook tests/case-study-type problems that test student knowledge of the key concepts presented in the core textbook.
- *Companion Website*: Every student will have open access to our online study guide, which contains helpful links, self-test questions, and an online glossary. Students will be able to submit their results for a score that can be sent to a professor or themselves for further evaluation. This resource, combined with the Student CD, gives students the opportunity to put into practice the skills they are being taught in the classroom.

The Instructional Package
- *Instructor's Resource Manual*: The Instructor's Resource Manual contains chapter learning objectives, lesson plans for each learning objective (with a customizable section for instructor notes), teaching tips, concepts for lecture, PowerPoint lecture slides that correspond to each concept for lecture, suggestions for classroom activities, and answers to all of the textbook exercises, including the three practice certification exams located in Appendix F.
- *CD-ROM*: The instructor's CD-ROM has a test generator and more than 3,500 test questions.
- *PowerPoint Slides*: The slides can be used during daily lectures.

About the Author

Mike Johnston is one of the most influential pharmacy technician leaders worldwide. In 1999, Mike founded the National Pharmacy Technician Association (NPTA) and led the association from 3 members to more than 20,000 in less than two years. Today, as Chairman/CEO of NPTA and Publisher of *Today's Technician* magazine, he spends the majority of his time meeting with and speaking to employers, manufacturers, industry leaders, and elected officials on issues related to pharmacy technicians.

Mike serves as the sole pharmacy technician delegate to the *United States Pharmacopeia* (USP) and is the only North American representative member of the Committee of European Pharmacy Technicians (CEPT). He is also a CPE administrator and field reviewer approved by the Accreditation Council on Pharmacy Education (ACPE).

Mike's background includes experience in community-based pharmacy practice, health-system pharmacy practice, and compounding, and as a pharmacy technician instructor. Mike has been nationally certified since 1997 (CPhT) and is also certified in IV/Admixture and Extemporaneous Compounding. He is the author of six previous textbooks on pharmacy technician education and *Rx for Success—A Career Enhancement Guide for Pharmacy Technicians*.

About NPTA

The National Pharmacy Technician Association (NPTA) is the world's largest professional organization specifically for pharmacy technicians. The association is dedicated to advancing the value of pharmacy technicians and the vital roles they play in pharmaceutical care. In a society of countless associations, we believe it takes much more than just a mission statement to meet the professional needs of and provide the necessary leadership for the pharmacy technician profession—it takes action and results.

The organization is composed of pharmacy technicians practicing in a variety of practice settings, such as retail, independent, hospital, mail-order, home care, long-term care, nuclear, military, correctional facilities, formal education, training, management, sales, and many more. NPTA is a reflection of this diverse profession and provides unparalleled support and resources to members.

NPTA is the foundation of the pharmacy technician profession; we have an unprecedented past, a strong presence, and a promising future. We are dedicated to improving our profession while remaining focused on our members.

Pharmacy technician students are welcome to join more than 30,000 practicing pharmacy technicians as members of NPTA.

For more information:
call 888-247-8706
visit www.pharmacytechnician.org

Acknowledgments

The author wishes to give special acknowledgment and thanks to the following individuals, who represent the greatest contributors to this text.

Joan Gill, for your strong leadership, guidance, and insight on this project as executive editor.

Jill Rembetski, for your persistence, dedication, and amazing talent as a developmental editor.

Bronwen Glowacki, for all of your assistance and responsiveness as associate editor.

Julie Alexander, for your ongoing commitment and support as publisher.

Mark Cohen, for your initial efforts in signing me with Pearson Education.

Julie Li, for your attention to detail and assistance.

Contributors

We wish to thank the following individuals for sharing their knowledge and expertise by providing content for specific sections of this textbook and learning package.

Karen Davis, CPhT
Pharmacy Technology Director/Instructor
Southeastern Technical College
Vidalia, GA

Michelle Goeking, BM, CPhT
Instructor
Black Hawk College
Moline, IL

Jeff Gricar, CPhT, MEd
Faculty, Pharmacy Technician Program
Houston Community College
Houston, TX

Michael M. Hayter, PharmD, MBA
Adjunct Instructor, Pharmacy Technology and Health Information
Virginia Highlands Community College
Abingdon, VA

Reviewers

We wish to thank the following individuals for reviewing this textbook for accuracy and providing invaluable suggestions and feedback.

Julette Barta, CPhT, BSIT
Pharmacy Technician Instructor
San Joaquin Valley College
Rancho Cucamonga, CA

Kathleen M. Beall, BS, RT (R)
Clinical Instructor
Pima Medical Institute
Mesa, AZ

Amy Elias, CPhT, RPhT
Instructor
Richland College
Dallas, TX

Michelle Goeking, BM, CPhT
Instructor
Black Hawk College
Moline, IL

Jeff Gricar, CPhT, MEd
Faculty, Pharmacy Technician Program
Houston Community College
Houston, TX

Michael M. Hayter, PharmD, MBA
Adjunct Instructor, Pharmacy Technology and Health Information
Virginia Highlands Community College
Abingdon, VA

Anne P. LaVance, BS, CPhT
Director
Pharmacy Technician Program
Delgado Community College
New Orleans, LA

Michele Benjamin Lesmeister, MA
Renton Technical College
Renton, WA

Chris Neer, CPhT
Lead Pharmacy Tech Instructor
Remington College—Memphis Campus
Memphis, TN

Vincent Range
Assistant Professor of Mathematics
ATS Math Chairman
Jefferson College
Hillsboro, MO

DeEtta Ryan, MBA
Basic Studies Instructor
Renton Technical College
Renton, WA

Paula Denise Silver, BS Biology, PharmD
Medical Instructor
Medical Careers Institute
Newport News, VA

Karen Snipe, CPhT Med
Department Head
Diagnostic and Imaging Services
Trident Technical College
Charleston, SC

Bobbi Steelman, CPhT, MEd, Specialist in School Administration
Pharmacy Technician Program Manager
Draughons Junior College
Bowling Green, KY

Benjamin Walker, CPhT
Program Director
ATI Career Center
Dallas, TX

LEARNING OBJECTIVES

After completing this chapter, you should be able to:

- Describe the health-system pharmacy practice setting.
- Describe the advantages of a unit-dose system.
- List the necessary components of a medication order.
- Compare the duties of a technician with those of a pharmacist in accep a medication order in a health-system setting.
- Compare centralized and decentralized unit-dose s
- Compare the duties of a technician with those of a medication order in a health-system setting.

◄ Learning Objectives

Each chapter opens with a list of **learning objectives**, which can be used to identify the material and skills the student should know upon successful completion of the chapter.

KEY TERMS

adjudication 124

Certified Pharmacy Technician (CPhT) 116

chain pharmacy 115

counseling 126

DAW 123

doctor of pharmacy (PharmD) 116

franchise pharmacy 115

front end 116

household system 125

neighborhood pharmacy 115

◄ Key Terms

The **Key Terms** section appears at the beginning of each chapter. The terms are listed in alphabetical order and the terminology appears in boldface on first introduction in the text. A feature in the margin gives the definition of the term so that students have definitions immediately available in the context of the chapter content.

INFORMATION

Voicemails and Patient Confidentiality

Patient confidentiality is a major issue in all pharmacy work, but you must take special care regarding confidentiality when leaving voicemail messages. If you are calling a doctor's office to get a refill authorization, at the patient's request, obviously you will need to provide detailed information, including the patient's name and the medication. If, however, you are leaving a voicemail for the patient, on either a home answering machine or a work voicemail, it is inappropriate to include any detailed or confidential information. A proper message would be: "Hello, this is Brad with Main Street Pharmacy calling to speak with Ms. Chan. You can call me back at 281-555-7900. Again, this is Brad at Main Street Pharmacy. The telephone number is 281-555-7900. Thank you."

◄ Information Boxes

Information boxes containing additional historical, technical, or interesting content related to the chapter appear throughout each chapter.

PROFILES IN PRACTICE

Tabitha works as a pharmacy technician at a chain retail pharmacy. A new patient arrived and requested to have a prescription filled, but was unable to complete the patient profile form when asked to do so. Tabitha's patient is illiterate.

- How can Tabitha assist without embarrassing the patient?

◄ Profiles in Practice

Profiles in Practice boxes in each chapter feature short scenarios that depict realistic pharmacy problems. Students use knowledge they have gained from the chapter to answer the critical thinking questions related to the scenario.

Workplace Wisdom Telephone Tips

Here are some tips on telephone-based communication:

- Use a pleasant and professional tone of voice.
- State your name and place of business.
- If answering a phone call, ask how you can help the caller.
- If making a phone call, explain your need or objective.
- If taking a message, document the items listed below under "Receiving a Voicemail."

◄ Workplace Wisdom

Workplace Wisdom boxes interspersed throughout each chapter offer helpful tips, comments, and additional resources and provide additional information the student might use on the job.

Chapter Summary

Each **chapter summary** is an excellent review of the chapter content.

Chapter Review Questions

Multiple-choice questions appear at the end of every chapter to measure the student's understanding and retention of the material presented in the chapter. These tools are available for use by the student or can be used by the instructor as an outcome assessment. Answers appear in the *Instructor's Resource Manual.*

> **CHAPTER REVIEW QUESTIONS**
>
> 1. Which of the following is not an example of an ambulatory or retail pharmacy?
>   a. franchise or chain pharmacy
>   b. nursing home pharmacy
>   c. privately owned pharmacy
>   d. all of the above are examples
> 2. The term *ambulatory pharmacy* refers to a setting in which:
>   a. the patient arrives by ambulance.
>   b. the patient lives at the facility where the pharmacy is located.
>   c. the patient "walks" into the pharmacy.
>   d. the pharmacy is part of a larger facility.
> 3. Which of the following need not be recorded on a prescription?
>   a. prescriber's signature
>   b. patient's age
>   c. medication quantity and strength
>   d. patient's complete name
> 4. A prescription must contain the following drug information:
>   a. name of the medication
>   b. strength
>   c. dosage form
>   d. all of the above
> 5. Which of the following is not the responsibility of a pharmacy technician?
>   a. verifying the patient's name, address, and telephone number
>   b. checking for drug name, quantity, strength, dose, and route
>   c. verifying the final prescription
>   d. entering and billing insurance

Critical Thinking Questions

Thought-provoking **critical thinking questions** appear at the end of chapters to test student comprehension on the chapter content. Students must rely on the content in the text and their own critical thinking skills to answer the questions. Answers appear in the *Instructor's Resource Manual.*

> **CRITICAL THINKING QUESTIONS**
>
> 1. List the Five Rights and discuss the potential consequences of not adhering to each.
> 2. In what ways are defense mechanisms and conflict connected?
> 3. Why are pharmacist consultations important, and why are they considered outside the scope of practice for pharmacy technicians?

Web Challenges

Web challenges at the end of chapters lead students to perform Internet research related to a chapter's content on the Internet, and then either answer questions related to their search, or prepare information about what they have discovered.

> **WEB CHALLENGE**
>
> 1. Go to http://thomas.loc.gov/ and search for the 2005 Patient's Bill of Rights. Print a copy of the complete act to read.
> 2. Go to http://www.funquizcards.com/quiz/personality/what-is-your-communication-style.php and take the online "What is Your Communication Style?" quiz. Print your assessment.

References and Resources

This listing at the end of each chapter provides additional information (organization contact information, Web sites, etc.) that is related to chapter content, as well as location information for references used in preparation of the text.

> **REFERENCES AND RESOURCES**
>
> Carrasquillo, O, Orav, EJ, Brennan, TA, & Burstin, HR. Impact of language barriers on patient satisfaction in an emergency department. *J Gen Intern Med.* 1999;4:82–87.
> Conflict Resolution Network: www.crnhq.org
> Gandhi, JK, Burstin, HR, Cook, EF, et al. Drug complications in outpatients. *J Gen Intern Med.* 1998;15:149–154.
> HPSO. Overcoming the language barrier. http://www.hpso.com/newsletters/1-2000flash.html
> Hu, DJ, & Covell, RM. Health care usage by Hispanic outpatients as a function of primary language. *West J Med.* 1998;144:490–493.
> Johnston, M. *Certification Exam Review.* Upper Saddle River, NJ: Pearson, 2005.
> Johnston, M. *Fundamentals of Pharmacy Practice.* Upper Saddle River, NJ: Pearson, 2005.
> Kirkman-Liff, B, & Mondragon, D. Language of interview: Relevance for research of Southwest Hispanics. *Am J Public Health.* 1991;81:1399–1404.
> Morales, LS, Cunningham, WE, Brown, JA, Honghu, L, & Hays, RD. Are Latinos less satisfied with communication by health care providers? *J Gen Intern Med.* 1999;14:400–407.
> National Assessment of Adult Literacy (NAAL). U.S. National Center for Education Statistics. 2005.
> U.S. Census Bureau, DP-2. *Profile of Selected Social Characteristics: 2000.* http://factfinder.census.gov
> UNESCO Institute for Statistics. *Data Centre Summary.* 2005.
> Weinick, RM, & Krauss, NA. Racial and ethnic differences in children's access to care. *Am J Public Health.* 2001;90:1771–1774.
> Woloshin, S, Schwartz, LM, Katz, SJ, & Welch, HG. Is language a barrier to the use of preventive services? *J Gen Intern Med.* 1997;12:472–477. [PubMed].
> Workman, TE, & Lombardo, NT. *Overcoming Language Barriers.* Binghamton, NY: Haworth Press, 2003.

PROCEDURE 9-1

Ordering Medications

1. Generate an order.
2. Review the order.
3. Confirm the order.
4. Submit the order.

◀ **Procedures**
Step-by-step **procedures** appear where relevant throughout the text to help students systematically work through processes and procedures they will perform on the job.

example 15.3

30 g of a compounded ointment contains 105 mg of neomycin sulfate. What is the final concentration (w/w)?

Let's look at the information that has been provided and is critical to solving the calculation:

0.105 g	amount of active ingredient
not provided	amount of base
30 g	total quantity

◀ **Examples**
Numerous **examples** appear in the Pharmacy Calculations chapters to help students visualize the most effective ways to work through different problem types.

PRACTICE Problems 13.1

Write the following metric measures using correct abbreviations denoting unit of measure.

1. five micrograms _____
2. two tenths of a milligram _____
3. sixteen grams _____
4. five hundredths of a kilogram _____
5. ten milliliters _____
6. three and one tenth liters _____
7. two tenths of a microgram _____
8. five hundred milligrams _____
9. six hundredths of a gram _____
10. one hundred milliliters _____
11. forty-one liters _____

◀ **Practice Problems**
Practice problems are also interspersed throughout the Pharmacy Calculations chapters to give students ample opportunities to apply the information they have learned in the chapter.

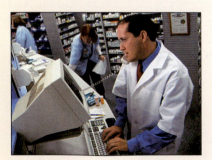

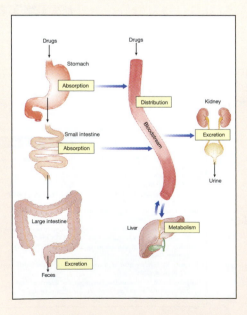

◀ **Illustrations and Photos**
Numerous **full color illustrations and photos** appear throughout the chapters to provide students with visuals and comparisons to reinforce the lesson.

Fundamentals of
Pharmacy Practice

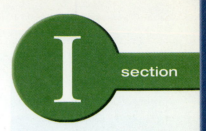

History of Pharmacy Practice

LEARNING OBJECTIVES

After completing this chapter, you should be able to:

- Describe the origins of the practice of pharmacy from the Age of Antiquity.
- Discuss changes in the practice of pharmacy during the Middle Ages.
- Describe changes in the practice of pharmacy during the Renaissance.
- List significant milestones for the practice of pharmacy from the 18th, 19th, and 20th centuries.
- Discuss the role biotechnology and genetic engineering could have on the future of pharmacy practice.

Introduction

Pharmacy is an ancient profession. Although the word *pharmacy* comes from the ancient Greek word *pharmakon*, meaning "drug," the actual origin of pharmacy practice has been traced back to ancient times, more than 7,000 years ago.

At first glance, the history of pharmacy practice may seem to be an unnecessary or nonsubstantive topic of study for someone who is preparing to become a pharmacy technician. However, if you are to understand many of the concepts, theories, and practices that are covered in the following chapters, you must understand the evolution of the profession. Many of the principles used in pharmacy thousands of years ago are still practiced today. In addition, you will be able to better appreciate the areas in which the profession has evolved and how professional guidelines and regulations have developed.

pharmacy the art and science of preparing and dispensing medication.

FIGURE 1-1 The Rx symbol.

The Age of Antiquity

The Age of Antiquity refers to the time span of 5000 BCE (BC) up through CE (AD) 499. This is the time of ancient humans and the great ancient empires.

Ancient Humans

The origin of pharmacy can be traced back to the crude and simple discoveries of ancient humans, who are most commonly referred to as cavemen (Figure 1-2). Ancient humans learned from observing their environment, as well as acting on instinct. They watched as both birds and beasts applied cool water, leaves, dirt, or mud to themselves; consequently, these became the first soothing remedies for humans as well. By trial and error, humans learned which plant and mineral remedies worked best, and eventually they began to share this knowledge with others.

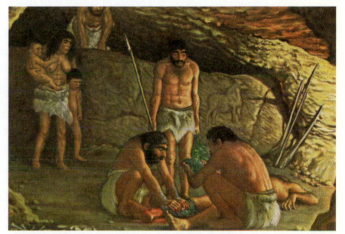

FIGURE 1-2 Ancient humans and medicine. (Used with permission of Pfizer, Inc. Images by Robert Thom. All rights reserved.)

Ancient Mesopotamia

Babylon, which is referred to as the cradle of civilization, provides the earliest known record of **apothecary** practice. Around 2600 BCE, healers were priest, pharmacist, and physician all in one. Archaeologists have found clay tablets that record the symptoms of illness, as well as prescriptions and instructions for **compounding**, or preparing, remedies.

apothecary Latin term for pharmacist; also used as a general term to refer to the early practice of pharmacy.

compounding producing, mixing, or preparing a drug by combining two or more ingredients.

Ancient China

According to legend, in 2000 BCE, Chinese Emperor Shen Nung took interest in and researched the medicinal value of several hundred herbs, testing many of them on himself. Additionally, he wrote the first *Pen T-Sao*, or native herbal, recording 365 drugs. In modern times, Shen Nung is still worshipped as the patron god of native Chinese drug guilds.

Ancient Egypt

The practice of pharmacy in ancient Egypt was conducted by two classes of workers: echelons and chiefs of fabrication. Echelons were gatherers and preparers of drugs, similar to the modern-day pharmacy technician, whereas chiefs of fabrication were the head pharmacists.

Although our knowledge of Egyptian medicine comes from records made as early as 2900 BCE, the most important Egyptian pharmaceutical document is the *Papyrus Ebers*, written in 1500 BCE. The *Papyrus Ebers* is a collection of 800 prescriptions that specifically mentions 700 unique drugs.

Ancient India

More than 2,000 drugs are recorded in the *Charaka Samhita,* an ancient Indian manuscript originating from as early as 1000 BCE. The *Charaka Samhita,* which means "compendium of wandering physicians," is the work of multiple authors and was written in Sanskrit, an ancient Indian language.

Ancient Greece

Terra Sigilata, or "sealed earth," was the first therapeutic agent to bear a trademark. Originating in ancient Greece prior to 500 BCE off the island of Lemnos, Terra Sigilata was a small clay tablet, similar in size to an aspirin. Each year, the people of Lemnos dug clay from a pit on a Lemnian hillside in the presence of political and religious leaders. The clay was washed, refined, shaped into uniform tablets, impressed with an official seal, sun-dried, and then distributed commercially. Thus, it is a precursor to today's modern branded and marketed drugs.

Theophrastus, one of the greatest early Greek philosophers and natural scientists, observed and wrote extensively on the medicinal qualities of herbs. He was known as the father of botany, and his observations and writings, which date back to about 300 BCE, were surprisingly accurate, as measured by present research and knowledge.

Hippocrates

Hippocrates of Cos (Figure 1-3) was an ancient Greek physician who lived between 460 BCE and 377 BCE. He was a third-generation physician, philosopher, and professor at the Cos School of Medicine. Known as the father of medicine, Hippocrates is commonly regarded as one of the most notable figures of all time in medicine. One of his writings, *Corpus Hippocraticum,* rejected the widely held view that illness was connected to mystical or demonic forces; instead, it positioned medicine as a branch of science.

Hippocrates developed the theory of humors, in which an individual's health was supposed to be connected to the harmony among or balance of four basic bodily fluids, known as *humors,* which also related to a mood or personality characteristic: blood (joyful/happy), phlegm (lethargic), yellow bile (irritable), and dark or black bile (angry).

In total, Hippocrates published more than 70 writings related to or referencing the practice of medicine and apothecary. Modern physicians still take the Hippocratic Oath, as part of which they pledge to "do no harm."

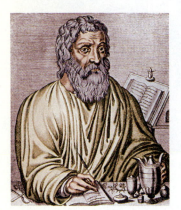

FIGURE 1-3 Hippocrates of Cos. (Stock Montage/Hulton Archive/Getty Images.)

Ancient Rome

Mithridates VI, King of Pontus, is known for developing poisons, as well as poison preventives and treatments around 100 BCE. He used himself and his prisoners as subjects on which to test poisons and antidotes.

During the first century of the common era, another Roman named Pedanios Dioscorides accompanied the Roman armies on their journeys throughout the known world, in order to study medicinal treatments. He recorded his observations and developed precise rules for collecting, storing, and using drugs. His writings, titled *De Materia Medica*, were used by medical professionals as late as the sixteenth century.

Galen practiced and taught both pharmacy and medicine in Rome during 130–200 CE. His principles for preparing and compounding medicines reigned in the Western world for 1,500 years, and his name is still associated with the class of pharmaceuticals compounded by mechanical means—galenicals.

The Middle Ages

The Middle Ages lasted from 500 CE through 1500 CE. Also referred to as the Dark Ages, this historic period is not noted for cultural or scientific progress. However, a number of significant developments took place in the practice of pharmacy.

Monasteries

During the Middle Ages, pharmacy and medicine were practiced and preserved in the monasteries; scientists are known to have been taught in the cloisters as early as the seventh century. The monks gathered herbs in the wild, or raised them in their own gardens and then prepared them according to the art of the apothecary to aid the sick and injured. Medicinal herb gardens can still be found today at many monasteries, in numerous countries.

The First Apothecaries

Late in the eighth century, the Arabs separated the arts of the apothecary and physician, establishing the first apothecaries (privately owned drug stores) in Baghdad (Figure 1-4). In addition to the Greco-Roman knowledge of apothecary, the Arabs used their natural resources to develop syrups, confections, conserves, distilled waters, and alcoholic liquids. As the Muslims traveled across Africa, Spain, and southern France, they brought this new system of pharmacy with them, and it was eventually adopted by Western Europe, where public pharmacies began to appear. However, it was not until 1240 CE, in Sicily and southern Italy, that pharmacy was separated from medicine. At the palace of Frederick II of Hohenstaufen, who was Emperor of Germany as well as King of Sicily, pharmacists were presented with the first European edict completely separating their responsibilities from those of medical practitioners.

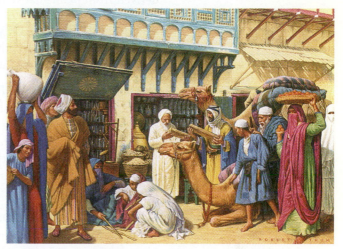

FIGURE 1-4 The first apothecaries. (Used with permission of Pfizer, Inc. Images by Robert Thom. All rights reserved.)

The First Pharmacopoeia

It was in Florence, Italy, that the idea of a **pharmacopoeia** with official status, to be followed by all apothecaries, originated (Figure 1-5). The *Nuovo Receptario*, as originally titled in Italian, was published and became the legal standard for the city-state of Florence in 1498. It was the result of collaboration between the Guild of Apothecaries and the Medical Society, marking one of the earliest manifestations of constructive interprofessional relations. The professional groups received advice and guidance from the powerful Dominican monk, Savonarola, who at the time was the political leader in Florence.

pharmacopoeia a compilation or listing of pharmaceutical products that also contains their formulas and methods of preparation.

The Renaissance

The Renaissance period, which includes the 16th and 17th centuries (1500–1600 CE), was filled with scientific advancements, a renewed interest in culture and the arts, and expanded exploration, which included the European discovery of the New World.

The First Anglo-Saxon Organization for Pharmacists

Trade in drugs and spices had been very lucrative during the Middle Ages. In the British isles, the Guild of Grocers, which represented shopkeepers, monopolized this trade and maintained jurisdiction over the apothecaries. After years of effort, the apothecaries found allies among court physicians; in 1617 King James I granted them a charter to form a separate company known as the "Master, Wardens and Society of the Art and Mystery of the Apothecaries of the City of London"—despite vigorous protests from the grocers. This marked the first organization of pharmacists in the Anglo-Saxon world.

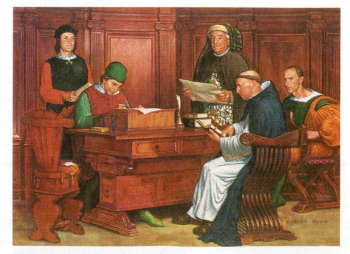

FIGURE 1-5 The first pharmacopoeia. (Used with permission of Pfizer, Inc. Images by Robert Thom. All rights reserved.)

The First Apothecary in the American Colonies

Many Europeans, particularly those who had some wealth and those who were religious nonconformists, were attracted to the opportunities presented by the American colonies. John Winthrop, the first governor of the Massachusetts Bay Colony and the founder of Boston, sought advice from English apothecaries and physicians when he was unable to persuade professionals to emigrate from Britain to the colony. In 1640, he began providing apothecary products by selling imported drugs, as well as those derived from plants native to New England.

The 18th Century

During the 18th century, the American colonies united, fought the British empire to gain their independence, and ultimately formed the United States of America.

America's First Female Pharmacist

In 1729, Christopher Marshall, an Irish immigrant, established an apothecary shop in Philadelphia. Over 96 years, the shop became a leading retail store, one of the first large-scale chemical manufacturers, a training school for pharmacists, and an important supply depot during the American Revolution. Eventually, management of the apothecary shop was taken over by Marshall's granddaughter Elizabeth, America's first female pharmacist.

America's First Hospital

Founded by Benjamin Franklin, colonial America's first hospital was established in Philadelphia in 1751, with the hospital's pharmacy beginning operations in 1752. Although Jonathan Roberts was the first hospital pharmacist in America, it was his successor, John Morgan, whose influence upon pharmacy and medicine made important changes to the development of professional pharmacy in North America. First as pharmacist, and later as physician, Morgan supported the use of written **prescriptions** and advocated for the independent practice of the two professions.

prescription an order, by an authorized individual, for the preparation or dispensing of a medication.

America's First Apothecary General

Andrew Craigie, a Bostonian, was the first man to hold the rank of a commissioned pharmaceutical officer in the American army. Appointed commissary of medical stores by the Massachusetts Committee of Safety, less than two months later Craigie was present at the Battle of Bunker Hill, on June 17, 1775, taking care of the sick and wounded. When Congress reorganized the Medical Department of the Army in 1777, Craigie became the first Apothecary General; his duties included procurement, storage, manufacture, and distribution of the Army's drug requirements. He also developed an early pharmaceutical wholesaling and manufacturing business.

The 19th Century

During the 1800s (the 19th century), America was a young country and the practice of American pharmacy was being established.

America's First College of Pharmacy

In the early 1800s, pharmacists were faced with two major threats: deterioration of the practice of pharmacy as they had known it, and a discriminatory classification by the University of Pennsylvania medical faculty. Pharmacists held a protest meeting in Carpenters' Hall on February 23, 1821, in Philadelphia. At a second meeting, on March 13, the pharmacists voted to form the Philadelphia College of Pharmacy, a school of pharmacy with a self-policing board, which became America's first educational institution for pharmacy.

The American Pharmaceutical Association

In October 1852, Daniel B. Smith, William Procter, Jr., and 20 delegates of the Philadelphia College of Pharmacy founded the American Pharmaceutical Association (APhA) to meet the needs for better communication among pharmacists, standards for education and apprenticeship, and quality control over imported drugs. Membership was opened to "[a]ll pharmacists and druggists of good character who subscribed to its Constitution and to its Code of Ethics."

Workplace Wisdom APhA

After more than 150 years, APhA continues to serve the profession, although it was recently renamed the American Pharmacists Association (APhA). For more information, go to **www.aphanet.org**

The Father of American Pharmacy

William Procter, Jr., is known as the father of American pharmacy (Figure 1-6). In 1837, he graduated from the Philadelphia College of Pharmacy; Procter operated a retail pharmacy, served the college as professor of pharmacy for 20 years, was a leader in founding the American Pharmaceutical Association, served that organization as its first secretary and later as its president, served 30 years on the USP Revision Committee, and was for 22 years editor of the *American Journal of Pharmacy*. In 1869, though retired, Procter continued to edit the *Journal* in a small publication office. He returned to chair the Philadelphia College of Pharmacy in 1872, before passing away in 1874.

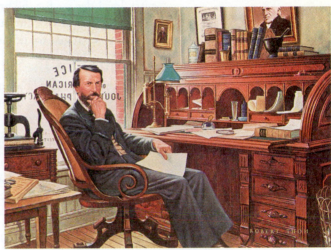

FIGURE 1-6 The father of American pharmacy, William Procter, Jr. (Used with permission of Pfizer, Inc. Images by Robert Thom. All rights reserved.)

The United States Pharmacopoeia

Published in 1820, the first *United States Pharmacopoeia* (USP) was the first book of drug standards to achieve acceptance by an entire nation. In 1877, the USP was in danger of discontinuation, because of a lack of interest from the medical profession, but Dr. Edward R. Squibb, a manufacturing pharmacist and physician, took the problem to the American Pharmaceutical Association, which formed a USP Committee on Revision. The publication quickly regained authoritative stature and continues to be published today.

Workplace Wisdom USP

To learn more about USP standards and publications, go to **www.usp.org**

INFORMATION

The Role of USP in Pharmacy Practice

After more than 150 years, the relevance of the USP to pharmacy practice continues to evolve and grow. Today, the USP is considered the official public standards-setting authority for all prescription and over-the-counter medicines, dietary supplements, and other healthcare products manufactured and sold in the United States. Currently, the National Pharmacy Technician Association (NPTA) serves as an official delegate member of USP, providing insights and a voice for pharmacy technicians.

The Father of Modern Genetics

Gregor Mendel (1822–1884) is known as the father of modern genetics. An Austrian priest and scientist, Mendel showed that the inheritance of traits follows particular laws, through his study of inherited traits in pea plants. The significance of Mendel's work was not recognized until his research was rediscovered at the turn of the 20th century.

The 20th Century

The 20th century (1900s) was a period of impressive scientific discoveries and advancement, including in the field of medicine. In addition, it was in the early 1900s that the federal government began to regulate the practice of pharmacy.

The American Council on Pharmaceutical Education

In 1932, multiple pharmacy-related associations co-founded the American Council on Pharmaceutical Education (ACPE) as an autonomous agency to establish standards for pharmacy education. ACPE initially established standards for the baccalaureate degree in pharmacy, and then added the doctor of pharmacy standards as an alternative. In the year 2000, it announced a conversion to the doctor of pharmacy (PharmD) as the sole entry-level degree for the profession of pharmacy. In 1975, ACPE developed standards for the approval of continuing pharmacy education providers. In 2003, the agency's name was changed to the Accreditation Council for Pharmacy Education (ACPE).

Evolution of the Pharmacist's Role

The 20th century saw the role of the modern American pharmacist evolve through four unique stages or eras: the traditional era, the scientific era, the clinical era, and the pharmaceutical care era.

The Traditional Era

From the early 1900s through the 1930s, pharmacists continued the traditional, pre-existing practice of pharmacy, in which their role consisted primarily of formulating and dispensing drugs derived from natural sources.

The Scientific Era

Beginning in the late 1930s, the practice of pharmacy began to take a significantly more scientific-based approach. This era was marked by the development of new drugs, scientific testing of the effects of drugs on the human body, new regulations pertaining to the efficacy of medications, and the mass production of synthetic drugs and antibiotics. Several factors caused this shift in practice. Both world wars required the production of massive quantities of drugs, both currently existing and newly developed, for the soldiers. A large number of new drugs were discovered and manufactured. In particular, the discovery and development of penicillin-based drugs saved countless lives during World War II. Unfortunately, during this time there were also many recorded incidents of fatalities and adverse reactions to nonregulated drugs.

The Clinical Era

In the 1960s, pharmacy again experienced a shift in practice: with the approval of numerous new medications, pharmacists were now expected to dispense not only medications, but also drug information, warnings, advice, and suggestions to their patients. This era transformed pharmacy into a cognitive-based profession, slightly before the United States as a whole entered the ongoing Information Age.

The Pharmaceutical Care Era

Toward the end of the 20th century, the practice of pharmacy shifted yet again. This time, however, it transformed into a combination of the three prior eras. The practice of pharmacy, and the role of the pharmacist, became focused on ensuring positive outcomes for drug-related therapies. This overarching philosophy, known as *pharmaceutical care*, is actually a combination of formulation and dispensing of drugs (traditional era), a scientific approach to evidence and outcome-based results (scientific era), and provision of expanded consultations and cognitive-based services (clinical era).

Evolution of the Pharmacy Technician

As previously discussed, the role of pharmacy technician can be traced back to the echelons in ancient Egypt. However, this role did not evolve significantly until the late 20th century.

In the early and mid-1900s, pharmacy technicians were referred to as clerks, assistants, or supportive personnel. Most pharmacy assistants were the children of pharmacists and worked at the family-owned pharmacy. Any training they received was informal and acquired on the job.

In the late 1900s, the United States military pioneered the evolution of the professional pharmacy technician, by developing standardized training and competency requirements and delegating more responsibilities to these better-educated technicians.

During the 1990s, the role and recognition of the pharmacy technician began to evolve significantly. Changes included the development of national competency-based examinations, a model curriculum for pharmacy technician training, and greater recognition of technicians in state pharmacy practice acts; in addition, the role of the pharmacy technician became more defined and technicians began to play a role in the governance of state pharmacy associations and state boards of pharmacy.

The Future

As we move further into the 21st century, the future of medicine and pharmacy practice appears to be poised for the greatest and most significant advancements to date.

Biotechnology

Biotechnology drugs are produced using living organisms such as yeast, bacteria, or mammalian cells. Although producing drugs from living organisms is not new, modern biotechnology has greatly expanded the number of different drugs that can be produced by using living organisms.

biotechnology a technique that uses living things to make or modify specific products.

The majority of biotechnology drugs are manufactured through a process called *recombinant DNA technology*, in which a human gene that is capable of triggering the production of a specific protein is inserted into a living organism that is then cultured in a laboratory (Figure 1-7). The organism incorporates the gene into its cell structure, and begins producing the desired protein (drug).

The proteins (drugs) produced by recombinant DNA technology are very fragile, and can be administered only by injection into the vein or under the skin. If taken orally, they would be destroyed by stomach acids and enzymes before they entered the patient's bloodstream.

Some of the drugs now produced by biotechnology were once made by different means. Insulin, for example, was once extracted from the tissue of animals. Most, however, are not producible by other methods.

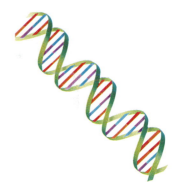

The majority of biotechnology drugs now under development are being tested for use in the treatment of cancer or cancer-related conditions, which could have a major impact on the future health care of cancer patients. Currently, the Food and Drug Administration (FDA) has approved 254 biotechnology drugs for 385 indications.

FIGURE 1-7 DNA and pharmacogenomics: The future of pharmacy.

Pharmacogenomics

It is not uncommon for patients to be given medications that either do not work effectively (for those patients) or that cause unwanted or dangerous side effects. These patients return to their doctors again and again, hoping to find a drug that will work for them. Enter **pharmacogenomics**, a very promising and appealing alternative.

pharmacogenomics the study of individual genetic differences in response to drug therapy.

Imagine that you go to your doctor's office. After a simple and rapid test of your DNA, your doctor changes her mind about the drug she was intending to prescribe for you because the genetic test indicates that you could suffer a severe negative reaction to that particular medication. Upon further examination of your test results, she finds that you would benefit greatly from a new or different drug, and that there would be little likelihood that you would react negatively to it. This is how the promise of pharmacogenomics is portrayed, and it is not as far off in the future as many expect.

According to the Biotechnology Industry Organization (BIO), "the topics of pharmacogenomics, the use of genomic or genetic information to predict [a] drug's efficacy, and personalized medicine, the tailoring of medical treatment to individuals, have been garnering increasing attention in Washington policy circles. BIO member companies are involved in using innovative pharmacogenomics and personalized medicine approaches across the full spectrum of drug development and commercialization. . . . [C]hanges in the regulatory review process and the healthcare reimbursement system are already underway, and will accelerate in coming months and years."

SUMMARY

The practice of pharmacy has deep, historic roots, in addition to an innovative and promising future. Although it has taken 7,000 years of progress, this profession has evolved from applying dirt and leaves to developing genetically tailored medications that are prepared specifically for each individual's unique DNA structure. The key concepts for this chapter include:

- The need for pharmaceutical products, services, and knowledge has existed since prehistoric times.

- As the profession gains new information and technology, pharmacy continues to evolve to better serve patients.

- The role of a pharmacy technician can be traced back to 2900 BCE in ancient Egypt; the responsibilities and opportunities for pharmacy technicians have evolved over time, just as the profession of pharmacy itself has.

CHAPTER REVIEW QUESTIONS

1. Which civilization provides the earliest known record of apothecary practice?
   a. ancient Egypt
   b. ancient China
   c. ancient Mesopotamia
   d. ancient Greece

2. The _____ is an ancient collection of prescriptions, mentioning more than 700 unique drugs.
   a. *Pen T-Sao*
   b. *Papyrus Ebers*
   c. Terra Sigilata
   d. *Charaka Samhita*

3. Which individual is recognized for shifting the view of medicine from the mystic to the scientific?
   a. Hippocrates
   b. Galen
   c. Savonarola
   d. Frederick II

4. Which individual is recognized as the father of American pharmacy?
   a. Christopher Marshall
   b. Benjamin Franklin
   c. William Procter, Jr.
   d. Dr. Edward R. Squibb

5. Which era of pharmacy practice in the 20th century is characterized by new regulations pertaining to medication efficacy?
   a. the traditional era
   b. the scientific era
   c. the clinical era
   d. the pharmaceutical care era

6. Which organization was established to autonomously set standards for pharmacy education?
   a. ACPE
   b. APhA
   c. BIO
   d. USP

7. Who is responsible for separating the practices of pharmacy and medicine?
   a. Savonarola
   b. King James I
   c. Hippocrates
   d. Frederick II

8. The first official pharmacopoeia originated in which country?
   a. England
   b. Greece
   c. Italy
   d. the United States

9. Colonial America's first hospital was founded by which individual?
   a. Benjamin Franklin
   b. John Morgan
   c. William Procter, Jr.
   d. Andrew Craigie

10. Biotechnology drugs are produced by using:
    a. bacteria
    b. mammalian cells
    c. yeast
    d. all of the above

CRITICAL THINKING QUESTIONS

1. In what ways has the practice of modern pharmacy remained consistent from the Age of Antiquity to today?

2. Describe the crucial differences in the practice of pharmacy during the Middle Ages and today.

3. With the evolution of biotechnology and pharmacogenomics, what might the practice of pharmacy look like in the 22nd century?

WEB CHALLENGE

1. Take The University of Arizona's History of Pharmacy Museum Virtual Tour: http://www.pharmacy.arizona.edu/museum/tour.php

2. What are "show globes" and what do most experts agree was their historic purpose? http://www.pharmacy.arizona.edu/museum/globes.php

REFERENCES AND RESOURCES

Accreditation Council for Pharmacy Education: www.acpe-accredit.org

Bender, GA. *Great Moments in Pharmacy*. Detroit: Northwood Institute Press, 1996.

Biotechnology Industry Organization: www.bio.org

Cowan, DL, & Helfand, WH. *Pharmacy: An Illustrated History*. New York: Harry N. Abrams, 1990.

Haggard, Howard W. *Devils, Drugs, and Doctors*. Blue Robon Books, 1929.

Washington State College of Pharmacy: www.pharmacy.wsu.edu

2 The Professional Pharmacy Technician

LEARNING OBJECTIVES

After completing this chapter, you should be able to:

- Summarize the educational requirements and competencies of both pharmacists and pharmacy technicians.

- Describe the two primary pharmacy practice settings and define the basic roles of pharmacists and pharmacy technicians working in each setting.

- Explain six specific characteristics of a good pharmacy technician.

- Demonstrate the behavior of a professional pharmacy technician.

- Explain the registration/licensure and certification process for becoming a pharmacy technician.

Introduction

A pharmacy technician is an integral part of the pharmacy staff and a member of the larger field of health occupations. These individuals are professionals, working within the most trusted profession in America. It stands to reason, then, that a pharmacy technician must maintain specific competencies, undergo specialized education and training, and exhibit key personal characteristics.

This chapter provides an overview of the pharmacy profession, the traits and characteristics of a good pharmacy technician, and the framework within which one prepares for a future as a professional pharmacy technician.

Overview of the Pharmacy Profession

A **profession** is an occupation that requires advanced education and training; each profession generally has a professional association, code of ethics, and process of certification or licensing. Historically, there were only three recognized professions: medicine, ministry, and law. **Pharmacy**, which evolved from the profession of medicine, is the profession of preparing and dispensing medications, as well as supplying drug-related information to patients and consumers.

By definition, a *professional* is any individual engaged within a specific profession. In pharmacy, there are two classifications of practicing professionals: **pharmacists** and **pharmacy technicians**. Pharmacists are educated, skilled individuals licensed to practice pharmacy and dispense medications, whereas pharmacy technicians are educated, skilled individuals who are trained to work in a pharmacy under the supervision of a pharmacist.

Educational Requirements

Pharmacy professionals are subject to regulations that impose educational and training requirements, so that they will have the knowledge base and competencies necessary to practice pharmacy.

Pharmacists

Pharmacists graduate from pharmacy school with a **doctor of pharmacy (PharmD)** degree, although up until the year 2000, the entry-level degree for pharmacists was the bachelor of science in pharmacy (BS Pharm) degree. A PharmD degree requires a minimum of six years of college, which include at least two years of pre-pharmacy study and four years of study at a college of pharmacy accredited by the Accreditation Council on Pharmacy Education (ACPE). Upon completion of the academic requirements, individuals must complete an extensive internship at a local pharmacy under the supervision of a licensed pharmacist. They must then pass a state board of pharmacy examination and register with their State Board of Pharmacy before they can practice as pharmacists.

Pharmacy Technicians

In the past, most pharmacy technicians were simply trained on the job, but on-the-job training (OJT), by its very nature, is employer-specific, and limited to the precise tasks required in the job for which the person was hired. In most cases, OJT does not provide instruction in or guarantee understanding of the theory or background surrounding pharmacy practice. Therefore, formal education requirements, competency exams, and registration with a State Board of Pharmacy are progressively replacing OJT.

Roles of Pharmacy Professionals

Although pharmacy is a collaborative practice, in which pharmacists and pharmacy technicians work as a team, there are specific—and even regulated—differences between their roles, responsibilities, and authority.

Pharmacists

The role of the pharmacist is extensive and varies significantly depending on the practice setting. For example, in a community pharmacy setting the pharmacist might counsel patients about over-the-counter remedies, whereas in a hospital pharmacy setting the pharmacist might advise physicians about the best drugs to prescribe for certain indications. The following information explores the basic duties of a pharmacist, and should not be considered absolute or exhaustive.

The primary jobs of all pharmacists are to dispense medications prescribed by authorized medical professionals and provide vital information to patients about medications and their use. Pharmacists also monitor the health and progress of patients in response to drug therapy to ensure that the medications being used are safe and effective.

Pharmacists in ambulatory (community-based) pharmacies counsel patients about prescription drugs and answer questions pertaining to possible side effects or interactions among various drugs. In addition, they provide information about and make recommendations of over-the-counter drugs and medical devices. Some pharmacists in community

profession an occupation that requires advanced education and training.

pharmacy the profession of preparing and dispensing medications, as well as supplying drug-related information to patients and consumers.

pharmacist educated, skilled individual licensed to practice pharmacy and dispense medication.

pharmacy technician educated, skilled individual trained to work in a pharmacy, under the supervision of a pharmacist.

doctor of pharmacy (PharmD) a doctoral degree in pharmacy practice.

pharmacies provide specialized services to help patients manage specific conditions, such as diabetes, and some are trained to administer vaccines.

health-system pharmacy common name for an institutional pharmacy.

Pharmacists who work in **health-system pharmacies**, such as in hospitals, nursing homes, and long-term care facilities, prepare and dispense medications for individual patients, as well as advising the medical staff on the selection and effects of drugs. They also assess, plan, and monitor drug regimens (see Figure 2-1). Pharmacists also may evaluate drug use patterns and outcomes for patients in hospitals or other institutional settings.

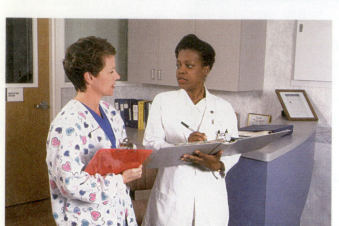

FIGURE 2-1 A pharmacist in a hospital setting often advises other medical personnel or monitors patient drug regimens.

Pharmacy Technicians

As with the pharmacist, the role of a pharmacy technician varies considerably depending on the practice setting and state regulations. The following information explores the basic duties of a pharmacy technician, and again should not be considered absolute or exhaustive.

Pharmacy technicians assist pharmacists to provide pharmaceutical care. It is common for technicians to perform routine tasks, such as computer entry, medication preparation and selection, counting, and labeling. The pharmacist is required to review and verify every prescription before it is dispensed to a patient. Technicians also are required to refer any patient questions regarding prescriptions, drug information, or related health matters to the pharmacist.

In **community pharmacies**, technicians also create and maintain patient profiles, handle insurance (third-party) billing, and manage the inventory.

In health-system pharmacies, technicians may review patient charts, prepare and deliver medications to nursing stations, perform unit-dose packaging, and, if trained and/or certified to do so, prepare sterile products such as intravenous (IV) antibiotics and chemotherapy (see Figure 2-2).

Practice Settings

There are two general classifications of pharmacy practice settings: ambulatory pharmacies and institutional pharmacies. **Ambulatory pharmacies** are community-based pharmacies, and include chain retail drugstores, grocery store pharmacies, home health care, mail-order facilities, and other pharmacies from which patients can obtain medications without living onsite (see Figure 2-3).

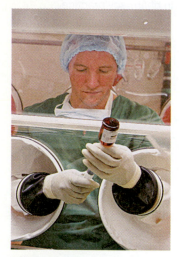

FIGURE 2-2 Trained or certified pharmacy technicians may prepare sterile products.

community pharmacy name commonly used for an ambulatory or retail pharmacy.

ambulatory pharmacy community-based pharmacy; includes chain retail drugstores, grocery store pharmacies, home health care, mail-order facilities, and other pharmacies from which patients can obtain medications without living onsite.

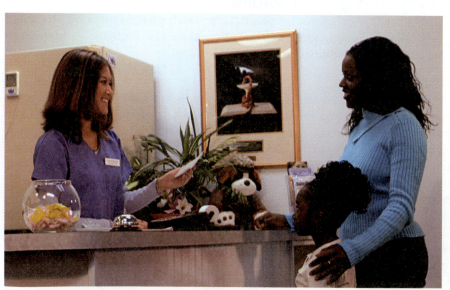

FIGURE 2-3 An ambulatory (community) pharmacy.

Institutional pharmacies, or *health-system pharmacies*, are found in places such as hospitals, long-term care facilities, extended-living facilities, and retirement homes (see Figure 2-4).

A good rule of thumb for telling which is which is that if patients can travel to the pharmacy or have the pharmacy travel to them, they are using an ambulatory pharmacy. If the patients and the pharmacy are housed in the same facility, it is an institutional pharmacy.

institutional pharmacy
a pharmacy found in places such as hospitals, long-term care facilities, extended-living facilities, and retirement homes, which require patients to reside onsite.

Working Hours

Schedules and shifts vary from pharmacy to pharmacy, depending on the practice setting and the hours of operation for each specific pharmacy. Pharmacy technicians routinely work evenings, weekends, and/or holidays; this is particularly true for newer technicians who have less seniority on the job.

The majority of chain retail pharmacies are open seven days a week. Table 2-1 shows an example of the hours and shift schedules for pharmacy technicians at a typical chain retail pharmacy.

Independently owned community pharmacies are typically open on weekdays only, although some may be open on the weekends as well. Table 2-2 shows an example of the hours and shift schedules for pharmacy technicians at a typical specialty pharmacy.

Most institutional pharmacies operate 24 hours per day, and many chain pharmacies now also operate a number of 24-hour pharmacies, dispersed geographically, within a specific city. Table 2-3 provides an example of the hours and shift schedules for pharmacy technicians at a typical 24-hour pharmacy.

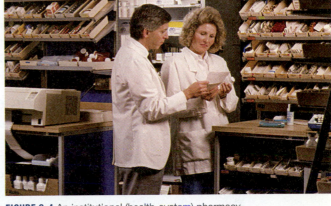

FIGURE 2-4 An institutional (health-system) pharmacy.

Table 2-1 Typical Chain Pharmacy Hours/Shifts

DAY	PHARMACY HOURS	1ST SHIFT	2ND SHIFT	3RD SHIFT
Monday–Friday	8:00 a.m.–10:00 p.m.	8:00 a.m.–4:00 p.m.	11:00 a.m.–7:00 p.m.	2:00 p.m.–10:00 p.m.
Saturday/Sunday	10:00 a.m.–6:00 p.m.	10:00 a.m.–6:00 p.m.	n/a	n/a

Table 2-2 Specialty Pharmacy Hours/Shifts

DAY	PHARMACY HOURS	1ST SHIFT
Monday–Friday	9:00 a.m.–5:00 p.m.	9:00 a.m.–5:00 p.m.
Saturday/Sunday	Often closed both days of the weekend, although this varies by pharmacy	n/a

Table 2-3 24-Hour Pharmacy Hours/Shifts

DAY	PHARMACY HOURS	1ST SHIFT	2ND SHIFT	3RD SHIFT
Monday–Friday	12:00 a.m.–12:00 p.m.	8:00 a.m.–4:00 p.m.	4:00 p.m.–12:00 a.m.	12:00 a.m.–8:00 a.m.
Saturday/Sunday	12:00 a.m.–12:00 p.m.	8:00 a.m.–4:00 p.m.	4:00 p.m.–12:00 a.m.	12:00 a.m.–8:00 a.m.

Staggered 30-minute lunch is included in this time block.

" Workplace Wisdom Work Shifts

First (1st) shift is commonly referred to as the "day shift."

Second (2nd) shift is also known as the "swing shift."

Third (3rd) shift is often referred to as the "graveyard shift."

"

Remember, the pharmacy hours and shift schedules outlined in this chapter are only examples. Each pharmacy will have its own specific hours of operation and schedules, including breaks and mealtime allowances. The schedules described here refer to full-time positions, but numerous part-time positions are available for pharmacy technicians. In addition, some pharmacy technicians work seven days on followed by seven days off, or work 10- or 12-hour shifts, similar to nurses.

Characteristics of a Good Pharmacy Technician

Pharmacy technicians must possess a wide range of knowledge and skills. Successful pharmacy technicians are intimately involved in providing critical health care to all types of people. They operate in strict compliance with written procedures and guidelines and answer directly to the pharmacist for the quality and accuracy of their work. The pharmacist is ultimately responsible for technicians' activities and performance and is their direct supervisor.

Because pharmacy technicians deal with private medical and insurance information as well as dangerous substances, they must act according to the highest ethical and professional standards. Breaches of this public trust can lead to serious consequences. When the one-hour-photo clerk makes a mistake, you lose your pictures and he could lose his job. When a pharmacy technician makes an error, the result can be serious health consequences and even death. Although the pharmacist is ultimately responsible for checking each technician's work, a technician can be held liable in court for errors of negligence or omission.

Display a Professional Manner and Image

"If you aren't managing your own professional image, others are," according to Harvard Business School professor Laura Morgan Roberts. She adds, "People are constantly observing your behavior and forming theories about your competence, character, and commitment, which are rapidly disseminated throughout your workplace. It is only wise to add your voice in framing others' theories about who you are and what you can accomplish."

As defined by Roberts, "Your professional image is the set of qualities and characteristics that represent perceptions of your competence and character as judged by your key constituents." As a pharmacy technician, your "key constituents" are your patients, customers, co-workers, and managers. Among the many attributes that contribute to a professional image, attitude, attire, and grooming consistently rank at the top.

Attitude

attitude a way of acting, thinking, or believing.

Attitude is a psychological concept. It can be positive, negative, or ambivalent, and generally it is a result of social learning from one's environment. When pursuing a professional image, however, a positive attitude is the only option. *Attitude* is technically defined as:

- the posture of the body in connection with an action or mood,
- a way of acting, thinking, or feeling, or
- the position of an aircraft in relation to the horizon line.

These definitions provide tremendous insight. Although most individuals recognize that attitude is a way of acting, thinking, or feeling, many forget the connection between attitude and the posture of the body—this is body language. You can say all the right things and take all the proper actions, but your body language cannot hide your true feelings and attitude (see Figure 2-5).

The last definition may at first seem inapplicable or inappropriate, but under the surface there is a great correlation. The attitude reading on a pilot's flight deck provides her with critical information relating the position of the aircraft in relation to the horizon. If the attitude is in check and correctly aligned, the pilot is then able to proceed safely and increase the altitude (height) of the plane. The same can be said about one's professional image and attitude: so long as it is in check and correctly aligned, the individual will be positioned to advance and grow within his or her profession.

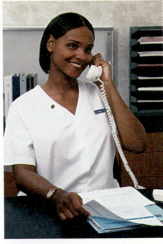

FIGURE 2-5 Displaying a positive attitude, whether in direct contact with customers, with co-workers, or while on the telephone, demonstrates your professionalism as a pharmacy technician.

Workplace Wisdom Tips on Having a Positive Attitude

- Create and maintain a "can-do" mindset.
- Approach and respond to others in a pleasant and upbeat manner.
- Maintain enthusiasm despite criticism.
- Express support, loyalty, and appreciation.
- Demonstrate an "I care" philosophy.

Attire

Attire, or clothing, refers to all items used to cover the body, including the hands, feet, and head. Attire has two primary purposes: function and image. Numerous attire elements are required and necessary when working in pharmacy environments; many (such as gloves, shoe covers, and face masks) are related to specific skills and practice settings (see Figure 2-6).

We discuss personal protective equipment and other items in later chapters. However, there is one common item that both serves as a functional attire element and relates to maintaining a professional image: the lab coat or smock. It is customary for pharmacy personnel to wear a lab coat in all practice settings and, interestingly, it serves both defined purposes for attire, function and image. The lab coat is functional in that it is a protective garment that keeps the individual's clothing from coming into contact with liquid medications, ointments, and chemicals. It also provides the individual wearing it with numerous, spacious pockets for storing reference booklets, notepads, calculators, and pens.

In addition to its functional purposes, the lab coat also contributes to a pharmacy technician's professional image. It is immediately recognizable by patients and customers, and inspires trust in the person wearing it. The public shares an unspoken expectation that a healthcare professional, such as a pharmacist or pharmacy technician, who is wearing a lab coat is knowledgeable and trustworthy.

attire clothing.

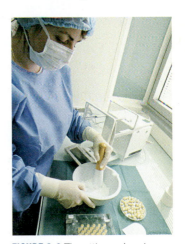

FIGURE 2-6 The attire and protective equipment you use on the job depends on your job function and the practice setting in which you work.

INFORMATION

General Lab Coat Guidelines

- White lab coat (short or long)—pharmacist
- Colored lab coat (short)—pharmacy technician
- White smock—pharmacy technician
- Sleeveless vest—pharmacy clerk/cashier

Most pharmacies also establish a specific dress code for their employees, for the primary purpose of maintaining a professional image. In general, pharmacies use one of two dress codes: business or scrubs.

Business

Pharmacy personnel are expected to dress above business-casual standards; however, the traditional definition of business attire is altered to be practical in the pharmacy environment. Men should wear slacks or dress pants, a button-down shirt, and a tie. Women can wear slacks, conservative skirts, blouses, shells, cardigans, or dresses. Most fabrics are appropriate, but denim is usually not acceptable. Business dress codes are most often adopted by retail-based pharmacies and management at health-system pharmacies.

Scrubs

Many pharmacies require personnel to wear scrubs, a medical uniform consisting of a pullover shirt and pants. The pharmacy will typically predetermine the color of scrubs required, and may or may not issue uniform scrubs to the staff. This dress code is most often adopted by health-system pharmacies.

Grooming

People present themselves to the public in a variety of ways. They may cut, dye, and style their hair; grow facial hair; use makeup or perfume and cologne; wear jewelry; mark their skin with tattoos; or have body piercings. All these options contribute to one's image, but do not constitute clothing per se; these elements are collectively classified as *grooming*.

Pharmacy professionals represent both their employer and the profession in the eyes of patients and customers, which is why it is important for each employee to use good judgment and good habits in grooming and personal hygiene.

Grooming standards will vary, and in some cases be regulated, by practice setting and employer. However, the following are basic grooming standards for professionals:

- Hair should be kept neat, clean, and professional; coloring should appear natural.
- Men should be clean shaven, or maintain a neat, trimmed mustache and/or beard.
- Makeup should be used in moderation and maintain a natural skin color.
- Fingernails should be kept trimmed and clean.
- A single pair of appropriate earrings may be worn.
- Additional piercing and tattoos should not be visible when one is in professional attire.
- Perfume/cologne should be used sparingly, or avoided altogether, at the workplace.

Demonstrate Initiative and Responsibility

Pharmacy technicians should be proactive within their role in the pharmacy and be accountable for the outcomes of their actions and behavior. In other words, a pharmacy technician should demonstrate initiative and responsibility within professional boundaries. The following are some practical examples of how to express these characteristics:

- Use professional resources and references effectively.
- Anticipate problems and develop solutions in advance.
- Become a valuable resource through personal research, knowledge, and networking.
- Brainstorm and suggest innovative ideas and solutions.
- Follow through on all promises and commitments.
- Take full responsibility for mistakes made and learn from them.

Work as a Team Member

The efficiency of a pharmacy depends directly on the effectiveness of its team-centered approach to practice. The best teams have strong leaders, committed members, a shared vision, and effective communication. Although the pharmacist-in-charge

(PIC) or pharmacy manager is the team leader of the pharmacy, your participation and attitude can greatly shape the work outcomes and stability of your team. Here are some specific examples of how to work as a team member:

- View yourself as an integral part of the team, not above nor below it.
- Build positive working relationships with all pharmacy staff members.
- Share information, knowledge, and experience openly with your co-workers.
- Cooperate with other staff members to achieve desired outcomes.
- Be open to feedback from your co-workers, and provide feedback when appropriate.
- Work to remove any barrier to your team's effectiveness.

PROFILES IN PRACTICE

Sharon is the lead pharmacy technician at her pharmacy, having worked there for nearly seven years, and she makes sure that everyone is mindful of her seniority. Sharon refuses to stock the vials, collect the trash, or check out customers, as she feels that she is above these duties.

- What impact does Sharon's perspective likely have on her co-workers?
- How can Sharon improve her professionalism and serve as a better role model for the other pharmacy technicians?

Adapt to Change

The practice of pharmacy is in a constant state of evolution and change. As the demand for pharmaceutical services grows, new drugs become approved, and advances in technology are implemented, the scope and standards of pharmacy practice change. It is imperative that, as a pharmacy technician, you anticipate changes with a positive attitude and a readiness to adapt. Here are some practical examples of demonstrating adaptability:

- Be flexible.
- View changes as progress or improvements.
- Adapt your own attitudes and behavior to work effectively with different people and situations.
- Accept and learn to work with changing priorities, strategies, procedures, and methods.
- Maintain work effectiveness in new or changing situations.
- Handle pressure and stress properly.

Enhance Skills and Knowledge through Continuing Education and Professional Development

The practice of pharmacy is in a constant state of change, especially in regard to updates of medical knowledge and drug information. Every year, new drugs are approved, new generics become available, new indications are issued, and new over-the-counter remedies are developed. Pharmacy professionals are required to undergo continuing education programs for these very reasons. In addition to continuing education (lifelong learning), continuous professional development is also important. Here are some recommendations regarding continuing education and professional development:

- Stay informed by reading trade journals and maintaining active membership in professional organizations.
- Attend pharmacy seminars and conferences.
- Take the initiative to learn new skills.
- Learn from and seek others' ideas, perspectives, and experiences.
- Seek feedback on performance.
- Adopt others' appropriate suggestions for improving your performance.
- Look for new ideas to improve personal, team, and pharmacy effectiveness.

Workplace Wisdom Continuing Education Resources

There are numerous resources with continuing education (CE) programs designed for pharmacy technicians. Typically, CE programs consist of an article with learning objectives and a multiple-choice test, which can be completed online or by mail. Additional types of CE programs include webinars, seminars, conferences, and podcasts. Here are some CE resources for pharmacy technicians:

- www.pharmacytechnician.org
- www.powerpak.com
- www.drugtopics.com
- www.continuingeducation.com

Treat Patients with Compassion and Empathy

compassion a deep awareness of and sympathy for another's suffering.

empathy a feeling of concern and understanding for another's situation or feelings.

It is a basic principle, but one often overlooked: pharmacy professionals serve patients who may be sick and/or in pain. With few exceptions, the customers or patients with whom a pharmacy technician interacts are seeking relief or treatment for an illness, disease, or other medical condition. It is important to treat all patients with **compassion** and **empathy**. Here are some points to keep in mind:

- Treat all people with dignity and respect.
- Be considerate, caring, and kind.
- Focus your efforts on helping the patient.
- Be understanding and forgiving of patients' behaviors and attitudes.
- Assume the best about others.
- Try to imagine yourself in the patient's situation.

Preparing for Your Future as a Pharmacy Technician

registration the process of listing, or being named to a list.

licensing permission granted by a government entity for an individual to perform an activity.

certification recognition granted by a nongovernmental agency attesting that an individual has met the required levels of competency.

Professionals are identified by several means, all of which are useful in the proper settings. Registration, licensing, and certification are some of the most common. It is important to understand these terms, as there has been much confusion in the pharmacy profession over their use.

- **Registration** is simply the process of listing, or of being named to a list.
- **Licensing** is permission granted by a government entity for an individual to perform an activity. The person has to meet certain standards, which are often set by law and are usually intended to protect the public.
- **Certification** is recognition granted by a nongovernmental agency attesting that an individual has met the required levels of competency.

Registration/Licensure for the Pharmacy Technician

Most states are now requiring pharmacy technicians to become either registered or licensed with the State Board of Pharmacy (SBOP). Each state decides whether it will register or license, and the baseline eligibility requirements for either also vary by state. Common eligibility requirements include:

- High school graduation or GED equivalent
- Attainment of a certain age, such as 18 years or older
- No felony conviction(s)
- Formal education or training as a pharmacy technician
- Passage of a State Board of Pharmacy competency exam
- Certification

These regulations and requirements vary by state, so you should consult your State Board of Pharmacy for specific information.

PROFILES IN PRACTICE

Terrance has been a pharmacy technician for two years and works in an out-patient hospital pharmacy. His state does not require certification, although registration is mandatory. Approximately half of the pharmacy technicians employed at the hospital are nationally certified; the others are not. Terrance is trying to decide whether to become certified.

- What advantages would Terrance have as a Certified Pharmacy Technician?

Certification for the Pharmacy Technician

When a pharmacy technician becomes certified, the certification agency verifies that the candidate has met the agency's or board's standards for skills and knowledge necessary to practice as a pharmacy technician. This signifies to employers, co-workers, and patients that a certain level of competence has been verified.

National certification for pharmacy technicians became possible in 1995 with the founding of the Pharmacy Technician Certification Board (PTCB). Although the PTCB continues to be the standard in technician certification, other agencies have recently emerged and achieved recognition. Of these newer agencies, the Institute for the Certification of Pharmacy Technicians (ICPT) has received the greatest recognition and acceptance of its certification exam, the ExCPT.

Workplace Wisdom Certification Exams for Pharmacy Technicians

ICPT (ExCPT exam) — www.nationaltechexam.org
PTCB (PTCE exam) — www.ptcb.org

ExCPT Certification Exam

The Exam for the Certification of Pharmacy Technicians (ExCPT) is offered by the Institute for the Certification of Pharmacy Technicians, based in St. Louis, Missouri. The ExCPT is nationally recognized and endorsed by the National Community Pharmacists Association and the National Association of Chain Drug Stores. The State Boards of Pharmacy in Connecticut, New Jersey, Minnesota, Oregon, and

Virginia have all officially recognized the ExCPT exam for registration/licensure eligibility.

The ExCPT is currently offered as a computerized exam on more than 300 days a year, at more than 1,000 locations. The exam consists of 110 multiple-choice questions, which must be completed within 2 hours. The criteria used by the ICPT measure the candidate in three areas of competence:

1. *Regulations and Technician Duties*, such as the role of pharmacists and pharmacy technicians, functions that a technician may and may not perform, prescription department layout and workflow, pharmacy security, the role of government agencies, inventory control, and pharmacy law (25% of exam).

2. *Drugs and Drug Products*, such as drug classification, mechanisms of action, dosage forms, and knowledge of the most commonly prescribed drugs (25% of exam).

3. *The Dispensing Process*, including preparation of prescriptions, dispensing of prescriptions, pharmacy calculations, sterile products, unit dosing, and repackaging (50% of exam).

Complete information on the ExCPT is available at www.nationaltechexam.org.

Candidates must meet certain qualifications in order to sit for the exam. For example, the candidate must be at least 18 years old, have a high school diploma or GED, and not have been convicted of a felony.

Renewal of certification, or *recertification*, is required every two years. To be recertified, individuals must have completed 20 hours of continuing education, including one hour of pharmacy law.

Pharmacy Technician Certification Exam

The Pharmacy Technician Certification Exam (PTCE) is offered by the Pharmacy Technician Certification Board, based in Washington, D.C. The PTCE is nationally recognized and endorsed by the National Association of Boards of Pharmacy, the American Pharmacists Association, and the American Society of Health-System Pharmacists. More than 300,000 individuals have passed the PTCE exam, which is officially recognized by more than 25 individual State Boards of Pharmacy. Only candidates who have successfully completed the PTCE may use the title Certified Pharmacy Technician (CPhT), which is a registered trademark of the PTCB.

The PTCE is currently offered each year during four testing "windows," each of which is five weeks long, in February, April, August, and November. The exam, which is computer-based, consists of 100 multiple-choice questions and must be completed within 2 hours.

The criteria used by the PTCB measure the candidate in three areas of competence:

1. *Assisting the pharmacist in serving patients*, such as by dispensing prescriptions, distributing medications, and collecting and organizing information. These responsibilities include screening prescriptions for accuracy and validity; counting, measuring, and compounding medications; and performing insurance billing (66% of exam).

2. *Maintaining medication and inventory control systems*, including placing and receiving drug orders, storing drugs correctly, removing outdated drugs from inventory, and organizing and monitoring pharmacy supply levels (22% of exam).

3. *Knowledge of general pharmacy operations*, including maintaining facilities, equipment, and information systems. This area includes servicing automated dispensing and refrigeration systems and performing computer maintenance (12% of exam).

Complete information on the PTCE is available at www.ptcb.org.

Candidates must meet certain qualifications in order to sit for the exam. For example, the candidate must be at least 18 years old, have a high school diploma or GED, and not have been convicted of a felony.

Renewal of certification, or recertification, is required every two years. To be recertified, individuals must have completed 20 hours of continuing education, including one hour of pharmacy law. The cost for recertification is $35 to $50.

Professional Organizations

In general, an **association**, or professional organization, is a group of individuals united for a specific purpose or cause. Associations are organized for various reasons, but typical recurring benefits they provide to their members include:

- Continuing education
- Professional development
- Information, research, and statistics
- Professional standards
- Networking
- Advocacy
- Professional recognition

association a group of individuals who voluntarily form an organization to accomplish a common purpose.

According to the American Society of Association Executives (ASAE), "Believing in the mission of an organization is a powerful incentive.... Associations have a responsibility to achieve results, not only for their members but for society at large."

There are four national organizations that are primarily focused on the practice of pharmacy, and which individual pharmacy technicians are permitted to join. Information on these four associations is outlined in Table 2-4.

In addition to the national pharmacy associations, there are also pharmacy organizations in individual states/cities, relating to specific practice settings, and targeted to race, religion, and other cultural variations. Research the various associations and determine which one(s) would be of greatest benefit to you—then get involved!

Career Opportunities

Being a pharmacy technician is among the best career opportunities that do not require a college degree. The National Pharmacy Technician Association reports that pharmacy technician ranks 60th in the 100 fastest-growing jobs in the United States and 19th in the 500 best jobs.

The U.S. Bureau of Labor Statistics confirms that pharmacy technician is among the most promising occupations, as they are forecasting an annual job growth rate of 28.8%, which equates to nearly 40,000 openings each year.

Pharmacy technicians are no longer limited to working in drugstores and hospitals. Numerous unique career-path options are now opening to pharmacy technicians, such as:

- Clinical practice
- Compounding
- Nuclear medicine
- Training/education
- Management
- Sales
- Research and development
- Consulting

Table 2-4 National Pharmacy Associations

ORGANIZATION	FOUNDED	MEMBER-SHIPS	BENEFITS[1]	DUES	MEMBER-SHIP SIZE[2]	CONTACT INFORMATION
AAPT American Association of Pharmacy Technicians	1970s	Technicians[3] Pharmacists Students	Newsletter with CE (4x); annual seminar; regional chapter seminars; member discounts	$50[4] $65[5] $25[6]	1,200	pharmacytechnician.com phone 877-368-4771 fax 336-333-9068
APhA American Pharmacists Association	1852	Technicians Pharmacists[3]	*Pharmacy Today*™ magazine (12x); annual meeting; CE—through pharmacist.com; member discounts; affinity programs	$57[4] $216[5]	50,000	aphanet.org phone 1-800-237-2742 fax 202-783-2351
ASHP American Society of Health-System Pharmacists	1942	Technicians Pharmacists[3] Students (RPh)	*ASHP Action Line* newsletter (12x); annual meetings; CE—TechTopics™ (10 hrs.); member discounts; affinity programs	$65[4] $225[5] $32[6]	30,000	ashp.org phone 301-657-3000
NPTA National Pharmacy Technician Association	1999	Technicians[3] Educators[7] Students	*Today's Technician*™ magazine (6x); annual and regional meetings; CE—unlimited/online; member discounts; affinity programs	$54[4] $54[5] $25[6]	30,000	pharmacytechnician.org phone 888-247-8700 fax 888-247-8706

[1]Benefits provided with listed technician membership dues, according to content published on website.

[2]Estimated total membership, including all categories.

[3]Primary membership category.

[4]Technician membership dues/year.

[5]Pharmacist/Associate membership dues/year.

[6]Student membership dues/year.

[7]NPTA does not offer membership to pharmacists unless they are full-time pharmacy technician educators.

SUMMARY

Pharmacy is an industry that consists of professionals: namely, pharmacists and pharmacy technicians. As with any profession, pharmacy requires an individual to be educated, trained, diligent, and ethical. You will have to study and work hard to attain your goal, but tremendous career opportunities await the professional pharmacy technician. The key concepts for this chapter include:

- The pharmacy profession includes both pharmacists and pharmacy technicians. Both groups have defined educational requirements and specific roles within the pharmacy.

- The professional pharmacy technician maintains a proper image, is responsible and a team player, adapts quickly and appropriately to change, seeks continuing education and development, and demonstrates compassion.

- The process of preparing for your future as a pharmacy technician includes formal education and training, registration/licensure, national certification, and involvement with a professional organization.

CHAPTER REVIEW QUESTIONS

1. Which of the following is classified as a health-system pharmacy?
   a. home health care
   b. chain drugstore
   c. mail-order facility
   d. extended-living facility

2. Pharmacists are required to complete _____ years of college-level education.
   a. 2
   b. 4
   c. 6
   d. 8

3. Which agency regulates registration and licensure?
   a. ACPE
   b. NABP
   c. PTCB
   d. SBOP

4. Attitude refers to a way of _____.
   a. acting
   b. feeling
   c. thinking
   d. all of the above

5. Which two agencies are recognized providers for national pharmacy technician certification?
   a. ICPT and PTCB
   b. APhA and ASHP
   c. NABP and NACDS
   d. ACPE and SBOP

6. Certified pharmacy technicians are required to complete _____ hours of continuing education every two years.
   a. 5
   b. 10
   c. 20
   d. 40

7. _____ refers to permission granted by a government entity for an individual to perform an activity.
   a. Certification
   b. Licensure
   c. Registration
   d. none of the above

8. Which of the following is a standard dress code used in pharmacies?
   a. business
   b. scrubs
   c. business-casual
   d. both a and b

9. Certified pharmacy technicians are authorized to:
   a. dispense medications.
   b. provide drug information.
   c. prepare and deliver medications to nursing stations.
   d. none of the above

10. Which professional organization publishes *Today's Technician* magazine?
    a. NPTA
    b. AAPT
    c. APhA
    d. ASHP

CRITICAL THINKING QUESTIONS

1. Why is it important that pharmacists and pharmacy technicians have specific and distinct competency requirements, roles, and responsibilities?

2. Which of the characteristics of a good pharmacy technician do you currently possess? Of the characteristics described in this chapter, which is your strongest area and which is your weakest area?

3. Why do you think that pharmacy has consistently been rated as the most trusted profession in America, even over doctors and clergy?

WEB CHALLENGE

1. Look up the website for your State Board of Pharmacy and then search the website for information and requirements for pharmacy technicians. Print out the information you find. (Hint: A list of SBOP contact information is available at www.nabp.net.)

2. Visit the website of each of the national pharmacy organizations listed here. Review the full list of membership benefits offered by each association.

AAPT—www.pharmacytechnician.com
APhA—www.aphanet.org
ASHP—www.ashp.org
NPTA—www.pharmacytechnician.org

REFERENCES AND RESOURCES

Accreditation Council for Pharmacy Education: www.acpe-accredit.org

American Association of Pharmacy Technicians: www.pharmacytechnician.com

American Pharmacists Association: www.aphanet.org

American Society of Association Executives: www.asaenet.org

American Society of Health-System Pharmacists: www.ashp.org

Bureau of Labor Statistics: www.bls.org

Johnston, M. *Certification Exam Review*. Upper Saddle River, NJ: Pearson, 2005.

Johnston, M. *Fundamentals of Pharmacy Practice*. Upper Saddle River, NJ: Pearson, 2005.

Michigan State University Human Resources: www.hr.msu.edu/hrsite

Roberts, LM. How to play to your strengths. *Harvard Business Review*. January 1, 2005.

Stark, M. *Creating a Professional Image*. Boston: Harvard Business School, 2005.

Communication and Customer Care

3 chapter

LEARNING OBJECTIVES

After completing this chapter, you should be able to:

- Describe and illustrate the communication process.
- List and explain the three types of communication.
- Summarize the various barriers to effective communication.
- List and describe the primary defense mechanisms.
- Describe specific strategies for eliminating barriers to communication.
- Summarize the elements of and considerations in caring for patients.
- List the Five Rights of medication administration.

Introduction

Communication is simply the process of transferring information—but it is not a simple process. The purpose of communication is to get your message across to others clearly and unambiguously. Communicating takes effort from everyone involved. During the process, errors can arise, resulting in confusion, misunderstandings, and sometimes a complete failure of the information transfer system. Customer service and pharmaceutical care both directly relate to the effectiveness of communication at the pharmacy. Thus, this topic is crucially important to the pharmacy technician.

The Communications Process

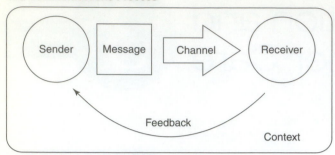

FIGURE 3-1 The communication process.

The Communication Process

Communication is a process (Figure 3-1). More specifically, it is a two-way process. Communication is more than just talking, or even just listening; there is an art to communication.

To better illustrate the communication process, let's use the following scenario: A patient, Mrs. Matthews, is at the pharmacy to pick up her son's medicine. After locating the prescription, the pharmacy technician, Rhonda, sees a note on the bag stating, "Insurance denied; must pay cash."

The Sender

sender the person who originates or imparts a communication message.

The communication process is initiated by the **sender**, the individual who has a statement to make or a question to ask. In our scenario, the pharmacy technician, Rhonda, becomes the sender and initiates the communication process, by explaining, "I am sorry, Mrs. Matthews, but apparently the insurance company denied the prescription. Your total is going to be $143.90."

The Message

message the substance, or information, being transferred in communication.

The **message** is the information that the sender provides, when making a statement, or requests, when asking a question. Although the concept of a message may seem elementary, many factors influence and create the full meaning of the message; these factors are discussed later in this chapter.

Rhonda's message was a statement; she provided information to Mrs. Matthews about the insurance company's action. In addition, Rhonda's message informed Mrs. Matthews how much money she needed to pay to receive her son's medication.

The Channel

channel a gesture, action, sound, written or spoken word, or visual image used in transmitting information.

The term **channel** simply refers to the mode by which the sender transmits the message. Communication occurs through written channels, such as letters and e-mails; verbal channels, such as phone calls; and nonverbal channels, such as the sender's body language. The channel of communication in our scenario is verbal. Both Rhonda and Mrs. Matthews are physically present at the pharmacy and they are speaking face to face.

The Receiver

receiver the person to whom a communication message is sent.

The **receiver** in the communication process is the individual to whom the sender is transmitting the message. In verbal communication, it is the person to whom the sender is speaking or questioning. In our scenario, Mrs. Matthews is the receiver as she hears Rhonda explain her message, "I am sorry, Mrs. Matthews, but apparently the insurance company denied the prescription. Your total is going to be $143.90."

Feedback

feedback the return of information, or a message, in the communication process.

Feedback is the aspect of communication that makes it a two-way process. The receiver provides the sender with feedback, which is a reaction—either verbal or nonverbal—to the communicated message. Feedback is critical to ensure that the receiver properly understood the message. Returning to our scenario, Mrs. Matthews lets out a loud sigh and shakes her head when she hears Rhonda's message. In a sense, feedback actually reverses the communication process, because in giving feedback the initial receiver becomes the sender and the initial sender becomes the new receiver. In effective communication, the process continues to reverse as it flows back and forth, creating a clear and useful conversation.

Context

Context refers to the situation, or environment, in which the message is delivered. In our scenario, one context is the pharmacy and the attitudes and beliefs related to pharmacy professionals. Pharmacy has for many years been cited as the most trusted and respected profession in the United States, ranking above medical practice, law, and ministry. This honor, however, comes with a responsibility to communicate in a trustworthy and professional manner.

Another context of our scenario is Mrs. Matthews's personal situation. It could be that her son is very sick, but she cannot afford the medication; therefore, her family's health and financial resources are also a part of the background to the feedback she is providing.

context the setting, or circumstances, in which communication occurs.

Communication Types and Methods

There are three primary types of communication: verbal, written, and nonverbal. As a pharmacy technician, you will need to communicate effectively in all three modes. Within the pharmacy practice setting (in fact, in any setting), we use a variety of methods for effective communication within any one type. To illustrate the types and methods of communication, we will continue to extend the scenario between Mrs. Matthews and Rhonda.

Verbal Communication

The first type of communication is **verbal communication** (Figure 3-2). Although this is an auditory-based type of communication, it encompasses much more than words alone. Verbal communication includes one's tone of voice, inflection, pitch, volume, and pronunciation and diction, as well as the specific words used.

verbal communication the imparting or interchanging of thoughts, opinions, or information through the use of spoken words.

The first, and most important, point to remember regarding verbal communication—or any type of communication, for that matter—is the accuracy and clarity of the message. Even if you handle every aspect of the communication process professionally, your efforts will not matter if the message you are sending is inaccurate.

The sender's tone of voice greatly influences the message and consequently the feedback received. Consider the message sent by Rhonda: "I am sorry, Mrs. Matthews, but apparently the insurance company denied the prescription. Your total is going to be $143.90." As words printed on a page, the message appears clear and professional, but what effect could Rhonda's tone of voice have?

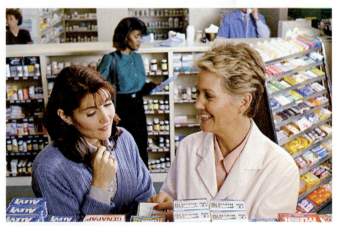

FIGURE 3-2 Verbal communication.

Read Rhonda's statement aloud, using a sympathetic, caring tone of voice: "I am sorry, Mrs. Matthews, but apparently the insurance company denied the prescription. Your total is going to be $143.90."

Now read her statement aloud again, using a monotone, impersonal tone of voice: "I am sorry, Mrs. Matthews, but apparently the insurance company denied the prescription. Your total is going to be $143.90."

Finally, read her statement aloud once more, using a condescending, annoyed tone of voice: "I am sorry, Mrs. Matthews, but apparently the insurance company denied the prescription. Your total is going to be $143.90."

Although not one single word was different, three entirely different messages were sent to Mrs. Matthews. It is easy to imagine how Mrs. Matthews's feedback would vary depending on the tone of voice Rhonda used.

Inflection is a change in the tone of voice, the emphasis or word stress used, or the pronunciation of a specific word or phrase. Inflection too can greatly influence a

inflection alteration in pitch or tone of the voice.

sender's message. To see the differences, repeat Rhonda's statement several times aloud, each time emphasizing a different word or phrase: "I am sorry, Mrs. Matthews, but apparently the insurance company denied the prescription. Your total is going to be $143.90."

pitch the property of sound that is determined by the frequency of sound-wave vibrations reaching the ear.

volume the loudness of a communication.

pronunciation the manner in which someone utters a word.

diction clarity and distinctness of pronunciation in speech.

The sender's voice **pitch** (how high or low the voice is in soundwave frequency), and the **volume** at which the sender speaks can affect the receiver's ability to properly understand the message. If Rhonda speaks to the client too softly, Mrs. Matthews might not be able to hear what Rhonda said and then become confused or agitated. In contrast, if Rhonda speaks too loudly, Mrs. Matthews might become embarrassed, self-conscious, uncomfortable, or defensive. This aspect of verbal communication is particularly important with geriatric patients, who may not hear very well, or may have specific ranges of hearing loss.

Finally, the sender's **pronunciation** and **diction** are critical to ensuring that the receiver properly understands the message. Incorrect pronunciation and/or the use of slang will both impair the message and reduce the receiver's perception of your credibility and professionalism.

There are two primary methods of verbal communication: face-to-face and by telephone.

Face-to-Face Communication

As a pharmacy technician, you will be involved in face-to-face communication nearly all day long, excluding a few specialty practice settings. This face-to-face communication will be with your pharmacists, your co-workers, and your patients and customers. Here are some tips for effective face-to-face communication:

- Smile. Be a pleasant individual to communicate with.
- Speak clearly and at an appropriate volume.
- Use professional and appropriate tones of voice, inflections, and diction.
- Actively listen when someone is speaking to you; acknowledge the speaker by nodding your head.
- Do not interrupt while someone is speaking. Wait until the speaker is finished.
- Ask questions to ensure that you both completely understand the conversation.

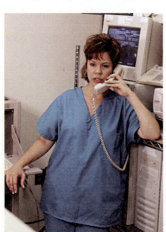

FIGURE 3-3 Telephone communication.

Telephone-Based Communication

Pharmacy technicians spend a great deal of time communicating on the telephone. They may use the phone to speak with patients, request refill authorizations from doctors' offices, or get assistance from an insurance company's help desk (see Figure 3-3). In any case, telephone-based communication can be more complicated than face-to-face communication because of the lack of additional information from nonverbal communication (discussed later in this chapter).

Workplace Wisdom Telephone Tips

Here are some tips on telephone-based communication:
- Use a pleasant and professional tone of voice.
- State your name and place of business.
- If answering a phone call, ask how you can help the caller.
- If making a phone call, explain your need or objective.
- If taking a message, document the items listed below under "Receiving a Voicemail."

PROCEDURE 3-1

Receiving a Voicemail

1. Record the date and time the message was left.
2. Record the caller's name and phone number.
3. Indicate the individual for whom the message was left.
4. Clearly document the request made on the voicemail.
5. Sign or initial the documentation.

PROCEDURE 3-2

Leaving a Voicemail

1. State your full name and the pharmacy's name.
2. Provide the pharmacy's phone number and hours of operation.
3. Indicate the purpose of your call.
4. Make any specific requests needed.
5. Give your name and the pharmacy's phone number a second time.

INFORMATION

Voicemails and Patient Confidentiality

Patient confidentiality is a major issue in all pharmacy work, but you must take special care regarding confidentiality when leaving voicemail messages. If you are calling a doctor's office to get a refill authorization, at the patient's request, obviously you will need to provide detailed information, including the patient's name and the medication. If, however, you are leaving a voicemail for the patient, on either a home answering machine or a work voicemail, it is inappropriate to include any detailed or confidential information. A proper message would be: "Hello, this is Brad with Main Street Pharmacy calling to speak with Ms. Chan. You can call me back at 281-555-7900. Again, this is Brad at Main Street Pharmacy. The telephone number is 281-555-7900. Thank you."

Written Communication

The second type of communication is **written communication**. Although many of the considerations concerning verbal communication apply to written messages as well, other factors come into play when you communicate in writing.

As a pharmacy technician, you will communicate in writing in a variety of ways, such as notes, messages, lists, reports, and other documentation. The most common written communications that pharmacy technicians receive are prescriptions and medication orders.

Just as with verbal communication, accuracy is fundamental with written messages. Legible handwriting and correct grammar both play a large role in creating accurate written messages. If your handwriting is illegible—that is, difficult or impossible to read—your communication will cause at the least delay, and possibly confusion or an outright error.

written communication the imparting or interchanging of thoughts, opinions, or information through the use of written words.

Nonverbal Communication

nonverbal communication the imparting or interchanging of thoughts, opinions, or information without the use of spoken words.

The final type of communication, and the most underestimated, is **nonverbal communication.** Research indicates that up to 80 percent of communication is nonverbal. However, most individuals are unaware of their nonverbal cues or, rather, do not realize that they are sending messages this way. Sometimes they inadvertently send nonverbal messages that contradict or oppose their verbal message.

There are many methods of nonverbal communication, some of which are used subconsciously. However, when you realize that more than three-fourths of human communication is nonverbal, you should also realize that it is imperative for you to take control over these cues if you are to be an effective and accurate communicator. The more prominent methods of nonverbal communication include:

- Facial expressions—communicate emotions, such as happiness, anger, or surprise.
- Gestures—can communicate thoughts, requests, or strong emotions.
- Eye contact—communicates interest in the dialogue. Looking away, or gazing, indicates disinterest in the communication.
- Posture—communicates confidence and energy level; good posture indicates a confident, professional, alert individual.
- Personal space—the distance one stands from another person when talking can communicate one's level of comfort and trust with the other individual. However, personal space can also simply be a cultural norm, as opposed to a nonverbal cue.
- Body movement—fidgeting with one's hands, or rocking back and forth, or swinging one's foot can communicate either disinterest in or agitation with the dialogue. Such movement often indicates a desire to end the communication as soon as possible.
- Silence—can deliver either positive or negative feedback, depending on the context of the communication.

Barriers to Communication

Problems with communication can arise at any stage of the communication process (sender, message, channel, receiver, feedback, or context). Any problems have the potential to create misunderstandings and confusion (see Figure 3-4).

To be an effective communicator, and to get your point across without misunderstanding or confusion, your goal should be to reduce the occurrence of problems at each stage of the process by using clear, precise, well-planned communications. If your message is too long, jumbled, or inaccurate, you can expect to be misunderstood or misinterpreted. Poor grammar and conflicting body language can also make a message unclear or send additional, unintended meanings. You must commit to breaking down the barriers that exist in each of the stages of the communication process. This section examines some common barriers to the communication process, their impact, and tips on how to eliminate them.

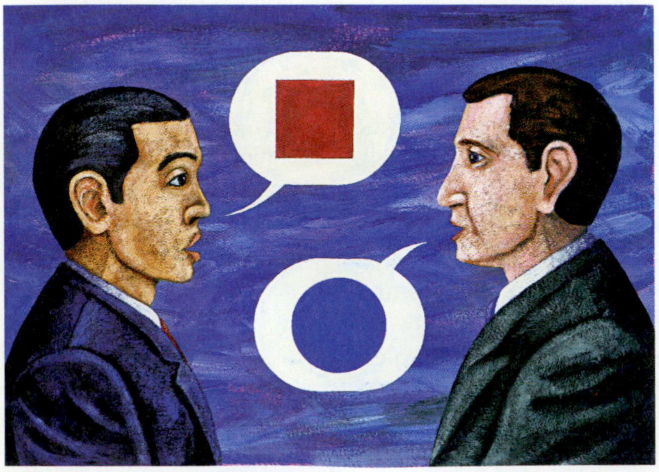

FIGURE 3-4 Language barriers.

Language Barriers

One of the leading barriers to communication in the United States is language. This barrier arises when a patient or co-worker is unable to speak or understand the English language. This communication barrier affects one out of every five people in the United States:

- 21 million people speak English less than adequately.
- 46 million people do not speak English as their primary language.

As a pharmacy technician, you must be prepared to deal with patients who speak little or no English. Although it is the role of the pharmacist to counsel patients on their prescriptions and medications, technicians are the frontline employees who communicate with patients directly about many important issues.

Workplace Wisdom   Bilingual Benefits

Bilingual pharmacy technicians are a valuable asset to any pharmacy and typically have a greater earning potential. There is a great need for pharmacy professionals who are fluent speakers of languages other than English, particularly Spanish, Vietnamese, Chinese, and French, across the United States. Be sure that you include details on your résumé pertaining to any other language(s) you speak.

Here are some tips on how to overcome a language barrier:

- **Use the client's native language, if possible.** Many pharmacy technicians are bilingual. If you can speak the patient's language, do so.
- **Offer to use a translator.** A translator could be a co-worker, a member of the client's family, another healthcare provider, or even an employee from a different department. In any case, it should be someone that patients feel they can trust.
- **Provide written instructions in the client's native language.** The computer systems in most pharmacies are able to print prescription labels and drug monographs in nearly any language. Offer this service to any patient for whom English is not the primary or native language.

Communication Impairments

Outside of language barriers, there are two primary communication impairments: hearing impairment and illiteracy. Both of these impairments can become significant obstacles in communicating with patients and customers, if you do not know how to properly address them.

Hearing Impairment

Hearing-impaired individuals have a relative insensitivity to sound in the speech frequencies, meaning that conventional speech, and language itself, become barriers to communication (see Figure 3-5).

Hearing impairment is categorized according to severity. The scale includes deafness, being "hard of hearing," and unilateral hearing loss.

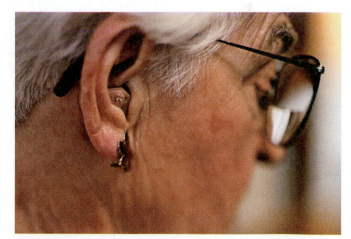

FIGURE 3-5 A hearing-impaired person will often wear a hearing aid.

- Deafness—little or no residual hearing capability; the patient is unable to hear.
- Hard of hearing—partially unable to hear; the patient typically requires hearing aids.
- Unilateral hearing loss—hear normally in one ear, but have trouble hearing with the other ear.

Here are some tips for communicating with clients who have hearing impairments:

- **Look directly at the patient when speaking.** Individuals who suffer from impaired hearing rely heavily on lip reading as people speak. To ensure that clients are able to read your lips, look directly at them as you speak. If you can see their lips, you know that they can see yours.
- **Speak louder.** Many people who are hard of hearing, or have unilateral hearing loss, need you to speak at a louder-than-normal volume to communicate effectively.

Keep in mind, however, the nature of your comments or questions. You must still protect your patient's confidential information. Be subtle when speaking loudly, because proper tone and inflection are still important.

- **Reduce background noise.** Background noise, which is common at most places of business, can further impair an individual's ability to hear you. When possible, particularly when communicating with those who have unilateral hearing loss, speak in a location with little or no background noise, such as in the patient consultation room.
- **Learn sign language.** The preceding tips probably will not help you communicate with totally or profoundly deaf patients. However, learning American Sign Language (ASL) may allow you to communicate effectively with these patients.

INFORMATION

An Internet-based resource for learning ASL online is available at www.signingonline.com.

Workplace Wisdom Hearing Impairment

Many persons in the deaf community reject the term *hearing impairment*, because the phrase implies a disability. Many are offended by the term *impaired*. Be sensitive to these patients and the effect of any labels you may have innocently used.

Illiteracy

According to the National Audit Literacy Survey (NALS), 40–44 million American adults, defined as Americans aged 16 or older, rank at Level 1, the lowest level of literacy. In other words, 20–23 percent of American adults have difficulty using certain reading, writing, and computational skills considered necessary for functioning in everyday life. This finding is consistent with a 2000 UNESCO Institute for Statistics report, which indicated a global adult illiteracy rate of 20.3 percent, or 862 million people worldwide who could not read their own language.

Illiteracy can have a significant impact on individuals receiving pharmaceutical services and taking prescription or over-the-counter drugs. Many individuals who lack sufficient reading and writing skills feel embarrassed and even ashamed of this problem, and often go to great lengths to hide their inability. They are often hesitant to reveal or communicate their struggle to others, including healthcare professionals. Because they cannot read directions and instructions, these patients are at significantly increased risk of improper medication use and serious adverse effects. Some tips for assisting patients with restricted literacy include:

- **Always have the pharmacist provide counseling on new prescriptions.** By ensuring that the pharmacist consults each patient on new prescriptions, you guarantee that, at a minimum, patients receive verbal instructions and warnings related to their medication(s).
- **Always ask patients if they have any questions.** Regardless of whether patients are picking up refills of existing prescriptions, dropping off new prescriptions, or purchasing over-the-counter medications, ask if they have any questions. This approach provides an opportunity for those with insufficient reading skills to gain information without feeling embarrassment or shame.
- **Watch for indicators of low-level literacy skills.** Although it is not appropriate to "profile" individuals according to their literacy skills, certain indicators can be useful. For example, if a patient seems to have difficulty reading or completing a new patient profile, this could indicate low literacy skills. If you suspect

that a patient may have literacy complications, ask him or her to write the address, date of birth, or other common profile information on the prescription as he or she drops it off to be filled. This allows you to screen for literacy problems and therefore better understand the patient's communication needs. Compassion and empathy are crucial when dealing with persons who cannot read. They may be embarrassed, but they still need to understand their medicines. It is up to you to help make them feel comfortable and receptive to important information.

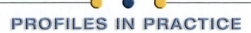

PROFILES IN PRACTICE

Tabitha works as a pharmacy technician at a chain retail pharmacy. A new patient arrived and requested to have a prescription filled, but was unable to complete the patient profile form when asked to do so. Tabitha's patient is illiterate.

- How can Tabitha assist without embarrassing the patient?

Defense Mechanisms

Another common barrier to communication is the utilization of **defense mechanisms**, which are unconscious behaviors or reactions that are generally prompted by anxiety. Pharmacy professionals serve individuals who are sick, ill, or fighting a disease, and most of these individuals are simultaneously experiencing anxiety and worry. When anxiety occurs, the mind initially responds with an increase in problem-solving thinking, seeking ways to escape the situation. At that point, a variety of defense mechanisms may be triggered.

All defense mechanisms share two common properties. First, they are often used unconsciously. Second, they tend to distort, transform, or otherwise misrepresent reality. Sigmund Freud, a pioneer of psychotherapy, identified nine primary defense mechanisms: denial, displacement, intellectualization, projection, rationalization, reaction formation, regression, repression, and sublimation. This section includes a brief overview of each one, to help familiarize you with these behaviors that you may see in customers or in yourself.

Denial

Denial is a defense mechanism whereby an individual avoids confronting a problem by denying the very existence of the problem. An example is the patient who is diagnosed with diabetes, but denies that she really has the disease and therefore decides not to take the prescribed medications and test her blood glucose levels.

Displacement

Displacement occurs when an individual transfers his own negative emotions to someone, or something, that is completely unrelated to the individual's feelings. An example of displacement is the patient who has been yelled at by his boss all day, and then transfers his anger and resentment to the pharmacy technician when at the pharmacy that evening.

Intellectualization

Intellectualization is the defense mechanism whereby an individual deals with conflict or stressors by making generalizations to minimize disturbing feelings. An example is the impatient customer who becomes irate when hearing that it will take an hour to fill her prescription—because, after all, "How long does it actually take to pour 30 tablets into a bottle and put a label on it?"

defense mechanisms unconscious mental processes used to protect one's ego.

denial a defense mechanism characterized by refusal to acknowledge painful realities, thoughts, or feelings.

displacement a defense mechanism in which there is an unconscious shift of emotions, affect, or desires from the original object to a more acceptable or immediate substitute.

intellectualization a defense mechanism used to protect oneself from the emotional stress and anxiety associated with confronting painful personal fears or problems; characterized by excessive reasoning.

projection a defense mechanism whereby one's own attitudes, feelings, or suppositions are attributed to others.

Projection

Projection occurs when an individual attributes his own thoughts or impulses to another person. For example, a patient who is prejudiced against minorities complains that both the African-American and Asian-American staff pharmacists treat him with disrespect, because they do not like him.

Rationalization

rationalization a defense mechanism whereby one's true motivation is concealed by explaining one's actions and feelings in a way that is not threatening.

Rationalization is a defense mechanism whereby an individual offers a socially acceptable and apparently logical explanation for an act or decision actually produced by unconscious impulses. An example is the patient who decides to take twice the prescribed dosage of her medication, believing that if 500 mg is good, then 1,000 mg would be even better.

Reaction Formation

reaction formation a defense mechanism characterized by action at the opposite extreme of one's true feelings, as overcompensation for unacceptable impulses.

Reaction formation occurs when someone goes to the opposite extreme of behavior, overcompensating for unacceptable impulses. Consider the patient who is confronted by his physician about requesting an unnecessary number of prescription drugs, and then stops taking any medications at all.

Regression

regression a defense mechanism characterized by reverting to an earlier or less mature pattern of feeling or behavior.

Regression is a defense mechanism in which an individual suffers a loss of some of the development already attained and reverts to a lower level of adaptation and expression. An example is the adult who suddenly becomes incapable of taking tablets or capsules, and requires all of her medication in liquid form.

Repression

repression a defense mechanism characterized by the exclusion of painful impulses, desires, or fears from the conscious mind.

Repression involves an involuntary exclusion of a painful thought, impulse, or memory from awareness. For example, a patient immediately changes the subject when asked how he is doing after the death of his spouse.

Sublimation

sublimation a defense mechanism in which unacceptable instinctual drives and wishes are modified to take more personally and socially acceptable forms.

Sublimation is a defense mechanism whereby individuals redirect their socially unacceptable impulses or emotions into a socially acceptable form. An example is the patient who has been diagnosed with a debilitating disease: to divert her attention, she begins to work excessively long hours at the office.

Conflict

Conflict will certainly arise in the pharmacy setting, just as it does in any workplace. Serious disputes, disagreements, and arguments are all considered conflict, and they may arise with your patients or your co-workers. Strategies on resolving conflict include:

- Get assistance from your pharmacy manager.
- Identify attitude shifts to show respect for others' needs.
- Transform problems into creative opportunities.
- Develop communication tools to build rapport. Use listening to clarify understanding.
- Apply strategies to attack the problem, not the person.
- Manage your emotions. Express fear, anger, hurt, and frustration wisely to effect change.
- Identify personal issues that may be involved in the situation.
- Evaluate the problem in its broader context.

The best strategy for pharmacy technicians to use in conflict resolution is to request the assistance of the pharmacist or pharmacy manager. It is important to remember your scope of authority and duties. Conflict that arises with a patient will often require the pharmacist to become involved or handle the situation. When conflict develops between co-workers, the matter should be taken to the pharmacy manager or supervisor.

Eliminating Communication Barriers

Throughout this section, we have explored various barriers to effective communication, in addition to strategies and tips on how to eliminate them. The universal keys to eliminating communication barriers include:

- Fully understanding the communication process
- Recognizing that numerous barriers to communication exist
- Knowing and effectively using strategies to overcome communication barriers
- Being willing to recognize and eliminate communication barriers as they arise

The final key—willingness to recognize and eliminate communication barriers as they arise—is the most important of the four. Unless you are willing to actively address communication barriers, they will continue to hinder and reduce the effectiveness of your communication.

Caring for Customers and Patients

In addition to dispensing prescription medications, pharmacy professionals provide comfort, care, advice, and instructions. They also guarantee specific rights, such as patient confidentiality.

Patient Rights

In pharmacy practice, patients are guaranteed five specific rights, known as the *Five Patient Rights*. These rights ensure that the *right* patient receives the *right* medication, at the *right* strength, by the *right* route, at the *right* time. By following the Five Rights, medication safety is ensured.

1. **Right patient.** The prescription must be labeled for, dispensed to, and billed to the right customer.
2. **Right medication.** The prescription for medication must be accurately interpreted and the correct medication dispensed.
3. **Right strength.** The dosage, or strength, prescribed must be accurately interpreted, and the medication accurately labeled and dispensed.
4. **Right route.** The intended dosage form or route of administration must be used.
5. **Right time.** The proper directions for administration must be correctly interpreted from the prescription, included in the medication labeling, and explained to the patient.

Workplace Wisdom The Five Rights

- Right patient
- Right medication
- Right strength
- Right route
- Right time

In addition to the long-standing (but unofficial) Five Rights, Congress passed the Patient's Bill of Rights in 2005. In general terms, the Patient's Bill of Rights guarantees that patients have the right to:

- The best care available for their health needs.
- Be treated with courtesy and respect.

- Know their illness, condition, and treatment.
- Give or refuse permission for care, treatment, or research.
- Plan and participate in their own care.
- Be examined and treated in private.
- Receive care in a manner that supports comfort and dignity.
- Have communications and records concerning their care treated in a confidential manner.
- Have their families and significant others treated respectfully.
- Know the names and positions of the persons caring for them.
- Make healthcare decisions by completing a living will, or by appointing a person to make healthcare decisions on their behalf.
- Take part in discussion of ethical issues that arise regarding their care.
- Spiritual care and religious support consistent with personal beliefs.
- Know how issues, complaints, and grievances about their care will be handled.
- Care that respects their growth and development.
- Effective assessment and management of pain.
- An interpreter or assistive devices when they have a communication impairment, or do not speak or understand the language of the healthcare team.
- Family involvement in decisions about organ, tissue, and eye donation.
- Leave the hospital or outpatient clinical site even if their physicians advise against it.
- Ethical business practices.

The Patient's Bill of Rights covers all aspects of medical and pharmaceutical care, so certain guarantees in it may not relate directly to the practice of pharmacy. It is essential, however, that pharmacy technicians familiarize themselves with the Patient's Bill of Rights and abide by its directives.

Greeting Customers

Pharmacy technicians are, most often, the frontline employees in the pharmacy, meaning that a technician is usually the first and last person to speak with a patient. In addition, as much as 75 percent, or more, of the communication and interaction the customer has at the pharmacy will be with you, the pharmacy technician.

It is important to remember that most patients who come to the pharmacy are sick or feeling badly. Customers may be confused about which OTC medication to purchase, or may be emotional because of news just received at the doctor's office. Whatever the situation, it is important to greet your customers in a timely, caring, and positive manner. Here are several keys to greeting your patients and customers effectively:

- Smile.
- Speak and act sincerely.
- Look at your customer attentively.
- Introduce yourself and ask for your customer's name.
- Build trust and establish a personal relationship with your patient over time.
- Refer customers to the pharmacist to address any questions outside your scope of practice.

Protecting Confidentiality

Confidentiality is essential in pharmacy practice, and is required by law. Although Chapter 4 outlines the legal aspects and requirements of patient confidentiality, it is appropriate to address the relationship of confidentiality to patient care here.

Generally speaking, every piece of data or information pertaining to a patient is considered confidential. In addition to their legal rights, patients have certain expectations regarding this information. They trust that any personally identifiable information will be kept safe and secure from personnel who do not need to know the information. They expect that patient profiles and medication histories will be kept private and used only for pharmacy-related issues. They also assume that any information regarding their medical conditions will not be released to anyone without their permission.

Confidentiality is vital because it is the foundation on which the patient's trust in the pharmacy and pharmacy staff is built. As a pharmacy technician, you will constantly work with private and confidential information. It is imperative that you always protect the confidentiality of your patients.

Pharmacist Consultations

Pharmacist consultations are one of the essential elements of providing pharmaceutical care (see Figure 3-6). Providing advice, instructions, and other clinical information falls outside the scope of practice for pharmacy technicians; these responsibilities are to be handled by the pharmacist on duty. It is the responsibility of the pharmacy technician, however, to ensure that patients and customers speak with the pharmacist when appropriate. A pharmacist consultation is required for any:

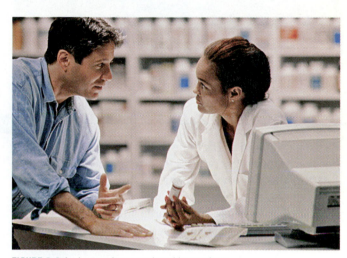

FIGURE 3-6 A pharmacist consults with a patient.

- new prescription that a patient has not previously taken.
- new prescription or refill when changes were made from previous dispensing.
- prescription or refill that flags a drug utilization review (DUR).
- request by a customer or patient to speak with the pharmacist.

There are certain exceptions to the rule that pharmacy technicians do not provide instructions to patients. Upon the authorization of the pharmacist, the technician may read the instructions or directions for a prescription. Also, after being trained and approved by the pharmacist, many pharmacy technicians assist patients with selecting and understanding OTC medical devices, such as blood glucose meters and nebulizers. These exceptions vary by state regulation and individual pharmacist approval. Under no circumstances, however, should a pharmacy technician ever provide verbal advice or clinical information.

Special Considerations

There are a number of special considerations in providing customer service and patient care, such as the patient's culture and age.

Cultural Differences

The United States is known as the melting pot; nowhere else on Earth will you find a greater diversity in ethnicity and cultural background. This becomes a special consideration at the pharmacy, as it is important to provide the highest quality pharmaceutical care while still respecting your patient's cultural differences. For example, different cultures accept different physical boundaries: persons from certain cultures prefer a greater distance from their conversation partners, whereas persons from other cultures prefer to stand very close to the person they are speaking with. In addition, different cultures have various methods of greeting, salutations, attire, and even medical beliefs. The key is to be attentive to your customers, learn what they find acceptable, and respect their preferences.

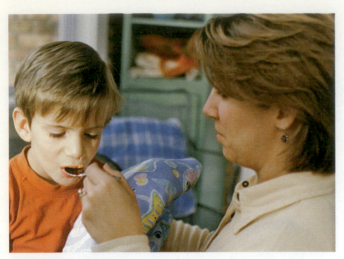

FIGURE 3-7 The age of a patient is a special consideration in pharmaceutical care.

Age

Another special consideration for providing pharmaceutical care is the age of the patient (see Figure 3-7). In general, this becomes a factor only when dealing with the extremes of age, for pediatric and geriatric patients. When providing care for pediatric patients (those under the age of 12), the communication process will be directed toward the parent or guardian. Geriatric (elderly) patients may themselves be the individuals with whom you communicate, or they may have a designated caregiver, such as a child, a person designated by a medical power of attorney, or a nurse.

SUMMARY

As you now know, communication is simply a process, but it is not a simple process. Pharmacy technicians work as frontline employees in the pharmacy, which means that both your management and your patients will rely on you to be an effective communicator.

Although barriers to effective communication can and will arise in the pharmacy, it is your responsibility to remain aware and take the initiative to eliminate those barriers or overcome defense mechanisms. This will require a concerted, proactive approach on your part.

In addition, it is important to remember that the practice of pharmacy no longer consists of just dispensing drugs. Rather, it involves dispensing pharmaceutical care, which includes customer service, pharmacist consultations, and other services.

CHAPTER REVIEW QUESTIONS

1. The most important key to eliminating barriers to communication is:
   a. fully understanding the communication process.
   b. recognizing that numerous barriers to communication exist.
   c. knowing strategies on how to overcome communication barriers.
   d. being willing to recognize and eliminate communication barriers as they arise.

2. A phone call is an example of which element of the communication process?
   a. channel
   b. context
   c. feedback
   d. message

3. How many Americans do not speak English as their primary language?
   a. 20.3 million
   b. 21 million
   c. 44 million
   d. 46 million

4. An involuntary exclusion of a specific thought or impulse is the defense mechanism referred to as:
   a. displacement.
   b. reaction formation.
   c. repression.
   d. sublimation.

5. _____ consists of serious disputes, disagreements, or arguments.
   a. Barrier to communication
   b. Conflict
   c. Defense mechanism
   d. none of the above

6. _____ is the condition in which an individual hears normally with one ear, but has trouble hearing with the other.
   a. Hard of hearing
   b. Deafness
   c. Unilateral hearing loss
   d. Selective hearing

7. Verbal communication methods include all of the following, except:
   a. diction.
   b. pitch.
   c. pronunciation.
   d. silence.

8. What percentage of Americans have difficulty reading and/or writing English?
   a. 20–23%
   b. 30–33%
   c. 40–44%
   d. none of the above

9. Offering a socially acceptable, or logical, explanation for an act is the defense mechanism known as:
   a. intellectualization.
   b. denial.
   c. projection.
   d. rationalization.

10. Pharmacists should be alerted for consultations in the following situations, except for:
   a. every new prescription.
   b. every refill.
   c. DUR prescriptions.
   d. OTC advice.

CRITICAL THINKING QUESTIONS

1. List the Five Rights and discuss the potential consequences of not adhering to each.

2. In what ways are defense mechanisms and conflict connected?

3. Why are pharmacist consultations important, and why are they considered outside the scope of practice for pharmacy technicians?

WEB CHALLENGE

1. Go to http://thomas.loc.gov/ and search for the 2005 Patient's Bill of Rights. Print a copy of the complete act to read.

2. Go to http://www.funquizcards.com/quiz/personality/what-is-your-communication-style.php and take the online "What is Your Communication Style?" quiz. Print your assessment.

REFERENCES AND RESOURCES

Carrasquillo, O, Orav, EJ, Brennan, TA, & Burstin, HR. Impact of language barriers on patient satisfaction in an emergency department. *J Gen Intern Med.* 1999;4:82–87.

Conflict Resolution Network: www.crnhq.org

Gandhi, JK, Burstin, HR, Cook, EF, et al. Drug complications in outpatients. *J Gen Intern Med.* 1998;15:149–154.

HPSO. Overcoming the language barrier. http://www.hpso.com/newsletters/1-2000flash.html

Hu, DJ, & Covell, RM. Health care usage by Hispanic outpatients as a function of primary language. *West J Med.* 1998;144:490–493.

Johnston, M. *Certification Exam Review.* Upper Saddle River, NJ: Pearson, 2005.

Johnston, M. *Fundamentals of Pharmacy Practice.* Upper Saddle River, NJ: Pearson, 2005.

Kirkman-Liff, B, & Mondragon, D. Language of interview: Relevance for research of Southwest Hispanics. *Am J Public Health.* 1991;81:1399–1404.

Morales, LS, Cunningham, WE, Brown, JA, Honghu, L, & Hays, RD. Are Latinos less satisfied with communication by health care providers? *J Gen Intern Med.* 1999;14:400–407.

National Assessment of Adult Literacy (NAAL). U.S. National Center for Education Statistics. 2005.

UNESCO Institute for Statistics. *Data Centre Summary.* 2005.

U.S. Census Bureau, DP-2. *Profile of Selected Social Characteristics: 2000.* http://factfinder.census.gov

Weinick, RM, & Krauss, NA. Racial and ethnic differences in children's access to care. *Am J Public Health.* 2001;90:1771–1774.

Woloshin, S, Schwartz, LM, Katz, SJ, & Welch, HG. Is language a barrier to the use of preventive services? *J Gen Intern Med.* 1997;12:472–477. [PubMed].

Workman, TE, & Lombardo, NT. *Overcoming Language Barriers.* Binghamton, NY: Haworth Press, 2003.

chapter 4

Pharmacy Law and Ethics

LEARNING OBJECTIVES

After completing this chapter, you should be able to:

- Classify the various categories of United States law.
- List the regulatory agencies that oversee the practice of pharmacy and describe their function(s).
- Summarize the significant laws and amendments that affect the practice of pharmacy.
- Recognize and use a drug monograph.
- Define ethics and moral philosophy.
- List and explain the nine ethical theories.
- Summarize the Pharmacy Technician Code of Ethics.

Introduction

Federal and state laws, as well as professional ethics, regulate the practice of pharmacy. The regulations on pharmacy practice in the United States have evolved and increased over the past 100 years, as legislators have responded to outcries from citizens to serve and protect the public interest. The government began to take the initiative in the regulation of pharmacy at the end of the 18th century. Over time, the profession of pharmacy has become subject to more regulations than were ever thought possible back in the 1800s. In the United States, a professional degree is a requirement for any individual who wishes to practice pharmacy. This requirement was established to protect the public and set minimum standards, so that citizens could rely on pharmacists having at least a standard level of education and competence.

This chapter focuses primarily on the major federal regulations pertaining to pharmacy practice. However, it does not list all federal laws pertaining to pharmacy, all the regulations included in or promulgated under the laws discussed, or state regulations. To learn more about these topics, contact your State Board of Pharmacy.

Overview of Law

There are four types of law in the United States: constitutional, statutes and regulations, administrative rules and regulations, and legislative intent.

Constitutional Law

The United States Constitution outlines the organization of the federal government. All laws passed must conform to the principles and rights set forth in the Constitution. The first 10 amendments to the Constitution are called the Bill of Rights; this is the source of the most fundamental rights, such as freedom of speech and religion, right to a jury trial, and protection against unreasonable searches and seizures.

Statutes and Regulations

Statutes are laws that are passed by federal, state, or local legislatures. Federal statutes are passed by the United States Congress and signed into law by the president. Regulations clarify and explain statutes, but they must also be consistent with the enacted statute because they have the same legal effect and power as the statute under which they were promulgated. Statutes often assign the power to create regulations, and delegate the responsibility for doing so, to a regulatory agency.

statute a law, decree, or edict.

State Law and Regulations

State constitutions establish the organization of state government. Any laws passed by a state must meet the standards of both the federal and state constitutions; state statutes must also remain consistent with the United States Code (U.S.C.) and the *Code of Federal Regulations* (C.F.R.), which are federal statutes and regulations. State statutes and regulations may provide additional rights to corresponding federal law, but states may not take away rights that are established by or guaranteed under federal law.

Legislative Intent

Statutory and regulatory laws are based on legislative intent. In many cases, the legal interpretation of a law, the meaning of a particular section, or the meaning of a specific word is studied to determine what the legislators wanted the law to do or to cover. Interpretations are influenced by the use of "may" instead of "shall," or even the location of a semicolon. Justices and judges are often called upon to determine legislative intent. The opinions and decisions they issue are commonly referred to as *case law*.

Criminal, Civil, and Administrative Law

Law can also be categorized as criminal, civil, or administrative.

Criminal Law

Criminal laws are those dealing with homicide, illegal drugs, theft, and other antisocial behavior. These laws are enforced by state agents against specific persons or corporations. The victim cannot prosecute the criminal case and does not have the right to determine if the state will prosecute the alleged criminal, because criminal law is designed to protect society as a whole rather than to compensate individuals who have been victims of criminal activity. This explains why criminal cases are titled "State versus John Smith" or "People versus Doe."

criminal law any law dealing with crime or punishment.

Civil Law

Civil lawsuits involve personal injuries, business disputes, land deals, libel and slander, and various other commercial interests and noncriminal matters. **Civil law** actions must be brought by an attorney hired by the injured party, known as the **plaintiff**, against the alleged wrongdoer, referred to as the **defendant**. The parties in a civil case may be individuals, corporations, or the state itself. **Medical malpractice** is a civil law action; therefore, pharmacies and pharmacy professionals are most often named in civil lawsuits, brought by plaintiffs claiming that professional errors or omissions were committed.

civil law any law dealing with the rights of private citizens.

plaintiff the party that initiates a legal action.

defendant the party against which a legal action is brought.

medical malpractice the negligent treatment of a patient by a healthcare professional.

Administrative Law

With the exception of the Defense Department and law enforcement agencies, the federal government conducts its activities through administrative agencies that enforce the laws. Examples of administrative agencies include the Internal Revenue Service (IRS), the Centers for Medicare and Medicaid Services (CMS), the Social Security Administration (SSA), and many others. States also operate through administrative agencies. Many of these, such as state equal employment opportunity commissions, correspond to federal agencies, whereas others, such as state boards of pharmacy, have no federal counterpart.

In addition to enforcing laws passed by the legislatures, administrative agencies refine these laws with regulations. Some laws, such as the Americans with Disabilities Act, leave agencies little room for interpretation. With other laws, such as those creating state boards of pharmacy, the enabling legislation is vague, giving the agency the authority to determine the scope and detail of any regulations. Agencies must satisfy specific procedural requirements when promulgating regulations, but once the regulations are established, they have the force of law.

Violations of the Law

misdemeanor an offense or infraction less serious than a felony.

felony a serious crime, such as rape or murder.

Any violation of the law is referred to as a *crime*, whether the law is criminal, civil, or administrative in nature. Crimes are further classified as either a **misdemeanor** or a **felony**. Misdemeanor crimes are considered less serious than felonies, and (depending on state law) are punishable by community service, parole, a fine, or imprisonment for 12 months or less. A felony, in contrast, is a serious crime, conviction of which typically results in imprisonment for more than a year.

Workplace Wisdom Professional Liability

As pharmacy technicians assume more responsibility, take on larger roles, and receive greater recognition in the pharmacy, they also become more subject to legal liability. Professional liability insurance coverage is now offered by a number of providers, including HPSO and Pharmacists Mutual.

PROFILES IN PRACTICE

Tim is a pharmacy technician who works at a local hospital preparing IVs and chemotherapy. One of the patients at the hospital dies from a medication error because Tim added the wrong medication to an IV bag. The hospital pharmacist is responsible for verifying the technician's work, including IV preparations.

- Who is responsible for the patient's death?
- What consequences can be expected?

Regulatory Agencies

A number of regulatory agencies, on both the federal and state levels, oversee the practice of pharmacy.

Centers for Medicare and Medicaid Services

The Centers for Medicare and Medicaid Services (CMS), formerly known as the Health Care Financing Administration (HCFA), is the agency that regulates the administration of Medicare, Medicaid, the State Children's Health Insurance Program (SCHIP), the Health Insurance Portability and Accountability Act, the Clinical Laboratory Improvement Amendments (CLIA), and several other health-related programs. The CMS conducts inspections to ensure compliance with its guidelines.

Drug Enforcement Administration

The Drug Enforcement Administration (DEA) regulates the legal trade in narcotic and dangerous drugs, manages a national narcotics intelligence system, and works with other agencies to prevent illegal drug trafficking. In 1982, coordinated joint jurisdiction over drug offenses was given to the Federal Bureau of Investigation (FBI) and the DEA. Agents of the two organizations work together on drug law enforcement, and the administrator of the DEA reports to the director of the FBI. The DEA has offices nationwide and in more than 40 foreign countries.

Food and Drug Administration

The Food and Drug Administration (FDA) is responsible for protecting the public health by ensuring the safety, efficacy, and security of drugs, biological products, medical devices, food, and cosmetics. The FDA is also responsible for reviewing and approving new drug applications, new generic equivalents, and new therapeutic indications for existing medications.

Joint Commission on Accreditation of Healthcare Organizations

The Joint Commission on Accreditation of Healthcare Organizations (JCAHO), now known simply as the "Joint Commission," evaluates and accredits nearly 15,000 health-care organizations and programs in the United States. Since 1951, JCAHO has established and enforced standards that focus on improving the quality and safety of care provided by healthcare organizations. JCAHO evaluates and accredits hospitals, hospice facilities, nursing homes, long-term care facilities, rehabilitation centers, and other healthcare organizations.

Occupational Safety and Health Administration

The Occupational Safety and Health Administration (OSHA) is a division of the U.S. Department of Labor that oversees the administration of the Occupational Safety and Health Act and enforces standards in all 50 states. The mission of OSHA is to ensure the safety and health of America's workers by setting and enforcing standards; OSHA establishes protective standards, enforces those standards, and reaches out to employers and employees through technical assistance and consultation programs.

State Boards of Pharmacy

The State Board of Pharmacy (SBOP) is the state agency that registers and regulates pharmacy facilities, pharmacists, and pharmacy technicians. Each state's Board of Pharmacy is responsible for establishing and maintaining a state pharmacy practice act that regulates the actual practice of pharmacy. The SBOP is granted the authority to monitor the activities of and, if necessary, reprimand licensed pharmacy professionals; it may also revoke the licenses of both pharmacy facilities and pharmacy professionals.

Overview of Pharmacy Law

Now that we have reviewed the various types of U.S. law and regulatory agencies, we can discuss legislation that specifically addresses the practice of pharmacy.

State and Federal Functions

Law and medicine are based on different, and sometimes opposing, professional paradigms. Medicine is a science-based profession; law is not based on a scientific paradigm. Nevertheless, the practice of pharmacy and medicine must conform to law.

The United States operates on a federalist system, in which there is a central government that has certain powers, but the state is the basic unit of political power. The distribution of power between the state and the federal government has always been a point of debate.

Historically, the states maintained power over their domestic matters. The federal government was given power over trade between the states and foreign policy issues. The federal government took greater power over domestic affairs during the Civil War, and has continued to expand its authority. The 1980s saw the federal government assume even more power through its mandate of entitlement programs such as Medicare and Medicaid, even while it reduced federal financial support for these programs.

It is the role of the federal government to determine the extent to which medical practice regulations are uniform among the 50 states, but in most areas of medical practice the states maintain the central regulatory role. States license pharmacies and pharmacy professionals, determine the standards under which pharmacists practice, and may add restrictions to federal laws, such as the food and drug laws.

The Pure Food and Drug Act of 1906

adulterated altered and causing an undesirable effect.

On June 30, 1906, Congress passed a law that provided for federal inspection of meat products, and forbade the manufacture, sale, or transport of **adulterated** food products or poisonous patent medicines. This law was called the Pure Food and Drug Act of 1906.

The Coca-Cola Company advocated for the 1906 Act so it could advertise that its soft drink was "Guaranteed under the Pure Food and Drug Act." In 1909, however, the federal government attempted to ban the soft drink, citing the Pure Food and Drug Act and Coca-Cola's caffeine and cocaine content. Coca-Cola ultimately settled the case out of court and altered the product ingredients.

Over time, the Pure Food and Drug Act proved to be inadequate, because it did not:

- cover cosmetics.
- grant the federal government authority to ban unsafe drugs.
- prohibit manufacturers from making false statements about their drugs.
- require labeling to identify the contents of a product.

INFORMATION

Disasters prompted the U.S. government to establish many of the original laws pertaining to pharmacy practice and the efficacy of medications. In 1937, a manufacturer decided to market a mixture of sulfanilamide and diethylene glycol as a remedy for sore throats. Diethylene glycol, known today as antifreeze, made the mixture into a deadly poison. This product caused 107 reported deaths, which became known as the Sulfanilamide Disaster of 1937 and prompted passage of the Food, Drug, and Cosmetic Act of 1938.

The Food, Drug, and Cosmetic Act of 1938

In 1938, U.S. legislators passed the Food, Drug, and Cosmetic Act, commonly referred to as the FDCA. The purpose of the FDCA was to limit interstate commerce in drugs to those that are safe and effective. Among the many major provisions of this legislation were the following:

- Manufacturers were required to submit evidence that new drugs were safe before they could market the drugs.
- All drugs had to have warnings and adequate directions for use.
- New drugs were required to be tested clinically before being marketed to the public.
- Drugs used as diagnostic agents, therapeutic devices, and cosmetics were regulated for the first time.

The FDCA established an agency within the U.S. Department of Health and Human Services to oversee the new policies: the Food and Drug Administration.

Many of the provisions of the FDCA pertain to requirements for the label of a drug. It is important to understand and recognize the difference between the *label* of a drug and the *labeling* of a drug. Although these sound the same, they are actually two uniquely different components regulated under the FDCA. The label of a drug is "a display of written, printed, or graphic matter upon the immediate container of any article"; it is the information on the outer portion of the package or container. The labeling of a drug refers to "all labels and other written, printed, or graphic[al matter] either upon or accompanying the drug." Thus, labeling is broader in scope than the label; the labeling of a drug includes the package and package inserts, as well as the label.

The FDCA also regulated who could prescribe *legend drugs*, those available by prescription only. The FDCA does not require that the prescriber be licensed in the state where the prescription is actually filled, as long as the prescription is valid in the state in which it was written. A prescriber is permitted to delegate an authorized individual to transmit a prescription; however, the prescriber cannot delegate the authority to prescribe or authorize a refill.

Legend Drugs

According to the FDCA, only a practitioner licensed to administer and prescribe legend drugs may do so. Such practitioners include physicians, surgeons, veterinarians, dentists, physician assistants, nurse practitioners, and even pharmacists in certain states and according to specific regulations.

These laws and regulations govern drugs dispensed for human use. Be aware that additional or modified requirements are in place for drugs dispensed for animal use.

Labeling requirements for dispensed prescriptions include the following (see Figure 4-1):

- Pharmacy name and address
- Serial number (Rx number)
- Date of fill
- Expiration date
- Prescriber's name
- Patient's name
- Directions for use
- Cautionary statements (if needed)

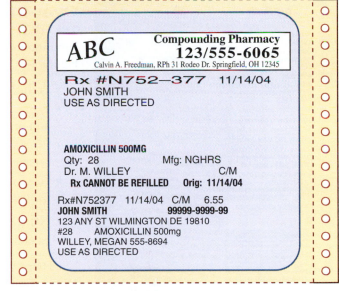

FIGURE 4-1 Sample prescription label.

The FDCA requires that legend drugs include the following information on the label of the drug (see Figure 4-2):

- Established name and quantity of each active ingredient
- Statement of new quantity
- Statement of usual dosage
- Federal legend
- Route of administration
- In the case of habit-forming drugs, a federal warning
- Name of all inactive ingredients, if intended for route of administration other than oral

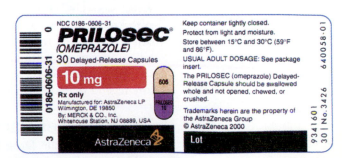

FIGURE 4-2 Sample legend drug label.
(Courtesy of Astrazeneca Pharmaceuticals LP.)

- Unique lot or control number
- Statement specifying the type of container to be used in dispensing
- The name and place of business of the manufacturer, packer, or distributor
- Expiration date, if applicable

Although the label is considered a component of the labeling of a drug, the FDA also requires additional information in the labeling that accompanies a legend drug. The following information is required by the FDA and is usually provided in the package insert:

- Description, which is usually a chemical structure
- Clinical pharmacology
- Indications and usage
- Contraindications—situations in which the drug should not be used
- Warnings of side effects and potential safety hazards
- Precautions—details as to special care that must be taken
- Adverse reactions
- Drug abuse and dependence
- Dosage
- Statement as to how the drug is supplied
- Date of the most recent revision to the labeling

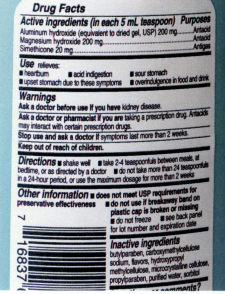

FIGURE 4-3 Sample OTC drug label.
(Courtesy of Fundamental Photographs, NYC.)

Over-the-Counter Drugs

The FDCA requires that drugs approved for over-the-counter (OTC) distribution include the following information on the label of the drug (see Figure 4-3):

- Product name
- Name and address of the manufacturer, distributor, repackager, and others in the chain of commerce
- Established name of all active ingredients and the quantities of certain other ingredients (active or inactive)
- Net contents
- Required cautions and warnings
- Name of any habit-forming drug contained in the formula
- Adequate directions for use

There have been numerous amendments to the original FDCA of 1938, as well as related legislative acts. This text cannot cover all of these amendments and acts, but the following subsections describe several of the most prominent ones.

The Durham-Humphrey Amendment of 1951

Also known as the Prescription Drug Amendment, the Durham-Humphrey Amendment of 1951 required that prescription drugs bear the legend, "Caution: Federal law prohibits dispensing without a prescription." This required legend is the reason why prescription drugs are referred to as *legend drugs*. Later amendments approved a substitute legend that simply reads "Rx only."

The Kefauver-Harris Amendment of 1962

Also known as the Drug Efficacy Amendment, the Kefauver-Harris Amendment of 1962 focused on drug manufacturers' accountability for the efficacy, or effectiveness, of drugs. Several provisions of this amendment are important to pharmacy practice:

- Good manufacturing practices (GMP) were established for manufacturers.
- Prior to marketing any new drug, manufacturers were required to supply proof of the effectiveness and safety of the drug.
- Advertising of prescription drugs was placed under the supervision of the FDA.
- Procedures for new drug applications and investigational drugs were established.

INFORMATION

The Kefauver-Harris Amendment was a legislative response to the thalidomide disaster of 1962, caused by a sedative, thalidomide, which had been developed and was widely available abroad, began to be used as an antinausea treatment in early pregnancy. Children of women who had taken the medication during their first trimester of pregnancy were often born with severe deformities, especially of the extremities.

The Comprehensive Drug Abuse Prevention and Control Act of 1970

In 1970, the Comprehensive Drug Abuse Prevention and Control Act essentially combined all of the federal laws dealing with narcotics, stimulants, depressants, and abused designer drugs.

More commonly referred to as the Controlled Substances Act of 1970, the Comprehensive Drug Abuse Prevention and Control Act established the Drug Enforcement Administration (DEA), which is an agency within the U.S. Department of Justice. It establishes a closed system, in which the distribution of controlled substances is permitted only between entities registered with the DEA.

The Controlled Substances Act (CSA) established five classes, referred to as *schedules*, of controlled substances. These schedules represent the potential for abuse of each drug. This legislation was enacted to help safeguard public safety. The schedules range from I to V, with Schedule I having the highest potential for abuse and Schedule V having the lowest (see Table 4-1).

Schedule I

Schedule I drugs have a high potential for abuse. They have no currently accepted medical use in the United States, or there is no accepted safety standard for use of the drug. Examples of drugs in Schedule I include heroin, LSD, and marijuana. C-I is the symbol for this class of drugs.

Schedule II

Schedule II drugs have a currently accepted medical use in the United States, but they also have a high potential for abuse, or the abuse of the drug or other substance may lead to severe dependence. Examples of drugs in Schedule II include cocaine, morphine, and Ritalin®. C-II is the symbol for this class of drugs.

Table 4-1 Controlled Drug Schedule

SCHEDULE	SYMBOL	EXAMPLES
Schedule I	C-I	heroin, LSD, marijuana
Schedule II	C-II	cocaine, morphine, Ritalin®
Schedule III	C-III	Vicodin®, Lortab®, Tylenol® #3, anabolic steroids
Schedule IV	C-IV	Valium®, Librium®
Schedule V	C-V	Lomotil®

Schedule III

Schedule III drugs have less potential for abuse than those in Schedules I and II and have a currently accepted medical use in the United States. Abuse of Schedule III drugs may lead to moderate physical dependence or high psychological dependence. Examples of drugs in Schedule III include Vicodin®, Lortab®, Tylenol #3®, and anabolic steroids. C-III is the symbol for this class of drugs. Schedule III substances may be refilled if authorized by the prescriber; however, refills are limited to five and all refills must be within six months of the date the original prescription was issued.

Schedule IV

Schedule IV drugs have a low potential for abuse, have a currently accepted medical use in the United States, or the abuse of these drugs may lead to limited dependence. Examples include Valium® and Librium®. C-IV is the symbol for this class of drugs. Schedule IV substances may be refilled if authorized by the prescriber; however, refills are limited to five and all refills must be within six months of the date the original prescription was issued.

Schedule V

Schedule V drugs have a low potential for abuse, have a currently accepted medical use in the United States, or the abuse of these drugs may lead to limited dependence in relation to all other controlled substances. An example of a Schedule V drug is Lomotil®. C-V is the symbol for this class of drugs. There are no additional requirements on refills of Schedule V substances, and a prescription can be refilled for up to one year according to the prescriber's directions.

Registration

Participation in any of the following activities requires registration with the DEA:

- Manufacturing controlled substances
- Distributing controlled substances
- Dispensing controlled substances
- Conducting research with controlled substances
- Conducting instructional activities with controlled substances
- Conducting a narcotic treatment program
- Conducting chemical analysis with controlled substances
- Importing or exporting controlled substances
- Compounding controlled substances

Those who engage in any of these activities must register with the DEA, using either Form 225 (to manufacturer or distribute), Form 224 (to dispense), or Form 363 (to compound or conduct a narcotic treatment program). Initial registration is granted for a period of 28 to 39 months, after which the registration period is every 36 months.

Registrants (those who are approved by the DEA) receive a unique identification number, referred to as their DEA number, to be used within the closed system.

Prescribing and Dispensing

According to the CSA, prescriptions for controlled substances must include the following:

- Full name and address of the patient
- Name, address, and registry number of the prescriber
- Date issued
- Manual signature of the prescriber

In addition, prescriptions for controlled substances are required to be written in ink, or with a typewriter or an indelible pencil.

There are additional requirements for prescribing a Schedule II substance. Most states require that these prescriptions be completed on a triplicate prescription form. Many states limit the validity of written prescriptions for C-II drugs to seven days only, and prescribers are prohibited from authorizing refills for these orders.

The dispensing of controlled substances is similar to the dispensing of legend drugs under the FDCA; however, there are several exceptions and additional regulations. In addition to the information required on the label for a noncontrolled legend prescription, controlled substances require a federal transfer warning; if the medication is a refill for a C-III or C-IV substance, the label must also include the date of initial filling, in addition to the date of the refill.

Ordering

To order Schedule I or Schedule II substances, a registrant must complete a triplicate form (DEA Form 222) or use the DEA Controlled Substance Ordering System (CSOS), which is electronic. However, registrants are not required to use the federal order form to obtain controlled substances in Schedules III, IV, or V, because of the lower potential for abuse of these substances (at least in comparison to the other schedules).

Recordkeeping

The CSA dictates that registrants keep records of the following items:

- "On-hand" inventory of controlled substances
- Biennial inventory, after the initial inventory of controlled substances

Additional records may be required depending on the activity of the registrant.

The DEA requires reporting of exact quantities of Schedules I and II substances; however, registrants are permitted to estimate quantity for Schedules III, IV, and V substances.

There are three approved filing methods for prescriptions of controlled substances:

1. Three-drawer—in which there is one file for C-II; one file for C-III, C-IV, and C-V; and one file for all other prescriptions.
2. Two-drawer—in which there is one file for all controlled substances and a different one for all other prescriptions. All prescriptions for substances on Schedules III through V must have a red "C" stamped in the lower right corner.
3. One-drawer—in which there is one drawer for C-II and one drawer for all other prescriptions, including those for Schedules III–V substances. Again, prescriptions for substances on Schedules III through V must have a red "C" stamped in the lower right corner.

Reporting

If theft of controlled substances is discovered, the registrant must report the theft to both the DEA and the local police. The disposal of controlled substances must be reported to the DEA on DEA Form 41.

Inspections

The DEA may inspect any location registered for controlled substances. It may inspect all records, reports, forms, physical inventories, prescriptions, containers, labels, and equipment pertaining to controlled substances. The DEA may also inspect security systems and/or take a physical inventory of all controlled substances.

The Poison Prevention Packaging Act of 1970

According to the Poison Prevention Packaging Act (PPPA) of 1970, all legend and controlled drugs, with some exceptions, must be dispensed in a childproof container. For patients such as the elderly, who do not wish to have their medications dispensed in such containers, a signed, written request to that effect should be kept on file at the pharmacy. Exceptions to the PPPA include sublingual doses of nitroglycerin, contraceptives, drugs dispensed to inpatients in hospitals, and certain emergency medications, among others.

" Workplace Wisdom PPPA Exceptions

- Sublingual nitroglycerin
- Sublingual/chewable isosorbide dinitrate (10 mg or less)
- Erythromycin granules for oral suspension
- Cholestyramine in powder form
- Unit-dosed potassium supplements
- Sodium fluoride (264 mg or less)
- Betamethasone tablets (12.6 mg or less)
- Pancrelipase preparations
- Prednisone tablets (105 mg or less)
- Mebendazole tablets (600 mg or less)
- Methylprednisolone tablets (84 mg or less)
- Colestipol in powder form (5 g or less)
- Erythromycin in tablet form (16 g or less)
- Drugs dispensed to inpatients in hospitals
- Upon request of the prescriber or patient

The Occupational Safety and Health Act of 1970

Congress passed the Occupational Safety and Health Act, commonly referred to as OSHA, to ensure worker and workplace safety. The goal was to make sure that employers provide their workers with a place of employment free from recognized hazards to safety and health, such as exposure to toxic chemicals, excessive noise levels, mechanical dangers, heat or cold stress, or unsanitary conditions.

To establish standards for workplace health and safety, the OSHA also created the National Institute for Occupational Safety and Health (NIOSH), a research institution for the Occupational Safety and Health Administration (OSHA).

The Drug Listing Act of 1972

The Drug Listing Act of 1972 amended the Federal Food, Drug, and Cosmetic Act to require drug establishments (manufacturers, repackagers, and distributors) to register their products and list all of their commercially marketed drug products with the Food and Drug Administration. This requirement includes establishments that repackage or otherwise change the container, wrapper, or labeling of any drug package in the course of distribution of the drug from the original place of manufacture to the person who makes final delivery or sale to the ultimate customer. The Drug Listing Act applies to all drug firms manufacturing or processing human drugs, veterinary drugs, and medicated animal feed premixes.

Each drug is assigned a unique and permanent product code, known as the National Drug Code (NDC), which identifies the drug establishment, the formulation, and the size/type of product packaging.

The Medical Device Amendment of 1976

The Medical Device Amendment of 1976 required, for the first time, that the safety and effectiveness of life-sustaining and life-supporting devices have premarket approval from the FDA.

The Orphan Drug Act of 1983

Congress passed the Orphan Drug Act of 1983 to stimulate the development of drugs for rare diseases (those that affect 200,000 people or fewer). Before passage of this legislation, private industry had little incentive to invest money in the development of treatments for small patient populations, because the drugs were expected to be unprofitable. The law provides three primary incentives:

1. seven-year market exclusivity to sponsors of approved orphan products,
2. a tax credit of 50 percent of the cost of conducting human clinical trials, and
3. federal research grants for clinical testing of new therapies to treat and/or diagnose rare diseases.

In 1997, Congress created an additional incentive when it granted companies developing orphan products an exemption from the usual drug application or user fees charged by the FDA.

The Drug Price Competition and Patent Term Restoration Act of 1984

Commonly known as the Hatch-Waxman Act, the Drug Price Competition and Patent Term Restoration Act of 1984 established the modern system of generic drugs. Manufacturers of generic drugs can file Abbreviated New Drug Applications (ANDAs) to seek FDA approval of generic versions of drugs for which patent protection is set to expire.

The Prescription Drug Marketing Act of 1987

The Prescription Drug Marketing Act was enacted to address certain prescription drug marketing practices that have contributed to the diversion of large quantities of drugs into a secondary "gray" market.

These marketing practices, including the distribution of free samples, the use of coupons redeemable for drugs at no cost or low cost, and the sale of deeply discounted drugs to hospitals and healthcare entities, helped create a multimillion-dollar drug diversion market that provided a portal through which mislabeled, sub-potent, adulterated, expired, and counterfeit drugs were able to enter the nation's drug distribution system.

The Anabolic Steroid Control Act of 1990

The Anabolic Steroid Control Act of 1990 placed anabolic steroids on Schedule III of the Controlled Substances Act. The CSA defines *anabolic steroids* as any drug or hormonal substance chemically and pharmacologically related to testosterone (other than estrogens, progestins, and corticosteroids) that promotes muscle growth.

The Omnibus Budget Reconciliation Act of 1990

Known as OBRA '90, the Omnibus Budget Reconciliation Act of 1990 focused on federal funding of the Medicare and Medicaid programs. This was the act that created an increased need for pharmacy technicians. While determining that funding, OBRA also mandated that the pharmacist perform drug utilization reviews (DURs) and offer counseling to patients, and even provided funding and set reimbursement fees for such activities. In addition to elevating the profession of pharmacist in the United States, OBRA, by its nature, created a real need for pharmacy technicians to assist pharmacists.

The Dietary Supplement Health and Education Act of 1994

The provisions of the Dietary Supplement Health and Education Act define dietary supplements and dietary ingredients; establish a framework for assuring safety; outline guidelines for literature displayed where supplements are sold; provide for use of claims and nutritional support statements; require ingredient and nutrition labeling;

and grant the FDA the authority to establish good manufacturing practice (GMP) regulations. The law also established an executive-level Commission on Dietary Supplement Labels and an Office of Dietary Supplements within the National Institutes of Health.

The Health Insurance Portability and Accountability Act of 1996

The Health Insurance Portability and Accountability Act of 1996, also known as HIPAA, was enacted to ensure patient confidentiality and privacy. Initially, HIPAA gave patients the right to review their medical records and established the requirement of patient consent for the transfer of medical records and for oral, written, and electronic communications regarding medical records. Today, patient consent is required for a pharmacist or pharmacy technician to fill a prescription.

HIPAA considers the following to be protected health information (PHI):

- Any information created or received by the pharmacy
- Information relating to a patient's health—mental or physical, past, present, or future
- Information that may identify a patient

The Combat Methamphetamine Epidemic Act of 2005

Known as the CMEA, the Combat Methamphetamine Epidemic Act of 2005 regulates, among other things, retail over-the-counter sales of ephedrine, pseudoephedrine, and phenylpropanolamine products. Retail provisions of the CMEA include daily sales limits and 30-day purchase limits, placement of product out of direct customer access, sales logbooks, customer identification verification, and employee training.

PROCEDURE **4-1**

Selling Methamphetamine-Related Products

1. Ensure that the request does not exceed daily or monthly limits.
2. Verify the customer's photo identification (e.g., driver's license).
3. Complete necessary paperwork and documentation of sale, including:
   - customer's name
   - customer's address and telephone number
   - customer's identification number (e.g., driver's license number)
   - product name
   - product strength
   - product quantity
   - date
   - customer's signature
   - your name and signature
4. Process the sales transaction at the pharmacy.

Adulteration versus Misbranding

According to the FDA, an *adulterated* drug is a drug that is in a condition contrary to the intentions of the manufacturer. Adulteration focuses on the physical condition of the drug or device. In contrast, *misbranding* focuses on the representations made by the manufacturer. Following are some criteria, any one of which is sufficient to constitute adulteration or misbranding.

misbranded drug a drug that has been misleadingly or fraudulently labeled.

Adulterated Drugs

Adulterated drugs:

- are prepared, packaged, packed, or held under unsanitary conditions.
- are manufactured in a way that does not conform to established GMPs.
- have a container composed of a poisonous or deleterious substance.
- contain an unsafe color additive.
- vary from an official compendium standard.
- are new, unsafe, animal drugs or animal feeds containing such drugs.
- are a Class III device without premarket approval (a banned device).
- are OTC drugs that are not packaged in tamper-resistant packaging.

Misbranded Drugs

Misbranded drugs:

- have false or misleading labels.
- have labels that fail to state the name and place of business of the manufacturer, packager, packer, or distributor and that lack an accurate statement of quantity.
- have labels with required information that is not prominently placed on them.
- have labels that do not state "Warning: May Be Habit Forming" in the case of habit-forming substances.
- have labels that, in the case of legend drugs, do not include the generic name or the names of ingredients, or have type on the label that is not less than one-half the size of the trade/brand name.
- are not listed in an official compendium (unless they are labeled and packaged by compendium standards).
- are in packages that are misleading.
- are subject to deterioration, and the label does not bear corresponding precautionary statements.
- endanger one's health if used in the manner suggested by the labeling.
- are composed of either insulin or an antibiotic drug and are not batch certified.
- contain a color additive and are not labeled accordingly.
- are produced by manufacturers who are not registered with the FDA and who do not list the drug as one they manufacture.
- are subject to the Poison Prevention Packaging Act of 1970 and are not packaged accordingly.
- are touted in advertisements that fail to mention the generic or established names (if they are prescription drugs) and that omit the side effects, warnings, contraindications, effectiveness, and quantitative formulas of the drugs.
- have labels with inadequate directions for use and inadequate warnings about the effects of the drugs.
- have labels that fail to bear the statement "Caution: Federal law restricts this drug to use by or on the order of a licensed veterinarian," in the case of veterinary drugs.

New Drugs

According to the FDCA, there are in essence only two ways in which drugs can be lawfully sold in the United States. The drug must either be exempted through the 1962 amendments or be approved by the FDA under the procedures for a new drug application.

The process by which the FDA approves new drugs includes the approval of an investigational new drug (IND) through the filing of a new drug application (NDA).

It can take years before approval is gained through this process, not counting the many years of research and development—and approval is never guaranteed.

Samples

The following is considered a drug sample by the FDA: any drug that is habit forming; bears the federal legend or is restricted to investigational use; or is not intended to be sold, but rather is purveyed to promote sale of the drug. The FDA permits manufacturers and distributors to distribute drug samples upon written request of a prescriber, under a system that requires the recipient to execute a written receipt for the sample and return the receipt to the manufacturer.

Medical Devices

medical device any instrument or apparatus used in the diagnosis, prevention, monitoring, treatment, or alleviation of disease.

A **medical device** is an instrument or machine that is recognized in either the National Formulary or *U.S. Pharmacopoeia*. It is intended for the diagnosis, cure, mitigation, treatment, or prevention of disease, or it is intended to affect the structure or any function of the body of a human or animal.

The FDCA categorizes medical devices into three classes. Class I devices are those that have relatively low potential to cause harm, such as scissors or needles. Class II devices are subject to specific performance standards established by a panel of experts. Examples of Class II devices are thermometers, hearing aids, and catheters. Class III medical devices are life-supporting systems whose failure could cause death or serious injury.

Monographs

monograph a detailed document pertaining to a specific drug.

Drug **monographs**, commonly known as *package inserts*, are a necessary component of a drug's labeling (see Figure 4-4). The monograph provides all the clinical information required by the FDA. Most monographs are similar in layout and style, and contain the following sections.

Description. This section provides a written description of the visual elements of the drug and packaging, as well as the basic chemical structure of the drug.

Clinical Pharmacology. Under this section, manufacturers provide information on the drug's mechanism of action, absorption, distribution, metabolism, elimination, and administration. They also include any notes relevant to specific patient populations, such as pediatric patients.

Indications and Usage. This section describes the specific conditions or symptoms that the drug has been approved by the FDA to prevent or treat.

Contraindications. This section lists the types of patients who should not use the medication, whether that is a class of patients (such as diabetics) or individuals taking another specific class of drug.

Warnings. This section details the serious side effects that can be caused by the medication and instructions on what the patient should do if these effects are experienced.

Precautions. This section lists all of the remaining possible, or potential, side effects that the patient should be aware of.

Drug Abuse and Dependence. This section provides notification if the medication has shown signs of a potential for abuse or dependence.

Adverse Reactions. This section covers reactions that are unexpected and potentially life-threatening.

Dosage. This section includes the recommended dosage of medication; dosages are typically categorized by patient age and/or weight.

How Supplied. This section describes how the medication is supplied, including strengths, dosage formats, and storage requirements.

PRESCRIBING INFORMATION

Sample package insert (figure content). Detected charts:

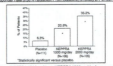
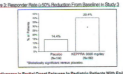
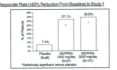

FIGURE 4-4 Sample package insert, or monograph, for Keppra® injection. (Courtesy of UCB, Inc.)

Ethics and the Pharmacy Technician

As in many professions, **ethics** is a factor in decision making for pharmacy professionals, including pharmacy technicians. Many situations can and will arise in which you or your colleagues will be required to make ethical decisions. Ethical decisions are required in those gray areas where there is no clear-cut, black-or-white, correct or incorrect response or choice. These decisions require an understanding of a professional code of ethics, as well as an understanding of moral principles and their application to your own life.

Ethics is not law, religion, or morals, but all of these can affect your ethical decisions. Ethics is as personal as your individual faith and influences much of your behavior. In a profession, members of that profession often adopt an ethical code. This code can serve as a guidepost or parameter to aid your reasoning process when a decision is

ethics a system of principles and duties; often associated with a profession.

required. Keeping your ethical decisions within the limits of an ethical code can also help protect you if you are called upon to defend your actions.

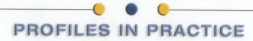

PROFILES IN PRACTICE

To better illustrate this topic, as well as later discussions on ethical theories, consider the following scenarios, which are commonplace situations in pharmacy practice.

- Mrs. Montgomery, a regular customer, arrives at your pharmacy and needs a refill for her Synthroid, a legend drug. While processing her order, you discover that she has no refills left on her prescription. It is 9:00 p.m. on Friday night, and Monday is the Fourth of July. You notify the pharmacist of the situation and await further instructions.
- A distribution problem arises when there is a vaccine or medication shortage. What factors must be considered when determining to whom those items will be dispensed or administered?

Defining Ethics

The term *ethics* derives from the Greek word *éthos*, referring to character. Ethics is commonly defined as the considered reflection and systematic analysis of the morality of certain behavior when required actions are unclear. An ethical decision is not an emotional, knee-jerk reaction, but something that has been weighed and measured carefully. **Medical ethics** is the discipline of evaluating the merits, risks, and social concerns of activities in the field of medicine.

> **medical ethics** principles and moral values of proper medical care.

Moral Philosophy

A *moral*, or *principle-based*, *philosophy* is an individualized set of values or value system. It is the moral reasoning process that guides you as you decide the rightness or wrongness of conduct. Such a philosophy will guide you in reaching ethical decisions that align with professional standards of conduct.

Practicing Ethics

Several moral principles concern pharmacy professionals. These principles are the basis for the theories of ethical practice discussed next. While reviewing the principles, keep in mind that there may be conflicts between them. For instance, beneficence may help the most people, but require you to abandon veracity. Here are the five principles:

> **beneficence** the quality of being kind or charitable.

> **fidelity** faithfulness to obligations and duties.

> **veracity** truthfulness; the quality of conforming with the truth.

> **justice** the principle of moral rightness and equity.

- **beneficence**—bringing about good
  Your role as a pharmacy technician places you in a position to benefit others (namely, your patients).
- **fidelity**—keeping a promise
  This is illustrated by a pharmacy technician who strictly fills prescriptions in the order in which they were dropped off, thereby keeping a promise to have patients' prescriptions ready by a certain time.
- **veracity**—telling the truth
  Pharmacy technicians demonstrate veracity when they report any inappropriate actions or behaviors occurring within the pharmacy, such as drug diversion or unreported medication errors.
- **justice**—acting with fairness or equity within the law
  An example of this occurred years ago, when a new OTC product was introduced: Cold Eze®. The product received extensive media coverage, and word-of-mouth testimonials caused the demand to quickly outgrow the supply.

Pharmacy technicians acted justly by limiting the quantities sold per individual and setting up waiting lists for new shipments.

- **autonomy**—acting with self-reliance
Pharmacy technicians demonstrate autonomy by working interdependently within the pharmacy; in other words, the technicians work by supporting the pharmacist, but also are reliable, dependable, and show appropriate initiative.

autonomy the condition or quality of being independent.

Ethical Theories

The following nine theories can help you measure possible ethical decisions. To better illustrate these theories, we will return to the ethical scenarios presented earlier.

Consequentialism

The theory of **consequentialism** states that the purpose of all actions should be to bring about the greatest good to the greatest number. Returning to Mrs. Montgomery's situation (mentioned previously), how does the theory of consequentialism treat her problem? What about restricting the use of flu vaccine in the case of a medication shortage? How could that decision be guided under this theory?

consequentialism the theory that the value of an action derives solely from the value of its consequences.

Nonconsequentialism

Nonconsequentialism is the study of actions themselves without regard to outcome. In other words, it is the argument that the ends justify the means. Could the pharmacist argue that Mrs. Montgomery having her medication is more important than the law that says legend drugs cannot be dispensed without a valid prescription? In the case of a shortage, could we say that first come–first served is the fairest way to distribute vaccine?

nonconsequentialism the theory that certain actions, in and of themselves, are wrong.

Social Contracts

Pharmacists, technicians, and patients recognize certain expectations of each other and act accordingly. Such expectations are called **social contracts**. Can Mrs. Montgomery argue that she entrusts the pharmacist with the responsibility to provide for her medication needs? Could the pharmacist in turn argue that her situation is not his problem, because Mrs. Montgomery has a responsibility to keep her prescriptions current and he in turn should be able to expect such behavior? How would this theory apply to the vaccine situation?

social contract an understood agreement between individual members of a society.

The Ethics of Care

The *ethics of care* is a "principle [that] requires the decision-maker to more clearly focus on such basic moral skills as kindness, sensitivity, attentiveness, tact, patience, and reliability." In the situation with Mrs. Montgomery, should the pharmacist ask herself what the kind and reliable action would be? Could she argue that "teaching" Mrs. Montgomery to be more conscientious by refusing to fill her expired prescription would be the better path? What is the most humane action in the face of a vaccine shortage?

Rights-Based Ethics

Rights-based ethics is a theory based on an understanding of human rights—the belief that an individual in a democratic society should be shielded from undue forces and allowed to enjoy and pursue personal projects; in short, the theory that each individual has certain moral rights as well as legal rights. Does Mrs. Montgomery have a right to receive her medication despite any rules or regulations? Could the pharmacist argue that she should fill Mrs. Montgomery's prescription because it is the patient's right? How would rights-based ethics apply to the vaccine shortage?

Principle-Based Ethics

Principle-based ethics state that moral principles are general, universal guides to action. This is a more personal approach. The pharmacist could say that going against a law is immoral for her. However, it could also be argued that refusing medication to anyone who needs it is also immoral. You could ask, "Is it ever moral to deny medication to someone in need?" How does that question, and your answer, change in a shortage situation?

Virtues-Based Ethics

Virtues-based ethics is the use of virtues, or the idealization of specific morals, establishing right reason in action. In Mrs. Montgomery's case, what would the most virtuous action be? What about in the vaccine shortage case?

Law

Law is closely related to the system of ethics and sometimes overlaps it, creating confusion and tension about the "right thing to do" in a given situation. Mrs. Montgomery is a good example. The laws governing prescriptions are very clear. They do not allow exceptions. The pharmacist could definitely quote the law to Mrs. Montgomery and refuse to fill her prescription, arguing that the law is the law and the pharmacist's hands are tied. Are there any laws governing the distribution of drugs? Would they apply to the vaccine case? Should there be new laws for just such a case?

Professional Code of Ethics

Pharmacy technicians are healthcare professionals who assist pharmacists in providing the best possible care to patients. The principles of this code, which apply to pharmacy technicians working in any and all settings, are based on the application and support of the moral obligations that guide the pharmacy profession in relationships with patients, healthcare professionals, and society.

An identifying benchmark for all professions is their sincere acceptance of the responsibility to maintain a standard of conduct beyond either an unthinking conformity to the law or the routine performance of technical skills. The code of ethics that follows is an example of the ninth ethical theory, virtues-based ethics. It was written by technicians for technicians and adopted by both the American Association of Pharmacy Technicians and the National Pharmacy Technician Association. Can you find an answer to Mrs. Montgomery's dilemma here that works for you?

The Pharmacy Technician Code of Ethics

Preamble

I. A pharmacy technician's first considerations are to ensure the health and safety of the patient and to use knowledge and skills to the best of his ability in serving others.

II. A pharmacy technician supports and promotes honesty and integrity in the profession, which includes a duty to observe the law, maintain the highest moral and ethical conduct at all times, and uphold the ethical principles of the profession.

III. A pharmacy technician assists and supports the pharmacist in the safe, efficacious, and cost-effective distribution of health services and healthcare resources.

IV. A pharmacy technician respects and values the abilities of pharmacists, colleagues, and other healthcare professionals.

V. A pharmacy technician maintains competency in his practice, and continually enhances his professional knowledge and expertise.

VI. A pharmacy technician respects and supports the patient's individuality, dignity, and confidentiality.

VII. A pharmacy technician respects the confidentiality of the patient's records and discloses pertinent information only with proper authorization.

VIII. A pharmacy technician never assists in the dispensing or distributing of medications or medical devices that are not of good quality or do not meet the standards required by law.

IX. A pharmacy technician does not engage in any activity that will discredit the profession, and he will expose, without fear or favor, illegal or unethical conduct in the profession.

X. A pharmacy technician associates with and engages in the support of organizations that promote the profession of pharmacy through the use and enhancement of pharmacy technicians.

SUMMARY

Many of the regulations pertaining to practice as a pharmacy technician are established and overseen by your specific state's board of pharmacy. In general, federal laws pertain to the manufacturing of pharmaceutical products, and state laws pertain to the actual dispensing of those products. It is imperative that you familiarize yourself with both the federal laws and the laws of your particular state pertaining to pharmacy practice. In addition, you should fully understand the basic ethical theories and the Code of Ethics for Pharmacy Technicians, in preparation for the ethical dilemmas and questions that will inevitably arise in the pharmacy setting.

CHAPTER REVIEW QUESTIONS

1. The _____ requires that prescription drugs bear the legend, "Caution: Federal law prohibits dispensing without a prescription."
   a. Drug Listing Act
   b. Kefauver-Harris Amendment
   c. Food, Drug, and Cosmetic Act
   d. Durham-Humphrey Amendment

2. _____ law cases may be initiated only by the state, not by victims.
   a. Administrative
   b. Case
   c. Civil
   d. Criminal

3. Which of the following is an example of a C-IV medication?
   a. Valium®
   b. Ritalin®
   c. Vicodin®
   d. Lomotil®

4. The chemical structure of a drug is listed within the _____ section of a drug's official monograph.
   a. adverse reaction
   b. clinical pharmacology
   c. description
   d. dosage

5. Which of the following moral principles refers to telling the truth?
   a. fidelity
   b. veracity
   c. beneficence
   d. autonomy

6. Which agency is responsible for registering and regulating pharmacy facilities and pharmacy professionals?
   a. CMS
   b. FDA
   c. OSHA
   d. SBOP

7. A hearing aid is classified as a Class _____ medical device.
   a. I
   b. II
   c. III
   d. IV

8. Which of the following is commonly referred to as the Drug Efficacy Amendment?
   a. Kefauver-Harris Amendment
   b. Durham-Humphrey Amendment
   c. Medical Device Amendment
   d. none of the above

9. Which of the following ethical theories states that pharmacists, technicians, and patients recognize certain expectations of each other and act accordingly?
   a. nonconsequentialism
   b. principle-based ethics
   c. social contracts
   d. virtue-based ethics

10. Which pharmacy-related law was determined to be inadequate because it did not require labeling to identify a product's contents?
    a. Controlled Substances Act
    b. Food, Drug, and Cosmetic Act
    c. Poison Prevention Packaging Act
    d. Pure Food and Drug Act

CRITICAL THINKING QUESTIONS

1. Contrast the role the federal government plays in the regulation of pharmacy practice with that of the state government.

2. An individual, who clearly abuses illegal drugs, asks to purchase a box of syringes at the pharmacy. On the one hand, if the pharmacy staff sells the syringes to the individual, they are in some way aiding in his addiction; on the other hand, they are ensuring that he does not feel obligated to share or reuse needles. What do you believe is the ethical thing to do? Why?

3. Why is it important that pharmacy technicians have a professional code of ethics?

WEB CHALLENGE

1. Pharmacy technicians can be, and have been, held liable in civil lawsuits related to medication errors. Several companies offer professional liability insurance designed for pharmacy technicians. Visit www.phmic.com and www.hpso.com and compare the policies they offer to technicians.

2. Using a search engine, search for "pharmacy technician sued" or "pharmacy technician lawsuit." While researching, print out information on three civil lawsuits in which a technician has been sued.

REFERENCES AND RESOURCES

Buerki, RA, & Voterro, LD. *Ethical Practices in Pharmacy: A Guidebook for Pharmacy Technicians.* Madison, WI: American Institute of the History of Pharmacy, 1997.

Johnston, M. *Certification Exam Review.* Upper Saddle River, NJ: Pearson, 2005.

Johnston, M. *Fundamentals of Pharmacy Practice.* Upper Saddle River, NJ: Pearson, 2005.

Nielsen, JR. *Handbook of Federal Drug Law* (2nd ed.). Philadelphia: Williams & Wilkins, 1992.

Richards, E, & Rathbun, K. *Law & The Physician: A Practical Guide.* Boston: Little Brown, 1993.

Terminology and Abbreviations

5 chapter

LEARNING OBJECTIVES

After completing this chapter, you should be able to:

- Identify selected root words used in pharmacy practice.
- Identify and correctly use selected prefixes and suffixes in conjunction with root words.
- Recognize and interpret common abbreviations used in pharmacy and medicine.
- List abbreviations that are considered dangerous and explain why.
- Recognize and list common drug names and their generic equivalents.
- Recall and define common pharmacy and medical terminology.

KEY TERMS

combining form 65

prefix 64

root words 64

suffix 65

Introduction

To understand the pharmacy industry and profession, you must learn the appropriate language, which consists of terminology and abbreviations. Most medical terms derive from Greek and Latin and consist of a root word, prefix, and/or suffix. By learning selected roots, prefixes, and suffixes, you will be able to understand words you may have never seen or heard before.

This chapter covers the most common words and phrases, as well as prefixes and suffixes, used to communicate in the practice of pharmacy. This chapter gives you an overview of the standard terminology that you will need to know if you are to succeed. The information is arranged by topic, and then alphabetically, for easier reference in the future. This chapter is not all-inclusive; you should continue to learn as much terminology as possible to increase your knowledge base.

root words words or parts of a word that identify the major meaning of a term.

Understanding Selected Roots

Root words are words or parts of a word that identify the major meaning of the term. Root words are the essential part of the whole word. More specifically, root words can identify the part of the body or condition to which a term relates. Table 5-1 lists some of the common root words used in various pharmacy settings.

Understanding Selected Prefixes

prefix a part of a word attached to the beginning of the root word that gives a specific meaning to the root.

A **prefix** is a part of a word attached to the beginning of the root word that gives a specific meaning to the root. For example, *bio-* means living organisms. If you recognize this prefix in a medical term, you will know that the term pertains in some way to living organisms. Prefixes are commonly used in the medical field to signify the meaning of a bigger word. Table 5-2 presents some of the common prefixes you will encounter as a pharmacy technician.

Table 5-1 Selected Roots

ROOT	MEANING	EXAMPLE
arter	artery	arterial
arthr	joint	arthritis
bronch	bronchus	bronchitis
carcin	cancer	carcinoma
cardi	heart	cardiac
cyst	bladder	cystoscopy
derma	skin	dermatology
enter	abdomen/intestine	enteral
gastr	stomach	gastric
gluco	sugar	glucose
hemo	blood	hematology
hepat	liver	hepatoma
my	muscle	myalgia
nasa	nose	nasal
nephr	kidney	nephrology
neur	nerve	neurology
oste	bone	osteoporosis
patho	disease	pathologist
phleb	vein	phlebotomy
pneum	lung	pneumonia
psych	mind	psychosis
procto	rectum	proctology
pulmo	lung	pulmonary
ren	kidney	renal
rhin	nose	rhinoplasty
thromb	blood clot	thrombosis
vas	(blood) vessel	vascular

Table 5-2   Common Prefixes

PREFIX	MEANING	EXAMPLE
a-, an-	without	anesthesia
ante-	before	anterior
anti-	inhibit, oppose	antibiotic
bio-	living organisms	biology
brady-	slow	bradycardia
con-	together	conception
contra-	against	contraindication
dia-	complete	diagnosis
dys-	abnormal, difficult	dyslipidemia
en-	in	enteral
ex-	out	external
hyper-	too much	hyperglycemia
hypo-	too little	hypoglycemia
inter-	between, among	interstitial
intra-	within	intradermal
macro-	large	macronutrients
mal-	abnormal	malabsorption
micro-	small	microscope
neo-	new	neonatal
para-	around	parasite
poly-	many, much	polydipsia
post-	after, behind	postmenopausal
pre-	before, in front	prenatal
sub-	below, underlying	sublingual
tachy-	fast	tachycardia

Understanding Selected Suffixes

A **suffix** is a part of a word attached to the end of the root word that gives a specific, new meaning to the root word. For example, *-logy* is a suffix that means "the study of." If you add *-logy* to the prefix *bio-*, you end up with *biology*, or the study of living organisms. Table 5-3 includes the common suffixes a pharmacy technician should be familiar with and understand.

suffix a part of a word attached to the end of the root word that gives a specific meaning to the root.

Understanding Combining Forms

A **combining form** is a root word with an added vowel. The vowel does not give a new meaning to the root word; its sole purpose is to make it easier to combine the root word with a suffix or another root. The combining form simply makes the new term easier to say, and does not change the meaning of the other word parts.

For example, *cardi-* is a root word meaning "heart." When the suffix *-ac* is added to the root, it becomes *cardiac*, which means pertaining to the heart. When the suffix *-logy*

combining form a root word with an added vowel.

Table 5-3 Common Suffixes

SUFFIX	MEANING	EXAMPLE
-ac	pertaining to	cardiac
-al	pertaining to	renal
-algia	pain	fibromyalgia
-ase	enzyme	protease
-cide	kill, killer	suicide
-cyte	cell	leukocyte
-dipsia	thirst	polydipsia
-ectomy	surgical removal	hysterectomy
-emia	blood condition	anemia
-ic	pertaining to	toxic
-itis	inflammation	rhinitis
-logist	specialist	oncologist
-logy	study of	biology
-oid	resembling	steroid
-oma	tumor	carcinoma
-osis	condition	histoplasmosis
-pathy	disease	neuropathy
-plasty	surgical repair	rhinoplasty
-rrhage	bursting of blood	hemorrhage
-rrhea	flowing discharge	diarrhea
-sclerosis	hardening	arteriosclerosis
-scope	instrument	microscope
-scopy	viewing of	colonoscopy
-stasis	control	homeostasis
-uria	urine	polyuria

is added to the root, we add an extra "o" to connect the root and suffix, producing *cardiology*, which means the study of the heart.

Pharmacy Abbreviations

As in the medical field, you will encounter numerous abbreviations, acronyms, and codes in the pharmacy setting. To completely understand the language of pharmacy, you must be able to understand and interpret these abbreviations. Although the abbreviations are not federally recognized, they are favored as substitutes, with a standard meaning, for a whole word or phrase. It is much easier to read a couple of symbols than to interpret several lines in a physician's poor handwriting. Symbols and abbreviations are also used as a time-saving measure for the physician and pharmacy staff. To prepare a prescription for dispensing correctly, you must be able to interpret the medication order as written by the physician. Tables 5-4 through 5-8 present the common abbreviations used in writing prescriptions, as well as those used in standard pharmacy practice. These include abbreviations related to pharmacy in general, directions and SIG codes, routes of administration, dosages and measurements, and medicines.

Table 5-4   General Pharmacy Abbreviations

MEANING	ABBREVIATION
adverse drug effect	ADE
adverse drug reaction	ADR
average wholesale price	AWP
compound	cmpd; cpd
concentration	conc
diagnosis-related group	DRG
discontinue	D/C; DC
dispense	disp.
dispense as written	DAW
Drug Enforcement Administration	DEA
drug utilization review	DUR
elixir	elix
enteric coated	EC
fluid	fl.
Food and Drug Administration	FDA
maximum allowable cost	MAC
no known allergies	NKA
nothing by mouth	NPO
ointment	oint; ung
over-the-counter	OTC
pediatric	ped
prescription	Rx
Schedule I	C-I
Schedule II	C-II
Schedule III	C-III
Schedule IV	C-IV
Schedule V	C-V
solution	soln
suppository	supp
syrup	syr
vitamin	vit
water	aq; aqua
wholesale acquisition cost	WAC

Table 5-5 Pharmacy Abbreviations—Directions/SIG Codes

MEANING	ABBREVIATION
after	p
after meals	pc
after meals and at bedtime	pc & hs
afternoon	pm
as desired	ad lib
as directed	u.d.
as needed	prn
as soon as possible	ASAP
bedtime	hs
before meals	ac
before meals and at bedtime	ac & hs
both ears	AU
both eyes	OU
by mouth	po; PO
daily	qd; QD
dispense as written	DAW
double strength	DS
every	q; Q
every day	qd; QD
every day at bedtime	qhs; QHS
every afternoon/evening	qpm; QPM
every hour	qh; QH
every morning	qam; QAM
every other day	qod; QOD
every week	qw
four times daily	qid; QID
hour	hr
left ear	AS
left eye	OS
may repeat	MR
right ear	AD
right eye	OD
three times daily	tid; TID
two times daily	bid; BID
weekly	w; wk
with	ć
without	s̄
while awake	W/A; WA
24 hours	24H

Table 5-6   Pharmacy Abbreviations—Routes of Administration

MEANING	ABBREVIATION
buccal	BU
by mouth	PO
External	EX
inhalation	IN
Injection	Inj
intradermal	ID
intramuscular	IM
intravenous	IV
intravenous piggyback	IVPB
intravenous push	IVP
intrauterine	IU
metered dose inhaler	MDI
mouth/throat	MT
nasal	NA
ophthalmic	oph; opth
oral	OR
otic	OT
rectally	PR; RE
subcutaneous	SC
sublingual	SL
tincture	tinct.
transdermal	TD
urethral	UR
vaginally	PV; VA

Table 5-7   Pharmacy Abbreviations

MEANING	ABBREVIATION
ampule	Amp
capsule	Cap
centimeter	Cm
cubic centimeter	Cc
drop	Gtt
drops	Gtts
each	aa; ea
fluid ounce	fl. oz.
grain	gr.
gram	g; gm

Table 5-7   Pharmacy Abbreviations (*continued*)

MEANING	ABBREVIATION
hour	H; hr
kilogram	Kg
liter	L
microgram	Mcg
milligram	Mg
milliequivalent	mEq
milliliter	ml; mL
millimeter	Mm
ounce	Oz
pound	lb; #
tablespoon	tbsp; TBS
tablet	Tab
teaspoon	Tsp
units	U
$\frac{1}{2}$	ss

Table 5-8   General Medical Abbreviations

MEANING	ABBREVIATION
acetaminophen	apap; APAP
acquired immune deficiency syndrome	AIDS
aspirin	asa; ASA
attention deficit disorder	ADD
attention deficit hyperactivity disorder	ADHD
autonomic nervous system	ANS
before surgery	pre op
birth control pills	BC; BCP
blood pressure	BP
blood sugar	BS
bowel movement	BM
calcium	Ca
carbohydrate	Carb
central nervous system	CNS
congestive heart failure	CHF
dextrose 5% in water	D5W
discontinue	D/C; DC
electrocardiogram	ECG; EKG

Table 5-8   General Medical Abbreviations (*continued*)

MEANING	ABBREVIATION
electroencephalogram	EEG
gastrointestinal	GI
genitourinary	GU
headache	HA
health maintenance organization	HMO
history	Hx
human immunodeficiency virus	HIV
hydrochlorothiazide	HCTZ
hydrogen peroxide	H_2O_2
intensive care unit	ICU
iron	Fe
magnesium	Mg
magnesium oxide	MgO; MagOx
managed care organization	MCO
milk of magnesia	MOM
multiple vitamin	MV; MVI
nausea and vomiting	N/V; N&V
nitroglycerine	NTG
nonsedating antihistamines	NSAs
nonsteroidal anti-inflammatory drugs	NSAIDs
normal saline	NS
penicillin	PCN
potassium	K
potassium chloride	KCl
preferred provider organization	PPO
sodium	Na
sodium chloride	NaCl
tetracycline	TCN
total parenteral nutrition	TPN
urinary tract infection	UTI

Dangerous Abbreviations

Effective January 1, 2004, the Joint Commission on the Accreditation of Healthcare Organizations (JCAHO) issued a list of dangerous abbreviations, acronyms, and symbols that are not to be used, known as the "Do Not Use" list. One of the major problems with certain abbreviations is that they may have more than one meaning. For example, "DC" could mean *discharge* in one instance and *discontinue* in another. Also, these abbreviations are prone to misinterpretation: poorly written, *QD* could look like *QID* to someone other than the writer.

With communication and use of medical records and documentation spanning various health care venues, abbreviations increase the risk of misinterpretation and error. In addition, some healthcare staff may be unfamiliar with certain abbreviations, which can cause a delay in getting appropriate health care to the patient. The primary benefit of excluding dangerous abbreviations is patient safety.

The following items are affected by this JCAHO initiative:

- medication orders
- clinical documentation
- progress notes
- consultation reports
- operative reports
- educational materials
- protocols
- other related

In 1999, the Institute of Medicine (IOM) issued a report stating that between 44,000 and 96,000 deaths each year may be attributed to medical errors. In light of this information, numerous healthcare entities are continuously evaluating and developing strategies for reducing these occurrences. One result has been the development of the "Do Not Use" list, which is based on the most commonly mistaken and misunderstood written abbreviations used in all forms of medical communication. As of January 1, 2004, a "minimum" list of dangerous abbreviations, acronyms, and symbols was approved by JCAHO (see Table 5-9). Beginning January 1, 2004, the items listed in Table 5-9 *must* be included on each accredited organization's "Do not use" list.

In addition to this basic list of items that must not be used, as of April 1, 2004, each organization had to identify at least three additional "Do not use" abbreviations, acronyms, or symbols (of its own choosing) to go on its mandatory "Do not use" list. Table 5-10 offers suggestions for items that should be considered for each facility's "Do not use" list.

Table 5-9   JCAHO's "Minimum" Do Not Use List

ABBREVIATION	POTENTIAL PROBLEM	PREFERRED TERM
IU (for international unit)	Mistaken as IV (intravenous) or 10 (ten)	Write "international unit."
MS, MSO_4, $MgSO_4$	Confused for one another; can mean morphine sulfate or magnesium sulfate	Write "morphine sulfate" or "magnesium sulfate."
Q.D., Q.O.D. (Latin abbreviation for once daily and once every other day)	Mistaken for each other. The period after the Q can be mistaken for an "I" and the "O" can be mistaken for "I"	Write "daily" and "every other day."
Trailing zero (X.0 mg), lack of leading zero (.X mg)	Decimal point is missed	Never write a zero by itself after a decimal point (X mg), and always use a zero before a decimal point (0.X mg) .
U (for unit)	Mistaken as zero, four, or cc	Write "unit."

Table 5-10   JCAHO's "Recommended" Do Not Use List

ABBREVIATION	POTENTIAL PROBLEM	PREFERRED TERM
µg (for microgram)	Mistaken for mg (milligrams) resulting in thousand-fold overdose.	Write "mcg."
A.S., A.D., A.U. (Latin abbreviations for left, right, or both ears); O.S., O.D., O.U. (Latin abbreviation for left, right, or both eyes)	Mistaken for each other (e.g., AS for OS, AD for OD, AU for OU, etc.).	Write "left ear," "right ear," or "both ears"; "left eye," "right eye," or "both eyes."
c.c. or cc (for cubic centimeter)	Mistaken for U (units) when poorly written.	Write "mL" for milliliter.
D/C (for discharge)	Interpreted as discontinue whatever medications follow (typically discharge meds).	Write "discharge."
H.S. (for half-strength or bedtime)	Mistaken for either half-strength or hour of sleep (at bedtime). q.H.S. mistaken for every hour. All can result in a dosing error.	Write out "half-strength" or "at bedtime."
S.C. or S.Q. (for subcutaneous)	Mistaken as SL for sublingual, or "5 every."	Write "Sub-Q," "subQ," or "subcutaneously."
T.I.W. (for three times a week)	Mistaken for three times a day or twice weekly, resulting in an overdose.	Write "3 times weekly" or "three times weekly."

In addition, the Institute for Safe Medical Practices (ISMP), has suggested other abbreviations, acronyms, and symbols that should be considered suspect. Optimally, all these terms should be prohibited also (see Table 5-11).

Further details are available on the following JCAHO and ISMP websites:

- www.jcaho.com
- www.ISMP.org

Table 5-11   ISMP's "Recommended" Do Not Use List

ABBREVIATION/ DOSE EXPRESSION	INTENDED MEANING	MISINTERPRETATION	CORRECTION
3	dram	Misunderstood or misread (symbol for dram misread as "3" and minim misread as "mL")	Use the metric system.
> and <	greater than and less than	Mistakenly used for the opposite of intended meaning	Use "greater than" or "less than."
/ (slash mark)	separates two doses or indicates "per"	Misunderstood as the number 1 ("25 unit/10 units" read as "110" units)	Do not use a slash mark to separate elements in doses. Use "per."
x3d	for three days	Mistaken for "three doses"	Use "for three days."
ARA°A ara-V	vidarabine	cytarabineARA°C (ara-C)	Write out drug name.
AU	aurio uterque (each ear)	Mistaken for OU (oculo uterque—each eye)	Do not use this abbreviation.
AZT	zidovudine (Retrovir)	azathioprine	Write out drug name.

Table 5-11   ISMP's "Recommended" Do Not Use List (*continued*)

ABBREVIATION/ DOSE EXPRESSION	INTENDED MEANING	MISINTERPRETATION	CORRECTION
BT	bedtime	Mistaken as "BID" (twice daily)	Use "hs."
cc	cubic centimeters	Misread as "U" (units)	Use "mL."
CPZ	Compazine (prochlorperazine)	chlorpromazine	Write out drug name.
D/C	discharge, discontinue	Premature discontinuation of medications when D/C (intended to mean "discharge") is misinterpreted as "discontinued" when followed by a list of drugs	Use "discharge" and "discontinue."
DPT	Demerol-Phenergan-Thorazine	diphtheria-pertussis-tetanus (vaccine)	
HCl	hydrochloric acid	potassium chloride (the "H" is misinterpreted as a "K")	
HCT	hydrocortisone	hydrochlorothiazide	
HCTZ	hydrochlorothiazide	hydrocortisone (seen in misinterpretation of HCT250 mg)	
IU	international unit	Misread as IV (intravenous)	Use "units."
m g	microgram	Mistaken for "mg" when handwritten	Use "mcg."
MgSO$_4$	magnesium sulfate	morphine sulfate	
MSO$_4$	morphine sulfate	magnesium sulfate	
MTX	methotrexate	mitoxantrone	
"Nitro" drip	nitroglycerin infusion	sodium nitroprusside infusion	
"Norflox"	norfloxacin	Norflex	
o.d. or OD	once daily	Misinterpreted as "right eye" (OD—oculus dexter), causing administration of oral medications in the eye	Use "daily."
per os	orally	The "os" can be mistaken for "left eye"	Use "PO," "by mouth," or "orally."
q6PM, etc.	every evening at 6 p.m.	Misread as every six hours	Use 6 p.m. "nightly."
q.d. or QD	every day	Mistaken for q.i.d., especially if the period after the "q" or the tail of the "q" is read as an "i"	Use "daily" or "every day."
qhs	nightly at bedtime	Misread as every hour	Use "nightly."
qn	nightly or at bedtime	Misinterpreted as "qh" (every hour)	Use "nightly."
q.o.d. or QOD	every other day	Misinterpreted as "q.d." (daily) or "q.i.d. (four times daily) if the "o" is poorly written	Use "every other day."
SC	subcutaneous	Mistaken for SL (sublingual)	Use "subcut." or write "subcutaneous."

Table 5-11 ISMP's "Recommended" Do Not Use List (*continued*)

ABBREVIATION/ DOSE EXPRESSION	INTENDED MEANING	MISINTERPRETATION	CORRECTION
ss	sliding scale (insulin) or ½ (apothecary)	Mistaken for "55"	Spell out "sliding scale." Use "one-half" or use ½.
sub q	subcutaneous	The "q" has been mistaken for "every" (e.g., one heparin dose ordered "sub q 2 hours before surgery" misinterpreted as every two hours before surgery)	Use "subcut." or write "subcutaneous."
TAC	triamcinolone	tetracaine, Adrenalin, cocaine	
TIW or tiw	three times a week.	Mistaken as "three times a day"	Do not use this abbreviation.
U or u	unit	Read as a zero (0) or a four (4), causing a 10-fold overdose or greater (4U seen as "40" or 4u seen as "44")	"Unit" has no acceptable abbreviation. Use "unit."
$ZnSO_4$	zinc sulfate	morphine sulfate	
Name letters and dose numbers run together (e.g., Inderal40 mg)	Inderal 40 mg	Misread as Inderal 140 mg	Always use space between drug name, dose, and unit of measure.
Zero after decimal point (1.0)	1 mg	Misread as 10 mg if the decimal point is not seen	Do not use terminal zeros for doses expressed in whole numbers.
No zero before decimal dose (.5 mg)	0.5 mg	Misread as 5 mg	Always use zero before a decimal when the dose is less than a whole unit.

Drug Names

Table 5-12 provides a comprehensive list of often-used brand-name drugs and their generic equivalents.

Table 5-12 Common Brand-Name and Generic Prescription Drugs

BRAND/TRADE NAME	GENERIC NAME
Abbokinase	urokinase
Accolate	zafirlukast
Accupril	quinapril HCl
Accutane	isotretinoin
Achromycin, Sumycin	tetracycline HCl
Aciphex	rabeprazole sodium
Aclovate	alclometasone dipropionate
Acthar, ACTH	corticotropin
Acticin	permethrin
Actifed, Triafed	triprolidine HCl & pseudoephedrine HCl
Actigall	ursodiol
Activase	alteplase

Table 5-12 Common Brand-Name and Generic Prescription Drugs (*continued*)

BRAND/TRADE NAME	GENERIC NAME
Actonel	risedronate sodium
Adenocard	adenosine
Adrenalin Chloride, Sus-Phrine	epinephrine HCl
Adrucil	fluorouracil
Advil, Motrin, Nuprin	ibuprofen
AeroBid, Nasalide	flunisolide
Aerosporin	polymyxin B sulfate
Afrin, Allerest, Dristan Long Lasting, Duration, Sinex Long Acting	oxymetazoline HCl (nasal)
Aftate, Tinactin	tolnaftate
Aggrastat	tirofiban
Agoral Plain, Kondremul	mineral oil emulsion
Akineton	biperiden
Alamast	pemirolast potassium
Albalon, Privine, Vasocon	naphazoline HCl
Albamycin	novobiocin
Albenza	albendazole
Aldactazide	hydrochlorothiazide & spironolactone
Aldactazide	spironolactone & hydrochlorothiazide
Aldactone	spironolactone
Aldomet	methyldopa
Aldoril	methyldopa & hydrochlorothiazide
Aleve, Anaprox	naproxen sodium
Alfenta	alfentanil HCl
Alkeran	melphalan
Allbee w/C, Stresscaps, Surbex-T	Vitamin B complex with C
Allegra	fexofenadine HCl
Alomide	lodoxamide tromethamine
Alphagan	brimonidine tartrate
Altace	ramipril
Alupent	metaproterenol sulfate
Amaryl	glimepiride
Ambien	zolpidem tartrate
Amerge	naratriptan
Americaine	benzocaine
A-Methapred, Solu-Medrol	methylprednisolone sodium succinate
Amicar	aminocaproic acid
Amidate	etomidate
Amikin	amikacin sulfate

Table 5-12   Common Brand-Name and Generic Prescription Drugs (*continued*)

BRAND/TRADE NAME	GENERIC NAME
Amoxil	amoxicillin
Amphojel	aluminum hydroxide gel
Amytal	amobarbital sodium
Anadrol-50	oxymetholone
Anafranil	clomipramine HCl
Ancef, Kefzol	cefazolin sodium
Ancobon	flucytosine
Androlone-D, Deca-Durabolin	nandrolone decanoate
Ansaid	flurbiprofen
Antabuse	disulfiram
Antagon	ganirelix acetate
Antilirium	physostigmine salicylate
Antivert, Bonine	meclizine HCl
Anturane	sulfinpyrazone
Anzemet	dolasetron mesylate
Aphthasol	amlexanox
Apresazide	hydralazine & hydrochlorothiazide
Apresoline	hydralazine HCl
Aquasol A	Vitamin A
Aquasol E	Vitamin E
Aquatensen, Enduron	methyclothiazide
Aralen HCl	chloroquine HCl
Aramine	metaraminol
Arava	leflunomide
Aredia	pamidronate disodium
Aricept	donepezil HCl
Arimidex	anastrozole
Artane	trihexyphenidyl HCl
Arthrotec	diclofenac sodium & misoprostol
Asacol, Pentasa, Rowasa	mesalamine
Ascorbic Acid	Vitamin C
Ascriptin, Bufferin	aspirin, buffered
Asendin	amoxapine
Aspirin	a.s.a (acetylsalicylic acid)
Astelin	azelastine HCl
Astramorph PF, Duramorph, MS Contin, Roxanol	morphine sulfate
Atacand	candesartan cilexetil
Atarax	hydroxyzine HCl

Table 5-12   Common Brand-Name and Generic Prescription Drugs (*continued*)

BRAND/TRADE NAME	GENERIC NAME
Ativan	lorazepam
Atromid-S	clofibrate
Atrovent	ipratropium bromide
Attenuvax	measles (rubeola) virus vaccine, live
Augmentin	amoxicillin & potassium clavulanate
Auralgan	antipyrine & benzocaine
Avapro	irbesartan
Aventyl, Pamelor	nortriptyline HCl
Avita, Renova	tretinoin
Axid	nizatidine
Aygestin	norethindrone acetate
Azactam	aztreonam
Azmacort, Kenalog, Nasacort	triamcinolone acetonide
Azo-Gantrisin	phenazopyridine HCl & sulfisoxazole
Azopt	brinzolamide
Azulfidine	sulfasalazine
Bacid, Lactinex	lactobacillus
Bactrim, Septra	sulfamethoxazole & trimethoprim
Bactroban	mupirocin
Beepen-VK, Pen-Vee K, Veetids	penicillin V potassium
Bemote, Bentyl, Antispas	dicyclomine HCl
Benadryl	diphenhydramine HCl
Benemid	probenecid
Benylin	dextromethorphan HBr
Benzedrex	propylhexedrine
Betadine	povidone-iodine
Betapace	sotalol HCl
Betoptic, Kerlone	betaxolol HCl
Biaxin	clarithromycin
Bicillin C-R	penicillin G benzathine & procaine
Bicitra	sodium citrate & citric acid
BICNU	carmustine (BCNU)
Blenoxane	bleomycin sulfate
Bleph-10, Sulamyd Sodium	sulfacetamide sodium
Blocadren, Timoptic	ticlopidine HCl
Brethine, Bricanyl	terbutaline sulfate
Bretylol	bretylium tosylate
Brevibloc	esmolol HCl

Table 5-12   Common Brand-Name and Generic Prescription Drugs (*continued*)

BRAND/TRADE NAME	GENERIC NAME
Brevital Sodium	methohexital sodium
Bumex	bumetanide
Buphenyl	sodium phenylbutyrate
Buprenex	buprenorphine HCl
BuSpar	buspirone HCl
Butisol Sodium	butabarbital sodium
Cafergot	ergotamine tartrate & caffeine
Calan, Isoptin, Verelan	verapamil HCl
Calciferol	Vitamin D
Calciferol, Drisdol	ergocalciferol
Calcijex, Rocaltrol	calcitriol
Calcium Pantothenate, Pantothenic Acid	Vitamin B_5
Camptosar	irinotecan HCl
Cantil	mepenzolate bromide
Capastat Sulfate	capreomycin
Capitrol	chloroxine
Capoten	captopril
Capozide	captopril & hydrochlorothiazide
Carafate	sucralfate
Carbatrol, Tegretol	carbamazepine
Carbocaine, Polocaine	mepivacaine HCl
Cardene	nicardipine HCl
Cardioquin	quinidine polygalacturonate
Cardizem, Dilacor XR	diltiazem HCl
Cardura	doxazosin mesylate
Carnitor	levocarnitine
Cartrol	carteolol HCl
Cataflam	diclofenac potassium
Catapres	clonidine HCl
Caverject	alprostadil
Ceclor	cefaclor
Cedax	ceftibuten
CeeNU	lomustine
Cefadyl	cephapirin sodium
Cefizox	ceftizoxime sodium
Cefobid	cefoperazone sodium
Cefotan	cefotetan disodium
Ceftin, Kefurox, Zinacef	cefuroxime

Table 5-12   Common Brand-Name and Generic Prescription Drugs (*continued*)

BRAND/TRADE NAME	GENERIC NAME
Cefzil	cefprozil
Celebrex	celecoxib
Celestone	betamethasone
Celexa	citalopram hydrobromide
Celontin Kapseals	methsuximide
Cerebyx	fosphenytoin sodium
Chirocaine	levobupivacaine
Chloroptic, Chloromycetin	chloramphenicol
Chlor-Trimeton	chlorpheniramine maleate
Choledyl	oxtriphylline
Chronulac, Cephulac	lactulose syrup
Cinobac	cinoxacin
Cipro	ciprofloxacin
Claforan	cefotaxime sodium
Claritin	loratadine
Cleocin	clindamycin
Climara, Estraderm	estradiol transdermal
Clinoril	sulindac
Clomid, Serophene	clomiphene citrate
Clorpres, Combipres	clonidine HCl & chlorthalidone
Cloxapen	cloxacillin sodium
Clozaril	clozapine
Cogentin	benztropine mesylate
Cognex	tacrine HCl
Colace, Diocto	docusate sodium (dss)
Colestid	colestipol HCl
Coly-Mycin M	colistimethate sodium
Coly-Mycin S	colistin sulfate (polymixin E)
Combivent	ipratropium bromide & albuterol sulfate
Combivir	lamivudine & zidovudine
Compazine	prochlorperazine
Copaxone	glatiramer acetate
Cordarone	amiodarone HCl
Corgard	nadolol
Corlopam	fenoldopam mesylate
Cortef, Hydrocortone	hydrocortisone
Cortisporin	neomycin, polymyxin B, hydrocortisone
Cortone	cortisone acetate

Table 5-12 Common Brand-Name and Generic Prescription Drugs (*continued*)

BRAND/TRADE NAME	GENERIC NAME
Cortrosyn	cosyntropin
Corvert	ibutilide fumarate
Corzide	bendroflumethiazide & nadolol
Cosmegen	actinomycin D
Cosmegen	dactinomycin
Cotazym, Viokase, Creon, Ilozyme, Pancrease	pancrelipase
Coumadin	warfarin sodium
Crixivan	indinavir mesylate
Cuprimine, Depen	penicillamine
Cutivate, Flonase	fluticasone propionate
Cyanocobalamin	Vitamin B_{12}
Cyclocort	amcinonide
Cyclospasmol	cyclandelate
Cycrin, Depo-Provera, Provera	medroxyprogesterone acetate
Cylert	pemoline
Cystadane	betaine anhydrous
Cystagon	cysteamine bitartrate
Cytadren	aminoglutethimide
Cytomel, Triostat	liothyronine sodium
Cytosar-U	cytarabine
Cytotec	misoprostol
Cytovene	ganciclovir sodium
Cytoxan, Neosar	cyclophosphamide
D.H.E. 45, Migranal	dihydroergotamine mesylate
Dalgan	dezocine
Dalmane	flurazepam HCl
Danocrine	danazol
Dantrium	dantrolene sodium
Daranide	dichlorphenamide
Daraprim	pyrimethamine
Daricon	oxyphencyclimine HCl
Darvocet-N	propoxyphene napsylate & acetaminophen
Darvon	propoxyphene HCl
Darvon Compound-65	propoxyphene HCl, aspirin, caffeine
Darvon-N	propoxyphene napsylate
DaunoXome	daunorubicin citrate liposomal
Daypro	oxaprozin
Decadron, Hexadrol	dexamethasone

Table 5-12 Common Brand-Name and Generic Prescription Drugs (*continued*)

BRAND/TRADE NAME	GENERIC NAME
Decholin	dehydrocholic acid
Declomycin	demeclocycline HCl
Delestrogen, Valergen	estradiol valerate
Delta Cortef, Prelone	prednisolone
Demadex	torsemide
Demerol HCl	meperidine HCl
Demser	metyrosine
Denavir	penciclovir
Depakene	valproic acid
Depakote	divalproex sodium
Depo-Medrol	methylprednisolone acetate
Depo-Testosterone	testosterone cypionate
Desenex	undecylenic acid
Desferal	deferoxamine mesylate
Desoxyn	methamphetamine HCl
Desquam, Persa-Gel	benzoyl peroxide
Desyril	trazodone HCl
Detrol	tolterodine tartrate
Dexedrine	dextroamphetamine sulfate
DiaBeta, Glynase, Micronase	glyburide
Diabinese	chlorpropamide
Diamox	acetazolamide
Dibenzyline	phenoxybenzamine HCl
Didrex	benzphetamine HCl
Didronel	etidronate disodium
Differin	adapalene
Diflucan	fluconazole
Digibind	digoxin immune FAB
Digitek, Lanoxin	digoxin
Dilantin	phenytoin
Dilaudid	hydromorphone HCl
Dilaudid Cough Syrup	hydromorphone HCl & guaifenesin
Dimetane	brompheniramine maleate
Dimetapp	brompheniramine maleate & phenyl-propanolamine HCl
Diovan	valsartan
Dipentum	olsalazine sodium
Diprivan	propofol
Diprosone	betamethasone dipropionate

Table 5-12 Common Brand-Name and Generic Prescription Drugs (*continued*)

BRAND/TRADE NAME	GENERIC NAME
Disalcid	salsalate
Ditropan	oxybutynin chloride
Diuril	chlorothiazide
Dobutrex	dobutamine HCl
Dolobid	diflunisal
Dolophine HCl	methadone HCl
Dolorac	capsaicin
Donnatal	belladonna alkaloids & phenobarbital
Dopar, Larodopa	levodopa
Dopram	doxapram
Doral	quazepam
Dostinex	cabergoline
Dramamine	dimenhydrinate
Drixoral	dexbrompheniramine maleate & pseudoephedrine sulfate
DTIC-Dome	dacarbazine
Dulcolax	bisacodyl
Durabolin, Hybolin	nandrolone phenpropionate
Duragesic	fentanyl transdermal
Duranest HCl	etidocaine HCl
Duricef	cefadroxil
Dycill, Dynapen, Pathocil	dicloxacillin sodium
Dymelor	acetohexamide
DynaCirc	isradipine
Dyrenium	triamterene
E.E.S., EryPed	erythromycin ethylsuccinate
Ecotrin	enteric coated aspirin
Edecrin	ethacrynic acid
Effexor	venlafaxine
Elavil	amitriptyline HCl
Eldepryl	selegiline HCl
Ellence	epirubicin HCl
Elmiron	pentosan polysulfate sodium
Elspar	asparaginase
Emete-Con	benzquinamide HCl
Emetrol	phosphated carbohydrate solution
Eminase	anistreplase, anisoylated PSAC
Emprin with Codeine	aspirin with codeine
E-Mycin, Eryc, Ery-Tab, Ilotycin, PCE	erythromycin base

Table 5-12 Common Brand-Name and Generic Prescription Drugs (*continued*)

BRAND/TRADE NAME	GENERIC NAME
Enbrel	etanercept
Enduronyl	methyclothiazide & deserpidine
Engerix-B, Recombivax HB	hepatitis B vaccine
Enlon, Reversol, Tensilon	edrophonium chloride
Entex LA	phenylpropanolamine HCl & guaifenesin
Epogen	epoetin alfa
Epsom Salt	magnesium sulfate
Equagesic	meprobamate & aspirin
Ergamisol	levamisole HCl
Ergocalciferol	Vitamin D_2
Ergomar, Ergostat	ergotamine tartrate
Ergotrate	ergonovine maleate
Erythrocin Stearate	erythromycin stearate
Estinyl	ethinyl estradiol
Estrace	estradiol
Ethmozine	moricizine HCl
Ethyol	amifostine
Eurax	crotamiton
Euthroid, Thyrolar	liotrix
Evista	raloxifene
Exosurf	colfosceril palmitate
Famvir	famciclovir
Fareston	toremifene citrate
Fastin, Zantryl	phentermine HCl
Felbatol	felbamate
Feldene	piroxicam
Femcare, Gyne-Lotrimin, Lotrimin, Mycelex	clotrimazole
Femiron	ferrous fumarate
Feosol, Fer-In-Sol	ferrous sulfate
Fergon	ferrous gluconate
Fioricet	butalbital, caffeine, & acetaminophen
Fiorinal	butalbital, caffeine, & aspirin
Flagyl, Metrogel, Protostat	metronidazole
Fleet Enema	sodium phosphate enema
Flexeril	cyclobenzaprine HCl
Florinef Acetate	fludrocortisone acetate
Floxin, Ocuflox	ofloxacin
Fludara	fludarabine phosphate

Table 5-12 Common Brand-Name and Generic Prescription Drugs (*continued*)

BRAND/TRADE NAME	GENERIC NAME
Flumadine	rimantadine HCl
Fluothane	halothane
Folex, Rheumatrex	methotrexate
Folvite	folic acid
Fortaz, Tazidime	ceftazidime
Fortovase, Invirase	saquinavir
Fosamax	alendronate sodium
FUDR	floxuridine
Fungizone	amphotericin B
Furadantin	nitrofurantoin
Gabitril	tiagabine HCl
Galzin	zinc acetate
Gamastan, Gammar	gamma globulin IM
Gamastan, Gammar	immune globulin IM
Gamimune N, Gammagard, Gammar-IV, Sandoglobulin	immune globulin IV (IGIV)
Gantanol	sulfamethoxazole
Gantrisin	sulfisoxazole
Gan-Xene, Tranxene	clorazepate dipotassium
Garamycin, Genoptic	gentamicin
Gastrocrom, Intal, Nasalcrom	cromolyn sodium
Gas-X, Mylicon, Phazyme	simethicone
Gemzar	gemcitabine
Geocillin	carbenicillin indanyl sodium
Geref	sermorelin
Glucophage	metformin HCl
Glucotrol	glipizide
Glyset	miglitol
Gonal-F	follitropin alfa
Grifulvin V, Grisactin, Fulvicin PG	griseofulvin
Habitrol, Nicoderm, Prostep	nicotine transdermal
Halcion	triazolam
Haldol	haloperidol
Halotestin	fluoxymesterone
Herplex	idoxuridine
Hespan	hetastarch
Hibiclens	chlorhexidine gluconate
Hiprex, Urex	methenamine hippurate
Hismanal	astemizole

Table 5-12 Common Brand-Name and Generic Prescription Drugs (*continued*)

BRAND/TRADE NAME	GENERIC NAME
Hivid	zalcitabine
Humalog	insulin lispro
Humatin	paromomycin
Humibid, Robitussin	guaifenesin (glycerol guaiacolate)
Humorsol	demecarium bromide
Hyalgan, Vitrax, Synvisc	sodium hyaluronate
Hycamtin	topotecan HCl
Hycodan	hydrocodone bitartrate & homatropine methylbromide
Hydeltra—T.B.A.	prednisolone tebutate
Hydeltrasol, Pediapred	prednisolone sodium phosphate
Hydergine	ergoloid mesylates
Hydrea	hydroxyurea
HydroDIURIL, Esidrix, Oretic, Microzide	hydrochlorothiazide
Hydromox	quinethazone
Hydropres	hydrochlorothiazide & reserpine
Hygroton	chlorthalidone
Hylorel	guanadrel sulfate
Hyperstat, Proglycem	diazoxide
Hyper-Tet	tetanus immune globulin
Hy-Phen, Vicodin	hydrocodone bitartrate & acetaminophen
Hytrin	terazosin
Idamycin	idarubicin HCl
Ifex	ifosfamide
Ilopan	dexpanthenol
Ilosone	erythromycin estolate
Imdur, ISMO	isosorbide mononitrate
Imitrex	sumatriptan succinate
Imodium	loperamide HCl
Imuran	azathioprine
Inapsine	droperidol
Inderal	propranolol HCl
Inderide	propranolol HCl & hydrochlorothiazide
Indocin	indomethacin
Infasurf	calfactant
InfeD	iron dextran
Innovar	fentanyl citrate & droperidol
Inocor	amrinone lactate
Integrillin	eptifibatide

Table 5-12 Common Brand-Name and Generic Prescription Drugs (*continued*)

BRAND/TRADE NAME	GENERIC NAME
Intropin	dopamine HCl
Inversine	mecamylamine HCl
Ismelin	guanethidine monosulfate
Isopto Carpine, Pilocar, Pilostat	pilocarpine HCl
Isordil, Sorbitrate	isosorbide dinitrate
Isuprel	isoproterenol
Kantrex	kanamycin sulfate
Kaon	potassium gluconate
Kaon-Cl, K-Dur, K-Lor, Klorvess, K-Lyte/Cl, K-Tab, Micro-K, Slow-K, Ten-K, Klor-Con, Klotrix	potassium chloride
Kaopectate	kaolin & pectin
Karidium, Luride, Pediaflor	sodium fluoride
Kayexalate	sodium polystyrene sulfonate
Keflex	cephalexin
Keflin	cephalothin sodium
Keftab	cephalexin monohydrate
Kemadrin	procyclidine HCl
Kenacort, Aristocort	triamcinolone
Ketalar	ketamine HCl
Kinevac	sincalide
Klonopin	clonazepam
Kristalose	lactulose (crystallized)
Kwell	lindane
Kytril	granisetron HCl
Lacril, Isopto Plain	methylcellulose drops
Lamisil	terbinafine HCl
Lamprene	clofazimine
Lariam	mefloquine HCl
Lasix	furosemide
Lescol	fluvastatin sodium
Leukeran	chlorambucil
Leukine	sargramostim
Leustatin	cladribine
Levatol	penbutolol sulfate
Levo-Dromoran	levorphanol tartrate
Levophed	norepinephrine (levarterenol)
Levsin, Cystospaz, Anaspaz	l-hyoscyamine sulfate
Lexxel Extended Release	enalapril maleate/felodipine

Table 5-12 Common Brand-Name and Generic Prescription Drugs (*continued*)

BRAND/TRADE NAME	GENERIC NAME
Librax	chlordiazepoxide HCl & clidinium bromide
Librium, Libritab	chlordiazepoxide HCl
Lidex	fluocinonide
Limbitrol	chlordiazepoxide HCl & amitriptyline HCl
Lincocin	lincomycin
Lioresal	baclofen
Lipitor	atorvastatin
Lithane, Lithobid, Eskalith	lithium carbonate
Lithostat	acetohydroxamic acid (AHA)
Livostin	levocabastine HCl
Lodine	etodolac
Lodosyn	carbidopa
Lomotil	diphenoxylate HCl w/atropine sulfate
Loniten, Rogaine	minoxidil
Lopid	gemfibrozil
Lopressor	metoprolol
Loprox	ciclopirox olamine
Lorabid	loracarbef
Lotemax	loteprednol etobonate
Lotensin	benazepril HCl
Lotrel	amlodipine/benazepril HCl
Lotrisone	clotrimazole & betamethasone dipropionate
Lovenox	enoxaparin sodium
Loxitane	loxapine succinate
Lozol	indapamide
Ludiomil	maprotiline HCl
Lufyllin	dyphylline
Luminal, Solfoton	phenobarbital
Lupron	leuprolide acetate
Luvox	fluvoxamine maleate
Lysodren	mitotane
Maalox	aluminum hydroxide, magnesium hydroxide suspension
Macrobid, Macrodantin	nitrofuratoin macrocrystals
Magan	magnesium salicylate
Milk of Magnesia (MOM)	magnesium hydroxide
Mandelamine	methenamine mandelate
Mandol	cefamandole naftate

Table 5-12   Common Brand-Name and Generic Prescription Drugs (*continued*)

BRAND/TRADE NAME	GENERIC NAME
Maolate	chlorphenesin carbamate
Marcain, Sensorcaine	bupivacaine HCl
Marezine	cyclizine
Marinol	dronabinol
Matulane	procarbazine HCl
Mavik	trandolapril
Maxair	pirbuterol acetate
Maxalt	rizatriptan benzoate
Maxaquin	lomefloxacin HCl
Maxipime	cefepime HCl
Maxzide, Dyazide	triamterene & hydrochlorothiazide
Mazanor, Sanorex	mazindol
Mebaral	mephobarbital
Meclan	meclocycline sulfosalicylate
Meclomen	meclofenamate sodium
Medrol	methylprednisolone
Mefoxin	cefoxitin sodium
Megace	megestrol acetate
Mellaril	thioridazine HCl
Mentax	butenafine HCl
Mepergan	meperidine HCl & promethazine
Mephyton, Aquamephyton, Phytonadione	phytonadione (Vitamin K_1)
Mepron	atovaquone
Meridia	sibutramine
Merrem IV	meropenem
Meruvax II	rubella virus vaccine, live
Mesantoin	mephenytoin
Mesnex	mesna
Mestinon, Regonol	pyridostigmine bromide
Methergine	methylergonovine maleate
Meticorten, Orasone, Deltasone	prednisone
Mevacor	lovastatin
Mexitil	mexiletine HCl
Mezlin	mezlocillin sodium
Miacalcin, Calcimar	calcitonin-salmon
Micardis	telmisartan
Micatin, Monistat-Derm	miconazole nitrate
Midamor	amiloride HCl

Table 5-12 Common Brand-Name and Generic Prescription Drugs (*continued*)

BRAND/TRADE NAME	GENERIC NAME
Milk of Magnesia (MOM)	magnesium hydroxide
Miltown, Equanil	meprobamate
Minipress	prazosin HCl
Minitran, Nitro-Bid, Nitrostat, Tridil	nitroglycerin
Minizide	prazosin HCl & polythiazide
Minocin	minocycline HCl
Miradon	anisindione
Mirapex	pramipexole
Mithracin	mithramycin
Mithracin	plicamycin
Mivacron	mivacurium chloride
Moban	molindone HCl
Moduretic	amiloride HCl & hydrochlorothiazide
Monocid	cefonicid sodium
Monopril	fosinopril sodium
Monurol	fosfomycin tromethamine
Mucomyst	acetylcysteine
Murine Plus, Tyzine, Visine	tetrahydrozoline HCl
Mustargen, HN_2	nitrogen mustard (mechlorethamine)
Mutamycin	mitomycin
Myambutol	ethambutol HCl
Mycifradin	neomycin sulfate
Mycobutin	rifabutin
Mycogen II, Mycolog II	nystatin & triamcinolone
Mycostatin, Nilstat	nystatin
Mylanta	aluminum hydroxide, magnesium hydroxide w/simethicone suspension
Myleran	busulfan
Myochrysine	gold sodium thiomalate
Mysoline	primidone
Mytelase	ambenonium chloride
Nalfon	fenoprofen calcium
Nallpen, Unipen	nafcillin sodium
Naprosyn	naproxen
Naqua, Metahydrin	trichlormethiazide
Narcan	naloxone HCl
Nardil	phenelzine sulfate
Naropin	ropivacaine HCl
Natacyn	natamycin

Table 5-12   Common Brand-Name and Generic Prescription Drugs (*continued*)

BRAND/TRADE NAME	GENERIC NAME
Navane	thiothixene
Nebcin, Tobrex	tobramycin sulfate
NegGram	nalidixic acid
Nembuta	pentobarbital sodium
Neo-Synephrine	phenylephrine HCl
Neptazane	methazolamide
Nesacaine	chloroprocaine HCl
Neumega	oprelvekin
Neupogen	filgrastim
Neurontin	gabapentin
Niacin, Nicotinic Acid	Vitamin B$_3$
Nicobid, Nicolar, Nicotinex	niacin (nicotinic acid)
Nilandron	nilutamide
Nimbex	cisatracurium besylate
Nimotop	nimodipine
Nitrek, Nitro-Dur, Transderm-Nitro	nitroglycerine (transdermal)
Nitropress	nitroprusside sodium
Nizoral	ketoconazole
Noctec	chloral hydrate
Nolvadex	tamoxifen citrate
Norcuron	vecuronium bromide
Norflex	orphenadrine citrate
Norgesic	orphenadrine citrate, ASA, & caffeine
Normodyne, Trandate	labetalol HCl
Noroxin, Chibroxin	norfloxacin
Norpace	disopyramide phosphate
Norpramin	desipramine HCl
Norvasc	amlodipine
Norvir	ritonavir
Novafed, Sudafed	pseudoephedrine HCl
Novantrone	mitoxantrone HCl
Novocain	procaine HCl
Nubain	nalbuphine HCl
Numorphan	oxymorphone HCl
Nuromax	doxacurium chloride
Nutropin	somatropin
Nydrazid, Laniazid	isoniazid
Ogen, Ortho-Est	estropipate

Table 5-12   Common Brand-Name and Generic Prescription Drugs (*continued*)

BRAND/TRADE NAME	GENERIC NAME
Omnicef	cefdinir
Omnipen, Principen, Totacillin, Polycillin	ampicillin
Oncovin, Vincasar	vincristine sulfate
Optimine	azatadine maleate
Oreton Methyl, Android, Testred	methyltestosterone
Organidin	iodinated glycerol
Orgaran	danaparoid sodium
Orinase	tolbutamide
Orudis, Oruvail	ketoprofen
Oxsoralen	methoxsalen
OxyContin	oxycodone HCl
Pamine	methscopolamine bromide
Paradione	paramethadione
Parafon Forte DSC, Paraflex	chlorzoxazone
Paral	paraldehyde
Paraplatin	carboplatin
Paregoric	camphorated tincture of opium
Parlodel	bromocriptine mesylate
Parnate	tranylcypromine suflate
Patanol	olopatadine HCl
Pavabid	papaverine HCl
Pavulon	pancuronium bromide
Paxil	paroxetine HCl
Paxipam	halazepam
PBZ	tripelennamine HCl
Pediazole	erythromycin ethylsuccinate/sufisoxazole
Peganone	ethotoin
Penetrex	enoxacin
Pentam 300, Nebupent	pentamidine isethionate
Penthrane	methoxyflurane
Pentothal	thiopental sodium
Pepatavlon	pentagastrin
Pepcid	famotidine
Percocet, Roxicet	oxycodone HCl & acetaminophen
Percodan	oxycodone HCl & aspirin
Periactin	cyproheptadine HCl
Peri-Colace	docusate sodium w/casanthranol (dss+)
Permax	pergolide mesylate

Table 5-12 Common Brand-Name and Generic Prescription Drugs (*continued*)

BRAND/TRADE NAME	GENERIC NAME
Permitil, Prolixin	fluphenazine HCl
Persantine	dipyridamole
Pfizerpen	penicillin G potassium
Phenergan	promethazine HCl
Pipracil	piperacillin sodium
Pitocin, Syntocinon	oxytocin
Pitressin	vasopressin
Placidyl	ethchlorvynol
Plaquenil Sulfate	hydroxychloroquine sulfate
Plasma-Plex, Plasmanate	plasma protein fraction
Platinol	cisplatin
Plavix	clopidogrel
Plendil	felodipine
Polaramine	dexchlorpheniramine maleate
Ponstel	mefenamic acid
Pontocaine HCl	tetracaine HCl
Prandin	repaglinide
Pravachol	pravastatin sodium
Precose	acarbose
Pregnyl	chorionic gonadotropin
Premarin	conjugated estrogens
Prempro	conjugated estrogens & medroxyprogesterone acetate
Prevacid	lansoprazole
Priftin	rifapentine
Prilosec	omeprazole
Primacor	milrinone lactate
Primaxin	imipenem-cilastatin
Prinivil, Zestril	lisinopril
Prinzide, Zestoretic	lisinopril & hydrochlorothiazide
Priscoline HCl	tolazoline HCl
ProAmatine	midodrine HCl
Pro-Banthine	propantheline bromide
Procardia, Adalat	nifedipine
Proleukin	aldesleukin
Proloprim, Trimpex	trimethoprim
Pronestyl, Procan-SR	procainamide HCl
Propacet, Wygesic	propoxyphene HCl & acetaminophen
Propecia, Proscar	finasteride

Table 5-12 Common Brand-Name and Generic Prescription Drugs (*continued*)

BRAND/TRADE NAME	GENERIC NAME
Propine	dipivefrin HCl
Propulsid	cisapride
ProSom	estazolam
Prostaphlin, Bactocill	oxacillin sodium
Prostigmin	neostigmine
Prostin E2	dinoprostone
Proventil, Ventolin	albuterol
Provigil	modafinil
Prozac	fluoxetine HCl
Pulmicort, Rhinocort	budesonide
Pulmozyme	dornase alfa
Purinethol	mercaptopurine (6-MP)
Pyridium, Urodine	phenazopyridine HCl
Pyridoxine HCl	Vitamin B_6
Quarzan	clidinium bromide
Quelicin, Anectine	succinylcholine chloride
Questran	cholestyramine
Quinaglute Dura-Tabs	quinidine gluconate
Quinora, Quinidex Extentabs	quinidine sulfate
Rapamune	sirolimus
Raplon	rapacuronium bromide
Raxar	grepafloxacin
Refludan	lepirudin (rDNA)
Regitine	phentolamine mesylate
Reglan	metoclopramide HCl
Regranex	becaplermin
Regroton	chlorthalidone & reserpine
Relafen	nabumetone
Relenza	zanamivir
Remeron	mirtazapine
Remicade	infliximab
Renagel	sevelamer
Renese	polythiazide
Requip	ropinirole HCl
Rescriptor	delavirdine mesylate
Restoril	temazepam
Retavase	reteplase
Retrovir	zidovudine (AZT)

Table 5-12 Common Brand-Name and Generic Prescription Drugs (*continued*)

BRAND/TRADE NAME	GENERIC NAME
Riboflavin	Vitamin B_2
Ridaura	auranofin
Rimactane, Rifadin	rifampin
Riopan	magaldrate
Risperdal	risperidone
Ritalin	methylphenidate HCl
Rituxan	rituximab
Robaxin	methocarbamol
Robaxisal	methocarbamol & aspirin
Robinul	glycopyrrolate
Rocephin	ceftriaxone sodium
Romazicon	flumazenil
Rubex, Adriamycin	doxorubicin HCl
Rythmol	propafenone HCl
Salutensin	hydroflumethiazide & reserpine
Sandostatin	octreotide acetate
Sansert	methysergide maleate
Seconal Sodium	secobarbital sodium
Sectral	acebutolol HCl
Seldane D	terfenadine & pseudoephedrine HCl
Selsun Blue, Selsun	selenium sulfide
Senokot, Senolax	senna
Ser-Ap-Es	hydralazine, hydrochlorothiazide, & reserpine
Serax	oxazepam
Serentil	mesoridazine
Serevent	salmeterol
Seromycin	cycloserine
Serzone	nefazodone
Silvadene	silver sulfadiazine
Sinemet	carbidopa & levodopa
Sinequan	doxepin HCl
Singulair	montelukast sodium
Solganal	aurothioglucose
Solu-Cortef	hydrocortisone sodium succinate
Soma	carisoprodol
Sonata	zaleplon
Sparine	promazine HCl
Spectrobid	bacampicillin HCl

Table 5-12   Common Brand-Name and Generic Prescription Drugs (*continued*)

BRAND/TRADE NAME	GENERIC NAME
Sporanox	itraconazole
Stadol	butorphanol tartrate
Stelazine	trifluoperazine HCl
Stilphostrol	diethylstilbestrol diphosphate
Streptase	streptokinase
Stromectol	ivermectin
Sublimaze	fentanyl
Sucraid	sacrosidase
Sufenta	sufentanil citrate
Sular	nisoldipine
Sulfamylon	mafenide acetate
Suprane	desflurane
Suprax	cefixime
Surfak	docusate calcium
Survanta	beractant
Sustiva	efavirenz
Symmetrel	amantadine HCl
Synalar	fluocinolone acetonide
Synercid	quinupristin/dalfopristin
Synthroid, Levothroid	levothyroxine sodium
Tagamet	cimetidine
Talacen	pentazocine & acetaminophen
Talwin	pentazocine
Tambocor	flecainide acetate
Tao	troleandomycin
Tapazole	methimazole
Tasmar	tolcapone
Tavist	clemastine fumarate
Taxol	paclitaxel
Taxotere	docetaxel
Temodar	temozolomide
Temovate	clobetasol propionate
Tenex	guanfacine HCl
Tenoretic	atenolol & chlorthalidone
Tenormin	atenolol
Tenuate	diethylpropion HCl
Terazol	terconazole
Terramycin, Uri-Tet	oxytetracycline HCl

Table 5-12 Common Brand-Name and Generic Prescription Drugs (*continued*)

BRAND/TRADE NAME	GENERIC NAME
Teslac	testolactone
Tessalon	benzonatate
Thalomid	thalidomide
Theo-Dur, Slo-Phyllin, Gyrocaps	theophylline
Thiamine HCl	Vitamin B_1
Thorazine	chlorpromazine HCl
Thypinone	protirelin
Ticar	ticarcillin disodium
Tigan	trimethobenzamide HCl
Tikosyn	dofetilide
Tilade	nedocromil sodium
Timentin	ticarcillin & clavulanate potassium
Timolide	hydrochlorothiazide & timolol maleate
TobraDex	tobramycin & dexamethasone
Tofranil	imipramine HCl
Tolectin	tolmetin sodium
Tolinase	tolazamide
Tonocard	tocainide HCl
Topamax	topiramate
Topicort	desoximetasone
Toprol XL	metoprolol tartrate
Toradol	ketorolac tromethamine
Torecan	thiethylperazine maleate
Tracrium	atracurium besylate
Transderm-scop	scopolamine HBr
Trecator-SC	ethionamide
Trental	pentoxifylline
Triavil	perphenazine & amitriptyline HCl
Tridione	trimethadione
Trilafon	perphenazine
Tritec	ranitidine bismuth citrate
Trobicin	spectinomycin
Tronolane, Tronothane HCl, Prax	pramoxine HCl
Trovan	trovafloxacin mesylate
Tums	calcium carbonate
Tussionex	chlorpheniramine polistirex & hydrocodone polistirex
Tuss-Ornade	caramiphen edisylate & phenylpropanolamine HCl

Table 5-12 Common Brand-Name and Generic Prescription Drugs (*continued*)

BRAND/TRADE NAME	GENERIC NAME
Tylenol, Tempra	acetaminophen
Tylenol #3	acetaminophen & codeine
Tylox	oxycodone HCl, acetaminophen, & sodium metabisulfite
Ultiva	remifentanil HCl
Ultram	tramadol HCl
Ultravate	halobetasol propionate
Unasyn	ampicillin sodium & sulbactam sodium
Uni-Cap Hexavitamin, Theragran	multivitamin
Unicap-T, Theragran-M	multivitamin w/minerals
Uniretic	moexipril HCl & hydrochlorothiazide
Urecholine, Duviod	bethanechol chloride
Urispas	flavoxate HCl
Urolene Blue	methylene blue
Valisone	betamethasone valerate
Valium	diazepam
Valstar	valrubicin
Valtrex	valacyclovir HCl
Vanceril, Beclovent, Beconase, Vancenase	beclomethasone dipropionate
Vancocin, Vancoled	vancomycin
Vansil	oxamniquine
Vantin	cefpodoxime proxetil
Vascor	bepridil HCl
Vaseretic	enalapril maleate & hydrochlorothiazide
Vasodilan, Voxsuprine	isoxsuprine HCl
Vasotec	enalapril maleate
Vasoxyl	methoxamine HCl
Velban	vinblastine sulfate
Velosef	cephradine
VePesid	etoposide
Vermox	mebendazole
Versed	midazolam HCl
Viagra	sildenafil citrate
Vibramycin, Doxychel, Doxy, Doryx, Monodox	doxycycline hyclate
Vicoprofen	hydrocodone bitartrate & ibuprofen
Videx	didanosine
Vioform	clioquinol (lodochlorhydroxyquin)

Table 5-12 Common Brand-Name and Generic Prescription Drugs (*continued*)

BRAND/TRADE NAME	GENERIC NAME
Vira-A	vidarabine
Viracept	nelfinavir mesylate
Viramune	nevirapine
Virazole	ribavirin
Visken	pindolol
Vistaril	hydroxyzine pamoate
Vistide	cidofovir
Vitamin B$_{12}$	cyanocobalamin
Vitamin C	ascorbic acid
Vitravene	fomivirsen sodium
Vivactil	protriptyline HCl
Voltaren	diclofenac sodium
Vontrol	diphenidol
Wellbutrin, Zyban	bupropion HCl
Wellcovorin	leucovorin calcium
Wycillin	penicillin G procaine
Wydase	hyaluronidase
Wytensin	guanabenz acetate
Xalatan	latanoprost
Xanax	alprazolam
Xeloda	capecitabine
Xylocaine, Nervocaine	lidocaine HCl
Yutopar	ritodrine HCl
Zaditor	ketotifen fumarate
Zagam	sparfloxacin
Zanaflex	tizanidine HCl
Zanosar	streptozocin
Zantac	ranitidine HCl
Zarontin	ethosuximide
Zaroxolyn	metolazone
Zebeta	bisoprolol fumarate
Zefazone	cefmetazole sodium
Zemplar	paricalcitol
Zenapax	daclizumab
Ziac	bisoprolol fumarate & hydrochlorothiazide
Ziagen	abacavir sulfate
Zithromax	azithromycin
Zocor	simvastatin

Table 5-12 Common Brand-Name and Generic Prescription Drugs (*continued*)

BRAND/TRADE NAME	GENERIC NAME
Zofran	ondansetron HCl
Zoloft	sertraline HCl
Zomig	zolmitriptan
Zosyn	piperacillin sodium & tazobactam sodium
Zovirax	acyclovir
Zyflo	zileuton
Zyloprim	allopurinol sodium
Zyprexa	olanzapine
Zyrtec	cetirizine HCl

Terminology

Terminology is the set of technical or special terms used in a business, art, science, or specific profession. Like many professions, pharmacy and medical professionals use a unique language and terminology. The following lists are not complete, but are a good reference when working in a pharmacy.

Pharmaceutical Terminology

A

Absorption is the time it takes for a drug to work after the drug has been administered; the rate at which the drug passes from the intestines into the bloodstream.

Acute refers to a disease or illness with a sudden onset and a short duration.

Active ingredient is the chemical in a medication that is known or believed to have a therapeutic effect.

Additive is a substance added to a liquid solution intended for IV use.

Admixture is a substance produced by mixing two or more substances.

Adverse reaction denotes an unwanted or unexpected side effect or reaction to a medication; it may also result from an interaction among two or more medications.

Aerosol is a medication dosage form that uses a gaseous substance consisting of fine liquid or solid particles.

Alcoholic solution is a solution that contains only alcohol as the dissolving agent.

Allergic reaction denotes a sensitivity to a specific substance that is absorbed through the skin, inhaled into the lungs, swallowed, or injected.

Allergy is a sensitivity of the immune system to a chemical or drug; an allergy causes symptoms ranging from rashes to more severe symptoms such as irregular breathing.

Amphetamines are substances that are frequently abused as stimulant medications; they can be used to treat the medical conditions of narcolepsy and eating disorders.

Analgesic refers to a substance used to relieve acute or chronic pain.

Analeptic refers to a substance that stimulates the central nervous system.

Anaphylactic shock is a hypersensitivity reaction to a substance.

Anesthetic refers to relief of pain by the process of interfering with the nerve transmission alerting the brain of pain.

Angiotensin-converting enzyme (ACE) inhibitors are used to treat hypertension (high blood pressure) and heart failure by blocking the enzyme that activates angiotensin—a natural substance that narrows the blood vessels and thereby raises blood pressure.

Anorectic refers to a substance that suppresses the appetite.

Antacid is a substance that relieves high acid levels in the gastric (stomach) area.

Antagonist refers to a substance that opposes the action of another drug or substance.

Antianxiety describes substances that reduce or relieve anxiety.

Antibiotic is a substance used to kill or stop the growth of bacteria in the body.

Antibody is a protein produced by the immune system to respond to foreign substances in the body.

Anticholinergic refers to a substance that inhibits hypersecretion and gastrointestinal motility.

Anticoagulant refers to a substance that stops blood clotting (also known as a blood thinner).

Anticonvulsant refers to a substance that stops brain nerve firing to suppress convulsive seizures.

Antidepressant is a substance that helps to maintain proper hormone balance levels to decrease depressive moods.

Antidiarrheal relieves and decreases gastrointestinal activity that produces diarrhea.

Antidote is a substance or remedy that counteracts the effects of a poisoning agent.

Antiemetic is a substance that relieves nausea and vomiting.

Antiflatulent refers to a substance that relieves the pressure of excess intestinal gas.

Antifungal refers to a substance that kills fungus growing in or on the body.

Antihistamine refers to a substance that stops the effects of histamine release, which causes sneezing, watery eyes, and congestion.

Antihypertensive substances work to lower blood pressure.

Anti-inflammatory substances reduce and relieve inflammation.

Antineoplastic substances are used to kill cancer cells.

Antioxidants are chemical substances that reduce or prevent oxidation (chemical binding of oxygen with other chemicals or molecules).

Antiplatelets are substances that reduce the ability of platelets to stick together and form a clot.

Antipruritic denotes a substance that relieves itching.

Antipsychotics are substances that block and inhibit the stimulatory actions of dopamine.

Antipyretic refers to a substance that relieves and lowers high fever.

Antispasmodics relieve stomach muscle spasms.

Antitussives relieve severe cough.

Antiviral refers to drugs that fight viral infections in the body.

Aqueous means "containing water."

Aseptic techniques are used to get rid of bacteria and other microorganisms and thus protect against infection.

Astringent refers to a substance that stops secretions or controls bleeding.

Auxiliary labels are placed on the medication package to provide information and instructions for use.

B

Beta-blockers are substances used in the treatment of hypertension, angina, arrhythmia, and cardiomyopathy; they may also be used to minimize the possibility of sudden death after a heart attack.

Binding agent is a substance that holds all of the ingredients in a tablet together.

Bioequivalence describes a substance acting on the body with the same strength and similar bioavailability as the same dosage of another substance.

Blood sugar level is the measure of glucose (sugar) level in the bloodstream.

Brand name is the proprietary name of a drug exclusive to a manufacturer for selling and distributing purposes.

Bronchodilator is a substance that relaxes the bronchial smooth muscles in the respiratory system.

Buccal tablet is a tablet that is dissolved in the lining of the cheek instead of being swallowed whole.

Bulk compounding is the process of compounding large quantities of a substance for dispensing or distributing.

Bulk manufacturing is the process of manufacturing large quantities of a substance for sale and distribution.

Bulking agent is a chemical substance required to produce a certain desired result.

C

Calcium-channel blockers are substances used to treat and reduce hypertension (high blood pressure) and disorders that affect the blood supply to the heart; also used in the treatment of irregular heartbeat.

Capsule is a solid dosage form of a medication; usually made of gelatin, which surrounds and holds fine particles of a solid or liquid.

Chewable tablets are meant to be chewed instead of swallowed whole.

Chronic refers to a disease or illness that has a long duration (e.g., lifetime).

Clinical trials are scientific experiments that test the effect of a drug in human test patients; required by the FDA for approval of a new medication.

Communicable refers to a disease or illness that can be transmitted to another person.

Compound refers to a substance made from a combination of two or more substances.

Contagious refers to the time period when an infectious person can transmit a disease to another person through direct or indirect contact.

Contraindication is an aspect of a patient's condition that does not fit with the proposed treatment.

Controlled release medications are released and metabolized over a period of time in the body.

Controlled substance refers to a drug with a high potential for abuse; manufacturing and distribution of these substances are regulated by the federal government to limit abuse and harm.

Corticosteroids are substances used to prevent minor asthma attacks or to treat severe attacks.

Cream is a dosage form of a medication that is a semisolid preparation, usually applied externally to soothe, lubricate, or protect.

Cure is the effective treatment of a disease or illness leading to elimination of all symptoms.

D

Decongestant refers to a substance that shrinks the mucous membranes that produce congestion.

Dehydration refers to excessive loss of water from the body.

Diagnosis is a process by which a healthcare professional (doctor, nurse, or technician) determines the patient's condition or disease, after tests and examinations.

Disease is a physical process in which the body or specific organs are being attacked or destroyed, causing harm and characteristic symptoms to the patient.

Distribution is the process following absorption by which a drug is passed to the cells of various organs.

Diuretic is a substance that increases the water output in the kidneys; reduces water retention in the body.

Dopamine is a neurotransmitter associated with the regulation of movement, emotions, pain, and pleasure.

Drops are a liquid dosage form of medication; they usually are placed in the eye or ear.

Drug is a chemical compound intended for use in the diagnosis, treatment, or prevention of a disease in human or animals; any substance that is intended to produce an alteration of the chemistry and/or functioning of the body.

E

Effervescent tablet is a tablet that is dissolved into a liquid before administration.

Electrolytes are salts that the body requires in its fluids; they are essential in nerve, muscle, and heart functions.

Elimination is the process following distribution by which a drug is broken down and the excess is excreted.

Elixir is a liquid dosage form that contains a flavored water and alcohol mixture.

Emulsion is a liquid dosage form of a mixture of two products that normally do not mix together.

Enema is the process by which a medicated fluid is injected into the rectum.

Esophagitis is a condition characterized by inflammation, swelling, and irritation of the esophagus.

Estrogens are hormones produced in the ovaries; they are responsible for the development and maintenance of female secondary sex characteristics.

Excretion is the process by which the body eliminates waste after metabolism and distribution.

Expectorants are substances that remove mucus from the upper respiratory system.

F

Food and Drug Administration (FDA) is the federal agency responsible for the approval, review, and regulation of drugs and dietary supplements.

Formulary refers to a list of preferred medications that insurance plans allow their members to get at a lower out-of-pocket expense.

Fungicide refers to a substance that kills fungi.

G

Generic name is the nonproprietary name of a drug.

Genetically engineered drugs are substances produced by organisms that have had foreign genes artificially inserted into their genetic codes.

Glucagon is a hormone produced in the pancreas that causes the automatic release of glucose.

Glucose is sugar found in the bloodstream; it is the primary energy source for bodily functions.

Glycogen is the principal substance the body uses for storing carbohydrates; stored in the liver, glycogen turns into glucose and is released into the bloodstream when the blood sugar level gets low.

H

Half-life defines the amount of time it takes for half of a substance to be broken down in the body and excreted.

Hazardous waste is any substance that is potentially dangerous and toxic to living organisms; these wastes must be disposed of properly.

Health is the physical, emotional, or mental well-being of a person.

Healthcare procedures, techniques, tests, and examinations are used to prevent, treat, and maintain a patient's health and well-being.

Histamine (H2) blockers reduce acid secretion by preventing histamine from reaching the H2 receptors.

Hydroalcoholic solutions contain water and alcohol.

Hypersensitivity is an exaggerated response to a given stimulus.

Hypnotic refers to a substance that relaxes the central nervous system to produce sleep.

I

Immediate-release medications are available to the body and metabolized immediately following administration.

Immunosuppressant refers to substances that are used to prevent the body from rejecting an organ transplant (also known as antirejection drugs).

Inactive ingredients are the ingredients found in a drug, other than the active ingredient; used to flavor, digest, color, and bind the whole substance.

Infusion is the process of slowly injecting a solution or emulsion into a vein or subcutaneous tissue.

Inhalation is the administration of a medication directly into the lungs via the mouth or nose.

Inhaler is a dosage form that uses a gaseous substance to force fine solid or liquid particles into the respiratory system through the nose or mouth.

Insulin is a hormone secreted by the pancreas that helps the body to digest sugars and starches; manufactured insulin is used when the patient's pancreas does not produce enough on its own.

Intolerance is an extreme sensitivity to a drug or other substance.

Intracardiac denotes the administration of a medication by injection directly into the heart.

Intradermal denotes the administration of a medication by injection into the skin.

Intramuscular refers to the administration of a medication within or into a muscle.

Intravenous refers to the administration of a medication within or into a vein.

Inventory refers to the supplies of medications that the pharmacy stocks for dispensing.

L

Labeling is the process of identifying a particular medication with the patient's and physician's information for dispensing.

Laxative is a substance that increases defecation.

Legend drug is a medication that requires a prescription written by a physician before it can be dispensed to the patient.

Local refers to a small area or single part of the body (e.g., local anesthetic).

Lotion is a liquid dosage form that contains a powdered substance in a suspension; used externally to soothe, cool, dry, and protect.

M

Medical devices are devices or products used for medical procedures or diagnostic tests.

Medication order is a prescription written in a hospital or other institutional setting.

Migraines are severe headaches caused by extreme changes in the blood vessels in the brain.

Muscle relaxants are used to treat involuntary, painful contraction of muscles by slowing the passage of nerve signals that cause pain to the muscles.

N

Narcotic is a drug for pain relief that has a high potential for abuse; can cause dependency and tolerance.

Narrow therapeutic range is the bioequivalence range of a brand-name drug and its generic counterpart where very small changes in dosage level could result in toxicity.

Nonaqueous means "contains no water."

Nonlegend drugs are medications that do not require a prescription before dispensing; more commonly referred to as over-the-counter medications.

Nonsteroidal anti-inflammatory agents are substances that inhibit the production of the enzymes necessary for the synthesis of prostaglandins, thereby reducing pain and inflammation.

O

Ointment is a semisolid (mixture of a liquid and solid) dosage form that is applied externally to deliver medication, lubricate, and protect.

Ophthalmic refers to administration of a medication through the eye.

Opiate is a drug derived from the opium poppy, such as morphine or codeine.

Opioid is a drug, hormone, or other substance that has sedative or narcotic effects similar to substances containing opium or its derivatives.

Oral refers to the administration of a medication into the mouth.

OSHA is the Occupational Health and Safety Association; responsible for developing safety guidelines for the workplace.

Otic denotes the administration of a medication into the ear.

Overdose is the action of, and condition resulting from, ingesting too much of a substance or drug; may result from one dose, or multiple doses over the course of time.

P

Package insert is a supplement, provided by the manufacturer, containing specific details, instructions, and warnings about the medication.

Parenteral denotes the administration of medication by any route other than oral; administration by injection.

Patch is a dosage form in which the medication is delivered through a solid application applied to the skin and absorbed into the bloodstream.

Patent is a federally granted, exclusive right to a product for a specific period of time (before other manufacturers can create and sell an identical product).

Pharmacist is a licensed, skilled healthcare professional who has been trained to dispense medications as ordered by physicians and to counsel patients on drug therapies.

Pharmacokinetics is the study of the rates at which drugs are metabolized, distributed, and excreted from the body after consumption.

Pharmacology is the study of drugs and their effects on the body.

Placebo is a pill-like preparation that contains no active chemical ingredients; usually given for its psychological effects (commonly referred to as a sugar pill).

Prescription includes a direction given by a physician for the preparation and use of a medication for a specific patient, to be dispensed by a pharmacist.

Progestins are female reproductive hormones; they cause menstruation as they trigger the shedding of the uterine lining.

Proton pump inhibitors are substances that reduce gastric acid buildup by blocking the release of protons in the stomach.

Psychotherapeutic drugs are substances used to relieve the symptoms of mental and psychiatric illnesses, such as depression, psychosis, and anxiety.

Psychotropic denotes a substance that affects a person's ability to distinguish the real from the imaginary.

R

Recreational drugs (usually illegal) are often used in a social setting for their pleasurable effects instead of their medicinal value.

Rectally refers to the administration of a solid or liquid medication given through the rectum.

S

Schedule I drugs are classified by the Drug Enforcement Administration as having a high potential for abuse and have no FDA approval for medicinal use (illegal drugs).

Schedule II drugs are classified by the Drug Enforcement Administration as having a high potential for abuse, with severe dependence liability (e.g., narcotics, amphetamines, stimulants).

Schedule III drugs are classified by the Drug Enforcement Administration as having less abuse potential than Schedule II drugs and moderate dependence liability (e.g., nonnarcotic stimulants, nonbarbituate sedatives, anabolic steroids).

Schedule IV drugs are classified by the Drug Enforcement Administration as having less abuse potential than Schedule III drugs and limited dependence liability (e.g., sedatives, antianxiety agents, nonnarcotic analgesics).

Schedule V drugs have limited abuse potential; they are available as prescription or over-the-counter drugs (e.g., cough syrups with small amounts of codeine, antitussives, antidiarrheals).

Sedatives relieve anxiety and tension, calm, and relax the patient.

Side effects are predicted, unwanted reactions to a substance or combination of substances.

Slow-release medications are released and metabolized over a period of time in the body.

Solution is a liquid dosage form in which the medication is completely dissolved in a liquid.

Sterilize means to cleanse (objects, wounds, burns, and so on) of microorganisms such as bacteria.

Stimulants are a class of medications that are intended to increase alertness and physical activity.

Subcutaneous refers to the administration of a medication given under the skin.

Sublingual tablet is a tablet that is dissolved under the tongue instead of being swallowed whole.

Suppository denotes administration through the vagina or rectum of a solid medication (also called a suppository).

Suspension is a liquid dosage form in which the solid particles are not completely dissolved.

Symptom is a condition that usually comes before the onset of a disease or illness; an abnormality that provides evidence of the existence of a disease or illness.

Syrup is a liquid dosage form that consists of water and sugar mixed with the medication.

T

Tablet is a solid dosage form in which the ingredients are compacted into a small, formed shape.

Tolerance is the condition in which the body has become unresponsive to a substance after prolonged exposure.

Topical refers to a substance used externally for relief of swelling, itching, or infection.

Transdermal refers to administration of a medication through the skin (e.g., patches).

U

U.S. Pharmacopoeia (USP) is a nonprofit organization, recognized by the FDA, that publishes standards on prescription drugs, over-the-counter medications, dietary supplements, and healthcare products.

V

Vaginal tablet is a tablet that is dissolved in the mucous lining of the vagina.

Vaginally denotes the administration of a solid or liquid medication through the vagina.

Vasodilator is a substance that causes the blood vessels to widen.

W

Withdrawal symptom is an effect that can occur as the result of suddenly stopping the use of a substance after prolonged use.

Medical Terminology

A

Acne vulgaris is a skin condition that occurs due to the overproduction of oil by the oil glands of the skin; results in pimples, blackheads, and whiteheads on the surface of the skin.

Addiction is physical or psychological dependence on a chemical substance, such as alcohol; any habit that cannot easily be given up.

Amnesia is a loss of memory (may be short- or long-term).

Anatomy is the study of the structures in living things.

Anemia is a condition in which the bloodstream has very few red blood cells that can carry oxygen to the tissues.

Anesthesiologists are physicians who specialize in administering drugs to anesthetize or sedate patients before surgical procedures; they monitor a patient's vital signs while the patient is under anesthesia.

Angina pectoris is a condition characterized by attacks of chest pain caused by an insufficient supply of oxygen to the heart.

Anorexia is an eating disorder characterized by a refusal to maintain body weight at a healthy range, low self-esteem, and an intense fear of gaining weight.

Arrhythmia is an irregular heartbeat.

Arteriosclerosis is a condition characterized by thickening and hardening of the arteries.

Arthritis is a condition characterized by inflammation of the joints.

Asthma is a condition that affects a patient's breathing by restricting the airways and oxygen supply due to inflammation, swelling, and irritation.

Attention deficit disorder (ADD) is a mental disorder characterized by developmentally inappropriate levels of attention, concentration, activity, distractibility, and impulsivity.

Attention deficit hyperactivity disorder (ADHD) is a mental disorder characterized by constant impulsive behavior, difficulty in concentration, and hyperactivity that decreases social, academic, or occupational functioning.

Autoimmune disorders are characterized by an immune response against the body's own tissues.

B

Bacteria are single-celled microorganisms that are abundant in most living things; may be beneficial or harmful to a person.

Benign refers to a condition or abnormal growth that is not cancerous (e.g., tumor, cyst).

Blood pressure measures the force exerted by blood against the walls of the arteries; measured when the heart contracts and relaxes.

Bloodstream is a general term for the area in which the blood flows; includes capillaries, veins, and arteries.

Body mass index (BMI) is the measurement of body fat relative to the patient's height and weight.

Bronchitis is a medical condition characterized by an acute inflammation of the bronchial tubes in the lungs.

C

Carcinogen is any agent capable of causing cancer.

Cardiologists are physicians who specialize in the treatment of heart disorders and illnesses.

Cardiovascular disease refers to conditions of the heart and circulation system.

Catalyst is a substance that speeds up a chemical reaction.

Cavity is a hollow space in a structure.

Cerebral refers to the brain.

Chemotherapy is the prevention or treatment of cancerous disease by the use of toxic chemical agents.

Cholesterol is a substance produced in the liver and used for normal body functions, including production of hormones, bile, and vitamin D.

Clinical refers to diagnostic tests, lab work, and procedures that require close observation of patients.

Congestive heart failure is a potentially fatal condition of the cardiovascular system wherein the heart has lost its ability to pump blood.

Contraceptives are drugs or devices used for the prevention of pregnancy; can also be used for hormone regulation.

Cranial refers to the skull or head.

Cystitis is a condition of inflammation of the urinary bladder.

D

Dementia is a disease characterized by progressive memory loss as well as learning and thinking disorders; it is often a symptom of Alzheimer's disease, though it may have other causes as well.

Dependency is physical and/or psychological reliance on a habit or chemical substance.

Depression is a mental disorder wherein the person feels sad and helpless; characterized by personality changes and a loss of socialization, communication, and energy.

Dermatologists are physicians who specialize in the treatment of skin disorders and illnesses.

Detoxification is the process by which the patient is medically supervised for withdrawal from alcohol or drug dependency.

Diabetes is a condition characterized by failure of the pancreas to produce insulin, which is essential for digestion and for retrieving energy from food.

Distal refers to the part that is farthest from the point of attachment.

E

Edema refers to abnormal swelling of the body or a body part caused by an increased buildup of fluids in tissues and organs.

Emergency medicine specialists are physicians who specialize in the treatment of emergency situations and trauma.

Emphysema is an irreversible disease (often caused by long-term smoking) in which there has been severe damage to the alveoli (tiny air sacs) in the lungs; results in a decrease in the ability of the lungs to exchange gases; symptoms are wheezing, coughing, shortness of breath, and difficulty in breathing.

Endorphin is a chemical or ingredient produced by the body that relieves pain and stress.

Erythrocyte is a red blood cell.

Esophagitis is an inflammation of the esophagus due to acid buildup.

Euphoria is a feeling of great happiness and well-being.

Excretion is the process by which waste is eliminated from the body.

External refers to the outer or outside part of a structure.

G

Gastric ulcer is a tear in the normal tissue lining of the stomach wall.

Gastritis is an inflammation of the normal tissue lining of the stomach wall.

Gastroenterologists are physicians who specialize in the treatment of digestive disorders and illnesses.

Gastroesophageal reflux disease (GERD) is a condition that occurs when food that has not been completely digested is forced back up the esophagus; the food is very acidic and irritates the esophagus, causing heartburn and other symptoms.

Gastrointestinal tract is the part of the digestive system that includes the mouth, esophagus, stomach, and intestines; aids in digesting and processing food in the body.

Geriatrics is the treatment of elderly patients.

Glaucoma is an eye condition in which pressure builds up in the eye because of reduced drainage of fluid from the eye; can result in the loss of vision in the affected eye.

Gynecologists are physicians who specialize in the treatment of disorders of women's reproductive organs.

H

Heartburn is a painful burning sensation in the throat (esophagus) just below the breastbone.

Hemorrhage refers to severe, uncontrollable bleeding (can be external or internal).

Hepatitis is a condition associated with inflammation of the liver.

Herpes simplex is an acute viral disease characterized by watery blisters on the skin and mucous membranes; commonly known as cold sores.

Hormone is a chemical substance that stimulates and regulates certain bodily functions.

Hormone replacement therapy (HRT) is a therapy developed for women to help increase estrogen levels that are declining during menopause.

Hyperglycemia is the condition of high blood glucose (sugar).

Hyperlipidemia refers to high cholesterol.

Hypertension refers to long-term high blood pressure.

Hypoglycemia is the condition of low blood glucose (sugar).

I

Immunity is the body's ability to fight off infections from bacteria and viruses.

Impotence is the inability to achieve and maintain penile erection.

Inflammation is any redness, swelling, pain, or heat in a body tissue or tissues caused by physical injury, infection, or irritation.

Influenza is a contagious viral infection of the nose, throat, and lungs, which often occurs in the winter season; also called flu.

Inpatient refers to a person who has been admitted to a hospital or other medical facility to receive treatment for a disease or injury.

Internal denotes the inner or inside part of a structure.

L

Leukemia is a condition characterized by elevated white blood cell counts.

Leukocyte is a white blood cell.

Lipids are organic compounds consisting of fats and other substances; used to measure cholesterol.

M

Malignant refers to an abnormal condition or growth in which a group of cells (e.g., cancerous cells) cause harm and destruction to other cells and tissues.

Metabolism consists of the physical and chemical processes of the body that convert consumed food into energy for use by the tissues and organs.

Metastasis is the spreading of a disease from one organ or part of the body to another organ or part of the body.

N

Narcolepsy is a rare, chronic sleep disorder characterized by constant daytime fatigue and sudden attacks of sleep.

Nausea is a feeling of sickness to the stomach, usually accompanied by the urge to vomit.

Neurologists are physicians who specialize in the treatment of disorders and illnesses within the brain and central nervous system.

Neuropathic relates to a disease of the nerves.

Neurotransmitter is a chemical substance released by one nerve cell that activates or inhibits a neighboring nerve cell.

O

Obstetricians are physicians who specialize in the care of pregnant women before and during the birth of the women's babies.

Oncologists are physicians who specialize in the treatment of cancer; they are usually expert in radiation therapy, chemotherapy, and other cancer treatments.

Ophthalmologists are physicians who specialize in the treatment of poor vision and eye disorders, using medication, corrective lenses, and surgery.

Organ is a part of the body made up of specialized tissues that performs a specialized function or functions; part of an organ system.

Orthopedists are physicians who specialize in the treatment of injuries and structural disorders of the bones and joints.

Osteoporosis is a medical disease characterized by a loss in total bone density; it can be the result of calcium deficiency, menopause, certain endocrine diseases, advanced age, medications, or other risk factors.

Otolaryngologists are physicians who specialize in the treatment of disorders and illnesses of the ear, nose, and throat.

Outpatient refers to a patient who receives treatment from a hospital or other medical facility on a scheduled basis without being admitted for overnight or continuous stay.

P

Pain is a feeling of slight or severe discomfort caused by an injury or illness.

Panic attack is a sudden, repeated episode of extreme fear, panic, and anxiety.

Parietal refers to the wall of a structure or cavity.

Pathogen is a microorganism (bacteria or virus) that causes disease.

Pathologists study the history, causes, and progress of diseases by examining specimens of body tissues, blood, fluids, and secretions.

Pathology is the study of the nature of disease(s).

Peripheral denotes a location at or toward the surface of the body or a body part.

Physiology is the study of the function of living things.

Prevention is the process of taking steps to keep a health condition or other abnormality from occurring or worsening.

Primary care is the medical care a person receives from a general practitioner or family physician.

Primary care physician is usually the internal medicine or family physician, who treats a variety of illnesses; this physician may refer a patient to a specialist if further specialized care or treatment is necessary.

Prognosis refers to the medical assessment of the expected outcome and course of a particular disease.

Proximal denotes the location of the part that is nearest to the point of attachment.

Psychiatrists are physicians who specialize in the treatment of mental, emotional, and behavioral disorders by the use of medications and psychotherapy.

Psychotherapy is the nondrug treatment of psychological disorders; usually performed as behavioral or cognitive therapy.

Pulmonary refers to the lungs and respiratory system.

R

Radiologists are technicians who use technologies such as X-rays, radiation therapy, and ultrasound machines to view and assess medical problems.

Receptor is the part of the nerve cell that recognizes the neurotransmitter and communicates with other nerve cells.

Respiration is the process by which gases are passed through the lungs and distributed throughout the body.

S

Seasonal affective disorder (SAD) is a type of depression that occurs during the fall and winter months, or during other times of the year or in parts of the world where exposure to natural sunlight is limited.

Secondary care is medical care that a person receives from a specialist after being referred by the primary care physician.

Serotonin is a neurotransmitter in the brain that regulates moods, appetite, sensory perception, and other central nervous system functions.

Spasm is an involuntary muscle contraction.

Specialists are physicians who are experienced in a certain area of medicine or study for treatment and prevention.

Surgeons are physicians who specialize in and are trained to perform surgical procedures and operations on patients to provide treatment or cure for an illness or injury.

Syndrome refers to a set of symptoms that are characteristic of a particular disease.

Systemic refers to the whole body.

T

Terminally ill refers to the condition of having an illness or disease for which no treatment or cure is available; the expected outcome is death.

Testosterone is a hormone produced in high amounts in males and that regulates certain characteristics of muscle-building, sexual organs, hair growth, and deepening of the voice during puberty.

Toxic refers to a poisonous substance.

U

Urinary incontinence is the inability to control the passage of urine from the bladder.

Urologists are physicians who specialize in the treatment of disorders in the urinary tract, as well as problems in the male reproductive organs.

V

Vaccine is a preparation that contains weakened or killed viruses and is administered to a person to activate immunity to the disease caused by that virus.

Vascular refers to the blood vessels and circulatory system.

Vertigo is a condition characterized by dizziness.

Virus is a very small infectious organism that requires a living cell host for reproduction.

Visceral refers to the structures inside the body.

SUMMARY

The ability to recognize and understand the language of pharmacy and medicine is necessary to practice as a pharmacy technician. This language includes terminology, abbreviations, and drug names. It is unlikely that you will immediately retain all of the information presented within this chapter, but over time and with experience you should gain a strong working knowledge of the information presented. This chapter will serve as a valuable reference as you continue your studies and begin practicing as a pharmacy technician.

CHAPTER REVIEW QUESTIONS

1. The root word "enter" refers to which of the following?
   a. intestines
   b. kidney
   c. mind
   d. nose

2. Which of the following is the generic equivalent for Cleocin®?
   a. loratadine
   b. flurazepam
   c. digoxin
   d. clindamycin

3. The prefix "hypo-" refers to which of the following?
   a. against
   b. large
   c. too little
   d. too much

4. The suffix "-algia" refers to which of the following?
   a. tumor
   b. pain
   c. inflammation
   d. control

5. Which of the following is the brand-name equivalent for furosemide?
   a. Lasix®
   b. Medrol®
   c. Paxil®
   d. Toprol XL®

6. The root word "pulmo" refers to which of the following?
   a. bone
   b. heart
   c. lung
   d. vein

7. What is the abbreviation for "after meals"?
   _____

8. What does the abbreviation "ADR" stand for?
   _____

9. What is the abbreviation for "four times daily"?
   _____

10. What does the abbreviation "DUR" stand for?
    _____

CRITICAL THINKING QUESTIONS

1. Why are some abbreviations, such as "d/c," considered dangerous and to be avoided?

2. How can recognizing root words, prefixes, and suffixes assist you in becoming and working as a pharmacy technician?

3. Why are abbreviations used on prescriptions?

WEB CHALLENGE

1. Go to www.jointcommission.org and print out JCAHO's Official Abbreviation "Do Not Use List," as well as tips on implementing the list in the pharmacy.

2. Visit Medic8's Online Medical Dictionary at http://www.medic8.com/MedicalDictionary.htm. Find three medical terms that are not listed in this chapter, and define them by using the root, prefix, and/or suffix.

REFERENCES AND RESOURCES

Fremgen, B & Frucht, S. Medical Terminology: A Living Language, 4th edition. Upper Saddle River, NJ: Pearson, 2009.

Johnston, M. *Certification Exam Review*. Upper Saddle River, NJ: Pearson, 2005.

Johnston, M. *Fundamentals of Pharmacy Practice*. Upper Saddle River, NJ: Pearson, 2005.

Rice, J. Medical Terminology: A Word Building Approach, 6th edition. Upper Saddle River, NJ: Pearson, 2008.

Turley, S. Medical Language. Upper Saddle River, NJ: Pearson, 2008.
http://www.aapmr.org/hpl/pracguide/jcahosymbols.htm

Community and Institutional Pharmacy

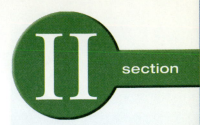

LEARNING OBJECTIVES

After completing this chapter, you should be able to:

- Explain the ambulatory pharmacy practice setting.
- Describe the two main types of retail pharmacies.
- List the various staff positions in retail pharmacies.
- Describe the typical work environment of a retail pharmacy.
- Discuss the two agencies that regulate retail pharmacy practice.
- List the legal requirements of a prescription medication order.
- Describe the different ways prescriptions arrive at a retail pharmacy.
- List the steps required for a prescription to be filled.
- Discuss the various job duties of technicians in retail pharmacies.
- Discuss the importance of confidentiality for personal health information.

Introduction

The two main types of pharmacy practice are ambulatory and institutional. If the patient resides where the pharmacy is located, it is considered an institutional setting. Examples of these are hospitals, nursing homes, hospices, and long-term care facilities. Most other pharmacies fall into the category of ambulatory. Examples of ambulatory settings, which are most commonly referred to as *community-based pharmacies*, are privately owned, chain, or franchise pharmacies, as well as clinics. These types of pharmacies are also known as *community* or *retail pharmacies* because they serve the local community in which they are located. It is well known that the retail pharmacy is one of the most accessible patient healthcare settings.

There are a vast number of career opportunities within ambulatory pharmacies. One such opportunity is a position in a retail setting, which is the focus of this chapter.

Retail Pharmacy

The best-known attribute of retail, or community, pharmacy is the face-to-face interactions among the pharmacist, technicians, and the patients. Many people rely on the pharmacy team's knowledge of **over-the-counter (OTC) products**, as well as prescription drugs. Also, when it comes to advice and information related to drugs, the retail pharmacy staff is usually more accessible to the general public than the staff in a doctor's office or clinic.

over-the-counter (OTC) products medications and devices that do not require a prescription for purchase and use.

Within the retail or community setting, ownership of the business can dictate the types of opportunities or tasks a pharmacy technician may have.

Independent Pharmacies

Most independent pharmacies are privately owned and relatively small in size, filling, on average, 100 to 300 prescriptions daily. This type of pharmacy is thought of as a **neighborhood pharmacy** (see Figure 6-1). Because of its smaller size and customer base, a neighborhood pharmacy can generally provide more personalized services to its customers, and pharmacy staff can become better acquainted with their patients.

Additionally, some of the independents can provide a wider range of care than the larger chain pharmacies. These expanded services may include offering compounded medications, home healthcare products, surgical supplies, a delivery service, and even patient charge accounts.

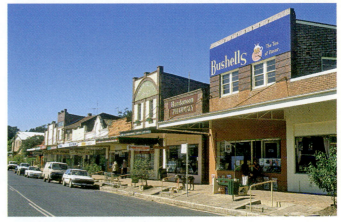

FIGURE 6-1 An independent pharmacy.

Most technicians choose to practice retail pharmacy first, because more job opportunities are available in that part of the field. Retail pharmacy allows a more hands-on approach to pharmacy practice. It involves reviewing, preparing, and recording prescription orders accurately, as well as compounding some special medications. In carrying out these tasks, the pharmacy team efficiently serves and cares for patients.

neighborhood pharmacy an independent pharmacy that is privately owned, small in size, and usually fills an average of 100 to 300 prescriptions per day.

Chain/Franchise Pharmacies

The other type of retail pharmacy is the **chain** or **franchise pharmacy**. This type of pharmacy consists of branches, or chains, of more than one store (see Figure 6-2). Chain pharmacies generally have a higher volume (number) of prescriptions than an independent pharmacy. Chain pharmacies are often larger and faster-paced. They can be further categorized as mass-merchandise stores, such as Wal-Mart; chain drugstores, such as CVS and Rite-Aid; or grocery store pharmacies, such as Krogers and Albertsons.

chain pharmacy a retail, or ambulatory, pharmacy that is owned by a corporation operating multiple pharmacy facilities at various locations.

Unlike independent pharmacies, chain drugstores can offer other career paths to their staff, including retail management and training opportunities. There is definitely room to grow within a chain pharmacy. Some offer to pay for the national certification exam, as well as offering scholarships and tuition grants to their employees for continuing education.

Chain pharmacies may be in operation 24 hours per day, 7 days a week, including holidays. In a chain pharmacy, there are usually three shifts: morning, afternoon, and evening. Volumes can differ on certain days, and also during specific hours of the day.

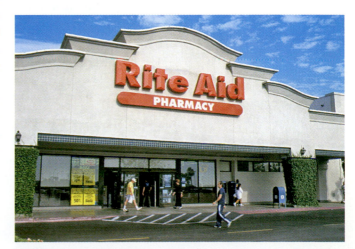

Retail Pharmacy Staff

The operations and management of a retail pharmacy require numerous staff members, each accountable and responsible for various job duties.

FIGURE 6-2 A retail pharmacy.

franchise pharmacy a retail, or ambulatory, pharmacy that consists of facilities at multiple locations, although each pharmacy may be separately owned.

Certified Pharmacy Technician (CPhT) an individual who is certified to assist pharmacists in providing pharmaceutical care, but is not permitted to dispense medication or counsel patients; certification is achieved by passing a national certification exam.

pharmacy clerk/cashier a noncertified/unlicensed individual who is authorized to do only nonpharmacy-related tasks, such as operating the cash register.

pharmacy manager an individual, almost always a pharmacist, who is appointed to supervise all aspects of the daily pharmacy operations.

doctor of pharmacy (PharmD) an individual who has completed a doctoral degree in pharmacy and is licensed to practice pharmacy in a specific state.

pharmacist in charge (PIC) an individual designated on the records of the State Board of Pharmacy as the primary, onsite pharmacist.

registered pharmacist (RPh) an individual who has completed a bachelor's degree in pharmacy and is licensed to practice pharmacy in a specific state.

store manager an individual appointed to supervise all aspects of the daily store operations, including the pharmacy department.

front end the over-the-counter (OTC) section of a retail pharmacy.

Certified Pharmacy Technician

A **Certified Pharmacy Technician (CPhT)** is an individual who is certified to assist pharmacists in providing pharmaceutical care, but is not permitted to dispense medication or counsel patients. Certification is achieved by passing a national certification examination.

Pharmacy Clerk/Cashier

A **pharmacy clerk/cashier** is a noncertified, unlicensed individual who is authorized to assist only with nonpharmacy-related tasks, such as operating the cash register.

Pharmacy Manager

A **pharmacy manager** is an individual, almost always a pharmacist, who is appointed to supervise all aspects of the daily pharmacy operations. The manager's duties may include inventory, scheduling, budgets and financial reports, human resources, customer service, and additional management tasks.

Doctor of Pharmacy

A **doctor of pharmacy (PharmD)** is an individual who has completed a doctoral degree in pharmacy and is licensed to practice pharmacy in a specific state.

Workplace Wisdom RPh versus PharmD

Both registered pharmacists (RPh) and doctors of pharmacy (PharmD) are commonly referred to as *pharmacists*.

Pharmacist in Charge

A **pharmacist in charge (PIC)** is an individual designated on the records of the State Board of Pharmacy as the primary, onsite pharmacist. The pharmacist in charge is responsible for ensuring that the pharmacy operates in accordance with state laws and regulations.

Registered Pharmacist

A **registered pharmacist (RPh)** is an individual who has completed a bachelor's degree in pharmacy and is licensed to practice pharmacy in a specific state.

Store Manager

A **store manager** is an individual who has been appointed to supervise all aspects of the daily store operations, including the pharmacy department.

Organization of Retail Pharmacies

The majority of retail pharmacies, regardless of type, are organized into eight sections or areas. The square footage, or space, allotted for each of these sections will vary depending on both the size of the pharmacy and the scope or focus of services offered.

OTC/Front End

The over-the-counter (OTC) section, which is referred to as the **front end** in retail terminology, provides customers with various medications, devices, and aids that they do not need a prescription to purchase (see Figure 6-3). Products commonly found in the OTC section include:

- analgesics
- antihistamines
- decongestants

- cough suppressants
- acid-reflux/heartburn medications
- laxatives and antidiarrheals
- vitamins and minerals
- appetite suppressants
- first-aid supplies and antiseptics
- antifungals
- feminine hygiene products
- contraceptives
- pregnancy tests
- nutritional supplements

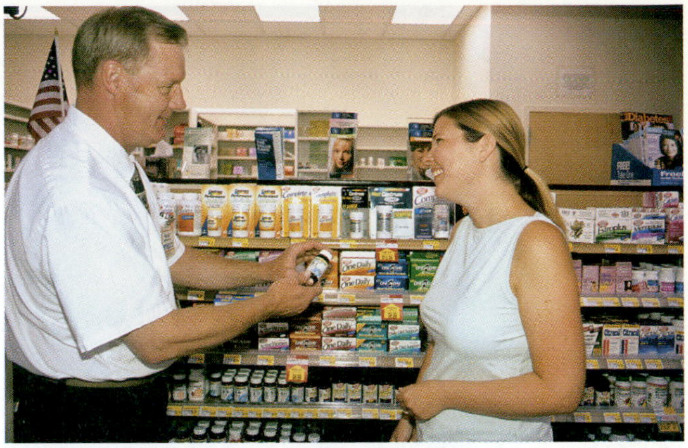

FIGURE 6-3 The front-end section of a pharmacy.

Behind-the-Counter OTC

In addition to the front-end section of OTC products, retail pharmacies also stock medications and devices, which are available without a prescription, behind the pharmacy counter (see Figure 6-4). These include special orders, restricted products, and higher-priced items. Common examples are:

- products containing pseudoephedrine
- blood glucose meters and test strips
- portable nebulizers
- blood pressure monitors
- smoking cessation products
- insulin and syringes
- support hosiery
- Plan B Contraception

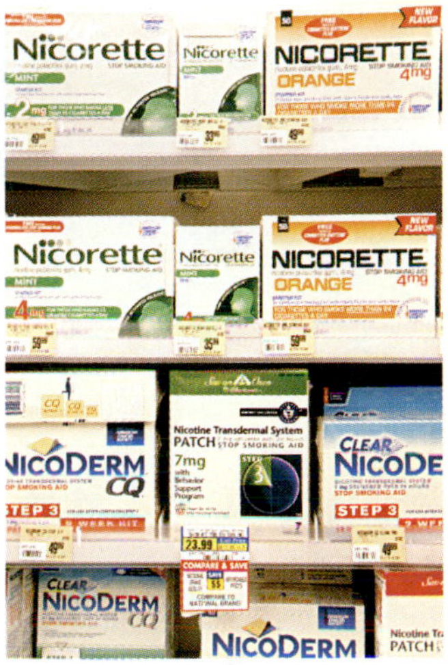

Prescription Drop-Off

Every retail pharmacy has one or more areas designated for "prescription drop-off," where patients can turn in their prescriptions to be filled (see Figure 6-5). This section typically includes a pharmacy computer to determine if the patient is already in the system and whether the patient's insurance information is up to date. In addition, new patient profile forms may be kept in this area; these are completed by any patient who is not already in the pharmacy computer system.

FIGURE 6-4 Examples of medications that are kept behind the counter.

Pharmacy Workstations

The pharmacy workstation is the area in which new prescriptions and refill requests are entered into the computer system, insurance claims are billed, and prescription labels and monographs are produced. Larger pharmacies may have five to six individual workstations, whereas smaller independent stores may have only one or two.

Pharmacy Counter

After a prescription has been dropped off, processed, and billed, and the paperwork has been printed, the prescribed medication is prepared and labeled at the pharmacy counter (see Figure 6-6). This is where pills are counted, liquids are measured, and compounds are prepared. After the prescription has been filled, labeled, verified by the pharmacist, and packaged, it is ready for pick-up.

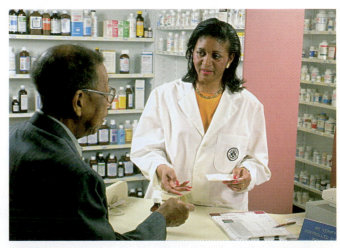

FIGURE 6-5 A customer dropping off a prescription at the pharmacy prescription drop-off area.

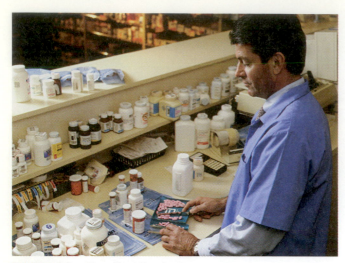

FIGURE 6-6 Counting pills at the pharmacy counter.

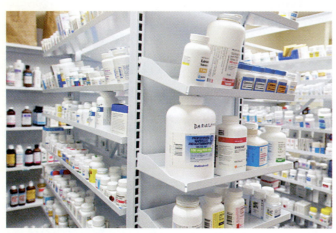

FIGURE 6-7 A typical storage area in a retail pharmacy.

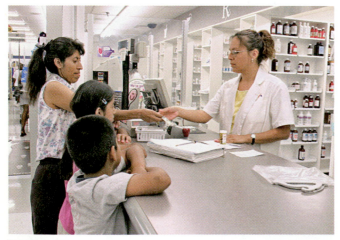

FIGURE 6-8 The pick-up area in a retail pharmacy.

Storage

Retail pharmacies have multiple storage areas to support the pharmacy operations (see Figure 6-7). Common storage areas are:

- medication storage, including shelves, cabinets, and a refrigerator/freezer
- filled prescriptions
- dispensing supplies, such as vials, bottles, labels, and bags
- prescription records

Pick-Up Area (Drive-Thru)

Just as every retail pharmacy has a designated prescription drop-off area, each pharmacy also has an area designated for prescription pick-up (see Figure 6-8). This section is typically located near the storage area for filled prescriptions and usually has a cash register for processing transactions. The pick-up window also houses a patient signature log, which records when and by whom each prescription was picked up. Some retail pharmacies have added a drive-thru window to enhance convenience for patients who are dropping off or picking up their prescriptions.

Counseling Area

HIPAA mandates that every retail pharmacy have an area designated for patient counseling. This section should be discrete and offer greater privacy than the general windows, so that the pharmacist may provide specific information and address an individual patient's questions. This area is designed for pharmacists and patients only, as pharmacy technicians are not permitted to counsel patients.

Regulatory Agencies

Retail pharmacies are regulated, primarily, by two agencies: the State Board of Pharmacy and the Centers for Medicare and Medicaid Services.

State Board of Pharmacy

The State Board of Pharmacy (SBOP) is the agency that registers and regulates retail pharmacy facilities, pharmacists, and pharmacy technicians. The practice of pharmacy is governed at the state level, whereas the pharmaceutical industry is governed at the national level.

The SBOP oversees compliance with the state's pharmacy practice act, and it is for this reason that the SBOP administers unannounced site inspections. The state's enabling legislation gives the state board the authority to require operational changes, and to suspend or revoke the license of a pharmacy, pharmacist, or pharmacy technician.

Centers for Medicare and Medicaid Services

The Centers for Medicare and Medicaid Services (CMS), formerly known as the Health Care Financing Administration (HCFA), is the federal agency that regulates the administration of Medicare, Medicaid, the State Children's Health Insurance Program (SCHIP), the Health Insurance Portability and Accountability Act (HIPAA), the Clinical Laboratory Improvement Amendments (CLIA), and several other health-related programs. Approval from the CMS is necessary to receive reimbursement from Medicare or Medicaid, and the CMS conducts inspections to ensure compliance with its guidelines.

The Prescription

Prescriptions are, in essence, orders, either written or verbal, for the dispensing of a medication made by authorized prescribers, such as medical doctors (MDs), physician assistants (PAs), nurse practitioners (CNPs), and dentists (DDS). Prescriptions are the main focus of retail pharmacy practice.

Elements of the Prescription

Every prescription has 10 basic elements (see Figure 6-9). It is the duty of the pharmacy technician to verify that the prescription is complete when it is dropped off or called in to be filled. Each element of the prescription is used in the computer entry, processing, and billing of the order. The 10 basic elements are:

1. *Prescriber information*—the name, address, telephone number, license number, and DEA number of the prescriber. (Note: DEA numbers are not required by law for noncontrolled medications.)

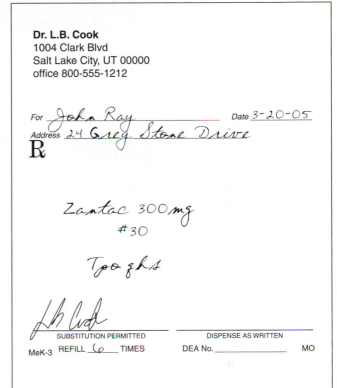

FIGURE 6-9 An illustration of a prescription.

INFORMATION

DEA numbers are license numbers provided by the Drug Enforcement Administration for registrants who are authorized to prescribe controlled substances. DEA numbers contain two letters followed by seven numbers (e.g., AB1234563). The first letter is typically an A or B; the second letter is typically the first letter of the registrant's last name. The numbers are designed so that the sum of the first, third, and fifth digits, added to twice the sum of the second, fourth, and sixth digits, will produce a number that contains the same last digit as the last (seventh) digit of the DEA number. If this formula does not work, the DEA number is fraudulent.

Example: Dr. Sarah Byer, DEA AB1234563

1. The B corresponds with "Byer."
2. The sum of the first, third, and fifth digits is 9.
3. The sum of the second, fourth, and sixth digits is 12; 12 doubled is 24.
4. 9 + 24 = 33. The last digit of 33 is 3, which matches the last digit of the DEA number.

PROCEDURE **6-1**

Verifying a DEA Number

1. Verify that the second letter corresponds to the first letter of the provider's last name.
2. Add the first, third, and fifth digits of the DEA number.
3. Add the second, fourth, and sixth digits.
4. Double the sum of the second, fourth, and sixth digits.
5. Add the sum of step 2 and step 4.
6. Verify that the last digit from step 5 matches the last digit of the DEA number.

2. *Patient name and address*—the name and address of the individual for whom the prescription was written.

" Workplace Wisdom Patient's Address

Most prescribers do not complete the patient's address, but this should be added when the prescription is dropped off to be filled. "

3. *Date prescribed*—the month, day, and year the prescription was written. This will determine the expiration date of the prescription and refills.
4. *Drug name and strength*—the name of the medication being prescribed and its strength, or the amount of active ingredient contained in manufactured prescription products.
5. *Dose and quantity*—the specific dose, or measured amount, of medication being prescribed and a total quantity to be dispensed.
6. *Route of administration*—the route by which the medication should be administered to the patient, such as PO (by mouth).
7. *Signa/Directions*—commonly referred to as the **SIG** or SIG code, these are specific directions for the patient to follow, such as dosage, schedule and frequency of dosage, and additional instructions.
8. *Number of refills*—the number of refills authorized by the prescriber, including zero.
9. *Product selection permitted*—the prescriber's authorization for the patient to select a less expensive generic equivalent (if available), or the prescriber's directive to dispense as written (no substitution permitted).
10. *Prescriber's signature*—a prescription is not considered valid unless it is signed by the prescriber.

SIG specific directions provided on a prescription for the patient to follow, such as dosages, schedule and frequency of administration, and additional instructions.

The Patient Profile

The **patient profile** is an electronic record, stored in the pharmacy computer system, that details the patient's personal and billing information, prescription records, and medical conditions (see Figure 6-10).

To generate a new patient profile, the pharmacy technician must first ask the patient to complete a paper patient profile form and provide the pharmacy with an insurance card. The patient profile form is used to collect the following critical information:

- patient's full name
- patient's address
- patient's telephone number(s)
- patient's Social Security number
- patient's date of birth
- patient's gender

patient profile an electronic record, stored in the pharmacy computer system, that details the patient's personal and billing information, prescription records, and medical conditions.

PATIENT PROFILE

Patient Name

_____   _____   _____
              Last   **First**   **Middle Initial**

- -

_____

_____
        Street or PO Box

_____   _____   _____
        City   State   Zip

- -

Phone   Date of Birth   Social Security No.
( )   _____   ☐ Male ☐ Female   _ _ _ _ _ _ _ _ _
             Month   Day   Year

☐ Yes, I would like medication dispensed in a child-resistant container.
☐ No, I do not want medication dispensed in a child-resistant container.
Medication Insurance   Card Holder Name _____

☐ Yes   ☐ No   ☐ Card Holder   ☐ Child   ☐ Disabled Dependent
                      ☐ Spouse   ☐ Dependent Parent   ☐ Full Time Student

MEDICAL HISTORY

HEALTH
		ALLERGIES AND DRUG REACTIONS
☐ Angina	☐ Epilepsy	☐ No known drug allergies or
☐ Anemia	☐ Glaucoma	reactions
☐ Arthritis	☐ Heart Condition	☐ Aspirin
☐ Asthma	☐ Kidney Disease	☐ Cephalosporins
☐ Blood Clotting Disorders	☐ Liver Disease	☐ Codeine
☐ High Blood Pressure	☐ Lung Disease	☐ Erythromycin
☐ Breast Feeding	☐ Parkinson's Disease	☐ Penicillin
☐ Cancer	☐ Pregnancy	☐ Sulfa Drugs
☐ Diabetes	☐ Ulcers	☐ Tetracyclines
Other Conditions _____		☐ Xanthines
		Other Allergies/Reactions _____

Prescription Medication Being Taken   OTC Medication Currently Being Taken
_____   _____
_____   _____

Would You Like Generic Medication Where Possible? ☐ Yes ☐ No

Comments
_____

Health information changes periodically. Please notify the pharmacy of any new medications, allergies, drug reactions, or health conditions.
_____ Signature _____ Date ☐ I do not wish to provide this information.

FIGURE 6-10 An illustration of a patient profile.

- known drug allergies
- drug sensitivities/reactions
- medical and health conditions
- preference on generic drug substitution
- preference on child-resistant lids

The following details from the patient's insurance card are also added to the patient profile (see Figure 6-11):

- name of insurance carrier
- identification (ID) number
- group code
- patient code—such as primary, spouse, or dependent

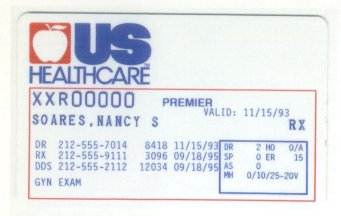

FIGURE 6-11 Example of a patient insurance card.

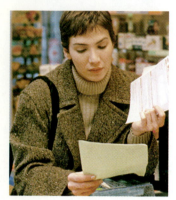

FIGURE 6-12 A patient brings a prescription to a pharmacy.

Processing Prescriptions

Multiple steps are required to process a prescription.

Receiving

Although most prescriptions are brought to the pharmacy in person, this is not the only way a prescription arrives at the pharmacy for processing (see Figure 6-12). For example, in many states faxes are considered legal documents, and it may be more convenient for a prescriber to fax a prescription directly to the pharmacy. A technician may remove a fax from the machine and fill the order because the pharmacist will be reviewing and checking the order. Most pharmacies do not give out their business fax numbers except to prescribers. If a technician is unsure of the source of a fax, he should immediately consult the pharmacist. C-II orders, which are prescriptions for Schedule II drugs (discussed in Chapter 4), are the exception because they must be handwritten original orders and, therefore, cannot be faxed, e-mailed, or phoned into the pharmacy.

Phoned-in prescriptions are also very common in ambulatory pharmacies. In most states, however, pharmacy technicians cannot accept a prescription over the phone. As we get closer to licensing and certification as federal requirements for pharmacy technicians, this may change; for now, though, when the prescriber calls in a prescription, the technician must refer the call to a pharmacist, depending on state law. If a patient calls in a refill of an existing order, the technician may take the refill order.

Computers are great communication tools and ambulatory pharmacies are no strangers to technology. Internet and mail-order pharmacies, among others, may accept prescriptions via e-mail or other Internet transmissions.

Reviewing

One of the first steps in providing medication for a patient is receiving and reviewing the order. Remember, legend drugs may not be dispensed without a legal prescription, because the government has decided the drug has potential for addiction or abuse, or is dangerous enough to require medical supervision during use. Pharmacy technicians are the front line in the prescription process. By reviewing an incoming prescription for legality and correctness, the technician is not just aiding the pharmacist and serving the patient, but also protecting the public.

Several pieces of information are required before the filling process can begin. It is up to the technician to screen orders to save time (both the pharmacist's and the patient's) and avoid waste.

The first piece of this puzzle is the patient's name. It is important to get the whole name, not just a nickname. You will need to match the patient's name to the names in your patient profiles, as well as to any possible insurance company records. It is the technician's responsibility to maintain current patient profiles, and this includes making name changes due to divorce or marriage.

The technician must verify the date on which the prescription was written. Remember, certain prescriptions are good for up to one year.

Current addresses and telephone numbers are also, for the reasons given earlier, important components of a valid prescription. This information need not be written on a prescription in order for the prescription to be legal, but the information has to be in the pharmacy's possession. This not only confirms the patient's identity but could save his life in the event of a problem or recall.

Once the technician verifies the patient for whom the order was written, the next step is to verify the medication being ordered. The correct dosage form, strength, and quantity must also be verified. If any of these components is missing, the technician should alert the pharmacist immediately and await further instructions.

Next, the technician should review the directions for clarity and precision. Does the prescriber allow generic substitution, or is this a dispense-as-written (**DAW**) prescription?

Are any refills available? Remember, according to federal law, a prescription for a C-II drug cannot allow refills; a C-III drug order can be refilled for six months, and prescriptions for C-IV and C-V medications may be refilled for up to a year.

Last, but certainly no less important, is the prescriber's signature. In many states, a prescriber's agent (physician's assistant or even nurse) may sign for the prescriber. Know your local laws to avoid making errors down the road.

Special circumstances apply to certain medications. For instance, prescriptions for C-II drugs must be original, bear no corrections or changes, and contain the prescriber's DEA number.

Errors common to ambulatory pharmacies can be avoided if the technician is knowledgeable and vigilant about accepting prescriptions. Some of the more common problems include:

- Improper patient identification
- Duplicate profiles for the same patient
- Therapeutic discrepancies due to time lapse between time of prescribing and time of dispensing
- Patients who waste time waiting only to find that their prescriptions cannot be filled without further instructions from the prescriber
- Inaccurate or missed insurance billing due to a lack of or incorrect information

One of the most basic services a pharmacy technician provides to a patient, a pharmacist, and society in general is the proper screening of prescriptions. Time, money, and even lives can be saved when this task is performed efficiently and correctly. What transpires in a few moments can affect the lives of many for a lifetime.

> **DAW** instructions from the prescriber to "dispense as written," without generic substitution.

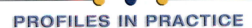

PROFILES IN PRACTICE

Jean is a pharmacy technician working at a retail pharmacy. A patient comes in with her sick child and drops off three prescriptions, asking how soon the medications will be ready. Jean indicates that the prescriptions will be ready in 15 to 20 minutes. After entering the prescriptions, printing the labels, and placing them in order to be filled, Jean realizes that the pharmacy is out of stock of one of the medications. The patient is due to return, expecting to pick up the prescriptions, in five minutes.

- What mistake did Jean make?
- What actions can Jean take to offset her mistake?

Translating

Verifying a prescription order is just the beginning of the pharmacy process. Remember, we have to get the right medication in the right strength and dose to the right patient at the right time! When reduced to a system of clearly defined and meticulously followed steps, the process should run efficiently and without errors.

Computer Entry

After a prescription has been reviewed and properly translated, the information on the prescription must be entered into the pharmacy computer system and the prescription label printed (see Figure 6-13). Nearly every retail pharmacy uses a different, or modified version of, a pharmacy software program. The good news, however, is that the essential elements of computerized prescription processing remain constant.

PROCEDURE 6-2

Entering a Prescription

The following is a general process for entering a prescription into the pharmacy computer system.

1. Perform a search for the patient, by last name then first name and date of birth.
   a. If the patient is already in the system and verified, go to step 2.
   b. If the patient is a new patient, cannot be found in the system, or has changes to the profile, have the patient complete a patient profile form and then create/edit the patient profile, including insurance information.
2. Select the correct patient profile and then select Fill/New Rx, which will prompt the prescription entry screen.
3. Perform a search for the prescriber by last name, then by first name and DEA number.
   a. If the prescriber is already in the system and verified, go to step 4.
   b. If the prescriber is new or cannot be found in the system, create a new prescriber profile using the information provided on the prescription.
4. Select the correct prescriber.
5. Enter the original date of the prescription.
6. Enter/select the drug prescribed and indicate if generic substitution should be used—based first on availability, then the prescriber's preference, then the patient's choice. Verify that the correct NDC number is selected for the prescription.
7. Enter the quantity prescribed.
8. Select/enter the directions for the prescription.
9. Enter the number of refills authorized.
10. Select/enter the correct DAW code.
    a. 0—product selection permitted
    b. 1—dispense as written
    c. 2—product selection permitted, but declined by patient
11. Verify/edit the day's supply quantity.
12. Notify the pharmacist of any DUR messages, for approval.
13. Transmit/submit for online adjudication by the insurance provider.
14. Approve the adjudication and print paperwork and labels.

adjudication the process of transmitting a prescription electronically to the proper insurance company or third-party biller for approval and billing.

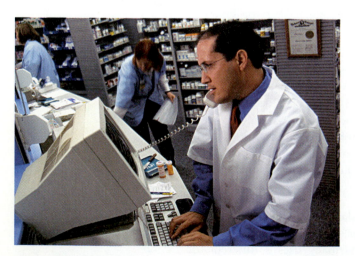

FIGURE 6-13 A pharmacy technician entering a prescription into the pharmacy computer system.

Adjudicating

Online **adjudication** is the process of transmitting a prescription electronically to the proper insurance company or third-party biller for approval and billing. Chapter 9 discusses insurance billing in detail.

Preparing

Inventory is a critical responsibility in pharmacy. When the exact medication prescribed is not on the pharmacy's shelves, patients are subjected to unnecessary delays and annoyance. Assuming that the right medication is available, a few extra checks made at this point can save valuable time and trouble later. The technician should check the lot number and/or the NDC numbers to ensure that the medication selected is the exact medication listed on the patient's label.

It is also important to check the expiration date at this point. The drug must not only be current on the day it is dispensed, but current throughout the entire course of therapy; that is, the expiration date must be far enough away to allow the patient to use all the drug as directed.

When selecting C-II drugs, the technician may be required to enter the medications into a log to aid in inventory control. Make sure you are aware of any state or employer policies before attempting to process a prescription for a C-II drug.

INFORMATION

NDC Numbers

National Drug Code, or NDC, numbers are identification numbers assigned to each unique drug product, similar to UPC codes for consumer goods. Each NDC number consists of three sets of numbers: the first set indicates the manufacturer; the second set indicates the drug, its strength, and its dosage form; the third and final set of numbers indicates the package size.

Example: NDC 51285-601-05

Counting/Measuring/Pouring

Workplace Wisdom

It is important that medications not be touched directly with the hands, because of the potential for contamination of the medicine and the person touching it.

Counting should always be done twice until the technician feels confident in her ability (see Figure 6-14). Prescriptions for C-II drugs should always be counted twice before they are given to the pharmacist for a final recount. Measuring and pouring can be a little more complicated because calculations may be involved. Technicians should not attempt to measure medications until they are comfortable with the metric system as well as the **household system**, which is the measurement system commonly used by Americans for general measuring and cooking. Consider the following prescription described in the Profiles in Practice scenario:

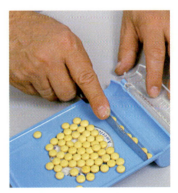

FIGURE 6-14 Counting pills.

household system the measurement system commonly used by Americans for general measuring and cooking.

PROFILES IN PRACTICE

Dr. Rizzo has prescribed Amoxil 250 mg suspension TID X 10D, but the pharmacy only has Amoxil 125 mg/5 mL in stock. Marcus, the pharmacy technician, not only has to know mg and mL, but also TID and 10D, to calculate the appropriate quantity to dispense. Marcus determines that the pharmacy will need to dispense 300 mL of the Amoxil 125 mg/5 mL, by using the following formula: 10 mL (dose) × 3 (frequency) × 10 (duration) = 300 mL

- What directions must be included on the label to ensure that the patient takes the correct dosage?

Packaging and Labeling

As simple as it sounds, labeling still requires attention to detail (see Figure 6-15). First, the label must go onto the correct medication container. This may sound silly, but in an assembly-line type of pharmacy, many errors occur over just this detail! For technicians, this is the last chance to check your work before submitting it to the pharmacist for a final check. Double-check the directions and drug strength, and affix any

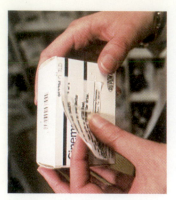

FIGURE 6-15 Labeling a prescription requires attention to detail.

auxiliary labels that may be appropriate. The drug label is usually generated by computer and will contain all the information required by law: that is, the name and telephone number of the dispensing pharmacy, the patient's name, the prescription number, the date the prescription was filled and the expiration date of the medication, the medication name and strength, directions, and the prescriber's name. The label also shows the quantity of medication inside, as well as the number of refills.

Final Check

The final check is the sole domain of the pharmacist. No medications may be dispensed without the pharmacist's final approval. In an ambulatory setting, this is a relatively simple process. The pharmacist will need the original prescription, the stock bottle used in filling the order, and the labeled container filled with the prescribed medication. Once the pharmacist approves it, the medication may be given to the patient.

Storing

After the final check has been performed by the pharmacist, the prescription is ready to be stored and then dispensed. The prescription is packaged in an appropriately sized prescription bag or box, and labeled with a patient prescription receipt and important drug information reports. Once the order is packaged, it is stored until either the patient comes to pick up the order or it is delivered.

For prescriptions that are scheduled to be picked up by the patient, most retail pharmacies store them alphabetically by the patient's last name in a system of bins, drawers, or shelves. Depending on the size of the pharmacy, and the volume it handles, the prescriptions may be alphabetized in groups of letters (e.g., bins labeled "A–C," "D–F," etc.) or by multiple bins per letter (e.g., bins labeled "Aa–Am," "An–Az," "Ba–Bo," "Br–Ce," etc.). Clearly, the more prescriptions an individual pharmacy fills, the more organized the storage has to be. Properly organized storage of prescriptions ensures that the prescriptions do not become lost and that they can be located quickly when the patient arrives for pickup.

Independent and specialty community pharmacies sometimes offer delivery of prescriptions to the home or office of the patient. Such delivery can be made by courier or mail, but, regardless of the mode of delivery, these prescriptions are stored in a separate area to be scheduled and prepared for delivery.

Dispensing

Technically speaking, the dispensing of a prescription is the process and time at which the medication is released from the pharmacy and given to the patient. For in-store pickups, a prescription is *dispensed* as soon as the pharmacy staff gives the medication to the patient. A delivered prescription is considered dispensed as soon as it leaves the pharmacy.

In other words, once the medication is no longer under the security and control of the pharmacy, it is considered dispensed, and once a medication has been dispensed it cannot be returned to the pharmacy. This is because the pharmacy is no longer able to guarantee the quality and integrity of the medication. Even if, for example, a patient picks up a prescription, walks out to his car, and then immediately comes back inside, the prescription has been dispensed and cannot be returned to stock.

Counseling

counseling the process of providing patients and customers with pharmaceutical and general health-related advice; provided only by registered pharmacists or doctors of pharmacy.

It is imperative that patients be counseled on all new prescriptions, and at any other time they have a question. **Counseling** refers to the professional, clinical advice given to a patient or caregiver by a pharmacist. Counseling can pertain to prescription medications, OTC medications, or even general health issues (see Figure 6-16).

Counseling is beyond the authorized scope of practice for pharmacy technicians. It is reserved only for pharmacists—without exception. Pharmacy technicians do, however, play an important role in the counseling process, in that they alert the pharmacist to the need to counsel patients on new medications, and by always asking patients—even if they are just picking up refills—if they have any questions for the pharmacist.

PROCEDURE 6-3

Dispensing a Prescription

1. Pharmacist must complete a final check of the prescription.
2. Verify whether the order is a new prescription or refill.
   a. If a new prescription, have the pharmacist come over to offer counseling.
   b. If a refill, ask the patient if he or she has any questions for the pharmacist.
3. Ring up the customer's order at the cash register.
4. Have the patient sign and date the prescription pick-up log.

Filing

The final step in processing a prescription is filing the actual hard copy of the prescription. Throughout the entire process, the hard-copy prescription will have been written upon, marked, initialed, and labeled. The label, which is generally placed on the back side of the prescription, will contain information generated by the pharmacy computer, including the information labeled on the patient's medication, insurance billing information, and a computer-generated serial number—commonly referred to as the prescription, or **Rx**, number.

The hard-copy prescriptions will be stacked throughout the workday, after the final check. At appropriate times and intervals the pharmacy technician will organize, verify, and file the hard copies.

The filing process will be determined by the method used by the individual pharmacy, but typically is set up as one series for legend prescriptions, one series for controlled prescriptions, and one series for Schedule II drug prescriptions.

Prescriptions will be divided by type, or series, and then organized in numerical order of the unique serial number generated by the pharmacy computer. Once the prescriptions have been placed in order, the pharmacy technician will verify that no prescriptions are missing and then file the hard copies—typically in batches of a hundred in specially made prescription file folders.

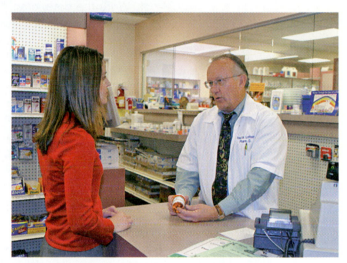

FIGURE 6-16 A customer receives counseling from the pharmacist about a new prescription.

Rx abbreviation for prescription.

Refills

Standard prescriptions can usually be refilled as many times as the prescriber orders within one year from the date the prescription was written; in other words, a prescription is good for one year. Exceptions to this rule, in most states, include controlled drugs, which are limited to a maximum of five refills, and C-II medications, which require a new, handwritten prescription for each fill.

In most pharmacies, pharmacy technicians are responsible for handling prescription refill requests. This task includes documenting patient refill orders, verifying prescription refills, processing orders with refills available, and contacting the prescriber to seek approval for additional refills past the number allotted on the original prescription.

PROCEDURE 6-4

Requesting a Refill Authorization

1. Ensure that there are no refills remaining on the prescription and that there are no prescriptions on hold, or logged, in the patient's profile for the medication.
2. Print out a copy of the patient's last refill.
3. Call the prescriber and request a refill by providing the following information, either on voicemail or to a nurse:
   a. Patient's name
   b. Patient's date of birth
   c. Drug name
   d. Drug strength
   e. Drug quantity
   f. Date of last fill
   g. Pharmacy's name and phone number
4. Write the date, time, "WCB" (will call back), and your initials on the form.
5. File the form, alphabetically by last name, with the other pending refills.

Note: This process can also be done electronically if the physician's office and pharmacy use an automated refill system.

Most pharmacies and insurance providers require that a prescription be 75 percent used before it may be refilled. For example, a patient with a prescription lasting 30 days cannot get a refill until after three weeks. There are exceptions to this rule, however. At her discretion, a pharmacist can provide up to a 72-hour supply of medication, until refills can be approved. Also, many insurance companies will override their refill policy for patients who are traveling overseas or taking extended trips, or in similar situations.

Transfer situation in which the patient would like to have the prescription refilled at a pharmacy other than where it was originally delivered or filled.

Transfers

Transfers are instances when the patient would like to have the prescription refilled at a pharmacy other than where it was originally delivered or filled (see Figure 6-17).

The laws governing the transfer of prescriptions between pharmacies differ from state to state and depend on the class of drug prescribed. When permitted, a prescription may be transferred for one fill only, or the entire prescription may be transferred. The critical factor is that there must be a paper trail for the DEA and State Board of Pharmacy.

The pharmacy's records must track that the prescription was indeed transferred, on a specific date and along with any available refills. If the prescription has already been filled and is being stored, the insurance claim must be reversed and the medication returned to stock. The new pharmacy will create a record showing that the prescription was a transfer; the new pharmacy is then responsible for any additional refills or transfers pertaining to that prescription.

In most states, a pharmacist is required to handle the process of transferring a prescription, either in or out. It is standard practice in the industry that the pharmacy that is to receive the transferred prescription should initiate the transfer request and phone call. In addition, most states restrict controlled medications with refills to a maximum of one transfer.

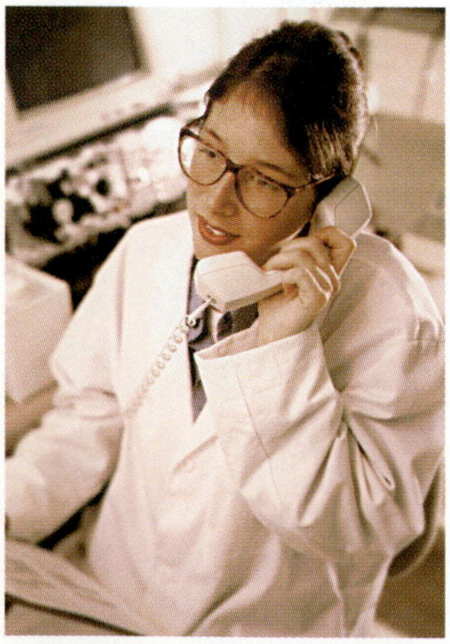

FIGURE 6-17 A pharmacy technician takes a call from a customer who is requesting a prescription transfer.

Pharmacy Technician Job Responsibilities

The daily duties of the pharmacy technician cover a vast number of tasks. One of the main responsibilities of a pharmacy technician in retail pharmacy is to assist the pharmacist in serving patients. Thus, the pharmacy technicians execute a variety of tasks under the supervision of the pharmacist. However, pharmacy technicians cannot counsel or give medical information or advice to patients. It is also the pharmacist's responsibility to perform the final check before a prescription is dispensed to a patient.

Other job responsibilities of the retail pharmacy technician include verifying drug deliveries, storing drugs, rotating stock, ordering drugs, and maintaining inventory records—and this is just the beginning. Pharmacy technicians also verify and accept new prescription and refill orders, as well as creating and maintaining patient profiles. Filling, compounding, and filing of medication orders are also within the scope of the pharmacy technician's practice. Technicians may also assist the pharmacist in the administration of the retail pharmacy, with duties that can include policy and procedure review, scheduling, and formulary issues. In short, a technician may perform any task that will assist the pharmacist in serving patients or pharmacy operations, with the exception of dispensing advice or drug-related information or dispensing legend drugs without a pharmacist's approval.

Becoming a pharmacy technician in a retail pharmacy setting is a very good career opportunity. Retail pharmacy is a great way to establish a position of status. Customers trust retail pharmacy technicians, and value the services they provide. Most people who come into a local community pharmacy think of the staff almost as members of their families, and trust the pharmacy team to provide the highest possible quality of service.

Over-the-Counter Medications and Pharmacy Technicians

The role of pharmacy technicians in relation to over-the-counter medications is a fine line. Legally, pharmacy technicians are not permitted to provide advice, or counsel, to patients regarding any medication, whether prescription or OTC. Pharmacy technicians do, however, assist patients in locating and purchasing OTC medications.

If, for example, a patient asks a pharmacy technician what is the best cough medication available over the counter, the technician must get the pharmacist. If a patient asks where to find the Robitussin® DM, the technician is permitted to assist the patient without interrupting the pharmacist.

There is debate over this topic within the industry. For example, customers can visit the local vitamin store and receive all sorts of advice from whomever may be working there—although that person may have no knowledge or training concerning OTC products. If the same customer goes to the local pharmacy, only the pharmacist can give them advice. The reasoning is this: When patients go to the vitamin store, they do not have an expectation that the employee is highly educated and trained on medications. When those same patients go to the pharmacy, though, they see someone who works in the pharmacy and wears a lab coat; most patients assume that every staff member is a pharmacist. They generally do not understand the difference in education and training between pharmacists and pharmacy technicians.

Medical Equipment and Devices

In contrast to the role of pharmacy technicians regarding OTC medications, the technician can provide detailed assistance to patients concerning OTC medical equipment and devices—as long as the technician is properly trained. Technicians educated on specific equipment can assist patients in product selection, operation of the device, and troubleshooting. Here are several examples of medical equipment and devices that pharmacy technicians can provide assistance with in community pharmacy settings:

- Nebulizers—used for delivering medication in a fine, particulate mist to a patient.
- Blood glucose meters—used for testing a patient's blood glucose level (normally used by patients with diabetes). In addition, technicians can assist patients with lancing devices used to draw blood for the glucose meter.
- Blood pressure monitors—used for determining an individual's systolic and diastolic blood pressure levels.

Patient Confidentiality and HIPAA

Patient confidentiality is an important concept for the pharmacy technician, who has access to large amounts of information that patients trust will not be exposed or released unless they grant permission. Electronic health information on a pharmacy's computer system, electronic prescribing data from physicians, transferred patient profiles from outside providers, prescription drug information, and payment records are all examples of information that pharmacy employees are required to maintain as confidential information.

A patient's confidential information is commonly referred to as *protected health information (PHI)*. PHI includes past, present, and future records or information pertaining to treatment or care received for physical or mental health, the rendering of that care, and payment for such services.

The question most commonly asked regarding PHI is, "When are you allowed to disclose or use a patient's confidential information in a pharmacy?" The short answer is that it is acceptable to do so when providing treatment to the patient or the patient's caregiver, when providing information to other healthcare providers who are caring for the patient, or while processing most payment and operational activities.

A more complex answer to the question requires background knowledge of the primary law governing pharmacies and their disclosure of PHI. The Health Insurance Portability and Accountability Act of 1996 (HIPAA) is a complex law that has greatly affected the entire healthcare system; it notably affects pharmacy practice because the privacy rules regulate the use of patients' health information.

On April 14, 2003, the HIPAA privacy regulations took effect. On and after that date, pharmacies were required to comply with all requirements relating to protection of patient confidentiality. You may have noticed significant changes in the way pharmacy technicians and pharmacists are now able to transfer and communicate a patient's PHI. New patients at any pharmacy will continue to be required to sign an acknowledgement of receipt of such privacy practices.

Your employer is also required to train all personnel on HIPAA requirements. In addition to the requirements set forth in HIPAA, any pharmacy may create its own systems to further protect and ensure patient confidentiality, as long as the requirements are equivalent to or stricter than those mandated by HIPAA. At the minimum, HIPAA set a standard for protecting patient information to prevent abuse of the privilege of having access to PHI.

Another common question relating to confidentiality of PHI is, "How much of a patient's confidential information can you disclose?" The standard of practice is known as the *minimum necessary standard*. This is interpreted to mean that you use or release the minimum amount of information needed to complete the task that requires you to use or disclose information. It can occasionally be difficult to judge when and where you can use a patient's PHI. Always ask for a second opinion if you feel uncomfortable releasing or revealing protected health information.

There are certain circumstances in pharmacy practice in which these requirements do not apply. This includes when you are communicating directly with the patient; there is no need to withhold the patient's personal information from the actual patient. Also, patients may waive their right to confidentiality or authorize you directly to use the information more freely. The most common situation in pharmacy practice in which the minimum necessary standard does not apply is when communicating with other healthcare providers who are involved in providing care for the patient. In this circumstance, the information is needed to provide congruent care. Finally, if you are ever required by court order or subpoena or government agency regulation to disclose information, you are authorized to do so.

An interesting feature of the HIPAA regulation is that patients were granted explicit rights relating to their PHI. For example, patients have the right to request additional restrictions on disclosure of PHI, obtain copies of their PHI, request changes to their PHI, or request information about who the pharmacy has disclosed their PHI to outside of the normal pharmacy communications. These are all examples of the affirmative rights provided to patients under the privacy rules enacted with HIPAA.

If you are ever uncertain about whether you are permitted to utilize confidential information, it is best to request permission, or at a minimum discuss the situation with a pharmacist or pharmacy manager. It is always best to be cautious when handling confidential information. It is also acceptable to request written patient authorization to ensure that disclosure or use of information is acceptable to the patient. Note that trash containing any privileged information (such as name, Social Security number, etc.) must be disposed of properly, such as by shredding or incineration. In addition, PHI should not be discussed around "the water cooler" or within earshot of bystanders, as this is also a violation of HIPAA.

Discretion is also pertinent now that specified consequences can result from improper use of PHI by a pharmacist, pharmacy technician, or other employee. In general, an investigation will occur if any allegations are made relating to violations of the HIPAA privacy rules. Penalties can range from $100 for a single violation to $250,000 and 10 years in jail for aggregate violations within a calendar year.

The HIPAA rules have certainly changed the practice of pharmacy. They have provided enhanced structure and guidance as to the manner in which, and the extent to which, pharmacy personnel can handle PHI. Pharmacy personnel will continue to improve their understanding of the privacy rules of HIPAA as more time elapses and further clarifications are issued concerning various practice settings. Until then, continue to use discretion when handling a patient's PHI and respect the fact that it certainly is a privilege for pharmacy personnel to use such information.

SUMMARY

Retail pharmacy is the largest category of pharmacy in the United States, and encompasses chain pharmacies, independent/franchise pharmacies, and clinic pharmacies, among others. Retail pharmacies are staffed by a pharmacist in charge, pharmacy manager, staff pharmacists, pharmacy technicians, and possibly pharmacy clerks. It is a fast-paced work environment, in which pharmacy professionals interact with and directly serve patients face to face.

Although pharmacy technicians cannot counsel patients, they can certainly take care of patients' insurance billing, help them locate OTC medications, and find prices for those medications. Pharmacy technicians also take care of inventory orders, rotations, returns, and billings. Of course, this is in addition to counting, measuring, filling, and labeling prescriptions. In ambulatory pharmacy, every day is another opportunity to serve the community.

CHAPTER REVIEW QUESTIONS

1. Which of the following is not an example of an ambulatory or retail pharmacy?
   a. franchise or chain pharmacy
   b. nursing home pharmacy
   c. privately owned pharmacy
   d. all of the above are examples

2. The term *ambulatory pharmacy* refers to a setting in which:
   a. the patient arrives by ambulance.
   b. the patient lives at the facility where the pharmacy is located.
   c. the patient "walks" into the pharmacy.
   d. the pharmacy is part of a larger facility.

3. Which of the following need not be recorded on a prescription?
   a. prescriber's signature
   b. patient's age

   c. medication quantity and strength
   d. patient's complete name

4. A prescription must contain the following drug information:
   a. name of the medication
   b. strength
   c. dosage form
   d. all of the above

5. Which of the following is not the responsibility of a pharmacy technician?
   a. verifying the patient's name, address, and telephone number
   b. checking for drug name, quantity, strength, dose, and route
   c. verifying the final prescription
   d. entering and billing insurance

6. Which of the following tasks may a pharmacy technician not perform?

   a. fill a prescription from a fax.
   b. accept a refill order from a patient.
   c. counsel patients about their prescriptions.
   d. call an insurer on behalf of a patient.

7. Before selecting the medication to fill an order, a pharmacy technician should:

   a. check the brand name.
   b. check the NDC and/or UPC code.
   c. check the contraindications.
   d. check with the pharmacist.

8. Which of the following does not appear on the patient's bottle?

   a. name of the medication being dispensed
   b. quantity of the medication being dispensed
   c. phone number of the prescriber
   d. phone number of the pharmacy

9. Which DAW code indicates that generics were permitted by the prescriber, but denied by the patient?

   a. DAW 0
   b. DAW 1
   c. DAW 2
   d. DAW 3

10. Which of the following is considered a chain pharmacy?

    a. Wal-Mart
    b. Walgreens
    c. CVS
    d. all of the above

CRITICAL THINKING QUESTIONS

1. Why do some pharmacies employ pharmacy clerks in addition to pharmacy technicians?

2. Why would retail pharmacies restrict access to certain OTC products, such as glucose meters and insulin syringes, by keeping them behind the pharmacy counter?

3. Why would retail pharmacies establish separate areas for dropping off and picking up prescriptions?

WEB CHALLENGE

1. Search the National Association for Chain Drug Stores (NACDS) website to find the current number of community pharmacies in the United States and the volume of prescriptions filled at retail pharmacies last year: http://www.nacds.org

2. Go to the National Community Pharmacists Association (NCPA) website and find the average number of prescriptions filled annually and per day at independent pharmacies: http://www.ncpanet.org

REFERENCES AND RESOURCES

Abood, R. *Pharmacy Practice and the Law* (4th ed.). Boston, MA: Bartlett Publishers, 2005.

American Medical Association. *Know your Drugs and Medications.* New York: Reader's Digest Association, 1991.

American Pharmacist Association. *Pharmacy Technician Workbook and Certification Review.* Englewood, CO: Morton Publishing, 2001.

American Society of Health System Pharmacists. *Manual for Pharmacy Technicians.* Bethesda, MD: ASHP, 1998.

American Society of Health System Pharmacists. *Pharmacy Technician Certification Review and Exam.* Bethesda, MD: ASHP, 1998.

Ansel, HC. *Introduction to Pharmaceutical Dosage Forms.* Philadelphia: Lea & Febiger, 1995.

Ballington, D. *Pharmacy Practice.* St. Paul, MN: EMC Paradigm, 1999.

Ballington, D. *Pharmacy Practice for Technicians.* St. Paul, MN: EMC Paradigm, 2003.

Cooperman, SH. *Professional Office Procedures.* Upper Saddle River, NJ: Pearson Education, 2006.

Cowen, D, & Helfand, W. *Pharmacy: An Illustrated History.* New York: Harry N. Abrams, 1990.

Crane, A. An overview of pharmacy automation. *Today's Technician.* 2004;5(4):26–37.

Facts and Comparisons. "Homepage" (accessed January 4, 2004): http://www.factsandcomparisons.com

Flaherty, J. Matters of privacy—Patient confidentiality. *Today's Technician.* 2005;6(2):8, 12.

Food and Drug Administration. "Homepage" (accessed January 4, 2004): http://www.fda.gov

Lambert, A. *Advanced Pharmacy Practice for Technicians.* Clifton Park, NY: Thomson Delmar Learning, 2002.

National Association of Chain Drug Stores, Inc., & Mintz, Levin, Cohn, Ferris, Glovsky and Popeo, P.C. *HIPAA Privacy Standards: A Compliance Manual For Pharmacies.* Alexandria, VA: NACDS, 2002.

Reifman, N. *Certification Review for Pharmacy Technicians* (6th ed.). Evergreen, CO: Ark Pharmaceutical Consultants, Inc., 2002.

U.S. Department of Health and Human Services: www.hhs.gov/ocr/hipaa

Health-System Pharmacy

7

LEARNING OBJECTIVES

After completing this chapter, you should be able to:

- Describe the health-system pharmacy practice setting.
- Describe the advantages of a unit-dose system.
- List the necessary components of a medication order.
- Compare the duties of a technician with those of a pharmacist in accepting a medication order in a health-system setting.
- Compare centralized and decentralized unit-dose systems.
- Compare the duties of a technician with those of a pharmacist in filling a medication order in a health-system setting.
- Define the tasks pharmacy technicians perform in health-system settings.

Introduction

Health-system pharmacy, or institutional pharmacy, describes the range of services provided to residents of long-term care facilities (nursing homes), hospitals, hospices, and other residential facilities (see Figure 7-1). In a health-system setting, the pharmacy department is responsible for all patients' medications; the pharmacists must ensure that drug therapies are appropriate, effective, safe, and used correctly. The health-system pharmacist also identifies, resolves, and prevents medication-related problems.

The pharmacy technician working in an institutional setting must be familiar with the policies and procedures of the particular institution as well as with state and federal law.

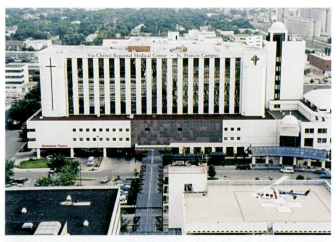

FIGURE 7-1 A health system pharmacy is often located within a hospital.

Health-System Pharmacies

health-system pharmacy classification of pharmacy setting in which patients reside onsite at the facility where the pharmacy is located (such as hospitals, nursing homes, and long-term care facilities).

The health-system pharmacy provides around-the-clock delivery service. Health-system pharmacists review patients' drug profiles to avoid possible duplications of treatment and adverse reactions. The health-system pharmacist is a principal defense against medication errors in the hospital.

institutional pharmacy another term for health-system pharmacy.

Health-system pharmacists often counsel patients on proper medication use, but they also provide drug information and recommendations to doctors and other caregivers. They review patient' drug regimens and oversee medication distribution throughout the institution. In long-term care settings, the pharmacists perform a drug therapy review for each patient on a monthly basis, or more frequently for special protocols. Health-system pharmacists often work with nurses, respiratory therapists, dietitians, laboratory personnel, physicians, and other professionals to discuss the drug therapy of patients, all with the aim of providing optimal pharmaceutical care.

Health-system pharmacy teams typically provide drug-related products and services 24 hours a day, 365 days a year. Health-system pharmacies also provide medications for emergency departments. Smaller hospitals may only be open for first and second shifts, with an on-call pharmacist after hours. Automated dispensing units are also frequently used to provide safe drug storage for medications required in emergency situations and/or after hours.

blister packs unit-dose packages.

Health-system pharmacists and technicians use controlled dispensing systems to ensure that patients have the right drugs at the right time and in the proper dosage and form. They may also provide prescription drugs in individually packaged **blister packs** (unit-dose packages) so that they are dispensed in a convenient and safe manner.

Health-system pharmacies allow unused, unopened products to be returned for credit (where permitted by state law). When unused, unopened drugs can be returned, medication changes do not result in unused products going to waste. This is very cost-effective.

Health-system pharmacy services are comprehensive in scope and intensity. Elderly, seriously ill, or chronically ill patients, who are often frail and have multiple conditions, need more attention than healthier ambulatory patients who are suffering from just one condition. Because the condition of an institutionalized patient constantly changes, frequent updating of drug regimens is required.

This section provides an overview of settings where health-system pharmacy services are typically found.

Long-Term Care Facilities

long-term care (LTC) facility facility that provides rehabilitative, restorative, or ongoing skilled nursing care to individuals who need assistance with activities of daily living.

Long-term care (LTC) facilities provide rehabilitative, restorative, or ongoing skilled nursing care to individuals, referred to as *patients* or *residents*, who need assistance with activities of daily living. The federal government acknowledged the distinctive features of the long-term care pharmacy when it passed laws and promulgated regulations to protect the health and well-being of institutional residents (OBRA 1987, OBRA 1990, HCFA'S 1990 nursing home regulations). These laws and rules recognize that drug therapy services for institutional patients are best delivered by long-term care pharmacists.

Hospices

hospice provides palliative care (care designed to help ease suffering) and supportive services to individuals at the end of their lives.

Hospices provide palliative care (care designed to help ease suffering) and supportive services to individuals at the end of their lives. Hospices also serve patients' family members and significant others. They operate 24 hours a day, 7 days a week, both in patients' homes and in facility-based settings. Hospices provide pharmaceutical, physical, social, spiritual, and emotional care to patients and their families during the last stages of an illness, the dying process, and the bereavement period.

Nursing Homes

Nursing homes offer skilled and custodial care to older Americans who do not need the intensive, acute care of a hospital but who can no longer manage independent living. Nursing homes are capable of caring for individuals with a wide range of medical conditions.

Nursing homes come in different sizes and have different names, such as health centers, havens, manors, homes for the aged, nursing centers, care centers, continuing care centers, living centers, or convalescent centers. The number of beds in a particular nursing home can range from approximately 25 to 500; the average number of beds per facility across America is 102.

Correctional Facilities

Correctional facilities, more commonly known as *prisons*, are places in which individuals are physically confined and usually deprived of a range of personal freedoms. Usually, these institutions are part of the criminal justice system. Correctional facility pharmacies oversee the provision of pharmaceutical services to those confined to the facility by operation of law (*inmates*).

Hospital Pharmacies

Hospital pharmacies are, by far, the most prevalent type of health-system pharmacy, with more than 5,750 registered hospitals operating in the United States.

Hospitals began as charitable institutions for the needy, aged, infirm, or very young. Today, though, they are institutions where sick or injured people receive many levels of medical or surgical care, ranging from outpatient services to long-term intensive care.

Hospital Classifications

The American Hospital Association (AHA) categorizes hospitals as community-based, federal government, psychiatric, long-term care, or institutional hospital units. Community-based hospitals, which include nonprofit, for-profit, and state/local government facilities, represent approximately 85 percent of the total number of registered hospitals. This chapter focuses primarily on the practices and standards of community-based hospital pharmacies, collectively.

Hospitals are also categorized by their location and size. Depending on their location, hospitals are referred to as either rural or urban. The bed capacity, or size, categories for hospitals are small (25–50 beds), medium-sized (50–100 beds), or large (more than 100 beds).

Hospital Staff

The operations and management of hospitals require numerous staff members, each accountable and responsible for various job duties.

Doctor of Osteopathy

A **doctor of osteopathy (DO)** is a licensed individual, trained to examine patients, diagnose illnesses, and prescribe and administer treatments using manipulative techniques on the musculoskeletal system in conjunction with conventional treatments.

Doctor of Medicine

A **doctor of medicine (MD)** is a licensed individual, trained to examine patients, diagnose illnesses, and prescribe and administer medication. In the hospital setting, the majority of medical doctors specialize in one particular field. For example, to name just a few, a cardiologist specializes in disorders of the heart and circulatory system. An oncologist specializes in diagnosing and treating patients with cancer. An OB/GYN specializes in both obstetrics and gynecology. Surgeons are trained in the treatment of injury or disease by manual or instrumental procedures.

---

nursing home facility that provides skilled and custodial care to older Americans who do not need the intensive, acute care of a hospital but who can no longer manage independent living.

correctional facilities more commonly referred to as *prisons;* places in which individuals are physically confined and usually deprived of a range of personal freedoms.

hospital pharmacy the most common type of health-system pharmacy; a pharmacy located within a hospital facility serving patients who have been admitted or are being discharged.

doctor of osteopathy (DO) a licensed individual, trained to examine patients, diagnose illnesses, and prescribe and administer treatments using manipulative techniques on the musculoskeletal system in conjunction with conventional treatments.

doctor of medicine (MD) a licensed individual, trained to examine patients, diagnose illnesses, and prescribe and administer medication.

physician assistant (PA) a licensed individual who is trained to coordinate patient care under the supervision of a medical or osteopathic doctor.

certified nursing assistant (CNA) an individual who is certified to assist RNs and LPNs in providing patient care, but is not permitted to administer medication.

licensed nursing assistant (LNA) an individual who is licensed to assist RNs and LPNs in providing patient care, but is not permitted to administer medication.

licensed practical nurse (LPN) an individual who is licensed to provide basic care, such as administering medication, under the supervision of a registered nurse.

nurse practitioner (NP) an individual who is licensed to work closely with a physician in providing patient care, and typically may prescribe medications under the supervision of a physician.

registered nurse (RN) an individual who is registered to assist physicians with specific procedures, administer medications, and provide patient care.

centralized pharmacy system system in which all pharmacy-related activities are performed from one location and medications are delivered to various patient care units throughout the facility.

decentralized pharmacy system pharmacy service system consisting of a central, or inpatient, pharmacy and multiple satellite pharmacies, as well as an outpatient pharmacy.

Physician Assistant

A **physician assistant (PA)** is a licensed individual who is trained to coordinate patient care under the supervision of a medical or osteopathic doctor. Although PAs are authorized to prescribe medications, there are certain restrictions on their ability to prescribe controlled substances.

Certified Nursing Assistant

A **certified nursing assistant (CNA)** is an individual who is certified to assist RNs and LPNs in providing patient care, but is not permitted to administer medication.

Licensed Nursing Assistant

A **licensed nursing assistant (LNA)** is an individual who is licensed to assist RNs and LPNs in providing patient care, but is not permitted to administer medication.

Licensed Practical Nurse

A **licensed practical nurse (LPN)** is an individual who is licensed to provide basic care, such as administering medication, under the supervision of a registered nurse.

Nurse Practitioner

A **nurse practitioner (NP)** is an individual who is licensed to work closely with a physician in providing patient care. In most states, nurse practitioners are authorized to prescribe medications under the supervision of a physician.

Registered Nurse

A **registered nurse (RN)** is an individual who is registered to assist physicians with specific procedures, administer medications, and provide patient care.

Organization of Hospital Pharmacies

Hospital pharmacies are structured and managed very differently than community-based pharmacies. A hospital pharmacy is organized either on the centralized pharmacy model or on the decentralized pharmacy model, with few exceptions (see Figure 7-2).

Centralized Pharmacy

A **centralized pharmacy system** is operated out of one primary location, the inpatient pharmacy (IP). In this organizational model, all pharmacy-related activities are performed at this one location and medications are delivered to various patient care units throughout the facility.

Decentralized Pharmacies

A **decentralized pharmacy system** can consist of a central, or inpatient, pharmacy with multiple satellite pharmacies, as well as an outpatient pharmacy. The disadvantage of this system is the necessary duplication of staff, inventory, and equipment; however, medium-size and large facilities often have to use this type of system.

Inpatient Pharmacy

The **inpatient pharmacy** is generally responsible for medication packaging, centralized inventory, sterile product preparation, and the preparation and delivery of medication carts. It provides pharmaceutical services to patients admitted to a facility.

Outpatient Pharmacy

The **outpatient pharmacy** is available to patients who are being discharged from the hospital, or who are being treated by a physician in the hospital but do not require overnight admission. It is, in a sense, a retail-style pharmacy located within the hospital facility.

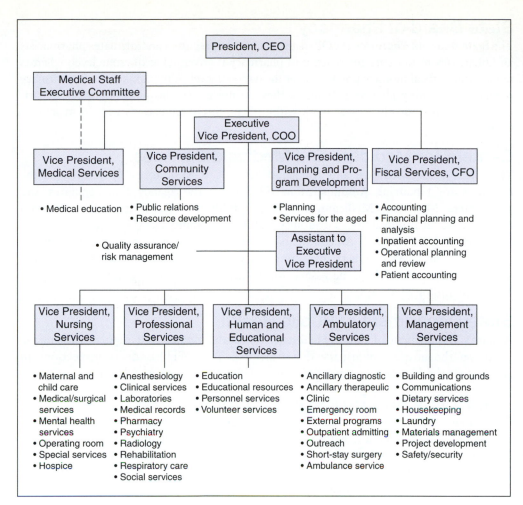

FIGURE 7-2 Typical hospital organization chart.

inpatient pharmacy (IP) portion of a facility that is responsible for medication packaging, centralized inventory, sterile product preparation, and the preparation and delivery of medication carts. It provides pharmaceutical services to patients admitted to a facility.

outpatient pharmacy a pharmacy that is available to patients who are being discharged from the hospital, or who are being treated by a physician without requiring overnight admission.

Satellite Pharmacies

Satellite pharmacies are responsible for receiving, processing, and dispensing medication orders for individual patients. Generally, satellite pharmacies provide initial doses and emergency medications, after which medications may be dispensed from floor stock. The number of satellite pharmacies varies by facility, as does their scope of service. In some hospitals, satellite pharmacies are established for specific patient care areas, such as operating rooms, oncology, or pediatrics. Other hospitals have satellite pharmacies spread throughout the facility based on location and access, as opposed to scope of services.

satellite pharmacies subunits of a central pharmacy, located near specific patient care areas in a facility, such as cardiology, operating rooms, and chemotherapy treatment centers.

Regulatory Agencies

Hospital pharmacies are regulated by a variety of agencies, including the Joint Commission on Accreditation of Healthcare Organizations, State Boards of Pharmacy, the Centers for Medicare and Medicaid Services, and state Departments of Public Health.

Joint Commission on Accreditation of Healthcare Organizations

The Joint Commission on Accreditation of Healthcare Organizations (JCAHO) surveys, inspects, and accredits health systems, such as hospitals, every three years. Site inspections, which include the pharmacy department(s), evaluate a facility's compliance with JCAHO standards and criteria. These intensive site surveys used to be scheduled in advance, but in 2006 JCAHO decided that inspections will now be unannounced. JCAHO accreditation is necessary for organizations to receive reimbursement from Medicare and many third-party insurance companies.

State Board of Pharmacy

The State Board of Pharmacy (SBOP) is the agency that registers and regulates pharmacists and pharmacy technicians; the practice of pharmacy is governed at the state level, whereas the pharmaceutical industry is governed at the national level. Although boards of pharmacy regulate community pharmacy facilities, they do not govern hospital pharmacy departments—just the individuals who work within them. SBOP regulations vary from state to state.

Centers for Medicare and Medicaid Services

The Centers for Medicare and Medicaid Services (CMS), formerly known as the Health Care Financing Administration (HCFA), is the agency that regulates and administers Medicare, Medicaid, the State Children's Health Insurance Program (SCHIP), the Health Insurance Portability and Accountability Act (HIPAA), the Clinical Laboratory Improvement Amendments (CLIA), and several other health-related programs. The CMS conducts inspections to ensure compliance with its guidelines; approval from the CMS is necessary for a facility to receive reimbursement from Medicare and/or Medicaid.

State Department of Public Health

A state's Department of Public Health (DPH) is the agency that regulates hospitals, including the hospital pharmacy department(s). The DPH conducts inspections to ensure that the facility is in compliance with DPH regulations and criteria.

The Policy and Procedure Manual

As do many other well-run organizations, a health-system pharmacy may develop a unique policy and procedure manual to establish specific guidelines and systems for the operations of the facility. *Policies* are definitive methods or courses of action, determined by an organization or department; *procedures* are the step-by-step directions provided to achieve an organization's policies.

The Need

The pharmacy department in a large health system generally has multiple levels of management and supervision, whereas rural health-system pharmacies tend to have smaller staffs and fewer managerial layers. The policy and procedure manual provides much-needed structure for the health-system pharmacy.

The Benefits

The policy and procedure manual (Figure 7-3) provides numerous benefits to a health-system pharmacy department. Primarily, it is being used as a resource to:

- ensure quality assurance throughout the department.
- implement quality control measures, which can reduce medication errors.
- reduce the time required to train employees.
- communicate job responsibilities and scope of authority.
- document compliance for regulatory agencies and accreditation organizations.

The Contents

The organization and contents of policy and procedures manuals will vary by facility, but there are several common methods that health-system pharmacies use to familiarize yourself with.

- *Alphabetical:* Policies and procedures are listed alphabetically according to their official titles.
- *Categorized:* Policies and procedures are divided into topical categories, such as organization, personnel policies, administrative policies, professional policies, and facilities/equipment.

**ADMINISTRATIVE PROCEDURES &
INFORMATION MANUAL
DEPARTMENT OF PHARMACY**

RE-REVIEW DATE:
(Assigned by Policy Review Committee)

SUBJECT: CLARIFICATION OF MEDICATION ORDERS

RESPONSIBLE DEPARTMENT, DIVISION OR COMMITTEE

EFFECTIVE DATE ORIGINAL POLICY: 8/29/xx	**EFFECTIVE DATE REVISED POLICY: 1/00 LAST REVIEW DATE: 3/05**	**SUPERSEDES POLICY NUMBER: DATED:**

POLICY: No prescription or order is to be filled if there is any doubt in the mind of the pharmacist as to what is called for: the dose, how it is to be given, or whether it is appropriate.

PROCEDURE:

1. Orders being questioned are to be entered on the patient profile as "pending" with documentation of the problem in the clinical notes and a statement in the Special Direction field "See Clinical Notes." The yellow copy of the order is to be placed in the "problem" box with a notation as to the problem. Orders with problems that could pose risk to the patient must contain the phrase "Do not dispense until clarified" on the yellow copy and in the Special Directions Field.

2. No medication is to be dispensed until the order is clarified.

3. It is the responsibility of the pharmacist to contact the prescriber.

4. In the event that the name of the prescriber cannot be determined from the signature or I.D. number, the nurse may be asked for the name of the prescriber.

5. The pharmacist will page the prescriber. If the prescriber is an intern and there is no response in 15 minutes, then page the resident. Repeat this procedure, if necessary. If still no response, contact the attending physician. This last step should be done when, in the pharmacist's professional judgment, the patient could be harmed by further delay.

6. If the matter has not been resolved by the end of the shift, the information must be communicated to a pharmacist on the next shift for follow-up and resolution.

7. Upon receipt of clarification, the pending order is cancelled and the corrected order is entered. Problem resolution is to be documented on the clinical notes.

8. If authorization to change an order has been obtained, a message is to be sent to the unit notifying the nurse of the change. (See "Change in Medication Order").

9. Documentation of a clarification/change will be made in the medical record by the authorized prescriber or the pharmacist.

J. Smith

Director of Pharmacy Services

FIGURE 7-3 Sample policy and procedures manual.

Dispensing Systems

Within a single health-system setting, there may be many types of medication distribution systems. This is especially true of a hospital setting, where there may even be multiple pharmacies. The common medication distribution systems are floor stock, patient prescription, and unit-dose.

Floor Stock

In the **floor stock** distribution system, medications are kept on each floor for distribution to patients (see Figure 7-4). This system is prone to errors, diversion, and employee theft. However, in recent times, computers have made this system much easier to monitor and

floor stock distribution system in which medications are kept on each floor for distribution to patients.

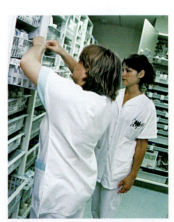

FIGURE 7-4 The floor stock distribution system.

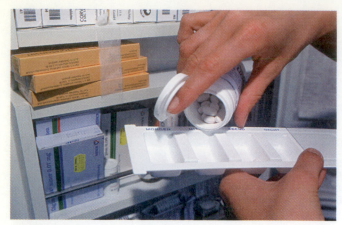

FIGURE 7-5 Filling a patient prescription.

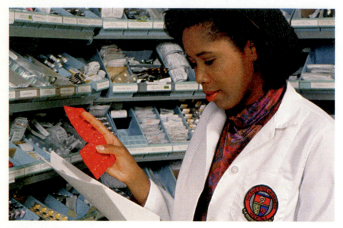

FIGURE 7-6 The unit-dose system makes it very easy to track a patient's medications.

patient prescription stock system a system in which medication orders are reviewed, prepared, and verified, and then the medications are taken to the floor and dispensed to the patient.

unit-dose a distribution system in which each medication order is filled in the pharmacy in a way that provides each dose in a package ready to administer to the patient. Usually, not more than a 24-hour supply is dispensed at one time.

medication order term for a patient prescription in a health system.

fill. The technician stocks the floor unit with a predetermined bulk supply after the pharmacist checks the order. The computerized system tracks the inventory, records who has accessed the unit, and even bills the patient. This system can generate refill orders to the technician, whereupon the process begins again. The floor stock dispensing system requires a great deal of floor space and imposes higher inventory requirements.

Patient Prescriptions

The **patient prescription stock system** is the most inefficient because of waste and the inability of the pharmacy department to properly monitor it. In this system, after reviewing medication orders for a floor, the technician takes the medications to the pharmacist for verification, and then takes the medications to the floor (see Figure 7-5). The orders are usually for several days' supply of the medication (typically three). Once opened, the medication cannot be returned to the pharmacy, since it is considered to have been dispensed and therefore to have left the control and closed system of the health-system pharmacy.

Unit-Dose

In contrast to the prescription system, the **unit-dose** system is the most efficient distribution system, and makes it very easy to track a patient's medications (see Figure 7-6). In this system, each medication order is filled in the pharmacy in as close to administration form as possible, meaning that not more than a 24-hour supply is dispensed at one time. Scanners may be used to track and bill for the medications when they are dispensed. Unit-dose systems centralize medication preparation in the pharmacy itself, cut the amount of time the nursing staff spends preparing medications, and greatly reduces waste.

Clearly, a unit-dose system requires more technician involvement. In a centralized pharmacy, technicians may have workstations for unit-dose medications (tablets, capsules, and liquids), IVs, sterile preparations, chemotherapy, injections, and compounding. Unit-dose systems can be centralized, decentralized, or a combination of both.

The Medication Order

In health-system pharmacies, prescribers order medications for patients on a **medication order** form, as opposed to the prescription pad used for retail pharmacies. The medication order form is a multipurpose tool for communication among various members of the healthcare team working within a health system. In addition to prescribed medications, this form can be used by the physician to order lab work, special diets, and X-rays or other medical procedures, so it is imperative that pharmacy personnel be able to properly distinguish and interpret medication orders.

Hospitals can choose to use physical, hard-copy medication order forms, a physician order entry system (**POE system**), or a computerized physician order entry (**CPOE**) system. The latter is a fully computerized system in which orders are entered electronically into the hospital's networked system.

Medication Order Components

There are some differences between the requirements for a medication order (see Figure 7-7) and those for a prescription. However, the reasons for the variations are pretty much self-evident.

- Patient information:
  - Name
  - Room/bed number
  - Hospital ID number
  - Birth date/age
- Medication information:
  - Name
  - Dose

POE system a point-of-entry computer system, networked within the health system to allow prescribers and nurses to enter medication orders directly for the pharmacy; sometimes referred to as a *computerized physician order entry (CPOE) system*.

16285
CH-7239
(FEB. 03)

PHYSICIAN'S ORDER WORKSHEET

NOTE: *Person initiating entry should write legibly, date the form using (Mo./Day/Yr.), enter time, sign, and indicate their title.*

USE BALL POINT PEN (PRESS FIRMLY)

Date	Time	Treatment
		③

 PHYSICIAN'S ORDER WORKSHEET Distribution: (Original) Medical Record Copy (Plies 3, 2, & 1) Pharmacy **T-5**

FIGURE 7-7 A sample medication order.

- Frequency of administration
- Route
- Signature of prescriber
- Date and hour the order was written

Types of Medication Orders

standing order a medication order used when a patient is to receive a specific medication at specific intervals throughout the day; also called a *scheduled order*.

PRN order a medication order used when a patient is to receive a medication only as necessary, as with pain medication.

STAT order a medication order used when a patient requires a medication immediately; this is an urgent order and thus takes priority over other orders and requests.

emergency medication order a specific type of STAT order for a medication that is required for a physician to be able to respond to a medical emergency.

investigational medication order an order for medication used in facilities that participate in research programs.

There are three main types of medication orders: **standing orders**, PRN orders, and STAT orders. A standing, or scheduled, order is used when a patient is to receive a specific medication at specific intervals throughout the day. A **PRN order**, which means an as-needed order, is used when a patient is to receive a medication only as necessary, as with pain medication. A **STAT order**, which stands for immediate order, is used when a patient requires a medication immediately. This is an urgent order that takes priority over other orders and requests.

INFORMATION

Standing order—to be dispensed routinely
PRN order—to be dispensed as needed
STAT order—to be dispensed immediately

In addition to these common types of medication orders, there are also emergency medication orders and investigational medication orders. An **emergency medication order** is a specific type of a STAT order for a medication that is required for a physician to be able to respond to a medical emergency. An **investigational medication order** is used in facilities that participate in research programs. Investigational drugs are ordered, prepared, and administered according to stringent protocols specific to the research program.

Receiving Medication Orders

Just as in an ambulatory setting, no medications are dispensed in a health-system setting without a prescription. In a health system, the medication order is not given to the patient to be filled; rather, it is entered, submitted, filled, billed, and delivered to the patient by facility staff.

The medication order may arrive in the pharmacy in several different ways:

- The order may be submitted electronically to the pharmacy, utilizing a POE, point-of-entry, or CPOE system.
- The order may be sent by way of a pneumatic tube device (see Figure 7-8).
- The order may be handed directly to the pharmacist.
- The order may be faxed to the pharmacy.
- Orders may be sent through the institutional computer system.
- A technician may be assigned to collect medication orders from many areas throughout the institution.

In addition, medication orders may be submitted directly to the nursing floors, in which case the orders are verified electronically by the pharmacist, and then administered by nurses using floor stock.

Processing Medication Orders

Health-system pharmacy settings are, basically, pharmacies that are located in the "homes" of the patients served there. The parent facility may be a hospital, nursing home, or hospice. Several differences distinguish a health-system pharmacy practice from an ambulatory pharmacy. The differences in institutional policies and procedures regarding the processing of medication orders can be challenging for technicians unless

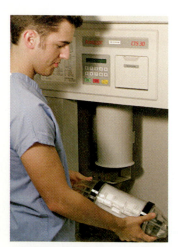

FIGURE 7-8 Receiving a medication order.

the technicians receive adequate training beforehand. This section briefly discusses the processing of medication orders and highlights these differences.

Order Entry

Hard-copy medication order forms may be entered into the computer system by pharmacy technicians, pharmacists, nursing clerks, nurses, or even physicians (see Figure 7-9). Regardless of who enters the order, the following items must be included:

- Patient name
- Patient hospital ID number
- Room number/bed number/location
- Drug name
- Drug strength
- Drug quantity (if a STAT order)
- Route of administration
- Frequency of administration
- Ordering physician
- Date and time of order

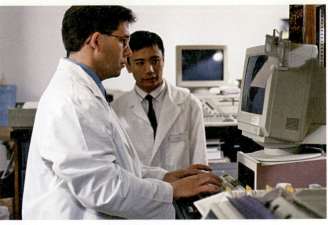

FIGURE 7-9 Entering a medication order.

Order Verification

Technicians practicing in health-system settings may be assigned to collect and accept medication orders. Technicians may even review the orders for completeness. These orders are called *unverified* and cannot be processed until they have been verified by a pharmacist. Each order must be screened by the pharmacist for correct order entry, potential interactions, allergies, drug utilization review, and formulary utilization.

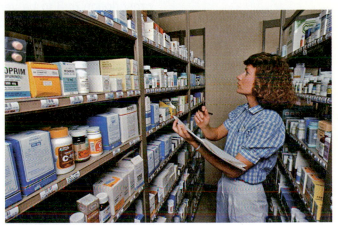

FIGURE 7-10 Preparing an order.

Order Preparation

Just as in an ambulatory setting, medications may be counted out in a health-system setting. The same care must be taken to match lot and UPC numbers, as well as to check expiration dates (see Figure 7-10). The technician performing this task needs to keep the spatula and counting tray clean at all times. Special care should be taken when counting cytotoxic or chemotherapy drugs.

❝ Workplace Wisdom Counting Medications ❞

A thorough technician will count twice, especially when counting C-II medications.

These facilities may also use automated counting machines that technicians are required to operate and maintain on a daily basis. These machines are popular because they are efficient, reduce errors, and can also reduce drug diversion. An important point to remember is that these machines are only as accurate as the technicians who operate them. At no time should a technician override a machine's built-in checking system. Technicians must also pay close attention to any policies or procedures pertaining to the operation of automated dispensing equipment.

| INFORMATION |

Some medications, such as parenteral nutrition, sterile products, and chemotherapy, must be compounded prior to dispensing/administration.

Dispensing Medication Orders

Filling prescriptions or medication orders is one of the most basic duties of a pharmacy technician in any health-system setting. However, filling consists of much more than just counting and basic measuring.

The final check is the sole domain of the pharmacist. No medications may be dispensed without the pharmacist's final approval. In a health-system setting, this is a relatively simple process. The pharmacist will need the original medication order and the labeled container filled with the prescribed medication. Once the pharmacist approves it, the medication may be sent to the proper ward or floor and dispensed to the patient.

Workplace Wisdom Tech-Check-Tech

Historically, any task performed by a pharmacy technician related to dispensing a prescription had to be verified and documented in writing by a pharmacist, but certain states have now approved Tech-Check-Tech, a policy which enables hospital pharmacists to spend more time on activities designed to reduce errors and to provide clinical support to physicians and nurses.

In general, hospitals that utilize Tech-Check-Tech employ specially trained pharmacy technicians to check medication cassettes and the work of other technicians. Tech-Check-Tech regulations vary by state and specific policies vary by institution. Because regulations change frequently, current information on Tech-Check-Tech regulations should be obtained from the State Board of Pharmacy.

Pharmacy Technician Job Responsibilities

To allow pharmacists to focus on the medication-related problems of their patients and provide the best pharmaceutical care, many tasks in the health-system care facility that were once performed by the pharmacist are now delegated to qualified support staff, including pharmacy technicians. The pharmacy technician, under the supervision of a pharmacist and according to the laws of the state in which the technician works, is permitted to perform a wide range of tasks. These tasks may involve a variety of the components of pharmacy practice, including, but not limited to:

- data collection and reporting (patient satisfaction assessments, compilation of continuous quality improvement data, drug inventory management, formulary maintenance, preparation of billing statements).
- surveys and inspections (conduct medication room inspections, conduct narcotic audits, check emergency boxes and replace outdated medications, check orders for completeness, inspect and service crash carts).
- education (assist in facility meetings, help organize and maintain the medical library, provide inservice training and continuing education for facility personnel).
- maintenance (assist in the maintenance of devices such as fax machines, automated dispensing systems, etc.).
- dispensing/inventory management (order medication stock, package medications, prepare intravenous solutions, fill and label prescriptions).

No task delegated to a pharmacy technician may involve performing a final check of a medication before it goes to the patient, nor may the technician perform any task that requires the professional judgment of a pharmacist.

To make sure that technicians are properly trained and their performance evaluated, the supervising pharmacist will provide a written job description of the functions performed by the pharmacy technicians, according to regulations of the state where the facility is located. The initial orientation and training for pharmacy technicians should include information about properly performing their assigned functions, the unique needs of institutionalized patients, and relevant regulations.

The pharmacy technician also needs to receive ongoing training and education. Technicians should be given periodic evaluations of their job performance.

Record Maintenance and Management

Technicians are responsible for maintaining accurate, complete, and updated records on patients, procedures, inventory, training, and regulatory compliance.

Unit-Dose Preparation

Pharmacy technicians are charged with maintaining the unit-dose systems in an institution (see Figure 7-11). This requires them to select medications and prepare medications for dispensing, much as they would in an ambulatory setting.

Medication carts are filled with the medications for each patient in their individual drawers. Because many medications do not come in unit-dose form, it is the pharmacy technician's responsibility to prepare all medications. The goal is to prepare each medication in a form as close to its dispensing form as possible. These doses are not labeled for a particular patient, but must be clearly labeled with the drug name and strength. As with any repackaging, strict attention to detail is essential. Each dose must be identifiable up to the time it is administered. All medications must remain sanitary, and in some cases, such as for IV or injection, sterile.

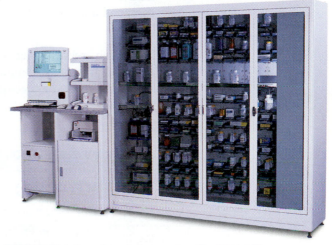

FIGURE 7-11 A view of a unit-dose system (the SP Unit Dispenser (SPUD). (Courtesy of ScriptPro.)

Some medications, such as drops, ointments, and creams, cannot be unit-dosed. In such cases, the medications must be labeled for the individual patient. The label must contain:

- patient's name
- location (floor, room, and bed number)
- drug (name and strength)
- date

Compounding

Compounding in health-system pharmacies refers to preparing custom-ordered medications, such as IVs, total parenteral nutrition (TPN), and nonsterile compounds. Technicians preparing orders for IV medications or TPN need specialized training. There are a plethora of machines and measuring systems available, but again, the equipment is only as good as the operator. Technicians filling these kinds of medication work with less supervision and do more calculations; therefore, they must be well trained. Several accreditations and certifications are available for technicians who wish to specialize in compounding. Technicians who want to perform this type of work should take advantage of those opportunities.

Workplace Wisdom USP <797>

The U.S. Pharmacopeia's (USP) Revised General Chapter <797> Pharmaceutical Compounding—Sterile Preparations sets practice standards to help ensure that compounded sterile preparations are of high quality. For more information on USP <797> go to www.usp.org.

Repackaging

Pharmacy technicians often repackage various medications in the pharmacy. Repackaging commonly consists of pharmacy technicians opening large containers of medicine and transferring the contents into smaller containers, including single or daily dosages. This requires the technician to be knowledgeable regarding appropriate containers and storage protocols.

Common containers used in repackaging include blister packs, vials, bottles, cups, and bags. Depending on the medication being repackaged, a light-sensitive container may be needed; these are usually brown or amber colored.

Workplace Wisdom Repackaging

Capsules and tablets are usually repackaged into blister packs or vials. Liquid medications are usually repackaged into cups or vials.

When repackaging medications, expiration dates must be determined and assigned. In general, expiration dates are established as either six months from the date of repackaging or one-quarter of the manufacturer's remaining expiration date, whichever is less.

PROCEDURE 7-1

Determining Expiration Dates

1. Locate the expiration date assigned by the manufacturer.
2. Calculate the total number of months remaining between today's date and the expiration date.
3. Divide the total number of months remaining by 4.
4. Add the result of step 3 to the current date.
5. Compare six months from today's date with the result of step 4 and select the lesser of the two.

PROFILES IN PRACTICE

Stephen is a pharmacy technician who works in the centralized pharmacy. He is mainly responsible for repackaging medications into unit-dosages. Currently, Stephen is repackaging docusate sodium, which bears a manufacturer's expiration date of 10/2012.

• What expiration date should Stephen assign to this medication?

Floor Stock Inspections

Most health systems utilize pharmacy technicians to inspect and maintain the floor stock. The technician inspects the inventory levels, expiration dates, stock condition, and storage conditions. *Floor stock* refers to medications that are located on the patient floors to be administered by nurses. These medications should be inspected daily.

Crash Carts

Pharmacy technicians are often responsible for stocking crash carts, which are sets of trays on a wheeled cart that are used in critical situations or for emergency medical care.

A crash cart typically contains a defibrillator and intravenous medications, plus a variety of medical supplies such as latex gloves and alcohol swabs. While the specific inventory of an institution's crash cart will vary, the following are the standard minimum equipment and medication requirements:

Equipment

Airways, all sizes
Forceps, large and small
Nasal Canulas, infant, pedi, adult
100% Non-rebreather Oxygen Face Masks, infant, pedi, adult
Ambu Bags, infant, pedi, adult
IV Start Paks
1000 cc bag Normal Saline Solution
IV Tubing (Burotrol for Pedi patients)
Angiocatheters
1cc syringes
3cc syringes
5cc syringes
10cc syringes
20cc syringes
Gauze
Alcohol Preps
Flashlight

Drugs

Aspirin 325 mg tabs
Nitroglycerin 0.4 mg sublingual tabs
Dextrose 50%
Narcan 1 mg Amps
Epinephrine 1 mg (1:10:000 conc)
Atropine Sulfate 0.1 mg/ml
Lidocaine 100 mg
EpiPen
EpiPen Jr.
SoluMedrol 125 mg Vial
Benadryl 50 mg Vial
Tagamet 300 mg Vial

SUMMARY

Health-system pharmacies are designed to serve patients who reside onsite, at the same facility where the pharmacy is located. Health-system pharmacies, also known as institutional pharmacies, include hospital pharmacies and pharmacies in long-term care facilities, nursing homes, correctional facilities, and other institutions. Hospital pharmacies are the most common.

Although filling a prescription and filling a medication order are basically the same, health-system pharmacy practice is more varied than community pharmacy practice. Health-system pharmacy technicians work with several distribution systems, repackage medications for specific patients, and also do bulk repackaging for floors and patient care areas. Health-system pharmacies commonly use unit-dose dispensing, in which patients receive no more than a 24-hour supply of the medications ordered. In hospitals, these medications are dispensed via a centralized pharmacy or a series of satellite pharmacies dispersed throughout the facility. Institutional technicians also deal in sterile and aseptic techniques, cytotoxins, and chemotherapy drugs, as well as a variety of automatic dispensing systems.

The practice of pharmacy in an institutional setting is evolving just as fast, if not faster, than practice in ambulatory settings. Innovations in medications, drug delivery systems, information systems, and patient care provide technicians opportunities for more training, education, and responsibility in the healthcare system.

CHAPTER REVIEW QUESTIONS

1. How often do pharmacists generally perform drug therapy review for each patient?
   a. weekly
   b. monthly
   c. semi-monthly
   d. quarterly

2. The federal government passed which of the following to protect the health and well-being of institutional residents?
   a. OBRA 1987
   b. FEDA 1981
   c. NOVA 1956
   d. OBRA 1945

3. What is the name for an adult care home that is licensed and governed by state and federal regulations?
   a. nursing home
   b. adult day care
   c. homeless shelter
   d. senior center

4. When labeling medications such as creams for specific patients, the label must contain:
   a. the patient's name.
   b. the patient's room number or location.
   c. the name and strength of the drug.
   d. all of the above

5. Once a medication order is packaged in a unit-dose container, it must be:
   a. rushed to the patient.
   b. taken to the attending nurse.
   c. properly stored until called for.
   d. checked by a pharmacist before being dispensed.

6. Pharmacy technicians may collect medication orders from:
   a. fax machines.
   b. the health-system computer system.
   c. prescribers throughout the institution.
   d. all of the above.

7. The most efficient medication delivery system in a health-system pharmacy is:
   a. individual.
   b. floor stock.
   c. unit-dose.
   d. bulk.

8. The benefit of an automated dispensing system is that it:
   a. is cost-effective.
   b. reduces errors when operated properly.
   c. helps reduce diversion.
   d. all of the above.

9. Which regulatory agency administers the State Children's Health Insurance Program?
   a. JCAHO
   b. SBOP
   c. CMS
   d. DPS

10. Which of the following cannot be repackaged as a unit dose?
    a. C-II medications
    b. liquid medications
    c. eye drops
    d. reconstituted powders

CRITICAL THINKING QUESTIONS

1. In what ways is health-system pharmacy practice different from community pharmacy practice?

2. What are the benefits of establishing satellite pharmacies within a health system?

3. Why do health-system pharmacies repackage and unit-dose medications?

WEB CHALLENGE

1. Go to the National Association for Public Hospitals and Health Systems (NAPH) website and research the definition and characteristics of a *safety net hospital*: http://www.naph.org

2. Visit the American Hospital Association (AHA) website and print out the "Fast Facts on US Hospitals" report: http://www.aha.org

REFERENCES AND RESOURCES

American Hospital Association. *2004 Hospital Statistic Report.* Chicago: AHA, 2004.

American Medical Association. *Know Your Drugs and Medications.* New York: Reader's Digest Association, 1991.

American Pharmacist Association. *Pharmacy Technician Workbook and Certification Review.* Englewood, CO: Morton Publishing, 2001.

American Society of Health System Pharmacists. *Manual for Pharmacy Technicians.* Bethesda, MD: ASHP, 1998.

American Society of Health System Pharmacists. *Pharmacy Technician Certification Review and Exam.* Bethesda, MD: ASHP, 1998.

Ansel, HC. *Introduction to Pharmaceutical Dosage Forms.* Philadelphia: Lea & Febiger, 1995.

Ballington, D. *Pharmacy Practice.* St. Paul, MN: EMC Paradigm, 1999.

Ballington, D. *Pharmacy Practice for Technicians.* St. Paul, MN: EMC Paradigm, 2003.

CareScout. "Nursing-Home" (accessed March 4, 2006): http://www.carescout.com

Cowen, D, & Helfand, W. *Pharmacy: An Illustrated History.* New York: Harry N. Abrams, 1990.

Facts and Comparisons. "Homepage" (accessed January 4, 2004): http://www.factsandcomparisons.com

Food and Drug Administration. "Homepage" (accessed January 4, 2004): http://www.fda.gov

Lambert, A. *Advanced Pharmacy Practice for Technicians.* Clifton Park, NY: Thomson Delmar Learning, 2002.

Medicare. "Homepage" (accessed March 4, 2006): http://www.medicare.net

National Hospice and Palliative Care Organization. *Hospice Standards of Practice.* Alexandria, VA: NHPCO, 2000.

Reifman, N. *Certification Review for Pharmacy Technicians* (6th ed.). Evergreen, CO: Ark Pharmaceutical Consultants, Inc., 2002.

Texas Tech University Health Sciences Center. "Minimum Crash Cart Supplies and Drugs" (accessed April 12, 2008): www.ttuhsc.edu/som/clinic/forms/ACForm2.03.A.pdf

United States Pharmacopeia. "Homepage" (accessed April 12, 2008): www.usp.org

chapter 8

Technology in the Pharmacy

LEARNING OBJECTIVES

After completing this chapter, you should be able to:

- List the hardware and software components used in pharmacy computers and summarize their purpose.
- Describe and discuss the use of automation and robotics in community pharmacies.
- Describe and discuss the use of automation and robotics in health-system pharmacies.
- Summarize the uses of personal digital assistants in medicine.
- Define and explain telepharmacy practice.
- Summarize the impact of patient confidentiality regulations on the use of technology in the pharmacy.

Introduction

Technology has revolutionized the practice of pharmacy, as it has so many other industries. Gone are the days of writing prescription instructions and labels by hand or with a typewriter, as was done as recently as the 1970s. Today, virtually every pharmacy uses computers, automated systems, and other technology platforms for its operations and management of pharmaceutical care. This is why a basic understanding of technology is necessary for the pharmacy technician.

Computers

A computer is, in essence, an electronic device used for inputting, storing, processing, and outputting information (see Figure 8-1). A computer system is comprised of both **hardware** and **software** components. This section describes some of the more common hardware and software components used in pharmacy.

Hardware

Three types of hardware are required for computers to operate effectively: input devices, processing components, and output devices. **Input devices** allow information, or data, to be entered into the computer system. Then, the **processing components** organize, manage, and store the data. Finally, the **output devices** produce and release the data in a visual or tangible, printed form.

Input Devices

Some familiar examples of computer input devices include:

- **Keyboard**: the primary input device of a computer system; used to enter information (both alphabetic and numeric) into the computer.
- **Mouse**: a device that rolls on a hard, flat surface and controls the movement of the cursor, or pointer, on the screen. Clicking the mouse buttons gives the user control of the computer; each mouse includes one to three buttons, with each one performing different functions. Figure 8-2 shows an example of a keyboard and mouse.
- **Scanner**: a device used to input a photographic image into the computer system (see Figure 8-3). Some pharmacies are now using scanners to input and store images of each hard copy, or physical, prescription.

hardware the mechanical and electrical components that make up a computer system.

software the programs and applications that control the functioning of computer hardware and direct the operation of the computer.

input devices hardware that allows information, or data, to be entered into a computer system.

processing components hardware devices used to organize, manage, and store data.

output devices hardware devices that produce and release data in a visual or tangible, printed form.

keyboard the primary input device of a computer system, used to enter information (both alphabetic and numeric) into the computer.

mouse a device that rolls on a hard, flat surface and controls the movement of the cursor, or pointer, on the screen.

INFORMATION

There are two main types of scanners. One works like a copy machine: you place a hard copy face down on the glass plate, close the lid, and press a button. The other type works more like a fax machine: you place a hard copy face down into a machine that feeds the document through after you push a button. The end result, which is the same with both types of scanning devices, is an electronic copy or image of the hard copy that can be stored, viewed, and retrieved within the computer system.

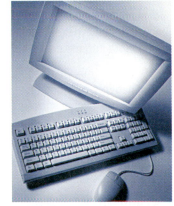
FIGURE 8-1 An example of a computer.

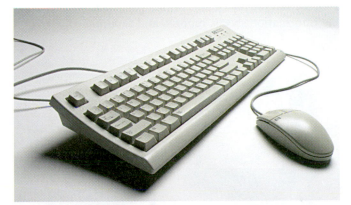
FIGURE 8-2 A computer keyboard and mouse.

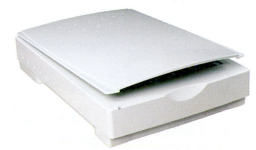
FIGURE 8-3 A computer scanner.

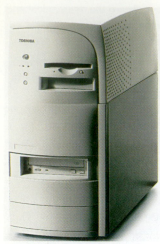

FIGURE 8-4 A central processing unit, or CPU.

scanner a hardware device used to input a photographic image into the computer system.

central processing unit (CPU) the brain of a computer system; it interprets commands, connects the various hardware components, runs software applications, and controls speed and use of memory space.

random-access memory (RAM) temporary memory used while information is being input into the computer.

read-only memory (ROM) permanent memory used for essential operating instructions for the computer system.

hard drive the main storage device of a computer; can be either external or internal.

modem hardware device used for connecting computer systems that are remotely located, via a telephone line or cable; can be installed either internally or externally.

monitor the visual display screen of the computer system.

printer the primary output device of a computer system, used to produce paper documents.

Processing Components

Some of the various computer processing components are:

- **Central processing unit (CPU)**: the brain of the computer system. The CPU is responsible for interpreting commands, connecting the various hardware components, running software applications, and controlling speed and use of memory space. Figure 8-4 shows a CPU.
- Memory and storage: all of the information and data being entered, or input, into a computer must be able to be stored. A computer's memory capacity is measured in kilobytes (Kb or K); 1 Kb equals 1,000 characters (bytes) of information. Storage is available through many different options, such as:
  - Memory chips/cards—CPUs contain two different types of memory chips: **random-access memory (RAM)** and **read-only memory (ROM)**. RAM is a temporary memory used while information is being input into the computer, whereas ROM is a permanent memory used for essential operating instructions for the system. RAM influences the speed of a computer system; the more RAM a computer has, the faster it will operate. In addition, memory chips and cards are now available in removable formats, such as cards, sticks, and "thumb" drives, all of which can store vast amounts of data on devices as small as keychains (see Figure 8-5).
- **Hard drives**: the main storage device of a computer; can be either external or internal. Hard drives are magnetic storage devices, usually referred to as the C drive. Many health-system pharmacies have multiple hard drives for their computers.
  - Tape, disk, CD-ROM, and DVD drives: in addition to memory chips and hard drives, computers may be equipped with various additional storage devices, including magnetic tapes, floppy disks, CD-ROMs, DVDs, and large-capacity disks, such as Zip or Jaz disks.
- **Modem**: a device used for connecting computer systems that are remotely located, via a telephone line or cable; can be installed either internally or externally. Modems are also used to connect computers to the Internet and company intranets.

Output Devices

Some of the various computer output devices available are:

- **Monitor**: the visual display component of the computer system (see Figure 8-6). The monitor is considered an output device; however, a touch-screen—a monitor that allows you to use your finger or a stylus as a mouse—is considered both an input and an output device. The monitor is often referred to as the *screen*.
- **Printer**: the primary output device of a computer system, used to produce paper documents (see Figure 8-7). Within the pharmacy, printers are used for preparing prescription labels, patient information sheets, reports, and receipts.

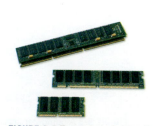

FIGURE 8-5 Examples of chips that store RAM.

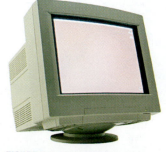

FIGURE 8-6 A computer monitor.

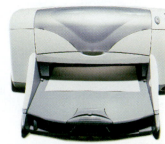

FIGURE 8-7 A printer is an example of a primary output device.

Software

In general, software can be thought of as the set or sets of instructions the computer follows to perform various functions. For example, a word-processing program is software that allows the user to type words into the computer to create letters, memos, and other types of documents. Examples of software include:

- **Operating system**: the primary software (program) used to connect the various hardware components of a computer and allow them to perform their essential functions. The most common operating systems are Microsoft® Windows®, Linux®, and Macintosh® OS®.

- **Applications**: software programs other than the operating system are referred to as *applications*; these are programs designed to perform specific functions, such as creating databases, spreadsheets, e-mail, or graphics, or performing word processing, to name only a few examples.

operating system the primary software program used to connect the various hardware components of a computer and allow them to perform their essential functions.

applications software programs designed to perform specific functions, such as creating databases, spreadsheets, e-mail, or graphics, or performing word processing.

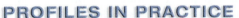

PROFILES IN PRACTICE

Pam is a pharmacy technician and works at an independent, community-based pharmacy. The pharmacy has a very small staff—one pharmacist and two pharmacy technicians. Pam is entering prescriptions into the computer system when she hears a loud boom of thunder during a storm. The entire system shuts down and the monitor goes blank.

- What should Pam do?

Computers in the Pharmacy

Within the pharmacy setting, computer systems are used to generate prescription labels, serial numbers, warning labels, and patient information (see Figure 8-8). They also function as massive collections of **databases** (which are simply lists of information, ordered in specific ways). With a few keystrokes, a pharmacy technician can pull up a specific prescription or a patient's whole profile of medications from a year ago. Technicians can even retrieve every prescription that has been written for a specific drug in a given period of time. It is easy to see how computer systems have forever changed (for the better) data management and accessibility for community pharmacies.

These systems also offer patient safety mechanisms. The software can alert the technician to potential drug interactions between the drug being filled and a drug or drugs on the patient's current profile. It can also alert the technician if the dose is too high or too low, based on the patient's age, and check new prescriptions against patient allergies.

Chains that have more than one pharmacy, or health-system pharmacies, can use their computer systems to electronically link their locations. This offers the pharmacy's customers greater flexibility when filling and refilling prescriptions, as many community pharmacies are able to access the patient's medication profile, insurance information, and personal details (e.g., date of birth, address, telephone number, allergies, and insurance information).

databases lists of information, ordered in specific ways.

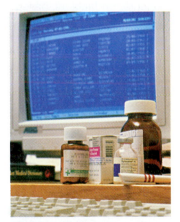

FIGURE 8-8 Within the pharmacy setting, computer systems generate prescription labels, serial numbers, warning labels, and patient information.

Automation and Robotics in Community Pharmacies

Prescription volume in community pharmacies is on the rise and is expected to continue to increase. Thus, the nation's retailers are facing a shortage of licensed pharmacists to fill these prescriptions. These facts present a formidable challenge to already overworked community pharmacies. Not only do these numbers indicate a substantial increase in the pharmacy workload, but, because of the lack of personnel in relation to the number of prescriptions filled, the potential risks to patient safety are alarming. Pharmacy staff members employed in community pharmacies are working as quickly as they can to keep up with current prescription demands. Pharmacies are increasingly turning to technology to assist pharmacy staff with managing day-to-day operations. Nowhere is the use of technology making a more obvious impact than in the community pharmacy.

One obvious solution is to increase the number of trained pharmacy technician employees in the pharmacy. Most states, in anticipation of the pharmacist shortages to come, are revisiting prior legislation that set a very low ratio of pharmacists to technicians (e.g., one pharmacist to one technician, or one pharmacist to two technicians). Several states have already adjusted this ratio. The other obvious solution, in today's age of computers and data management capabilities, is to add technology.

In years past, community pharmacies relied on typewriters to make labels for prescription bottles, manual stamps to generate prescription serial numbers, manual counting trays to aid in counting out tablets and capsules by hand, and a highly paid pharmacist to perform each and every one of these tasks. Today, nearly everything has changed in the community pharmacy. To begin with, pharmacists are no longer as involved with the actual mechanics of prescription filling; rather, they are becoming more involved in patient counseling and disease-state management. Pharmacy technicians are picking up the added responsibilities of prescription filling (although pharmacists are still required to check every prescription before it reaches the patient) and undertaking many of the day-to-day operations required to keep the pharmacy running.

In addition to hiring more technicians, community pharmacies are also employing technology to help to ease the burden of ever-increasing prescription volume. The following subsections discuss some examples of the types of technology commonly seen in community pharmacies.

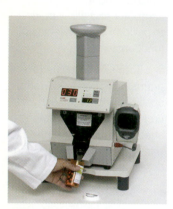

FIGURE 8-9 Example of a counting machine. (Courtesy of Kirby Lester.)

counting machines
electronic devices that automatically and precisely count capsules and tablets, based on weight.

Counting Machines

Pharmacies are using **counting machines** to cut down on the time it takes to manually count out oral solids like tablets and capsules. Medications that are poured in bulk into the counting machine fall past an electronic "eye" that counts the tablets. A digital display indicates how many have fallen into the receptacle. Some counters use even more complex technology. Based on the weight of a single tablet of a specific medication, and the number of tablets/capsules desired, the machine will determine how much the final number of tablets/capsules should weigh. This improves the accuracy of counting equipment to around 99.9 percent.

It is important to note that most pharmacies that use counting machines still require Schedule II (and sometimes Schedule III, IV, and V) narcotics to be counted out by hand, because of the stricter inventory and regulatory policies covering controlled substances. Additionally, because of the potential for allergic reactions due to cross-contamination, penicillin and sulfur-containing compounds should not be used in automated counters. Examples of counting machines include the Baker Universal 2010 (McKesson) and the KL15df (Kirby Lester) (see Figure 8-9).

Bar-Coding Equipment

Bar-code technology has finally come to pharmacy. In many community pharmacies, bar-coding is being used to increase accuracy and patient safety (see Figure 8-10). In much the same way that grocery stores use bar-coding (and have for years), pharmacies are now scanning the bar codes on medication bottles to make sure that the drug therein matches the drug called for on the prescription order. Each bar code contains embedded information that identifies the drug, dosage form, and strength. If the pharmacist or technician has pulled the wrong drug container from the shelf, the bar-code-reading machine will immediately alert the user to the error. Although this technology is somewhat expensive, when you consider what a company must pay to defend itself against a lawsuit, the cost-benefit analysis comes down squarely on the side of using this technology.

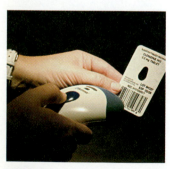

FIGURE 8-10 Bar-code technology is now used in many pharmacy applications.

Workplace Wisdom Bar Codes

The FDA also now mandates that all prescription medications contain a bar code.

Prescription Filling Robots

Community and outpatient pharmacies can also use robots and automation technology to fill prescriptions. Perhaps the most common form of this type of technology is the **cassette system**. These cassettes are essentially drug containers that can hold hundreds, and sometimes thousands, of tablets. The cassette that contains the correct drug is selected by the pharmacy technician and affixed to a counting machine. The user tells the machine how many tablets or capsules are needed, and the machine drops the correct number of tablets or capsules into a prescription vial. In some systems, each individual drug cassette includes its own counting mechanism. This system saves the time of shuttling the cassettes to the counter and placing them back in their original position when finished. Both systems are time savers in the pharmacy and take up a minimum amount of space, but both require human intervention.

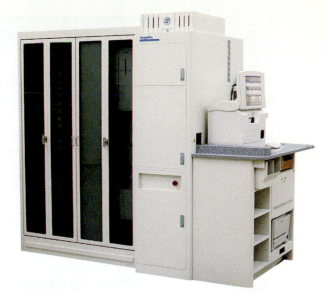

FIGURE 8-11 An example of a prescription filling robot: the SP Automation Center (SPace) SP 100 from ScriptPro. (*Courtesy of ScriptPro.*)

There are also true "robots" that are available to fill prescriptions, although these are much more prevalent in institutional pharmacies. Several companies make dispensing robots, like ScriptPro, PharmaCARE, and McKesson. These robots work in much the same fashion as a cassette system, except that they do not need a staff member to intervene. A robotic arm is placed in the center of many different cells (within reach of the arm). The arm then rotates and selects the correct medication automatically, based on data entered into the machine's computer system. These systems are very accurate. The largest of them can fill up to 130 prescriptions per hour and hold more than 200 different medications. The drawbacks to this type of robotic automation are the cost and size of the equipment. The cost of these machines is often prohibitive for pharmacies that fill a low (100 or less) to medium (100 to 300) number of prescriptions daily. Another drawback is that the size—the "footprint"—of the equipment is rather large. Even larger community pharmacies often do not have nearly enough floor space to accommodate a large prescription filling robot. Examples of prescription filling robots are the Baker Cassettes/Baker Cells® (McKesson) and the SP 200® (ScriptPro) (see Figure 8-11).

cassette systems drug containers that can hold hundreds or thousands of tablets and are affixed to a counting machine.

Automation and Robotics in Health-System Pharmacies

Health-system pharmacies are increasing their use of automation and robotics. Some automated systems operate completely free of staff intervention, whereas others require daily staff interaction and input. In fact, one company has developed a robot for use in hospitals. These robots have a map of the hospital or facility stored in memory, and are able to navigate to all areas of the hospital using sensors to avoid humans and obstacles. These robots make deliveries between hospital units, the pharmacy, and nursing stations. Some are even able to communicate with hospital staff via voice output. The robots use elevators to move between floors in the hospital, following an assigned route that can be programmed into the memory by the pharmacy.

Currently, it would be cost-prohibitive to install a whole fleet of robots to perform courier duties in a hospital. However, this is just one example of the types of automated systems that are available for institutional use.

There are so many types of automated systems available for health-system pharmacies that they cannot all be mentioned in this chapter. In the sections that follow, though, you will find descriptions of some of the types of technology most commonly used in health-system settings. Most of the focus is on automated medication delivery systems, because this is by far the most prevalent technology in hospitals today.

Automated Medication Delivery Systems

Automated medication delivery systems are found in hospitals and some long-term care facilities across the country. These systems allow much faster order turnaround time (the time it takes to fill an order from the time the order was written). They also allow meticulous inventory management of medications, hospital supplies, and narcotics. These systems can save hospitals tens and sometimes hundreds of thousands of dollars every year, simply by recouping lost charges and keeping track of medications and supplies.

Automated medication delivery systems are comprised of cabinets of various sizes. These cabinets contain drawers and compartments for different medications. The compartments and drawers maintain varying degrees of security, such as password protection or physical locks, based on the requirements of the institution or security needs dictated by the nature of the medication, such as controlled substances. The cabinet hardware also features a computer screen and keyboard that are physically attached to the cabinet. A nurse or other healthcare practitioner can access medications or other medical supplies by logging on to the computer at the cabinet. The items the individual can retrieve depend on that individual's preprogrammed level of access to the various items stored in the cabinet. For instance, in most healthcare facilities, respiratory therapists do not have access to any medications other than respiratory supplies. In this instance, the cabinet will deny this individual access to any medications or supplies other than respiratory supplies.

Medication Order—From Physician to Patient

Orders for patient medication are written by a physician in the hospital. A nurse then sends a copy of the order to the pharmacy department for computer order entry (usually done by a technician) and clinical review by a pharmacist. Then, someone from the pharmacy sends the medication back to the nursing unit for administration. Traditionally, with this system, it can take quite a while to get the medication to the patient. However, with the advent of automated delivery systems, the turnaround time for medication orders can be decreased dramatically.

The most time-consuming step in the process is usually the physical delivery of the medication to the nursing unit. With automated medication delivery systems in place, several things occur that speed up this process. The software that runs the automated cabinet is interfaced to the pharmacy/hospital computer system; consequently, information regarding the patient passes freely between the two systems within minutes of order entry. Additionally, a store of the most commonly used medications physically resides on the nursing unit, making it unnecessary for the pharmacy to take the medication to the unit. Instead, the nurse simply goes to the medication cabinet and selects the needed medication from the patient's available medication profile.

Decreased turnaround time for medication orders is only one of the advantages of having an automated medication delivery system in place. Here are several more benefits provided by this equipment.

Security

Many security issues surround the dispensing and handling of medication. Both controlled substances and other medications must be properly secured. Automated systems provide an extremely high level of security for hospitals and healthcare facilities via several components.

Every item within an automated cabinet can be password protected. This means that every individual who gains access to any particular medication or supply item is tracked by the computer system, based on that individual's personal password. There are also systems that use **biometrics**, such as fingerprints, to identify and track individual users on the system. Only licensed staff members within the facility are issued user identifications and passwords; thus, only they have access to medications and supplies.

    An additional level of security is available for controlled substances and/or items that have a high rate of theft or abuse. Some systems dispense medications one at a time. This is usually referred to as *unit-dose* or *unit-of-use dispensing technology*. This type of system allows users access only to the exact number of units of medication they asked for, instead of access to the whole inventory. As an example, think of the difference between a soda vending machine, which dispenses only the item that is paid for and selected by the user, and a newspaper vending machine, where the user pays for a paper but then has access to the machine's entire stock of papers.

biometrics technology that measures and analyzes human body characteristics, such as fingerprints, for authentication purposes.

Inventory Control

Automated systems can save healthcare facilities thousands of dollars a year by recouping lost charges and providing inventory usage reports. These systems can track and bill for hospital supplies and medications used by nursing units and patients. A completely integrated, interfaced system can tell a pharmacy director or materials manager exactly how much of each inventory item is in the hospital at any given point in time. The system can also pull historical data to determine usage rates at any given historical point or for any selected period of time. These reports, which can be generated within minutes, are invaluable tools for managing hospital inventory.

    Automated systems also cut down on the number of unexplainable inventory losses. Everyone using the automated supply and medication cabinets is required to log on to the system, via a username and password. This means that everyone who has access to any item in the inventory is tracked and can be identified easily via usage reports.

    These systems also are capable of automatic ordering from hospital suppliers and wholesalers. When the inventory of an item reaches a preset point, the system automatically reorders a preset amount of the item. No human intervention is required.

Patient Safety

The most important advantage of automated systems is increased patient safety, which comes about via a variety of mechanisms.

- **Patient profiles** Because of regulation changes by accrediting bodies, most hospitals using automated systems are either currently using patient medication profiling or are converting to it as quickly as they can. Profiling allows a nurse or other user to access only those medications that have been ordered for a particular patient. They do not select a medication for the patient from the entire drug inventory in the cabinet; rather, they select the desired medication from a list of patient-specific medications. This decreases the possibility of errors due to look-alike or sound-alike drugs. These patient medication profiles also display the details of the medication order and tell the nurse exactly how much of each drug to give the patient. Note, however, that there are certain nursing units within a hospital (such as emergency rooms and surgical units) where profiling is not and never will be used, because the patients are not there for long periods of time and usually need to receive medication on an emergency basis.

- **Drug information** Some automated systems are connected to drug information Internet sites. This allows users to look up clinical information about a particular drug while at the automated cabinet. Users can look up cautions, interactions, and side effects, and even print out patient information for any medication.

- **Pharmacist review** Because the automated medication dispensing machine is interfaced to the hospital/pharmacy computer system, a pharmacist has reviewed every order on a patient's medication profile for safety.

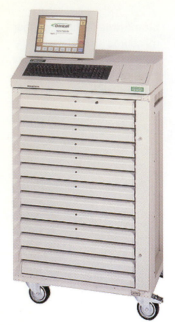

FIGURE 8-12 Example of an automated medication delivery system: the OmniRx Color Touch. (Courtesy of Omnicell, Inc.)

- **Administration times** Some systems allow nurse users to access a medication from the patient's profile only when that medication is due to be administered. This ensures that patients receive their medications at the proper times. This also ensures that a patient will not receive double doses of a medication. The system can track and alert users to missed doses.

- **Emergency override** Systems in place within the automated machines allow emergency removal of medication in an acute, critical situation.

Several companies make this type of equipment (see Figure 8-12). Examples of automated medication delivery systems include:

- OmniRx Color Touch® (Omnicell, Inc.)
- Omnicell® (unit-of-use dispensing) (Omnicell, Inc.)
- Pyxis MedStation® (Cardinal Health)
- AcuDose-Rx® (McKesson)

Automated Storage and Retrieval Systems

Just as the name indicates, automated storage and retrieval systems are used to store and retrieve inventories of medication kept in the pharmacy. Essentially, the companies that make this type of machinery have automated the pick list. Traditionally, pharmacists and technicians would walk through the pharmacy, manually selecting the items they needed to replenish medication inventories throughout the hospital. However, with the advent of medication carousel systems, the picking process is completely automated, thereby cutting down on pick errors. Because of computer interfaces, the storage and retrieval system knows exactly what items must be restocked on all the hospital units. Users simply tell the carousel system which unit they want to restock; the machine then physically locates all the medications that are needed and gives the user access to each location on the carousel, item by item. The carousel system can also automatically generate and send orders to the pharmacy's wholesale distributor to replenish pharmacy supplies. Examples of automated storage and retrieval systems include (see Figure 8-13):

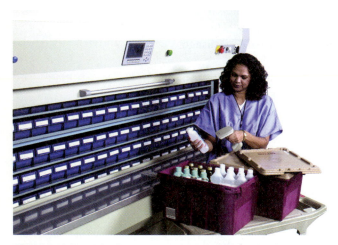

FIGURE 8-13 Example of an automated storage and retrieval system. (Courtes of McKesson.)

- PharmacyCentral® (Omnicell, Inc.)
- Pyxis Carousel System® (Cardinal Health)
- MedCarousel® (McKesson)
- MedSide® (S&S MedCart)

Bar-Coding

As mentioned previously, bar-coding technology is being used in all aspects of medication delivery and patient care. Once a medication order is received by the pharmacy, the order is input into the pharmacy computer system and that item is added to the patient's profile of ordered medications. The technician may then retrieve the medication. To ensure that the proper medication has been selected, the technician may use a handheld bar-code scanner on the item. If it is correct, the item is then labeled and sent to the nursing unit. The nurse receives the medication and takes it to the patient's bedside. The nurse then uses another scanner to scan the nurse's own bar-coded badge, the patient's armband, and the medication. This transaction is then logged in the computer system and given a time stamp. This process ensures that the Five Patient Rights are all electronically checked: the right patient receives the right drug in the right amount at the right time via the right route.

With the continuous growth in the use of automation and the number of drugs, the FDA deemed it necessary to create a method to reduce medication problems, through using state-of-the-art technology, and to reduce the number of medication errors in hospitals and other healthcare settings. Therefore, the FDA established a rule that bar-coding is mandatory on medications. This mandate applies to all prescription drug products, including biological products and vaccines (except for physician samples), and OTC drugs that are commonly used in hospitals and dispensed in a hospital. Standardized bar codes are also required on prescription drug products used in other settings, such as retail pharmacies.

The required bar code must contain the **National Drug Code (NDC) number** (unique identifying information about the drug that is to be dispensed) in a linear bar code as part of the drug label. Bar-coding will also allow for the addition of even more information as technology progresses.

National Drug Code (NDC) number a unique identifying number assigned to each drug by the manufacturer.

Personal Digital Assistants

Personal digital assistants, or PDAs, have become widely used in modern medical and pharmacy practice (see Figure 8-14). PDAs are handheld, battery-powered electronic devices that are approximately the size of one's palm. Despite their small size, PDAs are quite powerful; in fact, these devices can now run the same operating systems and software programs as personal computers.

personal digital assistant (PDA) handheld electronic device that is battery powered and operates like a computer.

Many physicians now utilize PDAs as electronic patient charts. Rather than retrieving an old-fashioned manila file folder with colored labels, physicians now pull up the patient's electronic chart on a PDA. They can review notes from previous visits, add new comments and diagnoses, and even enter the patient's prescriptions. The information entered into the PDA by the physician is electronically uploaded into the patient's electronic chart, which is stored on a server. From there, the prescriptions can either be sent electronically to the patient's pharmacy or be printed out.

Pharmacists are also utilizing PDAs as a valuable resource in providing timely and accurate pharmaceutical care and clinical advice. Although more commonly used by health-system pharmacists, PDAs can operate digital versions of clinical drug information books, such as Facts and Comparisons® and AHFS®. Rather than having to tote around heavy reference books or wait to access information from a single location, pharmacists can now use their PDAs as mobile reference centers.

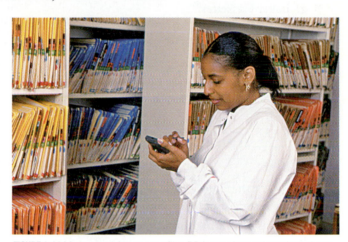

FIGURE 8-14 Many physicians now utilize PDAs as electronic patient charts.

Telepharmacy

Using advanced telecommunications technology, pharmacists can now provide pharmaceutical care to patients in rural and medically underserved areas at a distance. This is known as **telepharmacy**.

telepharmacy the practice of using advanced telecommunications technology to provide pharmaceutical care to patients in rural and medically underserved areas from a distance.

INFORMATION

In North Dakota, licensed pharmacists at a central pharmacy site can supervise a registered pharmacy technician at a remote telepharmacy site via teleconferencing. The technician prepares the prescription for dispensing, while the pharmacist communicates face-to-face in real time with both the technician and the patient. As of January 2006, North Dakota had more than 50 operational telepharmacies.

Pharmacy Technology and Patient Confidentiality

Patient confidentiality regulations, such as HIPAA regulations, apply to electronic data just as they do to written information. For this reason, pharmacy computer systems and technology applications must be configured to meet HIPAA privacy guidelines. Only authorized individuals should ever have access to confidential information, including information that is displayed on a computer monitor. Although technology has enabled numerous advances in the practice of pharmacy, it is imperative to keep patient confidentiality in mind, and use technology accordingly.

SUMMARY

Virtually every pharmacy today relies on computer systems. Computer hardware, such as the CPU, memory, monitor, keyboard, mouse, printer, modem, and scanner; and computer software, such as the operating system, pharmacy software program, and other applications, allow pharmacies to operate with increased accuracy and efficiency.

In addition to computer systems, both community pharmacies and health-system pharmacies are integrating automation and technology to improve their operations. Such automation and technology include automatic counters, dispensing systems, bar-coding, and even robots. In addition, both pharmacists and physicians have begun using PDAs for easy access to clinical resources and for electronic transmission of medication orders.

The advances in pharmacy practice are being driven by the development and use of computers, automation, robotics, and other technologies. The benefits of technology use are recognized in both community and health-system pharmacies. Pharmacy technicians must be computer literate and comfortable with using technology to practice modern pharmacy.

CHAPTER REVIEW QUESTIONS

1. Which of the following is an example of a prescription filling robot used in community pharmacies?
   a. Baker Cassettes®
   b. Kirby Lester KL15df®
   c. Baker Universal 2010®
   d. SureMed®

2. _____ is responsible for interpreting commands and running software applications in a computer.
   a. JAZ
   b. RAM
   c. CPU
   d. ROM

3. Which of the following is considered a benefit of using automation and robotics in pharmacies?
   a. decreased turnaround times
   b. increased patient safety
   c. better security
   d. all of the above

4. Microsoft Windows® and Linux® are both examples of:
   a. databases.
   b. operating systems.
   c. spreadsheets.
   d. word processors.

5. Pharmacies managed by a registered pharmacy technician, but supervised by a pharmacist at a central, offsite location, are known as:
   a. automated dispensing facilities.
   b. telepharmacies.
   c. satellite pharmacies.
   d. none of the above.

6. PDAs are used primarily by pharmacists working in _____ pharmacies.
   a. chain drugstore
   b. independent community
   c. health-system
   d. mail-order

7. Which of the following is considered a hardware output device?
   a. keyboard
   b. mouse
   c. printer
   d. scanner

8. Which of the following is an automated medication dispensing system?
   a. Acu-Dose Rx®
   b. MedCarousel®
   c. MedSide®
   d. Pharmacy Central®

9. _____ influence(s) the speed of a computer.
   a. Hard drives
   b. Modems
   c. RAM
   d. ROM

10. Which of the following is an automated storage and retrieval system?
    a. Acu-Dose Rx®
    b. Pyxis Carousel®
    c. Pyxis MedStat®
    d. SureMed®

CRITICAL THINKING QUESTIONS

1. How has technology such as the personal computer affected the evolution of pharmacy practice and pharmaceutical care?

2. In what ways could automation and robotics be a hindrance to the operation of a pharmacy?

3. What precautions can be taken to protect patient confidentiality and secure PHI against hackers and technology-driven identity theft?

WEB CHALLENGE

1. Go to www.computertalk.com and click on the link for Vendor Listings. Select any three vendors, visit their websites, and write a brief summary on the technology-based products/services they offer for pharmacies.

2. Go to www.asapnet.org, the website for the American Society for Automation in Pharmacy. Click on the button to "Download Presentations from Past Meetings," select a presentation, review the slides, and write a brief summary of the presentation.

REFERENCES AND RESOURCES

Abood, R. *Pharmacy Practice and the Law* (4th ed.). Boston: Jones and Bartlett Publishers, 2005.

American Medical Association. *Know Your Drugs and Medications*. New York: Reader's Digest Association, 1991.

American Pharmacist Association. *Pharmacy Technician Workbook and Certification Review*. Englewood, CO: Morton Publishing, 2001.

American Society of Health System Pharmacists. *Manual for Pharmacy Technicians*. Bethesda, MD: ASHP, 1998.

American Society of Health System Pharmacists. *Pharmacy Technician Certification Review and Exam*. Bethesda, MD: ASHP, 1998.

Ansel, HC. *Introduction to Pharmaceutical Dosage Forms*. Philadelphia: Lea & Febiger, 1995.

Ballington, D. *Pharmacy Practice*. St. Paul, MN: EMC Paradigm, 1999.

Ballington, D. *Pharmacy Practice for Technicians*. St. Paul, MN: EMC Paradigm, 2003.

Beaman, N, & Fleming-McPhillips, L. *Pearson's Comprehensive Medical Assisting*. Upper Saddle River, NJ: Pearson, 2007.

Cooperman, SH. *Professional Office Procedures*. Upper Saddle River, NJ: Pearson Education, 2006.

Cowen, D, & Helfand, W. *Pharmacy: An Illustrated History*. New York: Harry N. Abrams, 1990.

Crane, A. An overview of pharmacy automation. *Today's Technician*. 2004;5(4):26–37.

Facts and Comparisons. "Homepage" (accessed January 4, 2004): http://www.factsandcomparisons.com

Flaherty, J. Matters of privacy—Patient confidentiality. *Today's Technician*. 2005;6(2):8, 12.

Food and Drug Administration. "Homepage" (accessed January 4, 2004): http://www.fda.gov; http://telepharmacy.ndsu.nodak.edu/

Lambert, A. *Advanced Pharmacy Practice for Technicians*. Clifton Park, NY: Thomson Delmar Learning, 2002.

National Association of Chain Drug Stores, Inc., & Mintz, Levin, Cohn, Ferris, Glovsky and Popeo, P.C. *HIPAA Privacy Standards: A Compliance Manual for Pharmacies*. Alexandria, VA: NACDS, 2002.

Reifman, N. *Certification Review for Pharmacy Technicians* (6th ed.). Evergreen, CO: Ark Pharmaceutical Consultants, Inc., 2002.

U.S. Department of Health and Human Services: www.hhs.gov/ocr/hipaa

chapter 9

Inventory Management and Health Insurance Billing

LEARNING OBJECTIVES

After completing this chapter, you should be able to:

- List and describe the various purchasing systems used in pharmacies.
- List and describe the various methods of purchasing available to pharmacies.
- Define and describe prescription formularies.
- Describe and perform the steps necessary for placing orders.
- Describe and perform the steps necessary for receiving orders.
- Classify the reasons for product returns and describe the process of making returns.
- Describe and differentiate Medicare and Medicaid.
- Recognize and define terms commonly used in insurance billing.
- Describe and perform the steps in collecting data for insurance purposes.
- Describe and perform the steps necessary to transmit a prescription for insurance.
- List and explain common insurance billing errors and their solutions.

Introduction

Pharmacy technicians have many duties and responsibilities within a pharmacy practice setting; two of the most common duties include inventory management and processing of third-party, or insurance, billing claims. The importance of these two tasks is quite clear: The pharmacy cannot dispense prescriptions if the proper medications are not in stock, and the pharmacy must be reimbursed by insurance carriers in a timely fashion if the pharmacy is to operate. Both of these responsibilities, inventory management and insurance billing, require specific knowledge and training.

Purchasing Systems

Pharmacies must determine the most appropriate and advantageous **purchasing system**—the method for obtaining medications, devices, and products—for their organization. In general, there are two types of pharmacy purchasing systems: independent purchasing or group purchasing.

Independent Purchasing

In an **independent purchasing system**, the pharmacy, most often the pharmacy director or buyer, is responsible for establishing **contracts**, or written agreements, directly with each pharmaceutical manufacturer. Individual contracts set pricing and delivery terms, return policy, and dollar-volume requirements.

Group Purchasing

With a **group purchasing system**, the pharmacy joins a group purchasing organization (GPO), which contracts with pharmaceutical manufacturers collectively for all members of that GPO. In most circumstances, GPOs are able to obtain more competitive pricing and better terms than a pharmacy can get through independent purchasing.

Methods of Purchasing

In addition to the system of purchasing, each pharmacy must determine the method by which it will purchase pharmaceutical products. The three primary methods of purchasing are direct, wholesaler, and prime vendor.

Purchasing Direct

When purchasing direct, the pharmacy buyer places separate orders with each pharmaceutical company and receives separate shipments. Purchasing direct requires more time and resources, but can reduce expenses by eliminating markup percentages and fees charged by wholesalers and prime vendors.

Wholesalers

Wholesalers, such as Cardinal Health or Anda Generics, enable the pharmacy to purchase a large number of products, from various manufacturers, from a single source. It is common for wholesalers to offer next-day delivery service; however, their prices are almost always higher.

Primary Vendors

Contracting with a prime vendor, such as Amerisource Bergen, Cardinal, or McKesson, has all of the benefits of using a wholesaler, as well as better pricing and service terms. Prime vendors, however, require a dollar-volume commitment from the pharmacy and often contractually restrict the pharmacy's ability to enter into additional purchasing agreements.

Formularies

Formularies are, in essence, a listing of drugs approved for a specific purpose. Formularies can be used as a reference manual, as recommendations for prescribing, or even as strict parameters for the medications that are stocked and approved for reimbursement. Formularies are commonly used in health systems, and the listing of selected pharmaceuticals reflects the clinical judgment of the medical staff. Health-system formularies are established by the facility's Pharmacy and Therapeutics (P&T) committee, which is composed of physicians, pharmacists, nurses, administrators, and quality-assurance coordinators.

purchasing system an organization's strategy or procedure for obtaining medications, devices, and products.

independent purchasing system a purchasing system in which the pharmacy establishes contracts directly with each pharmaceutical manufacturer.

contracts written agreements.

group purchasing system a purchasing system in which a pharmacy joins a group purchasing organization (GPO), which contracts with pharmaceutical manufacturers collectively for all members of that GPO.

formularies a listing of drugs approved for a specific purpose.

The Ordering Process

The process of ordering medications will vary slightly based on the purchasing system and supplier(s) selected by the pharmacy, but the key steps of ordering are the same.

PROCEDURE 9-1

Ordering Medications

1. Generate an order.
2. Review the order.
3. Confirm the order.
4. Submit the order.

Generate Order

The first step of the ordering process is to generate an order. This can be done through an automated system, manually, or using a combination of both methods (see Figure 9-1).

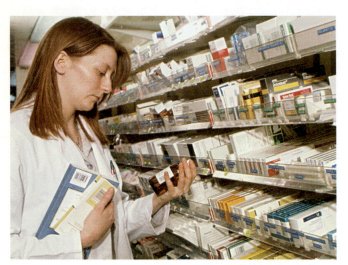

FIGURE 9-1 The first step in the ordering process is generating an order.

Automated

With an automated order, the computer system automatically generates a report (order) based on current inventory levels and preprogrammed reorder points. For example, if the system is programmed to keep a minimum of 200 Lasix® 20 mg, and the pharmacy inventory drops to 180 Lasix® 20 mg, the system will automatically add one bottle of Lasix® 20 mg to the next order.

Manual

In a manual ordering system, the pharmacy buyer reviews the inventory levels and creates an order based on current and forecasted stock needs. The manual method is not commonly used as the primary method of generating orders, as it has been almost entirely supplanted by technology and automated methods. In the manual system of ordering, it is common to use a "want book," which is simply a notebook in which pharmacy staff write down the inventory they need ordered.

Combination of Automated and Manual

The method of ordering most commonly used in modern pharmacy is a combination of the automated and manual methods. The computer system will generate an automated order, which is considered the primary order; then additional items are added manually by the buyer. This is the most efficient method, because it responds easily to changes. For example, restock levels may become outdated within the system, or physicians may suddenly be ordering a new drug in large volume, and so on. A combination method can easily handle such variations.

Confirm Order

Once an order has been generated, it must be reviewed and confirmed. It is not uncommon for the automated system to generate orders based on incorrect inventory levels or reorder points, so the buyer should review each order item to determine if it is really needed and that the appropriate quantity is being ordered. Any additions, deletions, or other changes must be entered into the system and then confirmed.

Submit Order

When the order is finalized and ready, it is electronically submitted to the supplier via phone or the Internet, depending on the vendor.

Supplier's Receipt of Order

Once the supplier has received the order, it will provide confirmation. Order confirmation can consist of a confirmation number given over the phone, sent in an e-mail, or as part of a confirmation report, again depending on the specifications of the vendor and the agreement with the purchaser.

Processing/Shipping of Order

The final step of the ordering process is the full responsibility of the supplier. After receiving and confirming the order, the supplier must process, package, and ship the order to the pharmacy department. Depending on the supplier, this can require anywhere from 12 hours to 2 weeks.

The Receiving Process

Just as with the ordering process, the procedures and process of receiving orders will vary by facility. However, the key steps remain the same.

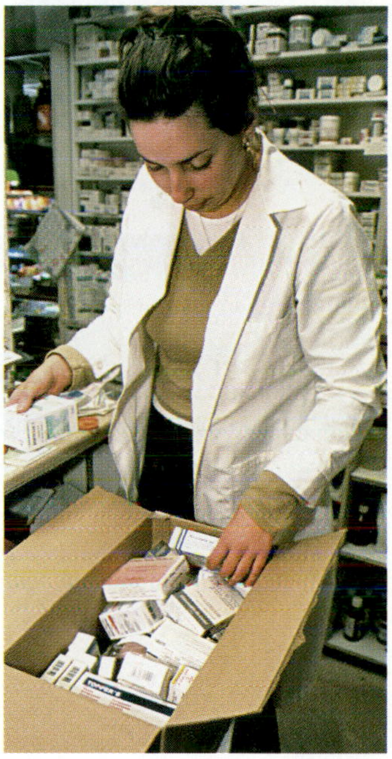

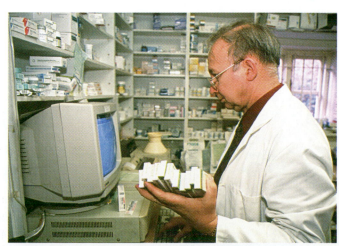

PROCEDURE 9-2

Receiving an Order

1. Accept delivery of the order.
2. Verify the order.
3. Adjust the inventory.
4. Stock the order.
5. File the paperwork pertaining to the order.

Order Delivery

The first step of the receiving process is delivery of the order. Depending on the supplier, the order may be delivered by a supplier-employed courier, FedEx, United Parcel Service (UPS), or the United States Postal Service (USPS). Orders are most often delivered via a supplier-employed courier using secured plastic totes.

FIGURE 9-2 Verifying an order.

Order Verification

After the order has been delivered, it must be verified (see Figure 9-2). Accuracy is an essential element of any inventory management and control system. It is important that the purchase order, the packing list, the invoice, and the actual order be reconciled against one another. Any errors or discrepancies should be addressed immediately.

Inventory Adjustment

Like the generation of an order, the adjustment of inventory based on a delivered shipment can be handled manually or electronically (see Figure 9-3).

FIGURE 9-3 The adjustment of inventory for a delivered shipment can be handled manually or electronically.

Automated

In an automated system, the computer system automatically updates the inventory levels based on the shipment delivered, not on the order placed. This is the most efficient and accurate method, since some items ordered may not have been shipped because of back ordering or shortages, for example.

Manual

In a manual system, the pharmacy buyer reviews the shipment and updates the inventory on hand, manually, into the computer system. Manual inventory methods are no longer common, as they too have largely been superseded by automated systems and newer technology.

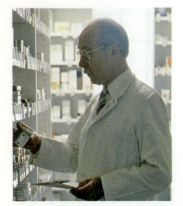

FIGURE 9-4 Stocking an order.

Stocking the Order

Once a shipment has been delivered and verified and the inventory has been updated, it is time to stock the order (see Figure 9-4). Medications must be stored according to the specifications of each manufacturer. Stored medications may be refrigerated, frozen, or kept at room temperature.

Most pharmacies organize stocked medications by route of administration, such as injectables, topicals, orals, and so on. Medications are then further organized by name, either alphabetically by brand name, in which case generic equivalents are stocked next to alphabetically organized brand-name drugs; or by generic name, in which case all drugs are alphabetically arranged by the generic drug name, whether the medication is a branded or generic product.

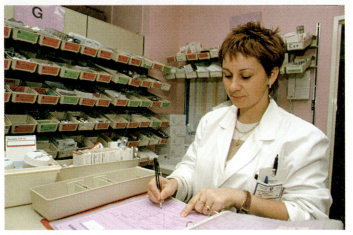

FIGURE 9-5 The pharmacy buyer maintains records for inventory management.

Recordkeeping

The pharmacy must keep records of each order placed and received, both for internal purposes and for regulatory accountability; regulatory agencies, such as the State Board of Pharmacy and the DEA, often carefully scrutinize pharmacy records and inventory. Although most pharmacies use an automated system to manage and track inventory, paper reports must still be generated and maintained. The specific format and frequency of reports will vary by facility; the task of generating reports is typically handled by a designated pharmacy buyer or the pharmacy manager.

In addition to inventory reports, the pharmacy should maintain copies of the packing slips for each order, as a manual backup to electronic files (see Figure 9-5).

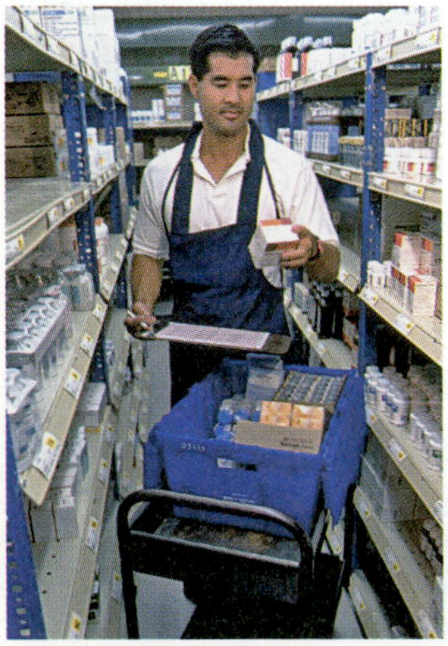

Returns

The last basic component of inventory management is handling returns (see Figure 9-6). In pharmacy, returns are typically made for one of the following reasons: expired drugs, manufacturer recalls, overstocked/undesired products, incorrect product sent by the wholesaler, or incorrectly ordered item.

FIGURE 9-6 Handling returns is part of inventory management.

● ● ●

PROFILES IN PRACTICE

Heather is a pharmacy technician who works in a long-term care facility. When reviewing her inventory order, Heather notices that a pint of liquid medication is damaged and leaked during shipment.

• How should Heather handle this matter?

Expired Drugs

Except for medical devices, every product in a pharmacy comes with an expiration date, which indicates when the product is no longer considered safe for use. Expiration dates must be monitored manually, which is typically done by checking the expiration date on all inventory regularly, such as once a month.

Inventory should be rotated so that drugs with shorter expiration dates are used before those with longer shelf lives. Drugs that are set to expire within six months are typically marked or labeled with an expiration sticker to draw the attention of pharmacy staff. **Expired drugs** must never be dispensed, so it is critical to monitor the stock and remove expired medications from the shelf.

Once a drug expires (reaches its expiration date), it must be returned to the manufacturer or destroyed, with proper documentation of the destruction. Most pharmacies opt to return expired drugs, because manufacturers provide a rebate or credit in most cases.

expired drugs drugs that have not been dispensed as of the manufacturer's printed expiration date.

INFORMATION

There are numerous companies, such as Guaranteed Returns, that can handle the entire return process on expired drugs for a pharmacy. Such a company will send employees to physically process the return and complete all the required paperwork. The company keeps a percentage of the refund as its fee for this service.

Recalls

Prescription and over-the-counter medications can be recalled directly by the manufacturer or by the FDA, as authorized by the Food, Drug, and Cosmetic Act. In most cases, manufacturers work closely with the FDA and therefore issue product recalls voluntarily.

Recalls are classified as Class I, Class II, or Class III. Class I recalls are the most dangerous and are designated for products that are defective and could cause serious adverse health conditions or death. Class II recalls are for products that could cause temporary or moderate adverse health conditions. Class III recalls are for products that would not cause harm, but have been mislabeled or are otherwise not in compliance with FDA regulations.

Recalled products are returned to their manufacturers directly from the pharmacy. Manufacturers prepare and distribute precise details and instructions on how pharmacies are to respond to a recall. Recalled products are identified by their NDC and lot numbers.

recall the process in which a drug manufacturer or the FDA requires that specific drugs or devices be returned to the manufacturer because of a specific concern about the recalled product.

Product Returns

Occasionally, a pharmacy needs to return products that have neither expired nor been recalled. It may be that the pharmacy has become overstocked with a particular product, or that an item was ordered accidentally, or even that the pharmacy is trying to reduce the amount of money invested in inventory sitting on its shelves. In any of these cases, to be returnable to the original supplier, the product must be in its original condition, meaning unopened and unmarked. Each supplier has its own specific procedure for handling returns, so the pharmacy technician must be familiar with each vendor's process.

Insurance Billing

We hear almost every day about the high cost of health care. Prescription costs are a contributing factor in that equation. To help defray the costs of prescriptions, many Americans have purchased or have employer-subsidized prescription insurance. One of the responsibilities of an ambulatory pharmacy technician is to process insurance claims for patients. Remembering a few basic points, along with some computer experience, will set technicians on their way to competence.

Types of Insurance

There are a number of health insurance options and many different insurers. This section discusses each type very briefly.

Health Maintenance Organizations

A health maintenance organization (HMO) is a type of health insurance coverage in the United States that is fulfilled through hospitals, doctors, pharmacies, and other providers with which the HMO has a contract.

Patients must select a primary care physician (PCP), who has contracted with the HMO, to be their first or primary point of medical care. To ensure benefit coverage, the PCP must make referrals to specialists in advance; the HMO usually has a list of approved specialists. HMO policies are generally the least expensive insurance plan option, because of their restrictions and conditions.

Workplace Wisdom HMOs

Common HMO providers include Aetna, Cigna, Humana, Kaiser, and TRICARE (CHAMPUS).

Preferred Provider Organizations

A preferred provider organization (PPO) differs from an HMO in that patients have greater choice in selecting their physicians and other care providers. Patients can choose to be seen by in-network providers, which have a direct contract with the PPO; or out-of-network providers, although it is more expensive to visit out-of-network providers. In addition, patients generally can elect to go to a specialist without a referral or prior authorization. A PPO may maintain lists of in-network specialists as well as primary care physicians.

Workplace Wisdom PPOs

Common PPO providers include BlueCross/BlueShield (BCBS), Pacificare, and United Healthcare (UHC).

Medicaid/Medicare

Medicaid the health insurance program for individuals and families with low incomes or disabilities.

Medicaid is the health insurance program for individuals and families with low incomes or disabilities; it is managed by the state and funded jointly by the states and federal government. Among the patients on Medicaid are eligible low-income parents, children, seniors, and persons with disabilities. Medicaid eligibility requirements are determined and vary by each state.

Medicare the health insurance program for individuals aged 65 or older, younger people with disabilities, and people with end-stage renal disease.

Medicare is the health insurance program for individuals aged 65 or older, younger people with disabilities, and persons with end-stage renal disease. It is funded by the federal government, in part through payroll taxes. Medicare is made up of several parts: Part A, which provides hospital insurance; Part B, which provides medical insurance; and Part D, which provides prescription drug insurance.

Patients who meet eligibility requirements may have both Medicaid and Medicare coverage.

Worker's Compensation

Worker's compensation is a form of insurance for employees who are injured while at work. Patients are not responsible for any payments, as all costs are covered by the employer. Worker's compensation, however, requires that providers complete extensive and tedious paperwork to receive payment.

Understanding the Insurance Billing Process

Most ambulatory pharmacies bill their patients' insurance carriers for them. The responsibility for collecting, maintaining, and transmitting insurance claims thus rests on the shoulders of the pharmacy technician (see Figure 9-7). The entire process is usually done by computer. Through the Internet, the pharmacy electronically submits a claim to the insurance provider's computer, or a third-party claims processor; after that (one hopes), there is an exchange of funds. This exchange takes mere moments in most cases, so the patients can be on their way.

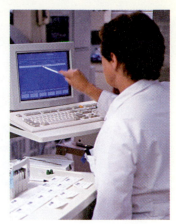

FIGURE 9-7 The insurance billing process is usually done by computer.

Insurance Terms

Just as in pharmacy, the insurance world has its own set of terms used in conducting its business. The following are some of the more common.

- **Adjudication**—the process of transmitting a prescription electronically to the proper insurance company or third-party biller for approval and billing.
- **Carrier/insurer/provider**—the insurance company.
- **Processor**—a company hired by the insurer to process claims.
- **Claim**—a request for reimbursement, for products or services rendered, from a healthcare provider to an insurance provider.
- **Co-pay**—a portion of the cost of a service or product that a patient pays out of pocket each time it is provided. For example, Mrs. Brown pays $5.00 for each prescription regardless of the actual cost of the medication.
- **Deductible**—a set amount a client pays up front before insurance coverage applies. This may be paid all at once or in increments. For example, Mrs. Brown has a $100 deductible. Her insurer may pay only 80 percent of each claim until she has paid $100; thereafter, her carrier pays 100 percent.
- **"Dispense as written" (DAW)**—a notation by the prescriber instructing the pharmacy to use the exact drug written (usually brand). Insurance providers may request the prescriber to state, in writing, the medical reasoning for this choice.
- **Days supply**—the number of days a dispensed quantity of medication will last.

Collecting Insurance Data

Just as the pharmacy keeps a confidential patient profile on all the clients it serves, so do insurance providers, whether public or private. When an insurance provider hires a third party to process claims, the insurer provides the necessary client information to the adjustors (see Figure 9-8). Whether it be the government (Medicaid and Medicare) or a private insurer (Blue Cross, Aetna, etc.), all providers keep records on their customers. These records contain much of the same information as the pharmacy patient profile.

Before a claim can be paid, the information in the claim has to match—exactly—the insurance company's information on file, starting with the correct name; the insurer may also provide an account number and possibly a personal code. Marriages, divorces, and births all can affect the continuation of insurance coverage. It is the technician's responsibility to collect all the current relevant information required for insurance billing for the pharmacy, but it is the patient's responsibility to keep the insurance provider's information updated.

Here is an example of this process: When Mary Smith got married, she changed her surname to Brown. The new Mrs. Brown dutifully changed her credit cards, address, and driver's license. When she came to the pharmacy, the astute technician also updated

adjudication the process of transmitting a prescription electronically to the proper insurance company or third-party biller for approval and billing.

carrier/insurer/provider the insurance company.

processor a company hired by the insurer to process claims.

claim a request for reimbursement, for products or services rendered, from a healthcare provider to an insurance provider.

co-pay a portion of the cost of a service or product that a patient pays out of pocket each time it is provided.

deductible a set amount that a client pays up front before insurance coverage applies.

"dispense as written" (DAW) notation by the prescriber instructing the pharmacy to use the exact drug written (usually brand).

days supply the number of days a dispensed quantity of medication will last.

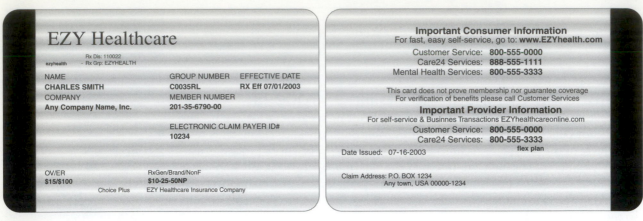

FIGURE 9-8 Insurance information.

her profile in the computer. However, when her insurance claim was submitted, it was refused! Why? Because Mrs. Brown neglected to update her records with her insurance provider; thus, the information submitted by the pharmacy, though correct, did not match the information in the insurance provider's records. *Claim denied*. For insurance billing to work, the two profiles (pharmacy and insurance) must match exactly.

Transmitting Prescriptions

Assuming that the patient profiles match, the billing technician's job is just starting. The insurance provider will need to know the name of the medication being dispensed. Providers may have formularies just as pharmacies do; in other words, the insurance provider will only pay for approved medications. Along with the strength and dose, there is the question of brand or generic.

Providers usually pay much more of the cost of a generic medication and shift more of the cost of a brand-name drug back to the patient. The exception to this rule is when a provider includes a DAW code for medical reasons. For example: Mrs. Brown requested a brand-name drug be used in filling her prescription. Her normal co-pay is $5.00, but this time it cost her $72.00. This is because Mrs. Brown's insurance will not pay for brand-name drugs unless her doctor states that it is medically necessary by placing "DAW" on her prescription.

If a technician writes the DAW code on a prescription, even in error, he could be charged with insurance fraud. If Mrs. Brown did not request the brand-name drug, but the prescriber did, and the technician forgot to put DAW in the claim, Mrs. Brown may end up paying way too much.

Workplace Wisdom Common DAW Codes

DAW Code	Meaning
0	Physician authorized generic substitution and (a) patient accepts the generic or (b) a generic is not available.
1	Physician requires that the prescription be filled exactly as written—no substitution permitted.
2	Physician authorized generic substitution and (a) a generic equivalent is available, but (b) the patient refuses generic substitution.

Troubleshooting Insurance

There are times when an insurance issue cannot be handled by computer. A good example is the case of an elderly woman whose doctor orders birth control pills as a hormone replacement. The insurance computer automatically refuses to pay for the prescription because birth control expenses are not covered. In this case, the technician may have to call the provider and explain that the medication is not being used for birth control, but for hormone replacement, which is a covered therapy.

As noted earlier, insurance computers simply match information coming in with the information in their databases. Twins are an insurance billing challenge because the computers simply match the parent's policy number with the eligible member number (example: Dad–01, Mom–02, and Children–3) and birth dates. Unfortunately, twins have the same birth dates. If they are both to receive a prescription, the provider may have to be contacted by phone before the proper payment can be made (see Figure 9-9).

Common Errors/Messages

The following are some of the error messages most commonly encountered in insurance billing rejections.

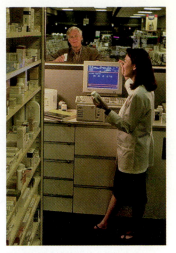

FIGURE 9-9 There are times when an insurance issue cannot be handled by computer.

- Incorrect name: may be due to use of a nickname, marriage, or divorce.
- Incorrect days supply: will affect refill times and insurance reimbursements.
- Incorrect provider: because of changes in employment or employer-provided benefits.
- Incorrect birth date: may be entered incorrectly for a number of reasons.

These errors will trigger the following refusal messages:

- "Patient not covered": the patient was not recognized, possibly because of incorrect name, wrong birth date, incorrect provider, or new coverage.
- "Too early to refill": the wrong days supply may have been entered.

A technician should never take these types of messages at face value or as the last word on the subject; rather, she should continue investigating. This is part of good patient service. There are times, however, when the insurance carrier will still refuse, even though you have done all you can to get a payment on behalf of your patient.

PROFILES IN PRACTICE

James is a pharmacy technician working in a retail pharmacy. He is processing a prescription for 90 Zoloft 100 mg tablets to be taken one at bedtime. The insurance company has rejected the prescription, citing "Incorrect Days Supply," but the patient insists that her paperwork stated she could get a three-month supply of her medications.

- How should James assist his patient?

Insurance billing is a wonderful customer service that pharmacy technicians provide for their patients each day. Insurance billing is done electronically. When machines talk to machines, they communicate only as well as the people operating them. Human intervention can save the day and humanize what can be a very cold process.

SUMMARY

Both inventory management and insurance billing are detailed tasks and big responsibilities.

Pharmacies obtain their inventory through a purchasing system, either as a member of a GPO or independently. Their inventory is often based on an organization's formulary or the formularies approved by insurance carriers. A pharmacy's inventory must be closely and regularly moni-

tored to ensure that adequate stock is available, that expired drugs are removed from the shelves, and that the pharmacy complies with any product recalls.

Insurance billing requires a comprehensive knowledge of billing terms, codes, and policies, such as DAW codes, authorized days supply, and formularies. Many insurance claim rejections can be prevented by ensuring that all information is correctly entered into the pharmacy's computer system before a claim is submitted.

When properly trained, pharmacy technicians are able to assist the pharmacist by handling these responsibilities and allowing the pharmacist to focus on more clinical aspects of providing pharmaceutical care. Both of these responsibilities vary by facility, but with time and experience, pharmacy technicians can effectively manage these aspects of pharmacy practice.

CHAPTER REVIEW QUESTIONS

1. Medicare is the federally funded insurance program for people:

   a. aged 65 or older.
   b. with disabilities.
   c. with end-stage renal disease.
   d. any of the above.

2. What is the correct DAW code for a prescription on which the physician does not permit generic substitution?

   a. 0
   b. 1
   c. 2
   d. 3

3. Which method of purchasing requires a dollar-volume commitment and may have restrictions on additional, outside agreements?

   a. primary vendor
   b. purchasing direct
   c. wholesale
   d. all of the above

4. Order confirmations are provided via:

   a. e-mail.
   b. telephone.
   c. reports.
   d. any of the above.

5. The most common method for delivery of orders is:

   a. a courier.
   b. FedEx.
   c. UPS.
   d. USPS.

6. An error code of "Patient Not Covered" means:

   a. the insurance coverage has been terminated.
   b. the name is entered incorrectly.
   c. the date of birth is incorrect.
   d. any of the above.

7. A _____ is a listing of preapproved drugs for specific purposes.

   a. formulary
   b. GPO
   c. purchasing system
   d. wholesaler

8. Which of the following actions can affect continuation of insurance coverage?

   a. a birth
   b. a divorce
   c. a marriage
   d. any of the above

9. The co-pay is the portion of the cost of a prescription that is paid by the _____.

   a. insurance carrier
   b. patient
   c. pharmacy
   d. wholesaler

10. Which of the following is a condition for which an outside company, such as Guaranteed Returns, will handle product returns?

    a. expired drugs
    b. drug recalls
    c. overstocked drugs
    d. any of the above

CRITICAL THINKING QUESTIONS

1. What are the advantages and disadvantages of each method of purchasing for a pharmacy?

2. Why must expired drugs be destroyed or returned to the manufacturer?

3. Why would January typically be the month with the most insurance rejections? What strategies could a pharmacy implement to reduce rejections?

WEB CHALLENGE

1. Visit Pharmacy Purchasing Outlook's website, click on the link for "PPO Reprints," and then read the article, "Those Secondary Vendors":
www.pharmacypurchasing.com

2. To learn more about both Medicare prescription drug coverage and formularies, review the CMS Medicare Formulary at http://www.cms.hhs.gov/PrescriptionDrugCovContra/Downloads/CY07FormularyGuidance.pdf

REFERENCES AND RESOURCES

Abood, R. *Pharmacy Practice and the Law* (4th ed.). Boston: Jones and Bartlett Publishers, 2005.

American Medical Association. *Know Your Drugs and Medications.* New York: Reader's Digest Association, 1991.

American Pharmacist Association. *Pharmacy Technician Workbook and Certification Review.* Englewood, CO: Morton Publishing, 2001.

American Society of Health System Pharmacists. *Manual for Pharmacy Technicians.* Bethesda, MD: ASHP, 1998.

American Society of Health System Pharmacists. *Pharmacy Technician Certification Review and Exam.* Bethesda, MD: ASHP, 1998.

Ansel, HC. *Introduction to Pharmaceutical Dosage Forms.* Philadelphia: Lea & Febiger, 1995.

Ballington, D. *Pharmacy Practice.* St. Paul, MN: EMC Paradigm, 1999.

Ballington, D. *Pharmacy Practice for Technicians.* St. Paul, MN: EMC Paradigm, 2003.

Cooperman, SH. *Professional Office Procedures.* Upper Saddle River, NJ: Pearson Education, 2006.

Cowan, DL, & Helfand, WH. *Pharmacy: An Illustrated History.* New York: Harry N. Abrams, 1990.

Crane, A. An overview of pharmacy automation. *Today's Technician.* 2004;5(4):26–37.

Facts and Comparisons. "Homepage" (accessed January 4, 2004): http://www.factsandcomparisons.com

Flaherty, J. Matters of privacy—Patient confidentiality. *Today's Technician.* 2005;6(2):8, 12.

Food and Drug Administration. "Homepage" (accessed January 4, 2004): http://www.fda.gov

National Association of Chain Drug Stores, Inc., & Mintz, Levin, Cohn, Ferris, Glovsky and Popeo, P.C. *HIPAA Privacy Standards: A Compliance Manual For Pharmacies.* Alexandria, VA: NACDS, 2002.

Reifman, N. *Certification Review for Pharmacy Technicians* (6th ed.). Evergreen, CO: Ark Pharmaceutical Consultants, Inc., 2002.

U.S. Department of Health and Human Services: www.hhs.gov/ocr/hipaa

Introduction to Compounding

LEARNING OBJECTIVES

After completing this chapter, you should be able to:

- Explain the purpose and reason for compounding prescriptions.
- Discuss the basic procedures involved in compounding.
- List and describe the equipment, supplies, and facilities required for compounding.
- List the major dosage forms used in compounding.
- Discuss the considerations involved in flavoring a compounded prescription.

Introduction

Webster's New World Dictionary defines the word *compound* as a verb meaning "1. to mix or combine, 2. to make by combining parts, and 3. to intensify by adding new elements." In pharmacy practice, the term *compounding* refers to the sterile and nonsterile preparation of many types of made-to-order suspensions, capsules, suppositories, topically applied medications, intravenous admixtures, and parenteral nutrition solutions. In essence, pharmaceutical **compounding** is the practice of extemporaneously preparing medications to meet the unique need of an individual patient according to the specific order of a prescriber. This differs from the traditional practice of pharmacy in that it involves a special relationship between patient, prescriber, and pharmacist.

Compounding medications for patients' specific needs is an integral part of the 5,000-year history of pharmacy. As recently as 1938, when the Food, Drug, and Cosmetic Act was introduced, 50 percent of prescriptions were compounded. During that time, pharmacists did most of the drug preparation and distribution. Today, as pharmacists become part of a multidisciplinary, multiskilled team to provide quality patient care, they rely more and more on pharmacy technicians. Technicians have now assumed many of the duties that were once performed by the pharmacist. One such duty is drug preparation: specifically, compounding and preparation of intravenous drugs.

INFORMATION

This chapter is just an overview of the specialty practice of compounding in community pharmacy. Specific techniques have not been included, as they are too advanced and detailed for the scope of this book. For an in-depth look at extemporaneous compounding and step-by-step procedures, please review *The Pharmacy Technician Series: Compounding* by Mike Johnston (Pearson/Prentice Hall, 2005).

Overview of Compounding

Pharmacy is the only profession that allows the extemporaneous compounding of chemicals for therapeutic care. Over the past 20 years, the need for compounded prescriptions has increased. Several reasons for this increase include the discontinuation of certain drugs by the original manufacturers, the removal from the market of some drugs by the Food and Drug Administration (FDA), and the unavailability of drugs in a strength or dosage form appropriate for a specific patient. Patients with sensitivities or allergies to preservatives or other certain **excipients** (substances) often must have their medications compounded, so that the offending agent or agents are omitted. A combination therapy that a prescriber desires, but that is not currently commercially available, can also be successfully compounded.

excipient any substance added to a prescription to confer a suitable consistency or form to the drug.

Pharmacy technicians, who have been adequately educated and trained, can play a vital role in the practice of extemporaneous compounding, including research, actual compounding of medications, and marketing (see Figure 10-1).

The physical properties of the prescribed drug and the dosage form desired by either the prescriber or the patient determine the level of difficulty in preparing the compounded prescription. In some cases, compounding will be a simple two-step process, whereas in others it will require extensive knowledge and the performance of many steps.

Regardless of the procedure, pharmacists must consider certain criteria for all compounded prescriptions. They must perform research on the active ingredient to determine cost-effectiveness, availability, solubility, stability, and possible dosage forms. Every pharmacy that compounds prescriptions should have access to quality reference resources. Some of these valuable resources include the following books and journals:

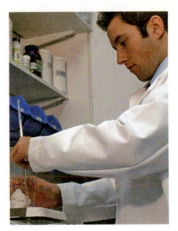

FIGURE 10-1 A pharmacy technician compounding a prescription.

- *Remington's Pharmaceutical Sciences*
- *The Merck Manual*
- *The Merck Veterinary Manual*
- *Trissel's Stability of Compounded Formulations*
- *Drug Facts and Comparisons*
- *United States Pharmacopeia*
- *Veterinary Drug Handbook*
- *International Journal of Compounding Pharmacists*

Compounding a Prescription

In addition to researching the active ingredients and excipients needed in a compounded prescription, the preparer must also know how to do pharmaceutical calculations. The potential for error is great in this area of compounding. Something as simple as a misplaced decimal point can have devastating results for the patient. Only a properly trained individual should perform the critical calculations involved in formulating a compounded prescription, and all calculations and measurements should be checked by the pharmacist.

The first step in compounding a prescription is to obtain a formula or recipe, prepared by a pharmacist, that includes all the necessary ingredients and explicit instructions for the preparer. The formula may be one that has already been published, or it may be created by the pharmacist in the compounding facility. If a formula is handwritten, it must be written legibly, with instructions communicated clearly to the preparer.

From the formula or recipe, the pharmacy technician then creates a worksheet that contains a list of active ingredients and excipients and the exact amounts needed of each to prepare the particular prescription. This worksheet should first be double-checked for error and then referred to as a checkpoint throughout preparation of the prescription. As the preparer weighs each ingredient, she can check it off the work-sheet. (This is especially necessary when a formula calls for multiple active ingredients and excipients.) The pharmacist should confirm the weights of all active ingredients. In some states, however, technicians may be allowed to check the work of other technicians during this step, with the authorization of the pharmacist.

Pharmaceutical compounding requires an extensive amount of equipment. When performing any task, you must be able to choose the appropriate tool needed to prepare a quality product. It is important for you as the compounding technician to be familiar with the tools available and their functions.

PROCEDURE 10-1

General Compounding Process

1. Obtain the recipe or formula.
2. Write up a compounding worksheet based on the formula.
3. Collect all ingredients and equipment necessary to prepare the compound.
4. Weigh each ingredient and have the measurements verified by the pharmacist.
5. Following the directions of the formula, prepare the compounded medication.
6. Package and label the compounded medication in an appropriate container.
7. Have the pharmacist do a final check on the compound.
8. Clean the workstation and equipment used.

INFORMATION

It is estimated that 1 percent of all prescriptions dispensed in the United States are compounded prescriptions; thus, this is a niche market. Most community pharmacies do basic compounding on occasion, but the majority of compounded prescriptions are dispensed by independent, niche pharmacies dedicated to compounding. Pharmacy technicians who are educated on and trained in the principles and skills of compounding have greater career opportunities available and typically earn higher salaries.

Equipment and Supplies

Table 10-1 shows a partial list of compounding equipment and the basic functions of each tool.

Compounding Facilities

An area suitable for compounding must be established before you begin preparing a compounded prescription (see Figure 10-2). The area should be separate from all other work areas and away from heavy traffic flow. The workspace should be large enough to accommodate all the necessary supplies. It should be clean and free of any clutter. Any object not directly involved in compound preparation should be removed. All tools and surface areas should be cleaned just prior to use and again when the compounding is complete. This can be accomplished by wiping everything down with 70-percent isopropyl alcohol or another suitable cleaning solution. This will safeguard

Table 10-1 Examples of Compounding Equipment

EQUIPMENT NAME	USE
balance	for measuring ingredients, can be either digital/electronic or manual
beakers	for measuring ingredients and for mixing or heating ingredients
capsule filling equipment	for preparing capsules
chopper/grinder	for breaking up solids or ingredients of large particle size
electronic mortar and pestle	for mixing creams and ointments and for reducing particle size
filter paper	for removing particulate matter from a liquid
funnels	for transferring liquids and powders
graduates	for measuring liquids
heat gun	for melting bases and smoothing the tops of troches and suppositories
homogenizer	for reducing particle size and evenly suspending liquids
hotplates	for melting bases
liquid blender	for mixing liquids
magnetic stir plate	for continuous stirring
magnetic stirrers	for continuous stirring
molds	for making troches and suppositories
mortars and pestles	for mixing powders and reducing particle size
glass	for liquids
Wedgwood	for powders
porcelain	for powders
ointment tile	for making creams and ointments
powder blender	for mixing powders
refrigerator	for storing ingredients and prescriptions that require cold temperatures
safety glasses	for protecting the preparer's eyes from debris
sieves in various mesh sizes	for reducing particle size
spatulas	for mixing creams and ointments and for retrieving chemicals from bottles
spray bottles	for dispensing cleaning solutions or distilled water
stirring rods	for stirring liquids by hand
strainers	for removing particulate from a liquid
thermometers	for controlling and checking temperature
tongs	for picking up items that should not be handled
tube crimper	for sealing ointment tubes
tubes	for dispensing creams and ointments
wash bottles	for washing
weigh boats/papers	for weighing ingredients on a balance
weights for calibration	for calibrating balances

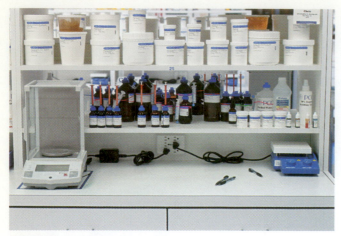

FIGURE 10-2 A typical compounding area.

geometric dilution technique of starting with the ingredient of the smallest amount and doubling the portion by adding the other ingredients, in order of quantity, until fully mixed.

the compounded prescription from possible cross-contamination, as well as preventing microbial growth within the final product.

When mixing the active ingredient(s) with the excipient(s), practice the principle of **geometric dilution**. This means that you start with the ingredient of which the smallest amount is needed and double the portion by adding the rest of the ingredients in ascending order of quantity. Each addition should result in a "doubled" amount until all the ingredients are mixed in. This process ensures even distribution of the active ingredient throughout the final product.

The most appropriate dosage form will depend not only on the drug that is being compounded, but also on the patient. The patient is probably the most important factor in the decision as to which dosage form to use for a compounded prescription. Some common dosage forms that can be effectively compounded are capsules, liquids, transdermal gels, creams, ointments, suppositories, and chewables. For each form, you must follow precise instructions if you are to prepare a quality, efficacious product. Although pharmacists can recommend an appropriate dosage form, the prescriber's approval is required.

Quality Assurance

quality assurance (QA) a program of activities used to ensure that the procedures used in the preparation of compounded products meet specific standards.

Although compounded products are prepared on an individual basis to meet the special needs of a patient or patient population, the pharmacy must have a good **quality assurance (QA)** program and maintain proper records to ensure that patients are receiving safe, stable, and properly compounded medications. In regard to compounding, quality assurance is a program of activities used to ensure that the procedures used in the preparation of compounded products lead to products that meet certain specifications and standards.

" Workplace Wisdom Quality Assurance Program

Typical components of a good quality assurance program include standard operating procedures (SOPs), formulation records, compounding worksheets, ingredient record forms, material safety data sheets (MSDS), documented training, and quality control (QC) tests for each compound. "

Dosage Forms and Basic Guidelines

capsule a solid dosage form in which the active ingredient and any excipients are enclosed in a soluble gelatin shell that will dissolve in the stomach.

There are many types of dosage forms. They include capsules, tablets, powders, lozenges, troches, sticks, suppositories, solutions, suspensions, emulsions, ointments, pastes, creams, gels, and ophthalmic, otic, and nasal preparations. This section briefly discusses each type.

Capsules

Capsules, as an oral dosage form, have been used for more than a century (see Figure 10-3). The capsule has an important role in drug delivery in that it is extremely versatile and offers a broad range of dosage options for patients. The capsule offers flexibility in dosing to the prescriber, as well as to the patient with specific needs.

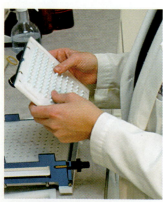

FIGURE 10-3 A capsule-filling machine.

Capsules can be prepared either by hand or by using a capsule machine. The method used will depend on the quantity needed and the physical characteristics of the powders included in the formula. Using a capsule machine saves time and produces a number of capsules at a time, depending on the size of the machine and the desired quantity. Capsules come in many sizes, as shown in Figure 10-4.

Tablets

Tablets are a solid dosage form that can be administered orally, **sublingually**, vaginally, or as an implant under the skin. Several different forms of tablets can be compounded.

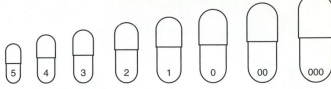

FIGURE 10-4 Capsule size chart.

Compressed tablets, made by pharmaceutical manufacturers, are the most commonly prescribed dosage form; they are convenient, portable, stable, and easy to administer. The single disadvantage of commercially made tablets is that they are available only in fixed dosage strengths and combinations.

The compounding pharmacy has always had the ability to compound molded tablets, and now, with the advent of pellet presses and single-punch tablet presses, compressed tablets can be prepared according to the requirements of specific patients (see Figure 10-5).

Powders

Powders are a solid dosage form made from a thoroughly blended mixture of one or more active ingredients and excipients (see Figure 10-6). As a pharmaceutical dosage form, powders may be used either internally (such as BC Powder®) or externally, like talcum powder.

Although the use of powders has declined, there is still an occasional need for a prescription powder. Patients who are either unable to swallow or have extreme difficulty in swallowing tablets or capsules (such as some pediatric and geriatric patients) can benefit from having their medication in powder form.

Lozenges and Troches

Lozenges and **troches** are both oral dosage forms that are placed in the oral cavity, either onto the tongue or into the cheek pouch, and allowed to dissolve; they are usually meant to disintegrate over time (see Figure 10-7). Recently, soft, chewable troches have been developed that are intended to be chewed and swallowed, to deliver medication to the gastrointestinal tract.

Some of the advantages of using troches and lozenges are that they are easy to handle and administer to a variety of patients. Because their base is made of sugar, troches generally have a pleasant taste, which makes them popular with pediatric, geriatric, and hospice patients.

Sticks

Medicated sticks are a unique dosage form used for topical application of local anesthetics, sunscreens, antivirals, antibiotics, and, of course, cosmetics. Sticks offer patients, physicians, and pharmacists a dosage form that is convenient, relatively

tablet a solid dosage form that may be administered orally, sublingually, vaginally, or under the skin.

sublingually under the tongue; preparations may be administered by placing them under the tongue and allowing them to dissolve.

powder a solid dosage form made from blended active ingredients and excipients.

lozenge a solid dosage form administered orally to be dissolved in the mouth.

troche interchangeable term for lozenge, but sometimes prepared in soft form.

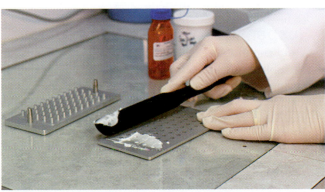

FIGURE 10-5 A technician prepares tablets using a mold.

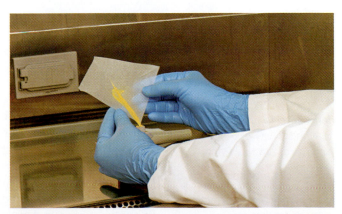

FIGURE 10-6 Powders are a solid dosage form made from a thoroughly blended mixture of one or more active ingredients and excipients.

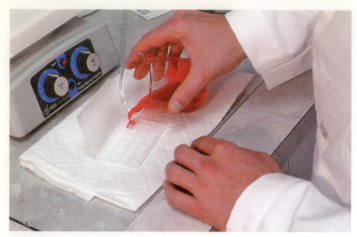

FIGURE 10-7 A technician makes troches using a mold.

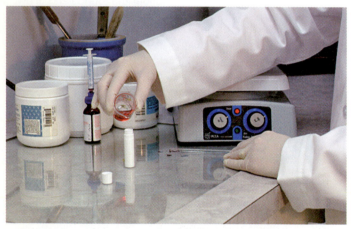

FIGURE 10-8 A technician prepares a stick.

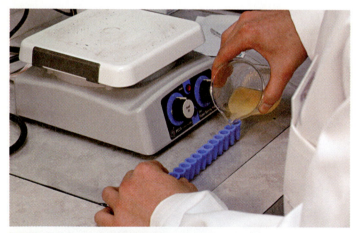

FIGURE 10-9 A technician prepares suppositories.

suppository a solid dosage form used to administer medication by way of the rectum, vagina, or urethral tract.

aqueous water-soluble.

suspension liquid containing ingredients that are not soluble in the vehicle.

stable, and fairly easy to prepare. Although relatively simple, the process of properly preparing medicated sticks can be a bit time-consuming (see Figure 10-8).

Suppositories

A **suppository** is a solid dosage form that is inserted into the rectum or vagina. The suppository melts and softens or dissolves at body temperature, thus allowing absorption of the medication into the surrounding tissues. Suppositories can have either a systemic effect or a local effect, depending on the desired effect expected by the prescriber or on the drug being used. Suppositories can be made in several different shapes and sizes, depending on the patient and the disease state being treated.

When determining which base is most appropriate to use in compounding a suppository, the pharmacy staff will have to consider the physical characteristics of the drug ordered as well as the patient (see Figure 10-9). Some of the common bases used for preparing suppositories include fattibase, polybase, and cocoa butter. A drug may be dissolved in the base, or it may have to be suspended, depending on the physical characteristics of the drug ordered. Whether the drug is dissolved or suspended, the active ingredients and excipients should be added in geometric proportion to ensure that the active ingredient is equally dispersed throughout the suppository product.

Solutions

In an **aqueous** solution, a water-soluble chemical is dissolved in the water phase of the compound. This may consist of just enough distilled or preserved water to dissolve the drug, or water may be as much as 50 percent of the final volume. After the drug is completely dissolved in the water, the preparer may complete the compound by adding flavoring agents and bringing it to the final volume with a sweetening agent such as Ora-Sweet, Simple Syrup, or Karo Syrup (see Figures 10-10 and 10-11). Although the drug is in solution, it may be necessary for the patient to shake the liquid before use to evenly distribute the flavor.

Suspensions

A **suspension** is a liquid preparation that contains insoluble solid particles uniformly dispersed throughout the vehicle. A suspension must be shaken prior to administration to ensure that the proper dose is dispensed. If a drug is to be suspended, a suspending agent such as Ora-Plus or Karo Syrup will be needed (see Figure 10-12).

Emulsions

An **emulsion** is another type of liquid or semisolid preparation that can be taken orally or applied topically. Emulsions are prepared whenever two immiscible liquids must be dispensed in the same preparation. An emulsifying agent is used to hold the two

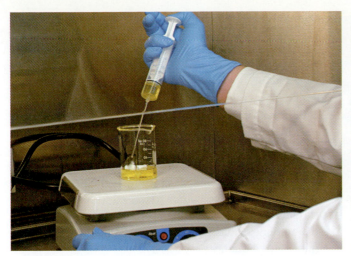

FIGURE 10-10 A technician prepares a sterile solution.

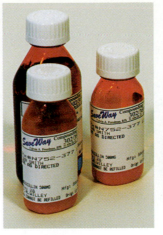

FIGURE 10-11 Examples of packaged liquids.

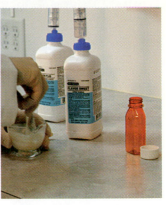

FIGURE 10-12 Working with a suspension.

together. One part is oil and the other part is aqueous. Emulsions are either water in oil or oil in water, depending on the external phase of the final product. Generally, emulsions that are to be used internally are of the oil-in-water type, whereas emulsions for topical use may be of either type.

As with a suspension, the patient should be instructed to shake an emulsion well before use to temporarily suspend the aqueous phase into the oil phase and equally distribute the active ingredient(s).

emulsion a suspension that consists of two immiscible liquids and an emulsifying agent to hold them together.

Ointments

An **ointment** is a semisolid preparation that is usually applied to the skin or to mucosal tissue. An ointment does not penetrate into the skin; rather, it stays on top of the skin. Ointments should be soft and easily spread. They should also be smooth in texture, not gritty. Common ointment bases used in compounding include white petrolatum, hydrophilic petrolatum, Aquaphor, hydrous lanolin, and PEG ointments.

To ensure a smooth ointment, the particle size of a powder being incorporated into the base should be reduced to an impalpable form by **comminuting** or **triturating**, which is the process of reducing particle size to a fine powder. This can be achieved by using a Wedgwood or porcelain mortar and pestle or by forcing the powder(s) through a size 100 mesh sieve (see Figure 10-13). Once the particle size is reduced, the powder can then be mixed into the base, using geometric dilution. At times it will be necessary to "wet" the powder with a solvent, such as glycerin, ethoxydiglycol, or propylene glycol, before incorporating it into the base. Other times the drug is dissolved in oil, such as mineral oil, before it is mixed with the base.

ointment a semisolid topical preparation that is applied to the skin or mucous membranes.

comminuting the process of reducing the particle size of a substance by grinding; also known as *trituration*.

trituration the process of reducing the particle size of a substance by grinding; also known as *comminuting*.

Pastes

Pastes are stiff, or very viscous, ointments that do not melt or soften at body temperature. They are intended to be used as protective coverings over the areas where they are applied, such as diaper rash preparations.

Creams

A *cream* is a soft, opaque solid that is usually applied externally (see Figure 10-14). Creams dissipate into the skin, healing the affected area from the inner layers of the dermis. Medications are usually suspended or dissolved

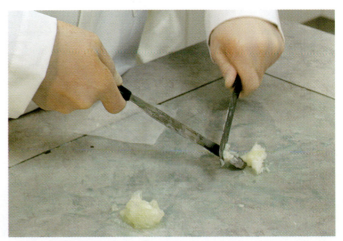

FIGURE 10-13 Preparing an ointment.

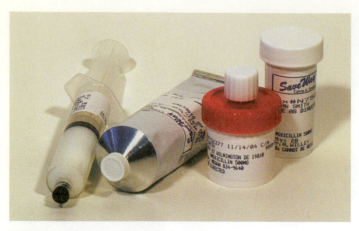

FIGURE 10-14 Examples of packaged topical creams.

in a water-soluble base when a cream is compounded (see Figure 10-15). A cream must be smooth, and the active ingredients should be dissolved completely so that they will be totally absorbed into the skin. Cream bases available for compounding include vanishing cream base and HRT base, as well as some commercially prepared creams such as Cetaphil, Eucerin, and Lubriderm.

When adding active ingredients to creams, it is critical to practice the principles of geometric dilution to ensure even dispersion. A wetting agent may be necessary; and, again, the volume required to wet the powder should be calculated into the formula when determining the amount of base needed to bring the product to the final desired quantity.

Gels

Gels are semisolid systems consisting of suspensions made up of small inorganic particles or of large organic molecules interpenetrated by a liquid.

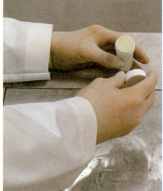

FIGURE 10-15 An example of a cream.

The **transdermal gel** is a unique, semisolid dosage form that is becoming increasingly popular. Transdermal gels have special absorption enhancers that "push" the medication through the layers of the skin so that the medication can be absorbed into the bloodstream. The transdermal gel is an especially desirable alternative for pediatric patients, animals that are difficult to "pill" or otherwise medicate, the elderly, and patients who are physically or mentally disabled.

The most common form of compounded transdermal gel therapy is a two-phase vehicle made from pluronic lecithin organogel. It consists of both an oil phase and an aqueous phase, making it a suitable choice for many chemicals. The oil phase, which is lecithin isopropyl palmitate, is generally used in a concentration of 22 percent; the balance is made of poloxamer. Oil-soluble drugs should be dissolved in the oil phase, whereas water-soluble drugs should be dissolved in the aqueous phase. The determined amount of drug is dissolved in the appropriate phase, and then the two components are mixed together using a shearing action (see Figure 10-16). This shear force is necessary for proper micelle formation in the gel. The poloxamer gel is a liquid, which is stored in the refrigerator. When brought to room temperature, it will form a gel. It is important for the final product to be stored at room temperature. Auxiliary labels to this effect (as well as other instructions for the patient, not included on the prescription label) should be placed on the package prior to dispensing.

transdermal gel a gel that penetrates the skin and allows the active ingredient to be easily absorbed into the body; also known as a *PLO gel*.

Ophthalmic Preparations

ophthalmic for or of the eye.

Ophthalmic preparations, or preparations for the eye, may be in the form of a solution, a suspension, or an ointment; all forms must be sterile (see Figure 10-17). Solutions, which must be clear and particulate-free, are the ophthalmic dosage form most commonly prepared in compounding pharmacies.

In addition to the active drug, ophthalmic preparations require several different ingredients to make them nonirritating to and compatible with the tissues of the eye. The eye generally tolerates a pH range of 4 to 11. Buffers are used in ophthalmic preparations to maintain the pH of the product within the desired range during storage and administration to the eye.

Preservatives are necessary when the ophthalmic preparation is intended for multiple uses. They prevent contamination of the preparation from microbial growth.

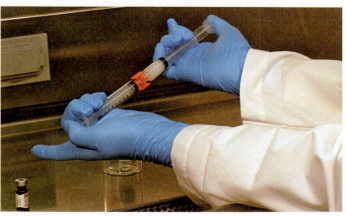

FIGURE 10-16 A technician loading a gel.

Otic Preparations

Preparations for the ear, or **otic** preparations, are made in liquid, powder, or ointment form (see Figure 10-18). Solutions and suspensions are instilled into the ear, whereas ointments are applied to the external ear. Powders are used infrequently, but are usually administered to the ear canal by a physician. Otic preparations are generally used to treat local infections and the pain associated with them. Other otic products are used to dissolve or remove blockages that can lead to infection.

The vehicles most often used when compounding otic liquids are propylene glycol, glycerin, polyethylene glycol, vegetable oil (especially olive oil), and, occasionally, mineral oil. It is necessary to use a viscous liquid such as one of these, because the compound should adhere to the ear canal. Water and alcohol may be used as a vehicle, but typically are used as solvents for the drugs being compounded or used in an irrigating solution. The physical characteristics of the ingredients used in otic preparations that must be considered include solubility, viscosity, and tonicity. Almost always, a preservative is used in an otic preparation. Although otic preparations need not be sterile, it is important for the pharmacy technician to follow quality control procedures to prevent cross-contamination or microbial growth in the compound. Many chemicals used in otic preparations are soluble in the vehicles used in compounding them. Because of the general viscosity of these products, a suspending agent is usually not necessary if the drug is insoluble.

When compounding a liquid for otic use, the drug and any preservatives or other excipients are accurately weighed and then dissolved or mixed with approximately three-quarters of the vehicle. When the drug is completely dissolved or evenly suspended, the preparation is then brought to final volume with more of the vehicle. When an ointment is being prepared, the drug and any other ingredients are accurately weighed and then mixed into the base using the principles of geometric dilution.

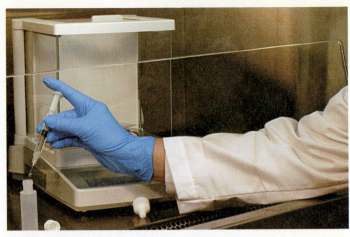
FIGURE 10-17 A technician prepares an ophthalmic preparation.

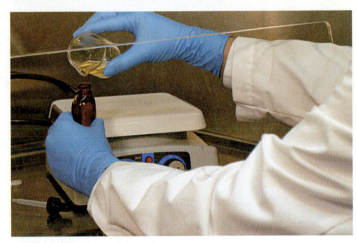
FIGURE 10-18 A technician prepares a liquid otic preparation.

otic for or of the ear.

Nasal Preparations

Preparations for nasal administration may take the form of solutions, suspensions, gels, or ointments. These preparations may be used locally or systemically, depending on the nature of the drug and the vehicle it is in.

In addition to the active ingredient, several excipients will most likely be used. These include the vehicle, buffers, preservatives, and tonicity-adjusting agents. Because nasal preparations are generally dispensed in multiuse containers, it is necessary to include a preservative. The pH must be adjusted so that maximum stability is obtained. Two common vehicles used for nasal solutions are sodium chloride 0.9 percent and sterile water for injection.

Ingredients for nasal preparations should be sterile, and aseptic technique should be used to make them. Sterility may be obtained by filtration or autoclaving (see Figure 10-19). If a drug is water soluble, it

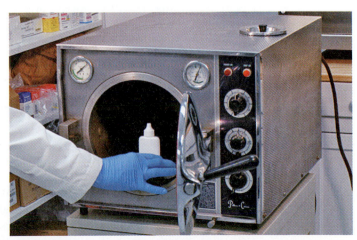
FIGURE 10-19 A technician places a nasal preparation in an autoclave for sterilization.

will be dissolved in a portion of the vehicle and the liquid will be brought to final volume with the vehicle. A suspension will require that the active ingredient and any excipients be mixed by using geometric dilution with a suspending agent and then brought to final volume with the appropriate vehicle. Nasal gels or ointments are made by mixing the active ingredient and any excipients with the base, using the principles of geometric dilution.

Quality assurance procedures should be observed when making nasal preparations. Before the compound is dispensed, the pharmacist should determine clarity, pH, and correct volume or weight.

PROFILES IN PRACTICE

Dan is a pharmacy technician who works in an independent, compounding pharmacy. A patient has called after seeing the pharmacy's ad in the phone book. She explains that her 14-year-old daughter cannot swallow pills, but the medication her doctor is prescribing is available only as a tablet. She asks if there is anything the pharmacy can do to assist.

• What suggestions might Dan make?

Veterinary Compounding

Veterinary compounding is one of the fastest growing areas of pharmaceutical compounding. Medication doses are usually calculated on the basis of milligrams per kilogram of body weight. Because of the vast differences in the sizes and physiology of animals, this makes appropriate dosing nearly impossible when using manufactured products.

The same principles used in compounding of human medications apply to veterinary compounding. Stability, solubility, drug availability, dosage form choices, cost-effectiveness of drug sources, and quality of final product are all factors to be considered before attempting to compound for animals.

In addition to capsules, flavored liquids, transdermal gels, and suppositories, the chewable treat is another dosage form available for veterinary pharmaceutical compounding. A chewable form, made from a base of ground food product and gelatin mixed with the active ingredient, is an excellent choice for animals. Some flavor choices for these chewable forms include liver, tuna, salmon, shrimp, chicken, and beef. Again, solubility is taken into consideration when preparing the treat form. If a drug is water-soluble, it can be incorporated into the gelatin phase of the compound. If insoluble, it will be mixed in geometric proportion with the solid, or food, phase of the compound and then mixed with the gelatin. The mixture is then forced into precalibrated molds by way of a syringe or other means. The final product is a soft, chewable form that can be offered to the animal as a treat, or mixed in with a small amount of the animal's favorite food, for consumption.

Medication Flavoring

Successfully flavoring a medication is a critical step in the process of properly preparing a prescription, especially when the taste of a particular drug is such that it will not be tolerated by the patient when administered orally.

Psychological Impact

Although no therapeutic benefit is evident, using the proper coloring and flavoring for medicinal substances is of considerable psychological importance. For example, a patient or the caregiver may think a liquid medication that is as clear as water and has no smell lacks the active ingredient(s). Conversely, a liquid that has been flavored, for example, with bubblegum and slightly tinged with a pink color will be thought to be more effective. A medication that is disagreeable, in appearance, texture, or taste, can be made more attractive and palatable by the careful choice of the most appropriate flavoring, sweetening, diluting, suspending, or coloring agent. Selection of the proper agent is important in preparing the best formulation and in ensuring patient compliance in medication administration. This selection is typically made by the pharmacist, or by the compounding technician subject to the pharmacist's review.

Sensory Roles in Flavoring

Taste, smell, sight, touch, and even sound are complex experiences that may influence the flavor sensation. In general, individuals are usually more sensitive to the aroma of a preparation than to the actual taste. Elderly patients may require added amounts of flavor to achieve the desired result. Females tend to be more sensitive to smell than males. Certain diseases will alter a patient's ability to taste and smell. For example, a patient suffering from a cold or influenza may have a dulled sense of smell and/or taste. When the nostrils are held closed, raw onions will taste sweet; likewise, bad-smelling medications will be much easier to ingest.

Psychological factors such as sight and sound play an important role in flavor experience, as certain reflexes become conditioned through association. In the classic experiments by Pavlov, the ringing of a bell caused the gastric juices of a habituated dog to begin to flow, even though no food was placed in front of the animal. Part of the enjoyment of eating crunchy foods, such as raw celery or carrots, is the sound they make as they are being chewed. Furthermore, the color of a preparation and the flavor should coincide. For example, cherry-flavored substances should be red and grape-flavored substances should be purple.

Flavoring Considerations

Consider each prescription that requires flavoring on an individual basis. It is important to be aware of any allergies or sensitivities a patient may have to particular ingredients, such as chocolate, peanuts, or possibly a particular preservative or dye. It is also helpful to know the patient's likes and dislikes, as well as any idiosyncrasies he or she may have. One should not rely on what is traditionally used or a flavor choice that is popular among a general group. For example, although most pediatric patients like flavors such as grape, bubblegum, and cherry, some patients may not tolerate the tannins or a specific dye contained in the flavoring agent, or they simply may not care for these flavors.

Pediatric Flavoring

Children have more taste buds than adults and, therefore, are more sensitive to taste. Infants and children tend to prefer sweet tastes, and do not respond well to bitter flavors. Appropriate flavor choices for children include raspberry, bubblegum, marshmallow, butterscotch, citrus, berry, and vanilla. The palate of a newborn or an infant typically has not been exposed to a wide variety of tastes; therefore, this young patient will not require as strong a flavor as an older patient. A patient who is required to take a medication for a long period of time may require a milder flavor to avoid flavor fatigue.

Adult Flavoring

Adults are usually more tolerant of bitter flavors, so with extremely bitter drugs a flavoring agent such as coffee, chocolate, cherry, anise, grapefruit, or mint will be acceptable. These bitter flavors are generally an acquired taste. Their own "bite" is helpful in cutting the bitterness of the drug.

Impact on Stability, Solubility, and pH

Other factors to be considered when choosing an appropriate flavoring agent include stability, solubility, pH, and the physical properties of the flavors available. Some flavors can negatively affect the compounded prescription, such as raising or lowering the pH of the final product, and possibly cause instability. Aqueous solutions should be flavored with water-miscible flavors, whereas oil preparations will require the use of an oil-based flavor. These factors may limit a patient's choice of available flavors. Some flavoring agents or the preservatives in the flavor may affect the active ingredient in the compound and cause degradation of the drug.

Compounded medications that are stable only at a certain pH should be flavored with an agent that will not affect the pH or one that will enhance the pH of the final product. Although pH values may be equal to or within close range from manufacturer to manufacturer, the exact pH should be obtained from the company that is the source of the flavoring agent. Most chemical companies that offer products for medicinal flavoring will be able to provide a list of their flavors and the relative pH values. This is a reference that every pharmacy that offers flavoring as a service should have.

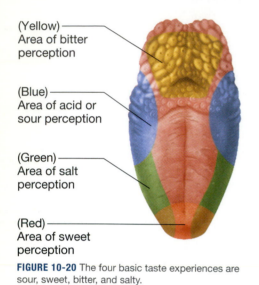

(Yellow)
Area of bitter
perception

(Blue)
Area of acid or
sour perception

(Green)
Area of salt
perception

(Red)
Area of sweet
perception

FIGURE 10-20 The four basic taste experiences are sour, sweet, bitter, and salty.

Four Taste Types

There are four basic taste experiences: sour, sweet, bitter, and salty (see Figure 10-20), plus a recently discovered fifth sense, called *umami*, which tastes glutamates and cannot be duplicated by the combination of any of the other four tastes. Each of these four taste types is experienced in a specific area of the tongue that contains taste buds with specialized functions. Taste receptors for all tastes are located in a narrow area surrounding the entire tongue. Sweet, salty, and sour taste receptors are in a region just inside the outer edge of the tongue. Salty and sour receptors are located in a small region toward the back of the tongue. Sour-only receptors are located approximately in the center of the tongue. There is an area toward the center and front of the tongue where no sensation of taste is experienced. Sweet and sour taste receptors are located just in front of this region, with bittersweet and sour tastes being experienced near the tip of the tongue just inside the area containing the receptors for all tastes. The brain, however, is not able to distinguish different taste components; rather, it perceives taste as a composite sensation.

Flavoring Techniques

Flavoring of medications can be seen as both a challenge and an opportunity. The challenge lies in the fact that there are no general or definite rules for what is right. There are no absolutes when it comes to flavoring, especially when working with an extemporaneously compounded prescription. Every formula that requires flavoring should be analyzed individually. The challenge of flavoring is further complicated by the individual preferences of each patient. The opportunity in flavoring lies in the ability to produce a quality product that the patient is willing to take or, at the very least, that the patient will tolerate.

Five basic flavoring techniques are used in preparing an acceptable product that minimizes a negative experience with regard to taste:

1. *Blending* uses a flavor that will blend with the drug taste. Citrus flavors blend with sour tastes; bitter tastes can be blended with salty, sweet, and sour tastes; salt reduces bitterness and sourness and increases sweetness. Chemicals such as vanillin, monosodium glutamate, and benzaldehyde are used for blending.

2. *Overshadowing* or *overpowering* involves the use of a flavor with a stronger intensity than the original product. Examples of intense flavoring vehicles are wintergreen, methyl salicylate, glycyrrhiza (licorice), and oleoresins.

3. *Physical methods* include the formulation of insoluble ingredients into a suspension; and emulsification of oils, where the offensive-tasting ingredient is placed in the oil phase and the flavoring or sweetening agent is placed in the aqueous phase. Effervescent additives are used in the preparation of salty-tasting drugs. The use of a high-viscosity fluid such as a syrup will limit contact of the offensive element with the tongue.

4. *Chemical methods* include absorption of the drug with an ingredient that eliminates the taste of the offensive drug.

5. *Physiological methods* involve using an additive such as menthol, peppermint, spearmint, or a spice such as cinnamon or clove to anesthetize the taste buds within the tongue. These flavor products reduce the sensitivity of the taste buds to bitterness.

In addition, flavor enhancers, such as monosodium glutamate (MSG), may be added to ensure intensity of flavor. It is important to note, however, that many patients are hypersensitive or allergic to MSG. The most-used flavor enhancer is vanilla. It can be added along with almost any flavoring agent to stimulate and intensify the desired flavor without altering the flavor or adding its own taste.

Coloring

Proper coloring of the prescription is equally important when making a compounded medication. The color should be appealing and appropriate for the dosage form. It is not always necessary to color a product, but if a coloring agent is used it should match the flavor of the product. Some patients may have sensitivities or allergies to certain dyes. This should be determined before compounding begins. There are sources of dye-free flavoring agents, and these should be considered for the patient who cannot tolerate a certain dye. In any case, the amount of color added to the formulation should be minimal, so that the final product is moderately light in color.

SUMMARY

Extemporaneous compounding is a special service provided by a number of community-based pharmacies. Additional training, skills, and practice are required for a pharmacy technician to assist in compounding, but compounding also provides a number of advanced professional opportunities for those who pursue these skills.

CHAPTER REVIEW QUESTIONS

1. What are some of the factors that must be considered before compounding a prescription medication?

   a. cost-effectiveness, availability, solubility, and stability
   b. suspending agent, profit margin, and ease of preparation
   c. proper tools, adequate support personnel, and time
   d. insurance reimbursement, available flavoring agents, active ingredient, and source

2. The extemporaneous compounding of prescription medications differs from traditional pharmacy in that it involves a relationship between:

   a. mother, father, and child.
   b. patient, practitioner, and pharmacist.
   c. pharmacist, patient, and insurance carrier.
   d. doctor, nurse, and patient.

3. Pharmacy is the only profession that allows the extemporaneous compounding of chemicals for:

   a. resale.
   b. veterinarians.
   c. therapeutic care.
   d. use in physicians' offices.

4. Of the following reference materials, which would not be necessary in a compounding facility?

   a. *Remington's Pharmaceutical Sciences*
   b. *The Merck Manual*
   c. *Drug Facts and Comparisons*
   d. *Pharmacy Times Magazine*

5. Which part of the compounding procedure has the greatest potential for error?

   a. pharmaceutical calculations
   b. retrieving the proper chemical
   c. selecting the proper vehicle
   d. choosing the best flavor

6. Who is responsible for checking the calculations performed for a specific formula?

   a. another technician
   b. the pharmacist
   c. the person who performs the calculations
   d. ancillary personnel

7. The compilation of ingredients and instructions is known as the:

   a. worksheet.
   b. menu.
   c. formula.
   d. list.

8. To avoid cross-contamination, the compounding area should be cleaned:

   a. before the procedure.
   b. after the procedure.
   c. daily.
   d. both before and after the procedure.

9. A transdermal gel in the form of a pluronic lecithin organogel is considered to be:

   a. an emulsion.
   b. an ointment.
   c. a cream.
   d. a suspension.

10. Which of the following types of mortar and pestle would be the ideal choice when working with liquids?

   a. porcelain
   b. glass
   c. Wedgwood
   d. any of the above

CRITICAL THINKING QUESTIONS

1. What are three reasons why extemporaneous compounding is important to pharmaceutical care?

2. Why is compounding considered a specialty?

3. Why does medication flavoring have an impact on patient compliance?

WEB CHALLENGE

1. Go to the following websites and print out information on obtaining advanced training, or certification, as a compounding pharmacy technician:

   http://www.gallipot.com

   http://www.pccarx.org

   http://www.pharmacytechnician.org

   http://www.spectrumrx.com

2. Go to http://www.compoundingtoday.com and print out an archived e-newsletter to discuss in class.

REFERENCES AND RESOURCES

Allen, LV Jr. A history of pharmaceutical compounding. *Secundum Artem.* 11(3): http://www.paddocklabs.com/secundum_artem.html:.

Allen, LV Jr. Pharmaceutical compounding calculations. *Secundum Artem.* 5(2): http://www.paddocklabs.com/secundum_artem.html.

Allen, LV Jr. Pharmacy compounding equipment. *Secundum Artem.* 4(3): http://www.paddocklabs.com/secundum_artem.html.

Allen, LV Jr. *The Art, Science, and Technology of Pharmaceutical Compounding.* Washington, DC: American Pharmaceutical Association, 1998.

Colbert, B, Ankney, J, & Lee, K. *Anatomy, Physiology, and Disease: An Interactive Journey for Health Professionals.* Upper Saddle River, NJ: Pearson Education, 2009.

Hoover, JE, ed. *Remington's Pharmaceutical Sciences* (15th ed.). *Pharmaceutical Necessities.* Easton, PA: Mack Publishing, 1975.

Introduction to Sterile Products

LEARNING OBJECTIVES

After completing this chapter, you should be able to:

- List the equipment and supplies used in preparing sterile products.
- List the routes of administration associated with sterile products.
- Discuss special concerns regarding chemotherapy and cytotoxic drugs.

Introduction

As pharmacy practice moves to a more patient-centered concept of pharmaceutical care, pharmacists rely on pharmacy technicians to take on new and expanded roles. Technicians have assumed many of the drug distribution responsibilities traditionally performed by pharmacists, to free pharmacists to provide direct patient care; however, technicians need proper training to be qualified to perform these responsibilities. This chapter introduces pharmacy technicians to sterile products and aseptic technique.

As you learned in Chapter 10, nonsterile compounding requires knowledge of numerous dosage formulations, such as capsules, solutions, suspensions, suppositories, and topicals. Sterile compounding requires, in addition, a command of aseptic technique. The more complex the compounding, the more precautions and steps must be added to guidelines to ensure proper aseptic technique.

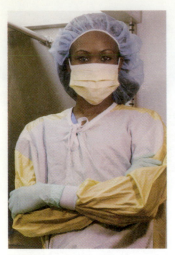

FIGURE 11-1 A technician dressed in sterile clothing.

aseptic technique the process of performing a procedure under controlled conditions in a manner that minimizes the chance of contamination of the preparation.

sterile free from bacteria and other microorganisms.

class 100 environment the classification of an airflow unit capable of producing an environment containing no more than 100 airborne particles of a size 0.5 micron or larger, per cubic foot of air.

laminar flow hood a device containing a HEPA filter; used for preparing sterile products.

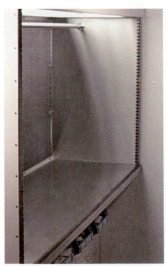

FIGURE 11-2 A laminar flow hood.

╭─ **INFORMATION** ─╮

This chapter is just an overview of this specialty practice in institutional pharmacy. Specific techniques are not included, as they are too advanced and detailed for the scope of this book. For an in-depth look at sterile products and step-by-step procedures for aseptic technique, review *The Pharmacy Technician Series: Sterile Products* by Mike Johnston, (Prentice-Hall Health, 2006).

Aseptic Technique

Aseptic technique is a way to perform a procedure under controlled conditions in a manner that minimizes the chance of contamination of the preparation (see Figure 11-1). Contamination can be caused by the following factors:

- Environment—conditions such as the air where the compounding is being performed must be controlled.
- Equipment—all objects that come in contact with the drug(s) must be sterile.
- Personnel—touch contamination is the most frequent cause of contamination.

We address each of these causes of contamination in detail, because each plays a key role in proper aseptic compounding.

The preparation of **sterile** drug compounds requires the utmost diligence to ensure final product integrity and sterility. Sterile products must be prepared with aseptic technique in a **class 100 environment**. This is a type of airflow unit capable of producing an environment containing no more than 100 airborne particles of a size 0.5 micron or larger, per cubic foot of air. Such an environment exists inside a certified horizontal or vertical laminar flow hood, a class 100 clean room, and a barrier isolator. A *barrier isolator* is a closed system made up of four solid walls, an air-handling system, and a transfer and interaction compartment.

Basic Equipment and Supplies

Basic equipment and supplies used in sterile compounding include laminar flow hoods, vertical flow hoods, biological safety cabinets, needles, syringes, and IV bags. This section introduces each one briefly.

Laminar Flow Hoods

Laminar flow hoods are designed to reduce the risk of airborne contamination during the preparation of **IV admixtures** by providing an ultra-clean environment (see Figure 11-2). The most important part of a laminar flow hood is a high-efficiency, bacteria-retentive filter, commonly called a **HEPA** (high-efficiency particulate air) filter. Room air is taken into the unit and passed through a pre-filter to remove relatively large contaminants such as dust and lint. The air is then compressed and channeled up behind and through the HEPA filter, which removes virtually all bacteria. The purified air then flows out over the entire work surface in parallel streams at a uniform velocity.

A laminar flow hood has three basic functions. The first is to provide clean air in the working area. This is done by passing room air through the bacteria-retentive filter to provide a continuous flow of clean air in the work area. Second, the constant flow of air out of the laminar flow hood prevents room air from entering the work area. Last, the air flowing out suspends and removes contaminants introduced into the work area by material (such as IV bags, syringes, or drug packaging) or personnel. Thus, a laminar flow hood provides an environment virtually free of airborne contaminants, in which sterile procedures can be safely performed. Laminar flow hoods may be used in the pharmacy to perform the following procedures:

- preparation of IV admixtures
- preparation of ophthalmic solutions
- reconstitution of powdered drugs
- filling of unit-dose syringes
- preparation of miscellaneous sterile products

Laminar flow hoods come in various sizes and models. One model, called a **console model**, sits on the floor. The other common model is called a **bench** or **countertop model**, because it sits on top of a counter; the space underneath it can be used for storage. Laminar airflow hoods are usually kept running continuously. If the hood has been turned off, it is recommended that it be run for at least 30 minutes before the work surface area is used again, so that the room air will be replaced with clean, filtered air. Laminar flow hoods should be inspected and certified every six months to ensure that the HEPA filter is intact, unclogged, and has no holes in it. The pre-filters in the hoods should be changed monthly.

Vertical Flow Hoods

Both console and bench models are available with vertical rather than horizontal airflow. With vertical flow, room air enters at the top of the unit, is channeled through the bacteria-retentive filter (which forms the ceiling of the unit), and down vertically across the work surface area. Neither of these models of laminar flow hoods should be used when preparing chemotherapy drugs. Although they protect the drug product from microbial contamination, they do not protect personnel or the environment from the hazards of these drug agents. These laminar flow hoods blow air across the work surface toward the operator and into the work environment. Drug particles or aerosols of these hazardous agents can easily contaminate both workers and the work environment.

Biological Safety Cabinets

Rather than a horizontal laminar flow hood, a **biological safety cabinet** is recommended to provide protection for the worker, the work environment, and the drug (see Figure 11-3). In a biological safety cabinet, air enters the unit at the top, where it passes through a pre-filter to remove large contaminants. Air then passes through a HEPA filter and is directed down toward the work surface, just as with a vertical laminar flow hood. The filter forms the ceiling of the work area in the biological safety cabinet and removes bacteria to provide ultra-clean air. Unlike the mechanism in a vertical laminar flow hood, however, as air approaches the work surface, it is pulled through vents at the front, back, and sides of the unit. A major portion of the contaminated air is recirculated back into the cabinet, and only a minor portion is passed through a HEPA filter before being exhausted into the room. Biological safety cabinets may also contain a partition on the front of the hood to help protect the user from exposure to hazardous substances.

Biological safety cabinets are of two basic types. A Class 2, type A, which was just described, represents the minimum recommended environment for preparing chemotherapy agents. Class 2, type B biological safety cabinets have greater intake flow velocities and are vented outside the building rather than back into the room. This type of safety cabinet is preferred, but the need to vent the filtered air to the outside can carry with it a substantial construction/installation cost.

It is important that biological safety cabinets run continuously. If turned off for any reason, such as for maintenance or filter changes, the cabinet must be thoroughly cleaned with a detergent, and the exhaust area must be covered with impermeable plastic and sealed to prevent any contaminants from escaping from the unit.

IV admixture a mixture of a solution and drug(s) prepared aseptically to be administered via a vein.

HEPA a high-efficiency particulate air filter; used in flow hoods.

console model a horizontal laminar flow hood that sits on the floor.

bench (countertop) model a horizontal laminar flow hood that sits on top of a counter; the space underneath it can be used for storage.

biological safety cabinet a vertical laminar flow hood used to provide protection for the worker, the work environment, and the drug.

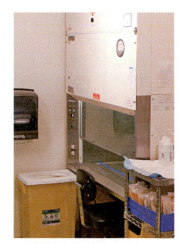

FIGURE 11-3 An example of a biological safety cabinet.

In January 2004, the *United States Pharmacopeia* published a set of new, stringent regulations regarding sterile product preparation facilities, referred to as *USP chapter 797*, or *USP 797*.

For facilities, USP 797 states that the surfaces of all ceilings, walls, floors, shelving, cabinets, and work surfaces in the buffer room and/or anteroom should be smooth, free from cracks and crevices, and nonshedding, so that they are easy to clean and sanitize. Junctures of ceilings and walls, walls and walls, and floors and walls must be covered or caulked to make them easier to clean. The areas may not have any dust-collecting ledges, pipes, or similar surfaces. Work surfaces must be durable, smooth, and made of stainless steel or molded plastic. Carts should be made of stainless-steel wire or sheet construction, with good-quality, cleanable caster wheels, and should be restricted to use in the controlled area only.

Needles

A *needle* consists of two parts: the shaft and the hub. The *shaft* is the long, slender stem of the needle that is beveled (diagonal cut) at one end to form a point. The cut end of the needle is the **bevel**. The hollow bore of the needle shaft is known as the **lumen**. At the other end of the needle is the *hub*, to which a syringe can be attached (see Figure 11-4).

Needle size is designated by length and gauge. The length of a needle is measured in inches from the juncture of the hub and the shaft to the tip of the point. Needle lengths range from $\frac{3}{8}$ inch to $3\frac{1}{2}$ inches or longer. The gauge of a needle, used to designate the size of the lumen, ranges from 27, the finest, to 13, the largest. The finer the needle, the higher the gauge number. In some disposable needles, the gauge is designated by the color of the hub (to facilitate recognition). One factor in choosing a needle size is the thickness (viscosity) of the solution to be injected. A fine needle with a relatively small lumen may be acceptable for most solutions, but a needle with a larger lumen and a smaller gauge number may be needed for more viscous solutions. Another factor in selecting the proper needle is the nature of the rubber closure to be penetrated. A fine needle with a smaller lumen may be preferred for rubber closures that core easily; *coring* means that part of the rubber closure gets carried into the drug solution when the needle penetrates the rubber closure. Needles are sterilized, individually wrapped, and disposable. Never reuse a used needle.

Filter needles are similar to other needles, except that they have a filter in the hub to catch any particles from an ampule or vial. They are used to vent small-volume vials. Dispensing pins, which can be attached to the syringe directly for multiple draws, rather than attaching multiple needles, are just one example of the various styles of equipment available from the many different distributors. Each works in the same fashion, by providing a venting system that traps any particles larger than the pores of the dispensing pin. A variety of different pore sizes are available. A 0.22-micron pore size is considered to be a sterilizing filter capable of removing all microorganisms. Other sizes commonly used in the pharmacy and suitable for clarifying solutions have porosities of 0.45, 1, 5, or 10 microns. The choice of which needle to use depends on your ability to manipulate the pin and the cost of the device.

bevel the sharp, pointed, diagonally cut end of a needle.

lumen the hollow space inside a needle.

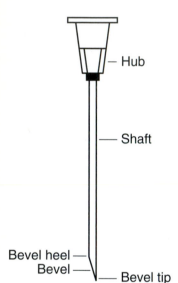

FIGURE 11-4 The parts of a needle.

Syringes

The two basic parts of a syringe are the barrel and the plunger (see Figure 11-5). The *barrel* is a tube that is open at one end and tapers into a hollow tip at the other end. The open end is extended radially outward to form a rim, or flange, to prevent the barrel from slipping through the fingers during manipulation.

The *plunger* is a piston-type rod with a slightly cone-shaped tip that passes inside the barrel of the syringe. The other end of the plunger is shaped into a flat knob for easy manipulation. The plunger must be able to move freely throughout the barrel, yet its surface must be so close to the barrel that the fluid cannot pass in between, even when under considerable pressure.

The tip of the syringe provides the point of attachment for a needle. The tip may be tapered to allow the needle hub to be slipped over it and held on by friction. With a system that uses this method, the needle is reasonably secure, but it may slip off if not properly attached or if considerable pressure is used to inject the solution. Locking devices have been developed to secure the needle more firmly onto the tip of the syringe; one such device has the trade name Luer-Lok. These devices incorporate a collar with a circular internal groove into which the needle hub is inserted. A half-turn locks the needle in place. This capability is especially valuable when pressure is required.

Graduation lines on the barrel of the syringe indicate the volume of solution inside. It is easier to make accurate readings if the color of the tip of the plunger is different from

FIGURE 11-5 The parts of a syringe.

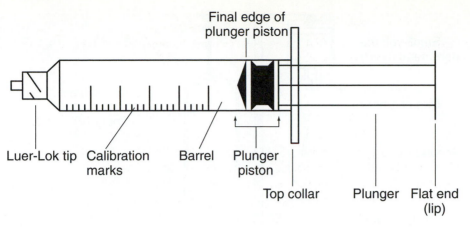

Final edge of plunger piston

Luer-Lok tip   Calibration marks   Barrel   Plunger piston   Top collar   Plunger   Flat end (lip)

that of the syringe itself. Syringes are disposable and have a capacity range of 0.5–60 mL. Graduation lines may be in milliliters or other measures, depending on the capacity and intended uses of the syringe; for example, the larger the capacity of the syringe, the larger the interval between graduation lines. Special-purpose syringes, such as insulin syringes, have graduation lines in both milliliters and insulin units to reflect their intended use.

To select an appropriate syringe, use the rule that the capacity of the syringe should be the next size larger than the volume to be measured. For example, use a 3 mL syringe to measure a 2.3 mL dose; select a 5 mL syringe to measure a 3.8 mL dose. This way, the graduation marks on the syringe will be in the smallest possible increments for the dose measured. Syringes should not be filled to capacity, because the plunger can easily be dislodged. It is recommended that syringes containing chemotherapy drugs not be filled to more than three-quarters of capacity.

Sterile, disposable syringes are discarded after one use and have the same advantages as disposable needles. Although syringes today are made of plastic, because it costs less, glass syringes are still available for drugs that are incompatible with plastic. Both syringes and needles must be disposed of in a sharps container. Do not recap needles after they have been used.

Prefilled Syringes

Some pharmaceutical manufacturers supply common doses of frequently used or emergency-use drugs in prefilled syringes. Prefilled syringes eliminate the need to measure doses, thus saving valuable time in compounding admixtures. Prefilled syringes are commonly placed in emergency carts, or are used in emergency rooms when it is critical to get medication to patients as quickly as possible.

Most prefilled syringes are supplied in a syringe that does not have a plunger. This is to prevent the drug from accidentally squirting out if pressure is applied to the plunger during storage or transferred. A device called a *tubex holder* is screwed onto the back of the syringe (where the plunger would have been), and a locking ring is then tightened around the end of the syringe.

IV Bags

Plastic bags are used for dilution of a solution, and are the most common containers used in administering intravenous (IV) medications to patients. Plastic bags are available in many different sizes, with 50, 100, 250, 500, and 1,000 mL being the most common. Special bags for compounding parenteral nutrition are available in 2,000 mL and 3,000 mL sizes. Most IV bags are made of polyvinyl chloride (PVC). More expensive than PVC bags are non-PVC bags, which are used for specific drugs (such as Taxol) that can adhere to the plastic of PVC IV bags. Figure 11-6 shows the parts of an IV administration setup.

At the top of the bag is a flat plastic extension with a hole to allow the bag to be hung on an administration pole. At the other end of the bag are two ports of about the same length. The administration set port has a blue plastic cover that maintains the sterility of

FIGURE 11-6 The parts of an IV.

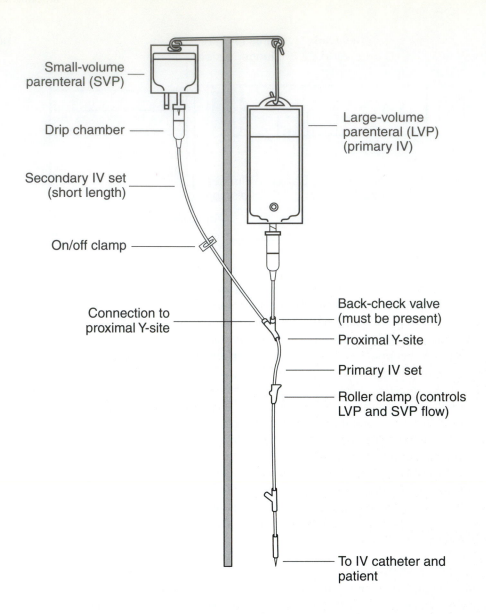

the port. The cover is easily removed by pulling on it. Once it is pulled off, the sterile port of the administration set is exposed. Solution will not drip from the plastic bag at this point because a plastic diaphragm about $\frac{1}{2}$ inch inside the port seals in the liquid. When the spike of the administration set is inserted into this port, it punctures the inner diaphragm, allowing the solution to flow from the flexible plastic bag into the administration set. When the solution has filled the administration set (this process is called *priming* the set), make sure to clamp the administration set so that the solution does not leak out. Once the inner diaphragm is punctured, it is not resealable.

The other port is the medication port. It is covered by a protective rubber tip. Medication is added to the solution through the medication port by means of a needle and syringe. The rubber tip is self-sealing, thus preventing solution from leaking when the needle punctures the tip.

Approximately $\frac{1}{2}$ inch inside this port is a plastic diaphragm that must be punctured for solution to enter the bag. The inner diaphragm is not self-sealing when punctured by a needle, so the rubber tip must stay attached to the bag. Graduation marks at 25–100 mL intervals, which indicate the volume of solution infused, are located on both sides of the front of some plastic bags, depending on the capacity of the bags.

When you label a plastic bag, it does not matter which side of the bag you place the label on; however, many institutions place the label on the printed side of the bag, beneath the solution name, and offset slightly to one side so that the graduation marks near the side can still be read. This procedure has the advantage of providing a convenient cross-check between the actual solution and the name appearing on the admixture label.

Some IV solutions, such as 5 percent dextrose injection and 0.9 percent sodium chloride injection, are available in minibags, or **piggyback bags**. These bags typically hold 50 mL or 100 mL of solution and are used to administer drugs (such as antibiotics) intermittently rather than continuously.

The plastic bag system is completely closed to air. It does not depend on air to displace the solution as it leaves the bag. The bag collapses as the solution is administered, so a vacuum is not created inside.

Routes of Administration

When drugs must be injected, any one of several routes can be used to administer them. Often, certain drugs can be administered only through specific routes, and this will be listed in the package insert. The most common injectable routes of administration are **intravenous** (in the vein), **intramuscular** (in the muscle), and **subcutaneous** (in the skin). Other, less frequently used routes include **intradermal** (in the dermis of the skin) and **intrathecal** (in the spine).

Intravenous administration of drugs has advantages over other routes because it provides the fastest route to the bloodstream. There are no barriers, like skin or muscle, to absorb the drug first, so the intravenous route allows the most rapid onset of action. If someone cannot take medication by mouth because he is unconscious or vomiting, then intravenous administration is the best route. Because the inner lining of a vein is relatively insensitive to pain, drugs that can be irritating if given by another route can be given intravenously at a slow rate without causing pain. Drugs that can be diluted to reduce irritation can be given only intravenously, because the tissues around the other routes cannot accommodate the large volume. Figure 11-7 shows some commonly used intravenous sites.

Intravenous Administration

There are two types of intravenous administration. The first, an IV push, is an intravenous injection in which the prepared medication is drawn up into a syringe and administered over a short time. The amount of medication is usually a small volume pushed through an IV line that is already in place on the patient. Before a medication is pushed into the vein, the syringe is pulled slightly back to draw blood out (*aspirated*) to make sure that the tip of the needle is in the vein.

The second type of administration is an IV **infusion**. Infusions are given to overcome dehydration, to build up depleted blood volumes, and to aid in the administration of medications. An infusion allows a larger volume of solution to be given at a constant rate (which depends on the drug being administered). Infusions can be administered continuously or intermittently. Continuous infusions are used to administer larger

piggyback bags minibags that hold 50 mL or 100 mL of solution and are used to administer drugs intermittently.

intravenous parenteral injection in the vein.

intramuscular parenteral injection in the muscle.

subcutaneous parenteral injection in the skin.

intradermal parenteral injection in the dermis of the skin.

intrathecal parenteral injection in the spine.

infusion a relatively large volume of solution given at a constant rate.

FIGURE 11-7 Intravenous administration sites.

Intravenous sites

Several sites on the body are used to intravenously administer drugs: the veins of the antecubital area (in front of the elbow), back of the hand, and some of the larger veins of the foot. On some occasions, a vein must be exposed by a surgical cut.

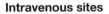
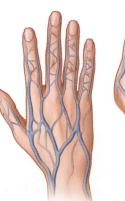
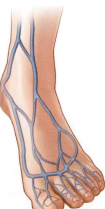

volumes of solutions over several hours at a slow, constant rate. Intermittent infusions are used to administer a relatively small volume over a short time at specific intervals.

Risks

There are some risks involved in intravenous administration. A primary problem is that if there is an error in the dose, it is difficult to stop the drug, because it is very quickly dispersed throughout the body and will start working within a few minutes. Another risk is the possibility of infection anytime the skin is punctured. These risks are why the pharmacy technician must have the knowledge and skills to prepare sterile products correctly.

Sterile Products

Sterile products, such as IV solutions and total parenteral nutrition (TPN), are medications compounded using aseptic technique. Sterility is the focus for making these products, because of the way they are administered. When a patient takes a capsule or tablet, the body has built-in defense mechanisms to filter the product before it enters the patient's bloodstream. IV solutions and TPNs, in contrast, are administered directly, bypassing many of these natural defense mechanisms. Use of aseptic technique ensures that products being administered directly into a patient's veins are sterile and do not introduce any particles or *pyrogens*, such as bacteria, fungi, or viruses, which can produce a fever or cause sepsis, a blood infection.

INFORMATION

The word *aseptic* comes from the Latin prefix *a*, meaning "without," and the Latin word *sepsis*, meaning "infection." When we use the term *aseptic*, we are talking about making or compounding a product without infection, also referred to as *sterile*.

Certain characteristics are desired in an IV solution. Some of the characteristics can be seen by visual inspection, whereas others cannot. The solution must be clear—which should not be confused with colorless—to indicate that the drug added has dissolved completely. IV fat emulsions (which are mostly used in conjunction with TPN solutions) are an exception to this rule, because they look like milk. A solution must also be free of any visible particulate matter (such as rubber cores from vials).

Sterility

Sterility is freedom from bacteria and other microorganisms. Solutions to be injected must be sterile. A product is either sterile or not sterile; products cannot be partially sterile. Sterility cannot be determined visually, but proper aseptic technique can maintain the sterility of solutions, drugs, and supplies during preparation.

pH

pH term describing the degree of acidity of a solution.

The term **pH** is used to describe the degree of acidity of a solution. pH values range from 0 to 14, with values below 7 representing greater acidity of the solution; values above 7 represent less acidity or greater alkalinity. A solution having a pH of 7 is neither acidic nor alkaline; it is considered neutral. Plasma in the human body has a pH of about 7.4, and solutions should be around that same pH. pH is another characteristic that cannot be seen, but it can be tested after a drug is prepared.

Tonicity

tonicity a state of normal tension of the tissues by virtue of which the parts are kept in shape, alert, and able to function properly.

isotonic containing the same tonicity concentration as red blood cells.

A final characteristic that cannot be determined visually is **tonicity**, which refers to a state of normal tension of the tissues by virtue of which the body tissues and parts are kept in shape, alert, and able to function properly. An **isotonic** solution has the same concentration as red blood cells. Isotonic IV solutions minimize patient discomfort and damage to red blood cells. The stinging caused by either a hypertonic solution (which may cause shrinkage of red blood cells) or a hypotonic solution (which may cause swelling of red blood cells) is not experienced with an isotonic solution. IV solutions should be as close to isotonic as possible. A good reference point to remember is that 0.9 percent sodium chloride injection and 5 percent dextrose injection are both approximately isotonic.

Storage

When storing sterile products, try to avoid places that are exposed to extreme hot or cold temperatures. Exposing products to cold could cause some drugs in a solution to **precipitate**. Solutions that contain drugs should also not be exposed to high temperatures, because the heat may accelerate decomposition of the drug. IV solutions should be kept at room temperature or in a cool place.

precipitate a solid that forms within a solution.

Common Products

Many different types of solutions are commercially available; however, three types are most frequently used: sodium chloride injection, dextrose injection, and Ringer's injection. These three most resemble the plasma in the blood. Sodium chloride 0.9 percent and dextrose 5 percent are isotonic, as mentioned earlier, but both provide a source of fluid and electrolyte replacement. Ringer's injection can be modified with the addition of sodium lactate to produce lactated Ringer's injection. Ringer's solutions are primarily used for fluid replacement and as a source of electrolytes.

Compatibility

Not all drugs are compatible with each other. The incompatibility may be between two drugs or between a drug and an IV solution. The possibility of an unexpected or undesirable combination is relatively low compared with the number of IV admixtures prepared, but incompatibility is always possible. An incompatibility can lead to a patient not receiving the full therapeutic dose of a medication or, even worse, to an adverse reaction. Some incompatibilities, such as a color change or hazy appearance, can be detected. Precipitate can form in the solution, or an evolution of a gas may even be smelled.

Be aware that sometimes when drugs are combined, an expected and harmless visible change may occur. Reading the package insert or checking with the pharmacist can confirm the reason for a change in appearance. Other incompatibilities cannot be detected visually. If two drugs are mixed that are incompatible with each other, one drug can cause the degradation of the other drug. Many factors can affect the compatibility and stability of drugs in IV admixtures. The following subsections describe each of the factors that may cause incompatibility.

Workplace Wisdom Handbook on Injectable Drugs

The Handbook on Injectable Drugs, by Lawrence A. Trissel, is an excellent reference book commonly used by pharmacy personnel when they are preparing sterile products. The text provides extensive compatibility information on the medications used in sterile products.

pH

pH is one of the most common causes of incompatibility. Combining two drugs that require two different pH values for the final solution can cause one or both drugs to either degrade or precipitate.

Light

Some drugs will start to break down and lose their therapeutic effect if exposed to light. Medications that are sensitive to light are supplied by the manufacturer in dark-colored (generally amber or brown), vials or ampules, and are dispensed in amber, light-sensitive bags.

Dilution

The concentration of a drug in solution may be a factor in its compatibility with other drugs. A problem can be avoided by ensuring that the drug in question is properly diluted before it is combined with the other drug.

Chemical Composition

The chemical composition of one drug can cause a change in the therapeutic effect of the other drug. When the two drugs combine, the new chemical combination may initiate adverse events.

Time

Most drugs start to degrade within a short time after being added to an IV solution.

Solutions

Some drugs require a specific solution or diluent to be used for reconstitution and further dilution. Choosing the wrong solution can cause the drug to break down more quickly, or can cause precipitate to form. Some drugs are packaged with a specific diluent for reconstitution; an example of this is Herceptin (trastuzumab).

Temperature

Heat increases the rate of most chemical reactions. Because the degradation of a drug in solution can be considered a chemical reaction, care must be taken to keep admixtures at a stable temperature. Some drugs remain more stable refrigerated than at room temperature. Some drugs, however, should never be refrigerated, because a precipitate can form. Not many experts recommend freezing drugs after reconstitution, and sometimes freezing actually reduces the stability of the drug.

Buffer Capacity

buffer capacity the ability of a solution to resist a change in pH when either an acidic or an alkaline substance is added to the solution.

Buffer capacity is the ability of a solution to resist a change in pH when either an acidic or an alkaline substance is added to the solution. Many drugs contain buffers to increase their stability. IV solutions in general do not have high buffer capacities. Therefore, when a drug with a high buffer capacity is added, the resulting solution will have a pH closest to the drug added.

Order of Mixing

The order in which drugs are added to a solution may be a factor in compatibility. Drugs that are concentrated and combined may react to form precipitate, whereas those same drugs in diluted solutions may be combined acceptably. This is very important when mixing parenteral nutrition solutions (discussed in detail later in this chapter). Electrolytes are commonly prescribed with phosphates, but this causes a problem with parenteral solutions if they are not mixed correctly. To avoid the problem, it is important to mix the solution well after each addition is made and to add the electrolytes last, after the phosphate has been well diluted.

Workplace Wisdom Calcium Gluconate

The additive calcium gluconate tends to precipitate easily when mixed with other electrolytes, so many facilities recommend adding this component last.

Plastic

As mentioned earlier, some drugs are incompatible with the plastic container that will hold the solution. Certain chemicals in PVC plastic can leach out of the bag, or the drug may adhere to the bag. It is recommended that one use a non-PVC container for these particular drugs.

Filters

Filters, also mentioned earlier, represent a possible problem in effective administration of a drug to a patient. Filters can cause a reduction in concentration of the drug to be administered.

Minimizing Incompatibilities

To minimize incompatibilities, follow these general guidelines:

1. Use solutions promptly after preparation to ensure administration of the most stable product; drugs tend to degrade in a relatively short time. If a newly made admixture is not to be used immediately, it should be placed in the refrigerator.

2. Minimize the number of drugs added to a solution. As the number of drugs added increases, the chance of an incompatibility rises. It becomes increasingly difficult to find information on compatibilities when more than two drugs are added to a solution.

3. Check incompatibility resources to verify which drugs have a very high or very low pH. Most drugs are acidic, so combining them with a drug having a very high pH is more likely to result in an incompatibility.

The most often used resources for information on incompatibilities are the manufacturers' drug package inserts. The package inserts have a wealth of information about the drug. Each package insert is developed by the manufacturer and approved by the FDA when the drug is marketed. The package insert generally is not as good a reference for incompatibilities; however, many other excellent resources are available, such as incompatibility charts, articles in professional magazines, reference books, and the Internet. These can give you more accurate and up-to-date information.

Incompatibility charts list drugs that can and cannot be mixed in particular solutions. Some charts list drugs horizontally across the top and vertically down one side. You find one drug in the top list and the other drug in the side list; then you follow along the lines for the two constituents of the admixture from the top and the side until the lines intersect. A notation in the space where the lines intersect denotes whether the mixture is compatible. (One problem with this kind of chart is that it does not list the reason the two drugs are incompatible.)

The *American Journal of Health-System Pharmacy* frequently has detailed research articles on intravenous incompatibilities. Some very useful reference books are the *Handbook on Injectable Drugs* and the *Drug Facts and Comparisons* book. Many pharmacy departments also maintain a file that categorizes drugs, to make looking up drug information quicker and easier. Some pharmacy computer systems screen IV admixture incompatibilities as well as drug interactions, alerting the pharmacist or pharmacy technician to these issues when the order is entered, before it is prepared.

Total Parenteral Nutrition

Parenteral nutrition solutions are complex admixtures used to provide nutritional support to patients who are unable to take in adequate nutrients through the gastrointestinal tract. These admixtures are composed of such things as fat, protein, dextrose, electrolytes, vitamins, and water. Parenteral solutions can be formulated and calculated to match an individual's nutritional requirements. Parenteral nutrition solutions are also referred to as *TPN solutions* or *TPNs*. Due to the complexity of and time needed to prepare a TPN solution, many pharmacies that compound a large number of parenteral nutrition solutions use high-speed compounders, Automixers, or Micromixers. These machines prepare complex solutions safely, accurately, and quickly. Automixers can hold from two to ten different components of the appropriate solution to be mixed. Figure 11-8 shows a technician preparing a TPN solution.

These compounders consist of two principal parts: the pump module and the control module. The pump module is placed in the laminar flow hood along with the components, which hang from hangers in the hood. A disposable transfer set is hooked up

parenteral nutrition complex admixtures used to provide nutritional support to patients who are unable to take in adequate nutrients through the gastrointestinal tract.

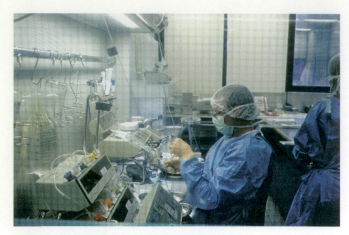

FIGURE 11-8 Preparing a parenteral nutrition solution.

to the machine, and then each tubing, or lead, is inserted into the source of each component. Each lead is color-coded to its specific spot on the compounder. All the leads come together at a junction and are connected to the final solution, which hangs from a hanger hooked up to an electronic scale that measures fluid by weight. This method is more accurate than measuring fluid volume because it is not adversely affected by air entering the system.

The control module is the computer that controls how much of each component goes into the final solution. The control module is kept outside the laminar flow hood and is controlled by using the keypad to enter data for each component. Some pharmacies have installed a bar-code system in their automixers to detect when a lead is not correctly attached to the right station. The bar code is scanned against the lead tubing and then scanned at the corresponding station; if they match, the correct attachment is assured. If the bar codes do not match when scanned, an alarm sounds and an error display appears on the control module.

Parenteral nutrition solutions must be administered with caution. There are two ways to administer parenteral nutrition solutions intravenously. The first is through a central vein; the second is through a peripheral vein. They are most commonly infused into a large central vein that leads directly to the heart. The subclavian vein, under the collarbone, is used most often. The route of administration may affect the concentration of certain ingredients in the TPN solution.

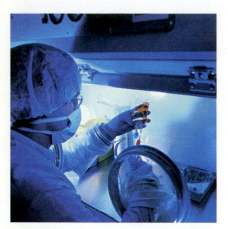

FIGURE 11-9 Preparing an antineoplastic drug.

chemotherapy drug therapy used to treat cancer and other diseases.

antineoplastics agents, such as medications, that prevent the growth of malignant cells.

Chemotherapy

The use of **chemotherapy** or **antineoplastics** to treat cancer began in the late 1940s. It was not until the late 1970s that health professionals became aware of potential hazards associated with the handling of antineoplastic drugs (see Figure 11-9). Concern has been mounting steadily over the risks incurred by pharmacy staff members who prepare and dispose of cytotoxic agents. Most of these agents were designed to damage the DNA of rapidly dividing cancer cells. However, because they lack specificity, any rapidly dividing cells in the body, whether normal or cancerous, become damaged. Repeated exposure to DNA-active drugs over a long period of time could potentially lead to irreparable DNA damage and might cause mutations, whether cancerous or not, to occur in unborn babies.

PROFILES IN PRACTICE

Karen is a certified pharmacy technician who works at an inpatient pharmacy preparing chemotherapy for her patients. Karen just confirmed that she is five weeks pregnant. She is concerned about the risks of being around chemotherapy agents while pregnant, but needs to keep working for financial reasons.

• What options should Karen consider?

cytotoxic poisonous or destructive to cells.

Health problems caused by acute exposure to **cytotoxic** agents include sensitivity, coughing, dizziness, headaches, caustic vesicant-like marks, and eye reactions. These can be caused by direct skin contact, inhalation, ingestion, or accidental injection of agents. The long-term consequences of low-dose exposure to antineoplastic agents are also a serious concern. To date, there is no conclusive proof that the potential problems associated with preparing these drugs will occur in professionals who have minimal exposure from handling these products. Furthermore, there is neither a known threshold of danger nor a reliable method of monitoring healthcare workers' exposure.

Workplace Wisdom Cytotoxic Agents

Personnel working with or around cytotoxic agents should always wear appropriate personal protective equipment (PPE), such as gloves, gowns, masks and face shields.

Several agencies, including the Occupational Safety and Health Administration, the National Institutes of Health, and the American Society of Health System Pharmacists have issued guidelines regarding the safe handling of drugs. Common sense dictates that, regardless of the type or size of the facility, practical measures are necessary for employee protection. Any organization handling cancer chemotherapy or other hazardous drugs must accept the following standards as essential components of occupational safety:

- written policies and procedures
- employee education
- certification
- continuing education
- proper aseptic technique
- access to medical attention for employees exposed to hazardous drugs
- appropriate documentation of exposure incidents

Employees must be informed of the possible risks and controversies at the time of hire and should be given the option of reassignment at vulnerable periods in their lives. For women, these times may include documented pregnancy and during breast-feeding. Some pregnant personnel choose to continue handling chemotherapeutic agents because they are confident that their workplace provides adequate protection. Some men may request a transfer away from drug preparation when planning a family, because of the possible impact on a male's sperm count.

An employee's competence and understanding of good work practices should be tested not only before hire, but also periodically throughout employment, through observation and written evaluation. Up-to-date policies and procedures for compounding sterile products should be written and available to all personnel involved in IV preparation. When policies and procedures are changed and additions or deletions are made, these updates should be communicated to all employees involved in drug preparation. The policies and procedures should address education and training requirements, competency evaluations, storage and handling of products and supplies, storage and delivery of final products, maintenance of facilities and equipment used in drug preparation, appropriate protective garments to be worn, validation of proper preparation technique, labeling of final products, documentation, quality control, and conduct for personnel working in the controlled area.

INFORMATION

Certain states require pharmacy technicians to be certified in aseptic technique before they may work in the clean-room environment, and some states require technicians who work with sterile products to complete a specific number of live, continuing education programs related to aseptic technique each year.

The National Pharmacy Technician Association offers a Sterile Products Certification course, which is valid nationwide and meets the most stringent of state requirements. In addition, NPTA offers live CE programs to aid technicians. For more information on either of these, contact NPTA via the Internet at www.pharmacytechnician.org or by calling 1-888-247-8700.

SUMMARY

Sterile products must be prepared using proper aseptic technique to ensure that all products remain free of bacteria, fungi, pyrogens, infections, and other microorganisms. To ensure sterility, these products are prepared in laminar flow hoods (including horizontal flow hoods and biological safety cabinets) that contain HEPA filters.

Sterile products are most commonly administered parenterally through various administration sites, such as veins (IV) and muscle tissue (IM). Other sterile products, however, are administered via other routes; these include total parenteral nutrition, ophthalmic preparations, and

otic preparations. Sterile product preparation can be a complex, high-risk process in the healthcare setting. Pharmacy technicians play an integral role in the procurement, storage, preparation, and distribution of these products. Training, education, and competency measurement are critical to ensure a safe chemotherapy process for patients and for employees. Increasing pharmacy technicians' awareness of safety standards for preparing sterile products will ensure a safe work environment and reduce potential medication errors.

CHAPTER REVIEW QUESTIONS

1. The following are the basic functions of the air flow in a laminar flow hood, except:
   a. preventing room air from entering the hood.
   b. providing clean air in the hood.
   c. suspending and removing contaminants introduced into the hood.
   d. providing personnel with protection from hazardous agents.

2. Laminar flow hoods may be used to perform the following procedures, except:
   a. reconstitution of powdered drugs.
   b. preparation of ophthalmic solutions.
   c. preparation of hazardous drugs.
   d. filling of unit-dose syringes.

3. What does HEPA stand for?
   a. huge effective particulate aerolizer
   b. high-efficiency particulate air
   c. highly effective particulate air
   d. high-efficiency particular airborne

4. What micron pore size is considered to be a sterilizing filter?
   a. 0.45
   b. 0.22
   c. 5
   d. 1

5. Which route of administration is given in the vein?
   a. intramuscular
   b. intradermal
   c. intrathecal
   d. intravenous

6. The desired characteristics of an intravenous solution include:
   a. sterility.
   b. clarity (except fat emulsions).
   c. freedom from particulates.
   d. all of the above.

7. When an intravenous solution is considered neutral, what is its pH?
   a. 0
   b. 7
   c. 14
   d. 7.4

8. The following are factors that can affect compatibility or stability of drugs, except:
   a. strength of the drug.
   b. dilution of the drug in a solution.
   c. chemical composition of the drugs.
   d. pH of the drugs.

9. The following are the essential components of occupational safety for any organization, except:
   a. proper aseptic technique.
   b. continuing education.
   c. DNA samples from all employees.
   d. certification.

10. Which of the following is not a form of personal protective equipment?
    a. prescription eyeglasses
    b. gloves
    c. gown
    d. face shield

CRITICAL THINKING QUESTIONS

1. What is the reasoning for requiring that certain compounded medications be sterile?

2. Can aseptic technique guarantee 100 percent sterility? Why or why not?

3. What risks are posed to pharmacy technicians who prepare sterile products?

WEB CHALLENGE

1. Go to the National Pharmacy Technician Association (NPTA) website and print out information regarding national IV certification: http://www.pharmacytechnician.org

2. Visit the American Society of Health-System Pharmacists (ASHP) website and search for their *Guidelines for Handling Hazardous Drugs*. Prepare a one-page summary of the information that you find: http://www.ashp.org

REFERENCES AND RESOURCES

American Society of Health-System Pharmacists. ASHP guidelines on quality assurance for pharmacy-prepared sterile products. *American Journal of Health-System Pharmacists*. 2000;57:1150–1169.

Attolio, RM. Caring enough to understand: The road to oncology medication error prevention. *Hospital Pharmacy*. 1996;31:17–26.

Ballington, D. *Pharmacy Practice for Technicians*. St. Paul, MN: EMC Paradigm, 2003.

Bergemann, DA. Handling antineoplastic agents. *American Journal of Intravenous Therapy and Clinical Nutrition*. January 1983:13–17.

Blecher, CS, Glynn-Tucker, EM, McDiarmid, M, & Newton, SA, eds. *Safe Handling of Hazardous Drugs*. Pittsburgh: ONS Publishing, 2003.

Buchanan, E. *Sterile Compounding Facilities. Principles of Sterile Product Preparation*. Bethesda, MD: ASHP, 1995.

Dorr, RT. *Practical Safety Precautions for Handling Cytotoxic Agents in Hospital Pharmacies*. Tucson, AZ: The University of Arizona Health Sciences Center, 1990.

Drug Facts and Comparisons® 2008. St. Louis, MO: Wolters Kluwer Health.

Hunt, ML Jr., ed. *Training Manual for Intravenous Admixture Personnel*. Chicago: Precept Press, 1995.

Johnston, M. *The Pharmacy Technician Series: Sterile Products*. Upper Saddle River, NJ: Prentice-Hall Health, 2006.

King, LD. Considering compounding. *America's Pharmacist*. September 2002: 16–20.

Talley, RC. *Sterile Compounding in Hospital Pharmacies*. Bethesda, MD: American Journal of Health-System Pharmacists, 2003.

Thompson, CA. USP publishes enforceable chapter on sterile compounding. Bethesda, MD: American Journal of Health-System Pharmacists. 2003;60:814–817.

Trissel, LA. (2005) *Handbook on Injectable Drugs* (13th ed.). Bethesda, MD: American Society of Health-System Pharmacists (ASHP).

Pharmacy Calculations

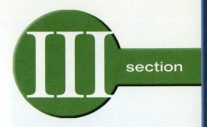

Basic Math Skills

LEARNING OBJECTIVES

After completing this chapter, you should be able to:

- Determine the value of a decimal.
- Add, subtract, multiply, and divide decimals.
- Recognize and interpret Roman numerals.
- Change Roman numerals to Arabic numerals.
- Change Arabic numerals to Roman numerals.
- Describe the different types of common fractions.
- Add, subtract, multiply, and divide fractions.
- Define a ratio.
- Define a proportion.
- Solve math problems by using ratios and proportions.

Introduction

Knowledge of basic arithmetic is essential for today's pharmacy technician. You must have basic skills in mathematics to understand and perform drug preparations. Nearly every aspect of drug dispensing requires a consideration of numbers. All advanced pharmacy calculations, which are explained throughout this text, rely on a solid understanding of basic math principles. This chapter will serve as a review of these general principles and as an assessment of your basic math skills.

Basic Math Pretest

The following diagnostic pretest will help guide your review and determine your strengths and weaknesses in basic math skills. The test should take you approximately one hour. Decimals should be rounded to the thousandths. You will need scratch paper.

Circle the decimal in each group with the highest value.

1.   4.1,   6.35,   0.31

2.   1.37,   1.33,   1.89

3.   0.4,   0.44,   0.41

Circle the decimal in each group with the lowest value.

4.   40.4,   40.0,   40.003

5.   0.15,   0.16,   0.016

6.   7.01,   7.71,   7.76

Add the following decimals.

7. $2.25 + 5.89 =$ _____

8. $62.36 + 1.755 =$ _____

9. $4.004 + 4.24 + 0.007 =$ _____

Subtract the following decimals.

10. $8.95 - 0.015 =$ _____

11. $6.665 - 0.007 =$ _____

12. $18.64 - 2.11 =$ _____

Multiply the following decimals.

13. $7.5 \times 0.23 =$ _____

14. $5.47 \times 1.15 =$ _____

15. $4.4 \times 3.875 =$ _____

Divide the following decimals.

16. $0.87 \div 0.2 =$ _____

17. $4.4 \div 0.3 =$ _____

18. $5.0 \div 5.5 =$ _____

19.   A jeweler had 12.5 oz. of gold in stock. Creation of a necklace required 1.8 oz. How much gold remained in stock after the necklace was made? _____

20.   Missy Jones earned $725.78 last week. Her payroll deductions totaled $169.47. How much remained after payroll deductions? _____

21.   Ray Wilhelm earned $371.64 for working 38 hours. How much did he earn per hour? _____

Identify the value of each of the following Roman numerals.

22.   X _____

23.   M _____

24.   L _____

Give the equivalent Arabic numbers for each of the following Roman numerals.

25.   XXIII _____

26.   MML _____

27.   XLVII _____

Add the following fractions. Reduce to the lowest possible terms.

28. $\dfrac{2}{3} + \dfrac{1}{8} =$ _____

29. $\dfrac{4}{9} + \dfrac{1}{5} =$ _____

30. $\dfrac{2}{7} + \dfrac{1}{3} =$ _____

Subtract the following fractions. Reduce to the lowest possible terms.

31. $\dfrac{1}{8} - \dfrac{1}{12} =$ _____

32. $\dfrac{4}{4} - \dfrac{1}{8} =$ _____

33. $\dfrac{6}{7} - \dfrac{1}{8} =$ _____

Multiply the following fractions. Reduce to the lowest possible terms.

34. $\dfrac{1}{10} \times \dfrac{2}{3} =$ _____

35. $\dfrac{250}{1} \times \dfrac{6}{9} =$ _____

36. $\dfrac{5}{20} \times \dfrac{6}{40} =$ _____

Divide the following fractions. Reduce to the lowest possible terms.

37. $\dfrac{1}{15} \div \dfrac{1}{10} =$ _____

38. $\dfrac{2}{5} \div \dfrac{4}{6} =$ _____

39. $\dfrac{1}{7} \div \dfrac{2}{3} =$ _____

40. A jigsaw puzzle contains 5,240 pieces. Joan estimates that the puzzle is $\frac{1}{4}$ completed. How many pieces have been put in place in the puzzle? _____

41. There were 10,240 attendees at a conference. If $\frac{3}{4}$ of the audience were women, how many women attended the conference? _____

42. A computer sells for $3,000. The company charges $\frac{1}{5}$ of the purchase price as a maintenance fee. How much is the maintenance fee for this computer? _____

Solve the following problems for x.

43. $\dfrac{3}{x} = \dfrac{5}{20}$ _____

44. $\dfrac{15}{1} = \dfrac{30}{x}$ _____

45. $\dfrac{6}{12} = \dfrac{x}{144}$ _____

Convert as indicated.

46. 0.08 to a percent _____

47. $\dfrac{4}{5}$ to a percent _____

48. 37% to a fraction _____

Table 12-1 Decimals as Fractions

DECIMAL NUMBER	READ	FRACTION
3.2	three and two tenths	$3\frac{2}{10}$
0.9	nine tenths	$\frac{9}{10}$
0.04	four hundredths	$\frac{4}{100}$
2.15	two and fifteen hundredths	$2\frac{15}{100}$
0.357	three hundred fifty seven thousandths	$\frac{357}{1000}$

49. $\frac{1}{3}$ to a ratio _____

50. $\frac{1}{500}$ to a ratio _____

Decimals

A clear understanding of decimals is critical to drug dispensing. A decimal point can mean the difference between a correct dose and a serious overdose or underdose. To determine the value of a decimal, you must first recognize that every digit in a decimal has a place value.

Decimals as Fractions

Decimals are fractions with a denominator that is a multiple of 10, such as 10, 100, 1000, and so on. The value of the denominator is determined by the number of digits to the right of the decimal point. **Decimal fractions** are written as a whole number with a zero and a decimal point in front of the value. For example, $\frac{8}{10}$ represents the decimal 0.8, $\frac{8}{100}$ represents the decimal 0.08, and $\frac{8}{1000}$ is equivalent to 0.008. It is often helpful to read decimals as their fraction equivalent.

decimal fractions fractions written as a whole number with a zero and a decimal point in front of the value.

Zeros placed either before or after a decimal number do not change the value of the number. For example, 0.8 could be written as 0.80, 00.8, or 0.80000; however, in healthcare professions such as pharmacy, you should always place a zero before the decimal point to avoid misreading a number. For example, .8 should be written as 0.8 to prevent it being read as the whole number 8. It is easy to miss a lone decimal point!

Key Points for Working with Decimals

Remember these points when working with decimals.

- Moving the decimal point one place to the right multiplies the number by ten. For example, 80.65 becomes 806.5 when you move the decimal point one place to the right, and $80.65 \times 10 = 806.5$
- Moving the decimal point one place to the left divides the number by ten. For example, 80.65 becomes 8.065 when you move the decimal point one place to the left, and $80.65 \div 10 = 8.065$

millions	hundred thousands	ten thousands	thousands	hundreds	tens	ones	.	tenths	hundredths	thousandths	ten thousandths	hundred thousandths	millionths

FIGURE 12-1 Place value.

• When calculating dosages, you only need to consider three places to the right of the decimal (thousandths), because drug dosages are not measured beyond this point.

PRACTICE Problems 12.1

Use the following problems to practice working with decimals.

Circle the number in each group with the highest value.

1. 2.4, 3.8, 3.1

2. 4.37, 6.05, 3.34

3. 1.4, 1.63, 11.19

4. 5.4, 3.86, 10.04

5. 6.23, 7.5, 12.19

Circle the number in each group with the lowest value.

6. 0.37, 0.11, 0.19

7. 7.53, 7.54, 7.05

8. 0.1, 0.32, 0.17

9. 1.125, 0.125, 1.1

10. 5.75, 2.95, 0.06

Rounding

As previously mentioned, in pharmacy practice decimals are considered at most to the thousandth, or third decimal, place, which means that some numbers must be rounded to the nearest tenth, hundredth, or thousandth for practical application. When rounding decimals, you should assume that you are rounding to the thousandth, unless instructed otherwise. Consider the following three steps:

1. Determine the appropriate decimal place to round to.
2. Look at the number directly to the right of the decimal place being rounded to.
3. If the number is 0, 1, 2, 3, or 4, the answer should be rounded down by simply removing the additional decimal places. If the number is 5, 6, 7, 8, or 9, the answer should be rounded up by removing the additional decimal places and increasing the number in the decimal place being rounded to by 1.

example 12.1

Round 24.2609 to the nearest:

thousandth   24.261

There is a 0 in the thousandth place and a 9 to its right—round up.

hundredth   24.26

There is a 6 in the hundredth place and a 0 to its right—round down.

tenth   24.3

There is a 2 in the tenth place and a 6 to its right—round up.

whole number   24

There is a 4 in the ones place and a 2 to its right—round down.

PRACTICE Problems 12.2

Use the following problems to practice rounding numbers.

Round 13.42891 to the nearest:

1. thousandth

2. tenth

3. hundredth

Round 0.96235 to the nearest:

4. whole number

5. thousandth

Adding and Subtracting Decimals

Although adding and subtracting decimals is a simple and basic skill, you must still pay attention to avoid making careless errors that can lead to significant adverse effects when dispensing medications. Consider the following three steps when adding or subtracting decimals:

1. Write the numbers vertically and line up the decimal points.
2. Add zero placeholders, if necessary.
3. Add/Subtract from right to left.

example 12.2

$0.89 + 0.76 = $ _____

$$
\begin{array}{r}
0.89 \\
+\ 0.76 \\
\hline
1.65
\end{array}
$$
  Add the 9 and 6 first, then the 8, the 7, and the 1 that was carried over.

So, $0.89 + 0.76 = 1.65$

example 12.3

Add 1.25 and 0.8 and 1.32.

$$
\begin{array}{r}
1.25 \\
0.80 \\
+\ 1.32 \\
\hline
3.37
\end{array}
$$
  Add a zero after the 8 as a placeholder to keep all of the numbers in line. Add the 5, 0, and 2; then the 2, 8, and 3; then the 1, 1, and the 1 that was carried.

So, $1.25 + 0.8 + 1.32 = 3.37$

example 12.4

4.45 − 2.25 = _____

$$\begin{array}{r} 4.45 \\ -\ 2.25 \\ \hline 2.20 \end{array}$$ Subtract the 5 from the 5, the 2 from the 4, and the 2 from the 4.

So, 4.45 − 2.25 = 2.20 or 2.2

example 12.5

Subtract 0.43 from 0.67

$$\begin{array}{r} 0.67 \\ -\ 0.43 \\ \hline 0.24 \end{array}$$ In word problems, the "from" figure should always be on top.
Subtract the 3 from the 7, then subtract the 4 from the 6.

So, 0.43 from 0.67 is 0.24

PRACTICE Problems 12.3

Use the following problems to practice adding and subtracting decimals.

Add the following decimals.

1. 3.65 + 1.27 = _____
2. 0.65 + 2.57 = _____
3. 1.32 + 4.01 = _____
4. 75.456 + 789.2 = _____
5. 5.002 + 7.28 + 0.012 = _____

Subtract the following decimals.

6. 402.89 − 2.9 = _____
7. 8.1 − 0.056 = _____
8. 68.22 − 4.026 = _____
9. 2.7 − 1.0024 = _____
10. 19.57 − 6.04 = _____

Multiplying Decimals

Multiplying decimals is a very simple process. The multiplication process is exactly the same as it is for whole numbers, with just one additional step at the end.

1. Multiply the numbers, ignoring the decimal points.
2. Add the total number of decimal places from the original numbers and then place a decimal point that number of places by moving from the right to the left of the answer. If there are not enough numbers for correct placement of the decimal point, add as many zeros as necessary.

example 12.6

$1.8 \times 2 =$ _____

$$
\begin{array}{r}
1.8 \\
\times\ 2 \\
\hline
36
\end{array}
$$
Multiply the top number by 2.

Now, add the total number of decimal point places in the original two numbers, which in this example is one.

Starting from the right, move one place to the left and add the decimal.

3.6

So, $1.8 \times 2 = 3.6$

example 12.7

$0.56 \times 0.12 =$ _____

$$
\begin{array}{r}
0.56 \\
\times\ 0.12 \\
\hline
112 \\
+\ 560 \\
\hline
672
\end{array}
$$

112   Multiply the top number by 2.

+ 560   Add a zero placeholder, then multiply the top number by 1.

Now, add the total number of decimal point places in the original two numbers—four.

Starting from the right, move four places to the left and add the decimal. A leading zero must be added, because the answer is only three digits.

0.0672

So, $0.56 \times 0.12 = 0.0672$

PRACTICE Problems 12.4

Use the following problems to practice multiplying decimals.

Multiply the following decimals.

1. $5.09 \times 0.5 =$ _____
2. $1.75 \times 3.4 =$ _____
3. $4.04 \times 2.25 =$ _____
4. $500 \times 0.015 =$ _____
5. $1.3 \times 4.7 =$ _____

Dividing Decimals

The division of decimal numbers requires several more steps than multiplication. This procedure must be done properly, and in order, to eliminate errors. The five steps you should follow to divide decimals are:

1. Place the dividend, or number to be divided, inside the division bracket.
2. Place the divisor, or number you are dividing by, outside the division bracket.

3. Change the divisor to a whole number by moving the decimal point all the way to the right.

4. Move the decimal point in the dividend the same number of places to the right as you did with the divisor.

5. Place a decimal point directly above the decimal in the dividend and divide as normal.

---

example 12.8

$10.08 \div 2.4 =$ _____

$2.4\overline{)10.08}$ Place the dividend in the division bracket and the divisor outside of it.

$24\overline{)100.8}$ Make the divisor a whole number by moving its decimal point to the right; then adjust the decimal point in the dividend by the same number of places.

$\overset{4.2}{\overline{}}$
$24\overline{)100.8}$ Place a decimal point above the decimal point in the dividend and divide as normal.
$\underline{96.}$
$\;\;48$
$\;\;\underline{48}$
$\;\;\;\;\underline{0}$

So, $10.08 \div 2.4 = 4.2$

PRACTICE Problems 12.5

Use the following problems to practice division of decimals.

Divide the following decimals.

1. $0.65 \div 0.4 =$ _____

2. $73 \div 13.40 =$ _____

3. $0.02 \div 0.006 =$ _____

4. $17.5 \div 2 =$ _____

5. $176 \div 2.2 =$ _____

Roman Numerals

Roman numerals letters and symbols used to represent numbers.

Roman numerals are used in health care to designate drug quantities. In the Roman system, letters or symbols are used to represent numbers. The symbols and their position are critical to your understanding and accurate deciphering of them. Study the Roman numerals and their Arabic equivalents shown in Table 12-2.

Rules for Roman Numerals

When working with Roman numerals, you must observe specific rules to ensure accuracy.

Rule 1.   Roman numerals are never repeated more than three times in a row.

Table 12-2 Roman Numerals

ROMAN NUMERAL	ARABIC EQUIVALENT
I	1
V	5
X	10
L	50
C	100
D	500
M	1000

example 12.9

Five is not represented as IIIII. It is represented as V.

Rule 2. When a Roman numeral is repeated, or when a smaller numeral follows a larger numeral, their values are added together.

example 12.10

$$III = 1 + 1 + 1 = 3$$
$$XXXI = 10 + 10 + 10 + 1 = 31$$
$$MDC = 1{,}000 + 500 + 100 = 1{,}600$$
$$VII = 5 + 1 + 1 = 7$$

Rule 3. When a smaller numeral comes before a larger numeral, the one of lesser value is subtracted from the larger value.

example 12.11

$$IV = 5 - 1 = 4$$
$$XL = 50 - 10 = 40$$
$$CM = 1{,}000 - 100 = 900$$
$$VL = 50 - 5 = 45$$

Rule 4. When a numeral of smaller value comes between two numerals of larger value, the subtraction rule is always applied first, then the addition rule.

example 12.12

$$XIV = 10 + (5 - 1) = 14$$
$$XLIX = (50 - 10) + (10 - 1) = 49$$
$$CVL = 100 + (50 - 5) = 145$$

" Workplace Wisdom Roman Numerals

- Ones (I) may only be subtracted from fives (V) and tens (X).
- Tens (X) can only be subtracted from fifties (L) and hundreds (C).
- Hundreds (C) may only be subtracted from five hundreds (D) and thousands (M). "

PRACTICE Problems 12.6

Use the following problems to practice converting Roman and Arabic numerals.

Convert the following Arabic numbers to Roman numerals.

1. 94 = _____

2. 367 = _____

3. 28 = _____

4. 2,650 = _____

5. 368 = _____

Convert the following Roman numerals to Arabic numerals.

6. XXXIX = _____

7. CCXIX = _____

8. DCCCXCVIII = _____

9. MCMXCIV = _____

10. XLIX = _____

Perform the indicated operations. Record the answers in Arabic numerals.

11. CCXX + CD = _____

12. MMXL − DCCIX = _____

13. XIII × IV = _____

14. LXVIII ÷ II = _____

15. XIX − IV = _____

proper fraction a fraction in which the value of the numerator is smaller than the value of the denominator.

common fraction a fraction written with a numerator that is separated by a fraction line and positioned above a denominator.

denominator the bottom value of a fraction; placed beneath the fraction line.

numerator the top value of a fraction; placed above the fraction line.

fraction line symbol representing the division of two values; placed between the numerator and the denominator of a fraction.

Fractions

A **proper fraction** is a quantity that is less than a whole number. There are two types of fractions: **common fractions**, such as $\frac{1}{2}$, $\frac{3}{8}$, and so on; and decimal fractions, such as 0.5, 0.78, and so on. We covered decimal fractions earlier in this chapter, so this section focuses on common fractions.

A common fraction consists of three parts: the **denominator**, which is the number below the fraction line; the **numerator**, which is the number above the fraction line; and the **fraction line**, which separates the numerator and denominator. Technically, the fraction line represents a division symbol, because $\frac{1}{2}$ translates to 1 ÷ 2.

$$\text{Numerator} \rightarrow \frac{1}{2} \leftarrow \text{Denominator}$$

The denominator indicates the total number of parts into which the whole is divided. The numerator indicates the number of parts used or being considered.

There are four basic types, or categories, of common fractions: proper fractions, improper fractions, simple fractions, and complex fractions.

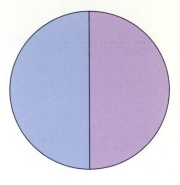

Proper Fractions

A *proper fraction* is a fraction in which the value of the numerator is smaller than the value of the denominator.

example **12.13**   **Proper Fractions**

$$\frac{1}{2}$$

$$\frac{4}{8}$$

$$\frac{9}{10}$$

Improper Fractions

An **improper fraction** is a fraction in which the value of the numerator is larger than the value of the denominator.

improper fraction a fraction in which the value of the numerator is larger than the value of the denominator.

example **12.14**   **Improper Fractions**

$$\frac{3}{2}$$

$$\frac{7}{3}$$

$$\frac{12}{11}$$

Simple Fractions

When a proper fraction is reduced to its lowest terms, it is considered a **simple fraction**.

simple fraction a proper fraction, with both the numerator and denominator reduced to lowest terms.

example **12.15**   **Simple Fractions**

$\frac{4}{8}$ is a proper fraction, but it can be reduced by dividing both the numerator and denominator by 4, producing $\frac{1}{2}$, which is a simple fraction. That is, it cannot be reduced any further.

complex fraction a fraction in which both the numerator and the denominator are themselves common fractions.

Complex Fractions

A **complex fraction** is a fraction in which both the numerator and denominator are themselves fractions.

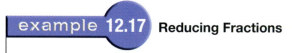

example **12.16** Complex Fractions

$$\dfrac{\frac{1}{6}}{\frac{1}{4}}$$

Rules for Calculating with Fractions

Certain rules must be observed when working with, and calculating, fractions. Understanding of these rules is a necessary foundation; you will use them when you later learn to solve ratios and proportions, and do most pharmacy calculations.

Rule: Reducing Fractions to Lowest Terms

To reduce a fraction to its lowest terms, thereby making it a simple fraction, you simply divide both the numerator and the denominator by the largest whole number that will go evenly into them both.

example **12.17** Reducing Fractions

Reduce $\frac{4}{16}$ to its lowest terms.

The largest whole number that will divide evenly into both 4 (the numerator) and 16 (the denominator) is 4.

$4 \div 4 = 1$

$16 \div 4 = 4$

So $\frac{4}{16}$ reduces to $\frac{1}{4}$.

Rule: Converting Improper Fractions

Improper fractions can be converted to an equivalent whole number or mixed number by dividing the numerator by the denominator. Any remainder should be expressed as a proper fraction and reduced to lowest terms.

example **12.18** Converting Improper Fractions

$\frac{21}{7}$ is an improper fraction.

If you divide the numerator (21) by the denominator (7), you get 3, a whole number.

$$\frac{21}{7} = 21 \div 7 = 3$$

$\frac{4}{3}$ is also an improper fraction.

The denominator (3) will only go into the numerator (4) one time, with a remainder of 1, which becomes $\frac{1}{3}$ when you place the remainder over the original denominator.

$$\frac{4}{3} = 4 \div 3 = 1\frac{1}{3}$$

Workplace Wisdom Converting Mixed Fractions

To convert a mixed fraction to an improper fraction, simply multiply the whole number by the denominator and add that number to the numerator. For example, $1\frac{2}{3}$ would be converted to $\frac{5}{3}$, by multiplying 1×3, which equals 3, and then adding that to the numerator, which is 2. Upon adding 3 to the numerator (3 + 2), the new numerator becomes 5, the denominator stays the same, and the whole number can be removed.

Rule: Adding and Subtracting Fractions

To add or subtract fractions, the fractions must all have the same denominator. If necessary, each fraction can be converted to a fraction with the least common denominator; then you can add or subtract the numerators.

example 12.19 Adding Fractions

$$\frac{1}{4} + \frac{1}{4} = \underline{\hspace{3cm}}$$

Because both fractions have the same denominator, simply add the numerators (1 + 1) and place this over the common denominator.

$$\frac{1}{4} + \frac{1}{4} = \frac{2}{4}$$

$\frac{2}{4}$ can then be reduced to $\frac{1}{2}$.

$$\frac{1}{2} + \frac{1}{3} = \underline{\hspace{3cm}}$$

These two fractions have different denominators, so the least common denominator must first be determined, which in this case is 6.

Now, both fractions must be converted to contain a denominator of 6.

$$\frac{1}{2} \times \frac{3}{3} = \frac{3}{6}$$

$$\frac{1}{3} \times \frac{2}{2} = \frac{2}{6}$$

$$\frac{3}{6} + \frac{2}{6} = \frac{5}{6}$$

example 12.20 Subtracting Fractions

$$\frac{9}{10} - \frac{7}{10} = \underline{\hspace{2cm}}$$

These two fractions have the same denominator, so you can subtract the numerators (9 − 7) to get 2.

$$\frac{9}{10} - \frac{7}{10} = \frac{2}{10}$$

$\frac{2}{10}$ can be further reduced to $\frac{1}{5}$.

$$\frac{4}{5} - \frac{1}{10} = \underline{\hspace{2cm}}$$

Because these two fractions do not have the same denominator, the least common denominator must be established, which in this case is 10.

$$\frac{4}{5} \times \frac{2}{2} = \frac{8}{10}$$

$$\frac{8}{10} - \frac{1}{10} = \frac{7}{10}$$

Rule: Multiplying Fractions

When multiplying fractions, multiply the numerators by the numerators and then the denominators by the denominators. Reduce to lowest terms.

example 12.21 Multiplying Fractions

$$\frac{4}{9} \times \frac{6}{8} = \underline{\hspace{2cm}}$$

$4 \times 6 = 24$

$9 \times 8 = 72$

So $\frac{4}{9} \times \frac{6}{8} = \frac{24}{72}$, which can be reduced to $\frac{1}{3}$

Rule: Dividing Fractions

To divide fractions, invert (flip upside down) the divisor, and then multiply the two fractions. Reduce to lowest terms.

Workplace Wisdom Reciprocals

The inverted fraction used when dividing fractions is referred to as the *reciprocal*.

example 12.22 Dividing Fractions

$\dfrac{2}{8} \div \dfrac{3}{7} = $ _____

$\dfrac{2}{8} \times \dfrac{7}{3} = $ _____

$2 \times 7 = 14$

$8 \times 3 = 24$

$\dfrac{2}{8} \div \dfrac{3}{7} = \dfrac{14}{24}$, which can be reduced to $\dfrac{7}{12}$

PRACTICE Problems 12.7 Calculating Fractions

Add the following fractions.

1. $\dfrac{1}{6} + \dfrac{3}{4} + \dfrac{2}{12} = $ _____

2. $\dfrac{2}{3} + \dfrac{1}{2} + \dfrac{1}{4} = $ _____

3. $1\dfrac{3}{8} + 1\dfrac{4}{5} = $ _____

Subtract the following fractions.

4. $\dfrac{5}{16} - \dfrac{1}{8} = $ _____

5. $6\dfrac{5}{12} - 3\dfrac{2}{12} = $ _____

6. $\dfrac{1}{2} - \dfrac{1}{5} = $ _____

Multiply the following fractions.

7. $\dfrac{3}{8} \times \dfrac{5}{12} = $ _____

8. $\dfrac{2}{3} \times \dfrac{5}{8} = $ _____

9. $1\dfrac{1}{5} \times \dfrac{2}{3} = $ _____

Divide the following fractions.

10. $\dfrac{7}{8} \div \dfrac{5}{6} = $ _____

11. $\dfrac{1}{4} \div \dfrac{1}{2} = $ _____

12. $7 \div \dfrac{2}{3} = $ _____

Ratios and Proportions

Ratios and proportions are basic math skills that can be effective in solving the majority of pharmacy calculations. The rest of the chapters in this book rely heavily on a solid comprehension of working with ratios and proportions, so it is very important that you understand the following information.

Ratios

ratio the expression of a relationship of two numbers, separated by a colon (:).

A **ratio** expresses the relationship of two numbers and is separated by a colon (:), just as a fraction expresses the relationship of two numbers and is separated by a fraction line. For example, if an ointment contained 1 g of active ingredient for every 10 g of ointment base, a relationship, or ratio, is established regarding the amount of active ingredient compared to the amount of inactive ingredient (1:10).

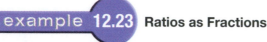 **example 12.23** Ratios as Fractions

1:2 is a ratio and is read as "1 to 2."

This ratio can be rewritten as a fraction, $\frac{1}{2}$, read as "1 over 2."

The ratio 3:8 can be rewritten as the fraction $\frac{3}{8}$.

PRACTICE Problems 12.8 Ratios as Fractions

Convert the following ratios to fractions and reduce to lowest terms.

1. 2:4 = _____
2. 6:8 = _____
3. 1:25 = _____

Fractions can just as easily be converted to ratios. Rewrite the numerator as the first number followed by a colon (:) and then the denominator as the second number in the ratio.

example 12.24 Fractions as Ratios

The fraction $\frac{5}{8}$, stated as 5 over 8, can be restated as 5:8, or 5 to 8.

PRACTICE Problems 12.9 Fractions as Ratios

Convert the following fractions to ratios.

1. $\frac{4}{5}$ = _____

2. $\frac{9}{10}$ = _____

3. $\frac{1}{400}$ = _____

To convert a ratio to a percentage, rewrite the ratio as a fraction, divide the numerator by the denominator, then multiply by 100 and add the percentage sign (%) to the answer.

---

example 12.25 **Ratios as Percentages**

$1 : 4 =$ _____%

$1 : 4 = \dfrac{1}{4}$

$1 \div 4 = 0.25$

$0.25 \times 100 = 25$

$1 : 4 = 25\%$

PRACTICE Problems 12.10 Ratios as Percentages

Convert the following ratios to percentages.

1. $4 : 5 =$ _____
2. $1 : 25 =$ _____
3. $1 : 200 =$ _____
4. $1 : 10 =$ _____
5. $4 : 16 =$ _____

Proportions

Proportions are two, or more, equivalent ratios or fractions that both represent the same value. The majority of pharmacy calculations are performed by establishing a proportion and then solving for the unknown. This can be illustrated by referring back to our previous example of the ointment that contains 1 g of active ingredient per 10 g of ointment base. If you know that you need 10 g of active ingredient, then you can use a proportion to determine the amount of inactive ointment base required.

Proportions are written as two ratios or fractions separated by a double colon symbol (::). The double colon symbol translates to "equals" or "is equal to," so the equal sign (=) is sometimes used in place of the double colon symbol.

proportion two, or more, equivalent ratios or fractions that both represent the same value.

---

example 12.26 **Samples of Proportions**

$1 : 4 :: 2 : 8$

$2 : 3 = 6 : 9$

$\dfrac{3}{5} :: \dfrac{6}{10}$

$\dfrac{4}{7} = \dfrac{8}{14}$

---

cross-multiplication a
principle used in solving
pharmacy calculations; you
set up two ratios or fractions
in relationship to each other
as a proportion and solve for
the unknown variable.

Solving for X

Cross-multiplication is a critical principle to understand in solving pharmacy calculations. Once you have set up two ratios or fractions in relationship to each other as a proportion, you can cross-multiply to solve for the unknown (X).

There are two approaches to using cross-multiplication to solve for X. You should practice using both methods and then use the approach you are most comfortable with.

In the first approach, you set the proportion up as fractions, making sure to keep units of measurement the same across from one another. Cross-multiply along the diagonal with two numbers and divide that value by the remaining number to solve for X.

example 12.27 Solving for X

$2 : 10 :: X : 30$

First, set up the proportion as fractions.

$$\frac{2}{10} = \frac{X}{30}$$

Multiply along the diagonal with two numbers (2 and 30).

$2 \times 30 = 60$

Divide that value by the remaining number to solve for X.

$60 \div 10 = 6$

$X = 6$

So, 2:10 :: 6:30

In the second approach, you again set the proportion up as fractions, making sure to keep units of measurement the same across from one another. This time, however, you cross-multiply along both diagonals to establish an equation, which you can solve for X.

example 12.28 Solving for X

$3 : 5 :: 12 : X$

First set up the proportion as fractions.

$$\frac{3}{5} = \frac{12}{X}$$

Then, cross-multiply both diagonals to establish an equation.

$3 \times X = 3X$

$5 \times 12 = 60$

$3X = 60$

Now you can use basic algebra to solve for X. In this example, that is done by dividing both sides of the equation by 3.

$$\frac{3X}{3} = \frac{60}{3}$$

X = 20

So, 3:5 :: 12:20

PRACTICE Problems 12.11 Solving for X

Using cross-multiplication, solve for X.

1. 1:2 :: X:14

2. 233:1 :: X:15

3. 4:9 = X:81

4. X:10 :: 25:50

5. 12.5:X = 75:600

INFORMATION

Consider the following tips for working with word problems.
RQWQCQ is a useful strategy when solving math word problems. Each of the letters in RQWQCQ stands for a step in the strategy.

Read—First read the entire problem to fully understand it. You may find it helpful to read the problem out loud, visualize the problem in your mind, or even draw a picture of the problem.

Question—Determine the question to be answered in the problem. Often the question is directly stated. When it is not stated, you will have to identify the question to be answered.

Write—List all of the facts provided in the problem. Then cross out any facts presented in the problem that are not needed to answer the question. Often, you will not need all of the facts presented in the problem to answer the question; the extraneous details can simply cause confusion.

Question—Ask yourself, "What computations must I do to answer the problem?"

Compute—Set up the problem on paper and do the computations. Check your computations for accuracy and make any needed corrections.

Question—Look at your answer and then ask yourself, "Is this answer possible?" You may find that your answer is not possible because it does not fit the facts presented in the problem. If this happens, go back through the steps of RQWQCQ until you arrive at an answer that is possible.

PROFILES IN PRACTICE

Paul is currently a pharmacy technician student. Although his grades are good, Paul is struggling with pharmacy calculations, as math was never his strongest point. Frustrated, Paul wonders why he needs to learn so much math to become a pharmacy technician.

- Why is it important for students, such as Paul, to have a strong knowledge of math to practice as pharmacy technicians?

SUMMARY

Although none of the material covered in this chapter should have been new to you, sometimes you need a solid, basic math review. As you prepare to learn and understand the calculations performed in pharmacy, remember that all the calculations you will learn are based on the basic skills covered in this chapter. If you find that you are still having difficulty with the problems presented in this chapter, you should continue to go over this material before proceeding.

CHAPTER REVIEW QUESTIONS

Carry answers to three decimal places and round to two places. Express fractions in lowest terms.

Circle the decimal in each group with the highest value.

1. 4.1, 4.01, 4.001

2. 6.0, 4.5, 2.8

3. 0.2, 0.5, 0.8

4. 0.2, 0.13, 0.26

5. 3.7, 3.6, 2.35

Circle the decimal in each group with the lowest value.

6. 1.233, 1.844, 1.999

7. 4.8, 7.8, 10.8

8. 0.05, 0.5, 0.115

9. 14.03, 16.03, 12.01

10. 1.25, 3.5, 1.26

Complete the operations indicated.

11. $1.233 + 12.01 =$ _____

12. $40.25 - 16.37 =$ _____

13. $0.65 \times 10.467 =$ _____

14. $13.2 \times 31.62 =$ _____

15. $1.25 \div 0.5 =$ _____

Convert to Roman numerals.

16. 7 _____

17. 25 _____

18. 84 _____

19. 67 _____

20. 472 _____

Convert to Arabic numbers.

21. XXIV _____

22. MMLV _____

23. LXXXVI _____

24. MCMXCV _____

25. LXXVIII _____

Complete the operations indicated.

26. $\dfrac{2}{4} + \dfrac{1}{3} =$ _____

27. $3\dfrac{1}{5} + 2\dfrac{2}{10} =$ _____

28. $\dfrac{4}{5} - \dfrac{1}{10} =$ _____

29. $\dfrac{6}{8} - \dfrac{1}{4} =$ _____

30. $\dfrac{5}{6} + \dfrac{3}{30} + \dfrac{3}{5} =$ _____

31. $\dfrac{2}{3} \times \dfrac{5}{8} =$ _____

32. $4\dfrac{2}{3} \times 3 =$ _____

33. $\dfrac{1}{15} \times \dfrac{6}{30} =$ _____

34. $4 \div \dfrac{3}{4} =$ _____

35. $\dfrac{25}{100} \times \dfrac{6}{10} =$ _____

36. $\dfrac{7}{8} \div \dfrac{5}{6} =$ _____

37. $8 \div \dfrac{1}{3} =$ _____

38. $\dfrac{3}{4} \div 20 =$ _____

39. $6\dfrac{1}{2} + 3\dfrac{2}{4} =$ _____

40. $4\dfrac{3}{8} \div 2\dfrac{2}{4} =$ _____

Solve the following word problems.

41. A patient is to take a medication that contains 0.6 mg per tablet. He is to take 1 tablet every 2 hours until pain is relieved. If it takes 5 tablets to obtain the desired effect, the patient took how many milligrams of drug? _____

42. Human blood has a pH of 7.4. A urine test shows a pH of 4.6 for the patient's urine. What is the difference in pH between the blood and the urine? _____

43. A patient takes 0.625 mg of drug twice a day for 7 days. What is the total dose? _____

44. A patient is taking 0.5 oz. of cough syrup per dose. If the bottle contains 20.5 oz., how many doses are in the bottle? _____

45. The cornerstone of the hospital shows the date when the hospital was built as MCMLXV. When was the hospital built? _____

46. A child is to receive X grains of a medication that is available in V-grain tablets. How many tablets should the child receive? _____

47. A laboratory technician uses $\frac{1}{4}$ oz., $\frac{2}{3}$ oz., and $\frac{3}{8}$ oz. of solution to prepare an IV admixture. How much total solution does she use? _____

48. A pediatric nurse measures a 1-year-old child and finds that the child is $40\frac{1}{4}$ in. tall. At birth she was $20\frac{3}{4}$ in. tall. How much did the child grow in one year? _____

49. A pharmacy technician uses a 240 mL bottle of cough syrup to fill unit-dose vials. If each vial holds $\frac{1}{15}$ of the volume of the stock bottle of cough syrup, how many milliliters of cough syrup are in each vial? _____

50. How many $\frac{1}{3}$ g doses can be dispensed from a stock bottle containing 12 g? _____

REFERENCES AND RESOURCES

Hegstad, LN, & Hayek, W. *Essential Drug Dosage Calculations* (4th ed.). Upper Saddle River, NJ: Pearson, 2001.

Johnston, M. *Pharmacy Calculations.* Upper Saddle River, NJ: Pearson, 2005.

Lesmeister, MB. *Math Basics for the Healthcare Professional* (2nd ed.). Upper Saddle River, NJ: Pearson, 2005.

Mikolah, AA. *Drug Dosage Calculations for the Emergency Care Provider* (2nd ed.). Upper Saddle River, NJ: Prentice-Hall, 2003.

Olsen, JL, Giangrasso, AP, & Shrimpton, D. *Medical Dosage Calculations* (8th ed.). Upper Saddle River, NJ: Pearson, 2004.

13 Measurement Systems

LEARNING OBJECTIVES

After completing this chapter, you should be able to:

- List the three fundamental systems of measurement.
- List the three primary units of the metric system.
- Define the various prefixes used in the metric system.
- Recognize abbreviations used in measurements.
- Explain the use of International Units and milliequivalents.
- Convert measurements between the household system and the metric system.
- Convert measurements between the apothecary system and the metric system.
- Perform temperature conversions.

Introduction

Three fundamental systems of measurement are used to calculate dosages: the metric, apothecary, and household systems. Pharmacy technicians must understand each system and how to convert from one system to another. Most prescriptions are written using the metric system.

The Metric System

The need for an international measurement system was recognized more than 300 years ago. In 1670, Gabriel Mouton proposed a measurement system based on the length of one minute of arc of a great circle of the earth. In 1671, Jean Picard suggested the length of a pendulum beating seconds as the unit of length. Other proposals were also made, but it was more than 100 years before any decisions were made.

In 1790, the National Assembly of France asked the French Academy of Sciences to deduce an invariable standard for all the measures and all the weights. The commission developed the **metric system**, a system that was both simple and scientific. The unit of length was set as a portion of the earth's circumference. Measures for volume and mass were derived from the unit of length, so that all units of measurement in the system would be related.

> **metric system** the international and scientific standard system of measurement; based on the meter, the gram, and the liter.

The metric system uses decimals to indicate tenths, hundredths, and thousandths; larger and smaller versions of each unit were created by multiplying or dividing the basic units by 10. This feature provides great convenience to users of the system. Similar calculations in the metric system can be performed simply by shifting the decimal point; therefore, the metric system is a *base 10* or *decimal* system.

The metric system is the most widely used system of measurement in the world today. It is more accurate than the household and apothecary systems and is preferred for healthcare applications because it is both more precise and the most common.

The metric system is based on these three primary units:

- **meter**, which measures length
- **liter**, which measures volume
- **gram**, which measures weight

> **meter** metric system's primary unit of length.
>
> **liter** metric system's primary unit of volume.
>
> **gram** metric system's primary unit of weight.

Prefixes are added when necessary to indicate larger or smaller units. The four prefixes most commonly used in pharmaceutical calculations are:

- kilo- = 1000, or one thousand of the base unit
- centi- = 0.01, or one-hundredth of the base unit
- milli- = 0.001, or one-thousandth of the base unit
- micro- = 0.000001, or one-millionth of the base unit

Tables 13-1 and 13-2 show the metric measurements and abbreviations you will encounter most frequently in everyday pharmacy practice.

Guidelines for Metric Notation

Use the following guidelines when working with metric notations.

1. Always place the number before the abbreviation. For example, write:

   4 mg, not mg 4

2. Place a zero to the left of the decimal when the decimal is less than 1. For example, write:

   Synthroid 0.2 mg, not Synthroid .2 mg

Table 13-1   Metric Units of Measurement

LENGTH	WEIGHT	VOLUME
meter (m)	gram (g or gm)	liter (l or L)
centimeter (cm)	milligram (mg)	milliliter (ml or mL)
millimeter (mm)	microgram (mcg)	
	kilogram (kg or Kg)	

Remember: A cubic centimeter (cc) is often used to denote a milliliter.

Table 13-2 Metric System Prefixes with Standard Measures

	UNIT	ABBREVIATION	EQUIVALENTS
Weight	gram	g or gm	1 g = 1,000 mg
	milligram	mg	1 mg = 1,000 mcg = 0.001 g
	microgram	mcg	1 mcg = 0.001 mg = 0.000001 g
	kilogram	kg	1 kg = 1,000 g
Volume	liter	L or l	1 L = 1,000 mL
	milliliter	mL or ml	1 mL = 1 cc = 0.001 L
	cubic centimeter	cc	1 cc = 1 mL = 0.001 L
Length	meter	m	1 m = 100 cm = 1,000 mm
	centimeter	cm	1 cm = 0.01 m = 10 mm
	millimeter	mm	1 mm = 0.001 m = 0.1 cm

This is a critical rule, as it will help prevent confusion and possible dosage error; in this case, 2 mg might be given if the decimal is not noticed.

3. Never place a zero to the right of the decimal place when you have a whole number. For example, write:

   a patient weighs 20 kg, not 20.0 kg

4. Always use decimals to reflect fractions when using the metric system. For example, write:

   6.5 mL, not 6 1/2 mL

5. Avoid unnecessary zeros. For example, write:

   3.2 g, not 3.20000 g

6. When converting from small units to larger units, make sure your number decreases proportionately. For example, write:

   2,000 mg = 2 g

7. When converting from large units to smaller units, make sure your number increases proportionately. For example, write:

   20 kg = 20,000 g

8. When multiplying metric values by multiples of 10, move the decimal point one place to the right for each zero in the multiplier.

9. When dividing metric values by multiples of 10, move the decimal point one place to the left for each zero in the divisor.

10. When in doubt, do not guess about the correct meaning. Always check when clarification is needed. A one-decimal-place error in dosing can be fatal to a patient!

━━━━━━━━━━━━━━ **INFORMATION** ━━━━━━━━━━━━━━

Here is a shortcut for converting between the most common units of the metric system.

kg	→	g	Move the decimal 3 places to the right
kg	→	mg	Move the decimal 6 places to the right
kg	→	mcg	Move the decimal 9 places to the right
g	→	kg	Move the decimal 3 places to the left
g	→	mg	Move the decimal 3 places to the right
g	→	mcg	Move the decimal 6 places to the right

mg → kg   Move the decimal 6 places to the left
mg → g   Move the decimal 3 places to the left
mg → mcg Move the decimal 3 places to the right

mcg → kg   Move the decimal 9 places to the left
mcg → g   Move the decimal 6 places to the left
mcg → mg   Move the decimal 3 place to the left

Please note that you can substitute liters or meters in place of grams for this chart.

PRACTICE Problems 13.1

Write the following metric measures using correct abbreviations denoting unit of measure.

1. five micrograms _____

2. two tenths of a milligram _____

3. sixteen grams _____

4. five hundredths of a kilogram _____

5. ten milliliters _____

6. three and one tenth liters _____

7. two tenths of a microgram _____

8. five hundred milligrams _____

9. six hundredths of a gram _____

10. one hundred milliliters _____

11. forty-one liters _____

12. seven tenths of a microgram _____

13. eight hundredths of a milligram _____

14. two thousand grams _____

15. four and one tenth milliliters _____

16. three hundred fifty liters _____

17. seven and four tenths grams _____

18. one thousand micrograms _____

19. fifteen hundred milligrams _____

20. one and one fifth kilograms _____

Convert the following metric units.

21. 25 mcg = _____ mg

22. 100 mg = _____ g

23. 0.6 g = _____ kg

24. 1.5 kg = _____ g

25. 0.22 g = _____ mg

26. 1,500 mg = _____ mcg

27. 1,000 mcg = _____ mg

28. 15.6 L = _____ mL

29. 1,500 mL = _____ L

30. 0.2008 kg = _____ mcg

31. 566.32 mL = _____ L

32. 988 mg = _____ g

33. 0.0125 g = _____ mg

34. 7,500 mL = _____ L

35. 0.789 L = _____ mL

36. 100 mcg = _____ g

37. 6,000,000 g = _____ kg

38. 105 L = _____ mL

39. 2,000 g = _____ mcg

40. 1 L = _____ mL

PRACTICE Problems 13.2

When solving the following problems, convert everything to the same units.

1. A newborn weighs 2,800 g. What is her weight in kilograms? _____

2. A patient receives a prescription for 3 g of an antibiotic. The tablets on the shelf are 250 mg. How many tablets should the patient take? _____

3. A patient is to receive 1.5 g of cephalexin per day divided into three equal doses.

   a. If the capsules are available in 100 mg, 250 mg, and 500 mg, which dosage should be used? _____

   b. If the dosage is increased to 2 g per day divided into four equal doses, what dosage should be used? _____

4. A pharmacy technician must combine four partially filled bottles of powder into one. How many grams of powder does she have if the bottles contain 240 g, 0.45 kg, 2,300 mg, and 22,000 mcg? _____

5. How many grams of aminophylline would be required to prepare 500 capsules of 7.5 mg each? _____

6. How many 180 mL bottles can be filled with 6.5 L of cough syrup? _____

7. A technician is preparing a compound. The prescription requires 350 mg of dextrose, 500 mg of sodium, and 150 mcg of potassium per 1,000 mL. What is the total weight in grams of the dry ingredients? _____

8. If the total dose is 0.85 g and the drug is given in four equal doses, what is the amount of each dose in milligrams? _____

9. A wholesaler is selling 250 g of a compounding powder for $8.52. How many grams can you get for $40? _____

10. You have acetaminophen tablets in 500 mg strength. If the prescription calls for 250 mg twice daily for five days, how many tablets would you give? _____

PROFILES IN PRACTICE

Sheba is a pharmacy technician who works in a mail-order pharmacy. When translating a prescription for data entry, she mistook 10 mcg for 10 mg.

- What effect will Sheba's mistake, if not caught, have on the patient?

International Units

A number of drugs, such as insulin, heparin, and penicillin, are measured in **International Units (IU)**. Therefore, pharmacy technicians must be able to recognize unit dosages and their official abbreviations. An International Unit measures a drug in terms of its action, not its physical weight.

When writing International Units, do not use commas in the unit value unless it has at least five numbers (for example, 25,000 units). Remember to write out the word *unit*(s) and do not use the abbreviation IU, as it could be easily misread as a Roman numeral or as an abbreviation for *intravenous*.

International Units (IU) measurement of a drug in terms of its action, not its physical weight.

PRACTICE Problems 13.3

Express the following unit dosages using the correct numeric notation and abbreviation(s).

1. twenty units _____

2. ten thousand units _____

3. one million units _____

4. fifty-three units _____

5. two hundred thousand units _____

6. twenty-three hundred units _____

7. one hundred units _____

8. one thousand units _____

9. sixty units _____

10. seven hundred units _____

Milliequivalent

A **milliequivalent (mEq)** is the number of grams of a drug in 1 mL of a normal solution. Potassium chloride is a common example of a drug expressed in milliequivalents. Dosages are written with the number followed by the abbreviation (for example, 20 mEq).

milliequivalent (mEq) unit of measurement based on the number of grams of a drug in 1 mL of a normal solution.

PRACTICE Problems 13.4

Express the following milliequivalent dosages using the correct numeric notation and abbreviation(s).

1. fifty milliequivalents _____

2. thirty milliequivalents _____

3. forty milliequivalents _____

4. five milliequivalents _____

5. fifteen milliequivalents _____

6. twenty milliequivalents _____

7. eighty milliequivalents _____

8. one hundred milliequivalents _____

9. ten milliequivalents _____

10. fifty-five milliequivalents _____

The Apothecary System

apothecary system an old English system of measurement of weight, based on the grain.

grain the primary unit of weight in the apothecary system.

The **apothecary system** is an old English system of measurement. Even though it will probably be replaced exclusively by the metric system within a few years, it is still used today for certain medications. The **grain** is the primary unit of weight in this system. The abbreviation for grain is *gr*. The basic units for volume or liquid measurement are the minim, the fluid dram, and the fluid ounce, as shown in Tables 13-3 and 13-4.

Table 13-3   Apothecary Weights

20 grains (gr) = 1 scruple
3 scruples = 1 dram = 60 grains
8 drams = 1 ounce (oz.) = 480 grains
12 ounces = 1 pound = 5,760 grains

Table 13-4   Apothecary Fluid Measures

60 minims = 1 fluid dram
8 fluid drams = 1 fluid ounce = 480 minims
16 fluid ounces = 1 pint
2 pints = 1 quart = 32 fluid ounces
4 quarts = 1 gallon = 128 fluid ounces

The Avoirdupois System

avoirdupois system the current American system of measurement of weight, based on a pound being equivalent to 16 ounces.

The **avoirdupois system** (see Table 13-5) is another system used only for measuring weight; it is also being replaced by the metric system. The name derives from the Old French term *avoir de pois*, meaning "goods of weight" and referring to goods sold by weight rather than by the piece. This system, which is based on 1 pound being equivalent to 16 ounces, is the weight system most commonly used in the United States, and it is still used extensively in Canada and the United Kingdom as well.

Table 13-5   Avoirdupois Weights

1 ounce (oz.) = 4,375 grains (gr) = 28.4 g
16 oz. = 1 pound (lb.) = 7,000 gr

The Household System

household system the system of measurement commonly used in American households, usually related to food and beverages.

Household units are used primarily to assist the patient with measuring while at home. Pharmacy technicians should be familiar with **household system** measurements so that they can explain medication directions easily in understandable terms, such as simply telling the patient to take 1 teaspoon (tsp.) instead of 5 mL (see Tables 13-6 and 13-7).

Table 13-6   Household Measure Equivalents

3 teaspoons (tsp.) = 1 tablespoon (Tbsp.)
2 tablespoons = 1 fluid ounce (fl. oz.)
8 fluid ounces = 1 cup
2 cups = 1 pint (pt.)
2 pints = 1 quart (qt.)
4 quarts = 1 gallon (gal.)

Table 13-7   Household Measures and Metric Equivalents

1 tsp. = 5 mL
1 Tbsp. = 15 mL
1 fl. oz. = 30 mL
1 cup = 240 mL
2.2 lb. = 1 kg
1 mL = 20 drops (gtt)

PRACTICE Problems 13.5

Express the following measurements using the correct abbreviation.

1. 50 milliequivalents _____

2. 10 teaspoons _____

3. 15 ounces _____

4. 10 tablespoons _____

5. one hundred units _____

6. seven drops _____

7. two pints _____

8. six quarts _____

9. three gallons _____

10. five hundred units _____

11. ten grains _____

12. one-half ounce _____

13. sixteen pints _____

14. two and one-half grains _____

15. thirty ounces _____

Converting Measurements

Although the metric system is used almost exclusively in pharmacy, the other systems of measurement, including the apothecary system, the avoirdupois system, and the household system, are used in certain cases. As a pharmacy technician, you will need to convert units of measure from one system of measurement to another.

Because pharmacies stock only a fraction of the drugs and dosage forms available, it is sometimes necessary to convert an order to match the stock on hand. Several conversion factors will help you convert apothecary and household values to the metric system (see Tables 13-8 and 13-9). However, these conversion factors are not absolute; the relationships are considered approximate equivalents. Therefore, you should choose the most direct route through a calculation. Remember, your job is to be sure the prescribed drug is delivered to the patient accurately calculated.

INFORMATION

If the system is not stated, assume that 16 oz. = 1 lb.

Converting the Household System

Converting between the metric and household systems is just a matter of memorizing the conversion factors and using them. Because the metric system is the most widely used (and preferred for accuracy), you should perform conversions to and from the metric system (see Table 13-10). Be aware that there are minor differences between the various systems. One example to note is the pound. In the apothecary system, 1 lb. = 12 oz., whereas in the household system 1 lb. = 16 oz.

You can perform conversions between the household and metric systems by setting up proportions as fractions and then multiplying the fractions to get the correct answer.

Formula: Conversion of Systems

This formula can be used to convert measurements between the various systems discussed.

$$\text{Units that you have} \times \frac{\text{Number of units that you want}}{\text{Units that you have}}$$

Table 13-8   Household Measure Equivalents

3 teaspoons = 1 tablespoon
2 tablespoons = 1 fluid ounce
8 fluid ounces = 1 cup
2 cups = 1 pint
2 pints = 1 quart
4 quarts = 1 gallon

Table 13-9   Household to Metric Conversions

HOUSEHOLD MEASURE		METRIC EQUIVALENT
1 teaspoon	=	5 mL
1 tablespoon	=	15 mL
1 fluid ounce	=	30 mL
1 pint	=	480 mL
1 gallon	=	3,840 mL
1 cup	=	240 mL
1 ounce	=	28.4 g
1 pound	=	454 g
1 pound	=	16 oz.

Table 13-10   Apothecary to Metric Conversion

APOTHECARY MEASURE		METRIC EQUIVALENT
15 minims	=	1 mL
1 fluid dram	=	4 mL
1 fluid ounce	=	30 mL
1 ounce	=	8 drams
1 dram	=	60 grains
6 fluid ounces	=	180 mL
8 fluid ounces	=	240 mL
16 fluid ounces	=	500 mL
32 fluid ounces	=	1,000 mL
1 grain	=	65 mg
1 ounce	=	140 grains
15 grains	=	1 g
1 pound	=	12 oz.
2.2 pounds	=	1 kg

example 13.1

Convert 5 tsp. to milliliters.

$$5 \text{ tsp.} \times \frac{5 \text{ mL}}{1 \text{ tsp.}} = 25 \text{ mL}$$

example 13.2

Convert 3 Tbsp. to milliliters.

$$3 \text{ Tbsp.} \times \frac{15 \text{ mL}}{1 \text{ Tbsp.}} = 45 \text{ mL}$$

example 13.3

Convert 4 oz. to milliliters.

$$4 \text{ oz.} \times \frac{30 \text{ mL}}{1 \text{ oz.}} = 120 \text{ mL}$$

example **13.4**

Convert 6.5 cups to milliliters.

$$6.5 \text{ cups} \times \frac{240 \text{ mL}}{1 \text{ cup}} = 1{,}560 \text{ mL}$$

example **13.5**

Convert 60 mL to teaspoons.

$$60 \text{ mL} \times \frac{1 \text{ tsp.}}{5 \text{ mL}} = 12 \text{ tsp.}$$

PRACTICE Problems 13.6

Convert the following measurements.

1. 3 tsp. = _____ mL

2. 4 pints = _____ mL

3. 1 Tbsp. = _____ mL

4. 3 fl. oz. = _____ mL

5. 3 gal. = _____ mL

6. 8 mL = _____ tsp.

7. 7 pt. = _____ mL

8. 5 lb. = _____ g

9. 2,365 mL = _____ pt.

10. 90 Tbsp. = _____ mL

11. 4.5 gal. = _____ pt.

12. 45 mL = _____ fl. oz.

13. 60 kg = _____ lb.

14. 20 mL = _____ tsp.

15. 6 oz. = _____ mL

16. 3 qt. = _____ pt.

17. 5 cups = _____ oz.

18. 1.5 gal. = _____ qt.

19. 12 oz. = _____ cups

20. 2 cups = _____ tsp.

21. You need to give 4 mg of a drug. The drug on hand has a concentration of 15 mg per ounce. How many teaspoons will you give? _____

22. The prescription calls for a dosage of 2 teaspoons. Your stock bottle contains 16 oz. How many teaspoons are in this bottle? _____

23. You are to reconstitute a particular drug. Each vial will get 6 oz. of sterile water. You have 2 gal. of sterile water. How many vials can you prepare? _____

24. You need to prepare three prescriptions containing the following volumes: 1 gal., 2 qt., and 10 oz. How many tablespoons were dispensed in the three prescriptions? _____

25. How many teaspoons are in a pint? _____

Converting the Apothecary System

The apothecary system is an ancient system of measurement based on grains of wheat, and it produces more approximate than exact values. Some prescribers still order medications using the apothecary system. The most commonly used apothecary measures are grains for solids and drams for liquids.

Workplace Wisdom Apothecary-Unit Applications

The majority of apothecary-unit applications are with older drugs, such as codeine, phenobarbital, and aspirin.

example 13.6

Convert 180 gr to ounces.

Using the conversion value, set up a proportion to solve for the number of ounces:

1 oz. = 480 gr

$$\frac{1 \text{ oz.}}{480 \text{ gr}} \quad \frac{X \text{ oz.}}{180 \text{ gr}}$$

Then cross-multiply and solve for X.

$$480X = 180$$

$$X = \frac{180}{480} = 0.375$$

So, 180 gr = 0.375 oz.

PRACTICE Problems 13.7

Convert the following measurements.

1. 5 gr = _____ mg

2. 20 mL = _____ drams

3. 15 gr = _____ mg

4. 4 oz. = _____ g

5. 600 mg = _____ gr

6. $\frac{1}{2}$ oz. = _____ mL

7. 7 drams = _____ oz.

8. 9 kg = _____ lb.

9. $\frac{1}{6}$ gr = _____ mg

10. 40 mL = _____ drams

11. 240 mL = _____ oz.

12. 50 gr = _____ mg

13. 3.5 kg = _____ lb.

14. 60 drams = _____ oz.

15. 150 lb. = _____ oz.

16. 680 g = _____ lb.

17. 99 lb. = _____ kg

18. 0.5 gr = _____ mg

19. 300 mg = _____ gr

20. 1 dram = _____ mL

21. A child weighs 45 lb. and is to receive 2 mg/kg/day. How much of the drug should the child receive per day? _____

22. A medication order calls for a potassium supplement to be administered in at least 150 mL of juice. How many ounces of juice should the patient pour? _____

23. A baby weighs 16 lb. What is the baby's weight in kilograms? _____

24. A doctor orders codeine $\frac{1}{5}$ gr. How many milligrams is this dose equivalent to? _____

25. A cancer patient is given $\frac{1}{4}$ gr of morphine sulfate every 2 hr. How many milligrams of morphine does he receive in 8 hr? _____

26. A pharmacy technician is to fill a prescription for aminophylline 10 gr. Tablets are available in 500 mg. How many tablets should the technician give? _____

27. A bottle of medication contains 45 drams. How many milliliters does it contain? _____

28. A prescription calls for the patient to take 6 drams. How many ounces is that? _____

29. Twenty-three grains equals how many grams? _____

30. How many milliliters of cough medicine are in 12 drams? _____

Temperature Conversions

Celsius (centigrade)
international unit of measurement for temperature.

Fahrenheit American unit of measurement for temperature.

Another important conversion in health care involves **Celsius** and **Fahrenheit** temperatures. The temperature measurement most commonly used in the United States is the Fahrenheit (°F) scale. In most other countries, the metric measurement of Celsius (°C) or **centigrade** is used. In the Fahrenheit system, the freezing point is 32° and the boiling point is 212°. In the Celsius system, the freezing point is 0° and the boiling point is 100°.

Simple formulas are used to convert between the two temperature scales. There is a 180° difference between the boiling and the freezing points on the Fahrenheit thermometer, and a 100° difference between the boiling and freezing points on the Celsius thermometer. Therefore, each Celsius degree is 180/100 or 1.8 the size of a Fahrenheit degree.

Workplace Wisdom Calculating Temperature Conversions

You may find it easier to calculate temperature conversions using the following formula. It can be used with basic algebra to solve for either °C or °F.

9C = 5F − 160

To convert from Fahrenheit temperature to Celsius, use the following formula:

$$°C = \frac{°F - 32}{1.8}$$

example 13.7

Convert 80°F to °C.

$$°C = \frac{80 - 32}{1.8}$$

$$°C = \frac{48}{1.8}$$

$$°C = 26.7°$$

To convert Celsius temperature to Fahrenheit, multiply by 1.8 and add 32.

$$°F = 1.8 × °C + 32$$

example 13.8

Convert 60°C to °F.

$$°F = 1.8 × 60 + 32$$

$$°F = 108 + 32$$

$$°F = 140°$$

PRACTICE Problems 13.8

Convert the following temperatures. Round your answers to tenths.

1. 59°F = _____ °C

2. 99°F = _____ °C

3. 100°F = _____ °C

4. 80°F = _____ °C

5. 130°F = _____ °C

6. 4°C = _____ °F

7. 32°C = _____ °F

8. 19°C = _____ °F

9. 38.4°C = _____ °F

10. 10°C = _____ °F

11. The normal temperature of hot water is 115°F. What is the temperature in Celsius? _____ °C

12. The normal range for body temperature is 96.8° to 100°F. What is the range in Celsius? _____ °C to _____ °C

13. The normal oral temperature is 37°C. What is the temperature in Fahrenheit? _____ °F

14. If a child has a fever of 100°F, what is his temperature in Celsius? _____ °C

15. If a drug is to be kept at 56°F, what is the storage temperature in Celsius? _____ °C

Workplace Wisdom Converting Temperatures Using the 9C = 5F − 160 Formula

Another option for converting temperatures is the formula 9C = 5F − 160. This algebraic formula works for converting to/from either unit. Simply replace the "C" or "F", where C = Celsius and F = Fahrenheit, with the known temperature and solve algebraically.

SUMMARY

Regardless of your practice setting, a solid knowledge of the systems of measurement and their units and abbreviations is the foundation for all pharmacy calculations. You must have a comprehensive understanding of this material before attempting pharmacy calculations.

Every practice setting is individual and unique; the conversions that you need to calculate on a regular basis at your practice setting will become second nature to you. Until such time, use the charts and formulas from this chapter. Although miscalculation of a conversion may seem to be a minor issue, it could have drastic and irrevocable effects on a patient's health.

CHAPTER REVIEW QUESTIONS

1. 800 g = _____.
   a. 1.8 lb.
   b. 18 lb.
   c. 8 lb.
   d. 0.8 lb.

2. 2 cups = _____.
   a. 120 mL
   b. 240 mL
   c. 480 mL
   d. 160 mL

3. 160 oz. = _____.
   a. 1 pt.
   b. 10 pt.
   c. 2 pt.
   d. 20 pt.

4. 2.5 cups = _____.
   a. 2.0 oz.
   b. 20 oz.
   c. 3.0 oz.
   d. 30 oz.

5. 2°F = _____.
   a. 32.4°C
   b. 28.6°C
   c. −12.4°C
   d. −16.7°C

6. How many 8 oz. bottles can be filled from 5 gal. of medicine? _____
   a. 80
   b. 20
   c. 30
   d. 110

7. A child weighs 45.9 kg. What is his weight in pounds?
   a. 128 lb.
   b. 87 lb.
   c. 74 lb.
   d. 101 lb.

8. A medication has 300 mg in 50 mL. How many milligrams are in 3 oz.?
   a. 900 mg
   b. 1,500 mg
   c. 540 mg
   d. 450 mg

9. If there are 30 mg in a teaspoon, how many grams are in a fluid ounce?
   a. 6.0 g
   b. 1.5 g
   c. 0.18 g
   d. 0.15 g

10. If a prescription reads "Take 3 tablespoons 4 times a day for 10 days," how many total tablespoons will the patient take?
    a. 240 Tbsp.
    b. 120 Tbsp.
    c. 80 Tbsp.
    d. 60 Tbsp.

CRITICAL THINKING QUESTIONS

1. Why is proper decimal notation so critical in pharmacy calculations?

2. Why does pharmacy continue to use both the metric system and the household system of measurement extensively?

3. When would a pharmacy technician need to calculate temperature conversions?

REFERENCES AND RESOURCES

Hegstad, LN, & Hayek, W. *Essential Drug Dosage Calculations* (4th ed.). Upper Saddle River, NJ: Pearson, 2001.

Johnston, M. *Pharmacy Calculations.* Upper Saddle River, NJ: Pearson, 2005.

Lesmesiter, MB. *Math Basics for the Healthcare Professional* (2nd ed.). Upper Saddle River, NJ: Pearson, 2005.

Mikolah, AA. *Drug Dosage Calculations for the Emergency Care Provider* (2nd ed.). Upper Saddle River, NJ: Prentice Hall, 2003.

Olsen, JL, Giangrasso, AP, & Shrimpton, D. *Medical Dosage Calculations* (8th ed.). Upper Saddle River, NJ: Pearson, 2004.

14 Dosage Calculations

LEARNING OBJECTIVES

After completing this chapter, you should be able to:

- Calculate the correct number of doses in a prescription.
- Determine the quantity to dispense for a prescription.
- Calculate the amount of active ingredient in a prescription.
- Determine the correct days supply for a prescription.
- Perform multiple dosage calculations for a single prescription.
- Calculate accurate dosages for pediatric patients.
- Convert a patient's weight from pounds to kilograms.
- Perform dosage calculations based upon mg/kg/day.

dosage calculations
pharmacy calculations pertaining to the number of doses, dispensing quantities, and/or ingredient quantities.

Introduction

Proper dosing of medications is important to ensure patient safety. **Dosage calculations** include calculation of the number of doses and dispensing quantities and ingredient quantities. These calculations are performed in the pharmacy on a daily basis. The pharmacy technician must have a full working knowledge of how to perform these calculations.

To perform dosage calculations, you will utilize the information and principles introduced in previous chapters of this book. You can solve these calculations by setting up ratios and proportions, keeping like units consistent, and cross-multiplying to solve for the unknown.

SIG Code Refresher

qd = every day

qod = every other day

bid = twice a day

tid = three times a day

qid = four times a day

q4h = every 4 hours, or six times a day

q6h = every 6 hours, or four times a day

q8h = every 8 hours, or three times a day

q12h = every 12 hours, or twice a day

q4–6h = every 4 to 6 hours, or four to six times a day

prn = as needed

Calculating the Number of Doses

Determining the correct number of **doses** to be dispensed, or available in stock, is an important dosage calculation. In this section, you will learn how to calculate the number of doses.

dose the amount of medication prescribed to be taken at one time.

example 14.1

How many 1 tsp. doses are in a 4 oz. bottle of Prozac® Liquid Solution 20mg/5mL? (See Figure 14-1.)

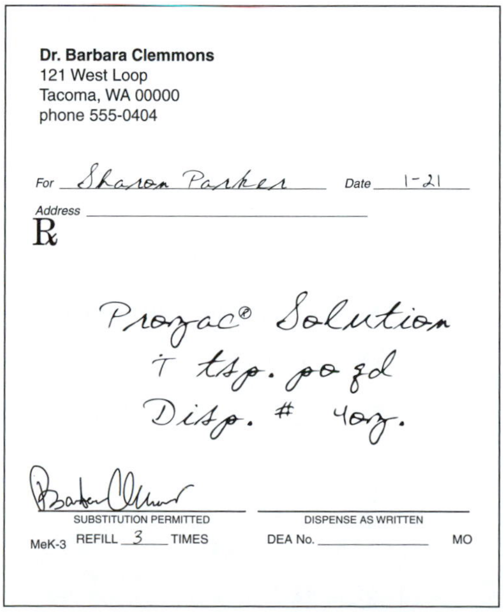

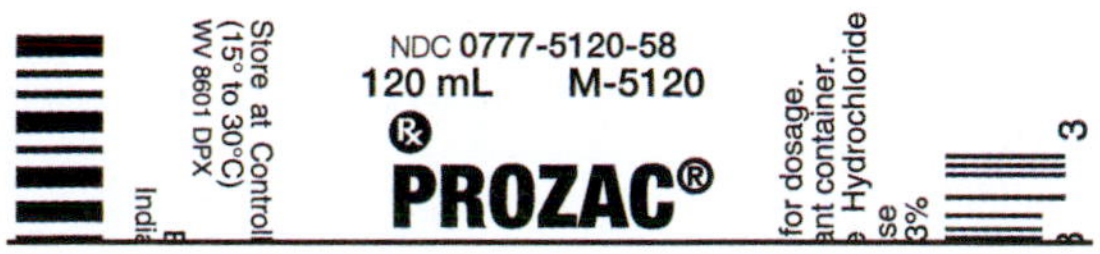

Dr. Barbara Clemmons
121 West Loop
Tacoma, WA 00000
phone 555-0404

For _Sharon Parker_   Date _1-21_

Address _____

℞

Prozac® Solution
ꞁ tsp. po qd
Disp. # 4oz.

Barbara Clemmons
SUBSTITUTION PERMITTED   DISPENSE AS WRITTEN

MeK-3   REFILL _3_ TIMES   DEA No. _____ MO

NDC 0777-5120-58
120 mL   M-5120
℞
PROZAC®

Store at Controlled
(15° to 30°C)
WV 8601 DPX

for dosage.
ant container.
Hydrochloride
se 3%

FIGURE 14-1 Drug label for Prozac®.
(Courtesy of Eli Lilly and Company.)

To calculate the number of doses, you should first determine which information presented is actually applicable to the question. Too often we make mistakes in dosage calculations because we overcomplicate them.

Let's look at the information that has been provided:

✓   1 tsp. po: *the dose*

✗   qd: *the frequency*

✓   4 oz.: *the quantity dispensed*

✗   Prozac® Solution 20 mg/5 mL: *the drug name and strength*

✗   120 mL: *the quantity of the stock bottle*

The question is simply asking how many doses make up the total amount being dispensed. The strength of the drug, frequency of dosage, and quantity of the stock bottle have no relevance in performing this calculation.

So now we know that we are working with 1 tsp. doses and a total quantity of 4 oz. To solve this calculation using a ratio/proportion, we have to have similar units of measure—in this case mL.

We know that 1 tsp. = 5 mL and we should also know that 4 oz. = 120 mL, but if you do not know this, you could also solve the problem by using a ratio/proportion.

$$\frac{1 \text{ oz.}}{30 \text{ mL}} = \frac{4 \text{ oz.}}{X \text{ mL}}$$

Cross-multiply and solve the equation for X.

$30 \cdot 4 = 120$ and $1 \cdot X = (1)X$
$(1)X = 120$

Now that we have both quantities converted to units in mL, we can set up our ratio/proportion and solve.

$$\frac{1 \text{ dose}}{5 \text{ mL}} = \frac{X \text{ doses}}{120 \text{ mL}}$$

Cross-multiply.

$5 \cdot X = 5X$ and $1 \cdot 120 = 120$

Now set up your equation and solve for X.

$5X = 120$

To solve for X, divide both sides by 5.

$$\frac{5X}{5} = \frac{120}{5}$$
$120 \div 5 = 24$

$X = 24$

So, there are 24 doses (of 5 mL each) in a 4 oz. (120 mL) bottle.

example 14.2

How many doses are provided in the prescription shown in Figure 14-2?

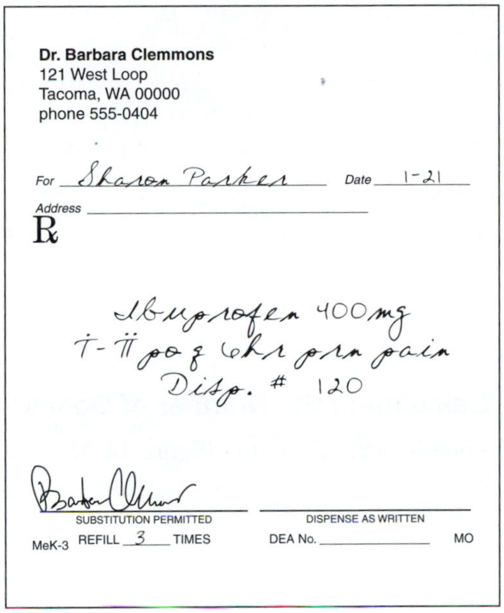

Dr. Barbara Clemmons
121 West Loop
Tacoma, WA 00000
phone 555-0404

For _Sharon Parker_   Date _1-21_

Address _____

℞ _____

Ibuprofen 400 mg
ⅰ-ⅱ po q 6hr prn pain
Disp. # 120

_____
SUBSTITUTION PERMITTED   DISPENSE AS WRITTEN

MeK-3   REFILL _3_ TIMES   DEA No. _____   MO

FIGURE 14-2

Let's look at the information that has been provided:

✓   1–2 po: *the dose*

✗   q 6hr prn pain: *the frequency*

✓   120: *the quantity dispensed*

✗   Ibuprofen 400 mg: *the drug name and strength*

Workplace Wisdom Conservative Calculations

Always use the higher dosage amount when performing dosage calculations on prescriptions that have a range for the dose, as in Example 14.2. This will provide the most conservative solution and ensure the most accurate potential for days supply.

Using the information provided, set up the ratio/proportion and solve.

$$\frac{1 \text{ dose}}{2 \text{ tabs}} = \frac{X \text{ doses}}{120 \text{ tabs}}$$

Cross-multiply.

$2 \cdot X = 2X$ and $1 \cdot 120 = 120$

Now set up your equation and solve for X.

2X = 120

To solve for X, divide both sides by 2.

$$\frac{2X}{2} = \frac{120}{2}$$

120 ÷ 2 = 60

X = 60

So, a minimum of 60 doses has been prescribed.

PRACTICE Problems 14.1 Calculating the Number of Doses

1. How many dosages are provided in the prescription shown in Figure 14-3?

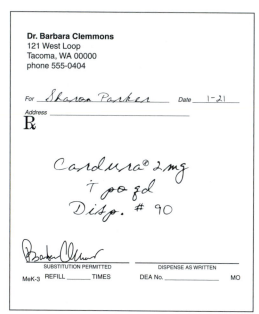

Dr. Barbara Clemmons
121 West Loop
Tacoma, WA 00000
phone 555-0404

For _Sharon Parker_   Date _1-21_

Address _____

℞

Cardura® 2mg
_ī po qd_
Disp. # 90

SUBSTITUTION PERMITTED   DISPENSE AS WRITTEN

MeK-3   REFILL _____ TIMES   DEA No. _____   MO

FIGURE 14-3

2. How many dropperfuls (at a 2.5 mL dosage) are in a 50 mL bottle of EryPed®
   Drops? (See Figure 14-4.)

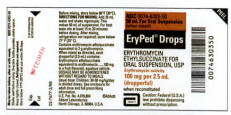

FIGURE 14-4 Drug label for EryPed Drops®.
(Reproduced with permission of Abbott Laboratories.)

3. How many doses are provided in the prescription shown in Figure 14-5?

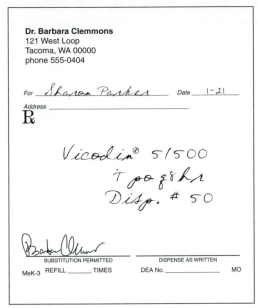

Dr. Barbara Clemmons
121 West Loop
Tacoma, WA 00000
phone 555-0404

For _Sharon Parker_ Date _1-21_

Address _____

Rx

Vicodin® 5/500
_ī po q8hr_
Disp. # 50

_____
SUBSTITUTION PERMITTED   DISPENSE AS WRITTEN

MeK-3 REFILL _____ TIMES   DEA No. _____   MO

FIGURE 14-5

4. How many 1 tsp. doses are in each bottle of Zithromax® 200 mg/5 mL, as shown in Figure 14-6, when mixed?

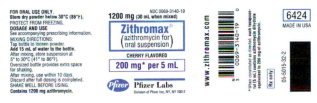

FIGURE 14-6 Zithromax® (azithromycin).
(Registered Trademark of Pfizer, Inc. Reproduced with permission.)

5. How many doses are provided in the prescription shown in Figure 14-7?

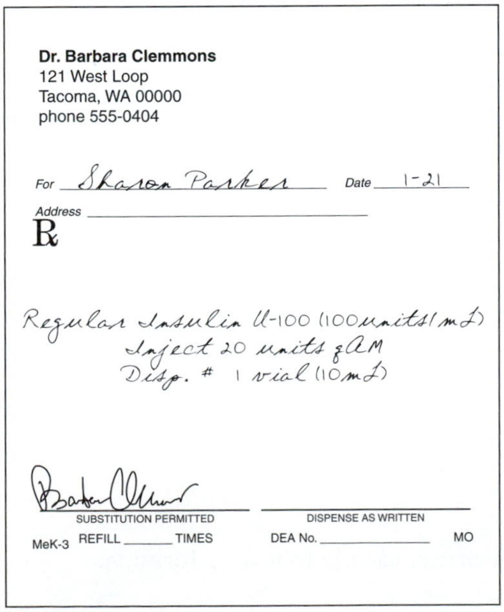

Dr. Barbara Clemmons
121 West Loop
Tacoma, WA 00000
phone 555-0404

For _Sharon Parker_ Date _1-21_

Address _____

Rx

Regular Insulin U-100 (100 units/mL)
Inject 20 units q AM
Disp. # 1 vial (10mL)

_____
SUBSTITUTION PERMITTED   DISPENSE AS WRITTEN

MeK-3 REFILL _____ TIMES   DEA No. _____   MO

FIGURE 14-7

Calculating the Quantity to Dispense

Determining the proper quantity to dispense is another critical dosage calculation, and is similar to calculating the number of doses. In this section, you will learn how to calculate **dispensing quantities**.

dispensing quantity the total amount of medication to be dispensed.

example **14.3**

How many Biaxin® 250 mg tablets should be dispensed, according to the prescription in Figure 14-8?

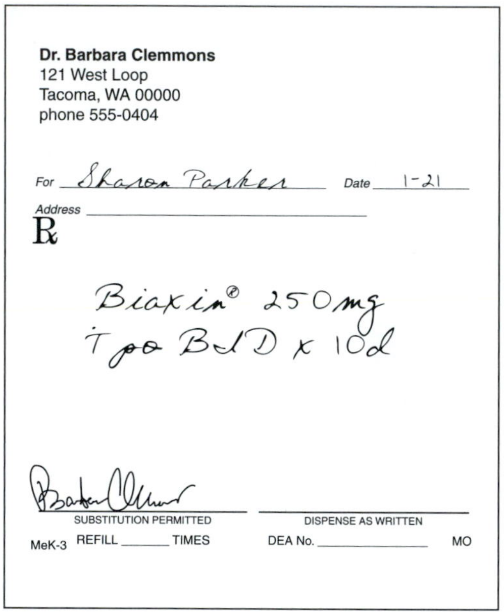

Dr. Barbara Clemmons
121 West Loop
Tacoma, WA 00000
phone 555-0404

For _Sharon Parker_   Date __1-21__

Address _____

℞

Biaxin® 250mg
T po BID x 10d

___Barbara Clemmons___   _____
SUBSTITUTION PERMITTED   DISPENSE AS WRITTEN

MeK-3   REFILL _____ TIMES   DEA No. _____   MO

FIGURE 14-8

Again, to solve this dosage calculation it is important first to determine which information is necessary; it is also critical to know the common SIG codes to perform dosage calculations. Let's look at the information that has been provided:

✓   1 po—*the dose*

✓   BID—*the frequency*

✓   x 10d—*the duration*

✗   Biaxin® 250 mg—*the drug name and strength*

✗   100 tablets—*the quantity of the stock bottle*

To calculate the appropriate quantity to dispense, use the following formula:

dose × frequency × duration = quantity to dispense

Using the information provided in the prescription, you can set up the calculation as follows:

$$1 \cdot 2 \cdot 10 = X$$

dose × frequency × duration = quantity to dispense

$1 \cdot 2 \cdot 10 = 20$

$20 = X$

So, 20 tablets of Biaxin® 250 mg should be dispensed.

---

example   14.4   Calculating the Quantity to Dispense

How much Promethazine w/Codeine Syrup should be dispensed, according to the prescription in Figure 14-9?

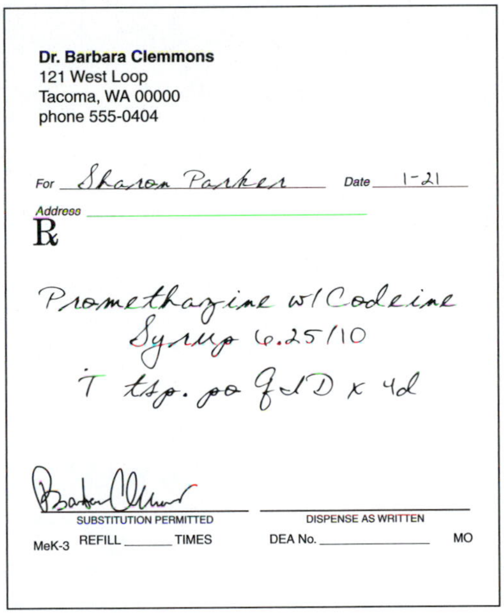

Dr. Barbara Clemmons
121 West Loop
Tacoma, WA 00000
phone 555-0404

For _Sharon Parker_   Date _1-21_

Address _____

℞

Promethazine w/Codeine
Syrup 6.25/10
ī tsp. po QID x 4d

SUBSTITUTION PERMITTED   DISPENSE AS WRITTEN

MeK-3 REFILL _____ TIMES   DEA No. _____   MO

FIGURE 14-9

Let's look at the information that has been provided:

✓   1 tsp. po—*the dose*

✓   QID—*the frequency*

✓   x 4d—*the duration*

✗   Promethazine w/Codeine Syrup 6.25/10—*the drug name and strength*

To calculate the appropriate quantity to dispense, use the following formula:

dose × frequency × duration = quantity to dispense

Using the information provided in the prescription, you can set up the calculation as follows:

$$1 \text{ tsp.} \cdot 4 \cdot 4 = X$$

dose × frequency × duration = quantity to dispense

$1 \cdot 4 \cdot 4 = 16$

$16 = X$

So, 16 teaspoonfuls, or 80 mL, of Promethazine w/Codeine should be dispensed.

PRACTICE Problems 14.2 Calculating the Quantity to Dispense

1. What quantity should be dispensed for the prescription shown in Figure 14-10?

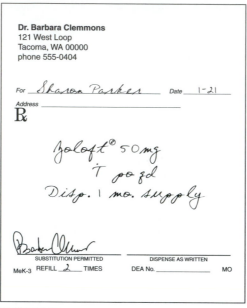

Dr. Barbara Clemmons
121 West Loop
Tacoma, WA 00000
phone 555-0404

For *Sharon Parker*   Date *1-21*

Address _____

℞

Zoloft® 50mg
ī po qd
Disp. 1 mo. supply

SUBSTITUTION PERMITTED   DISPENSE AS WRITTEN

MeK-3   REFILL *2* TIMES   DEA No. _____   MO

FIGURE 14-10

2. What quantity should be dispensed, using the stock medication shown in Figure 14-11, to provide 20 mg of diazepam prior to the procedure and 10 mg following?

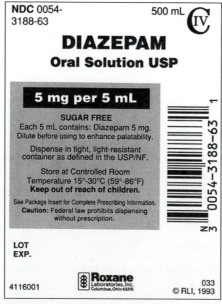

NDC 0054-3188-63   500 mL   C-IV

DIAZEPAM
Oral Solution USP

5 mg per 5 mL

SUGAR FREE
Each 5 mL contains: Diazepam 5 mg.
Dilute before using to enhance palatability.

Dispense in tight, light-resistant
container as defined in the USP/NF.

Store at Controlled Room
Temperature 15°-30°C (59°-86°F)
Keep out of reach of children.

See Package Insert for Complete Prescribing Information.
Caution: Federal law prohibits dispensing
without prescription.

LOT
EXP.

4116001   **Roxane**
Laboratories, Inc.
Columbus, Ohio 43216   033
© RLI, 1993

FIGURE 14-11 Drug label for diazepam.
(© Copyright Boehringer Ingelheim Roxane, Inc. and/or
affiliated companies 2009. All Rights Reserved.)

3. What quantity should be dispensed for a three-month supply of the prescription shown in Figure 14-12?

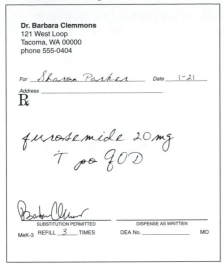

Dr. Barbara Clemmons
121 West Loop
Tacoma, WA 00000
phone 555-0404

For _Sharon Parker_   Date _1-21_

Address _____

Rx

furosemide 20mg
T po QOD

SUBSTITUTION PERMITTED   DISPENSE AS WRITTEN
MeK-3 REFILL _3_ TIMES   DEA No. _____   MO

FIGURE 14-12

4. What quantity should be dispensed when 50 mg of amitryptyline has been prescribed daily for 3 weeks, if the medication shown in Figure 14-13 is all that is available?

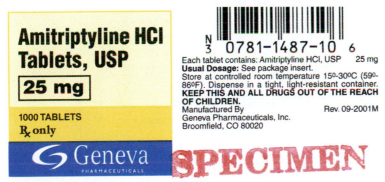

Amitriptyline HCl Tablets, USP
25 mg
1000 TABLETS
Rx only
Geneva PHARMACEUTICALS

N3 0781-1487-10 6
Each tablet contains: Amitriptyline HCl, USP   25 mg
Usual Dosage: See package insert.
Store at controlled room temperature 15º-30ºC (59º-86ºF). Dispense in a tight, light-resistant container.
KEEP THIS AND ALL DRUGS OUT OF THE REACH OF CHILDREN.
Manufactured By   Rev. 09-2001M
Geneva Pharmaceuticals, Inc.
Broomfield, CO 80020
SPECIMEN

FIGURE 14-13 Drug label for amitriptyline HCL.
(Courtesy of Sandoz.)

5. What quantity should be dispensed for a 30-day supply of the prescription shown in Figure 14-14?

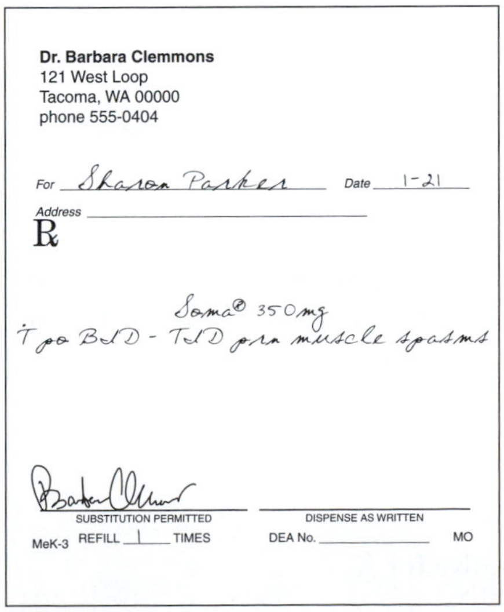

Dr. Barbara Clemmons
121 West Loop
Tacoma, WA 00000
phone 555-0404

For _Sharon Parker_   Date _1-21_

Address _____

Rx

Soma® 350mg
T po BID - TID prn muscle spasms

SUBSTITUTION PERMITTED   DISPENSE AS WRITTEN
MeK-3 REFILL _1_ TIMES   DEA No. _____   MO

FIGURE 14-14

Calculating the Quantity of Ingredient

It is sometimes necessary to calculate the amount, or quantity, of active ingredient required, particularly when preparing compounded preparations. In this section, you will learn how to accurately determine the quantity of active ingredient.

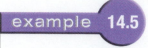

How much codeine is in each dose of Codeine Phosphate Oral Solution 15 mg/mL? (See Figure 14-15.)

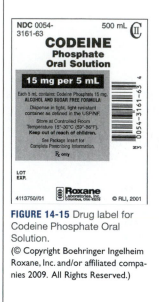

FIGURE 14-15 Drug label for Codeine Phosphate Oral Solution.
(© Copyright Boehringer Ingelheim Roxane, Inc. and/or affiliated companies 2009. All Rights Reserved.)

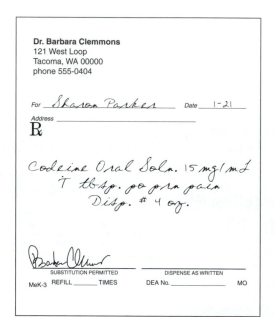

Let's first look at all of the information provided to determine which facts we will use in solving the problem:

✓   1 tbsp. po—*the dose*

✗   prn—*the frequency*

✗   4 oz.—*the quantity to dispense*

✓   Codeine Phosphate Oral Solution 15 mg/mL—*the drug name and strength*

✗   500 mL—*the quantity of the stock bottle*

To solve this problem, we need to set up a ratio/proportion using the dose and strength—but remember that units of measure must be the same. The dose (1 Tbsp.) is equivalent to 15 mL (you should know this by memory).

Now we can set up the ratio/proportion.

$$\frac{15 \text{ mg}}{1 \text{ mL}} = \frac{X \text{ mg}}{15 \text{ mL}}$$

Cross-multiply and then set up the equation to solve for X.

$15 \cdot 15 = 225$ and $1 \cdot X = 5X$

$1X = 225$

$X = 225$

So, there are 225 mg of codeine in each 1 Tbsp. dose.

---

example 14.6   **Calculating the Quantity of Ingredient**

How many mL of stock dopamine must be added to the IV solution? (See Figure 14-16.)

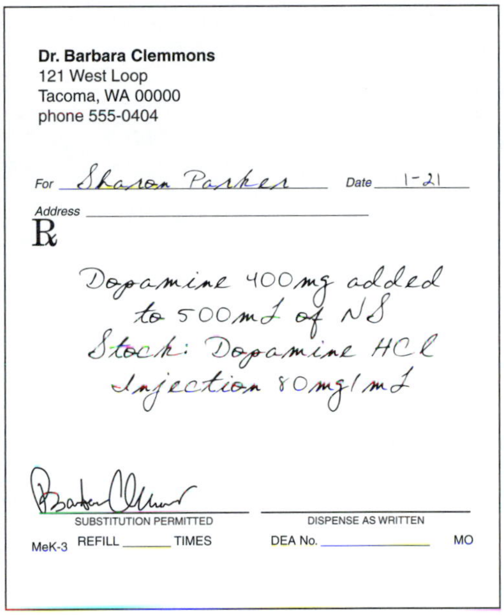

Dr. Barbara Clemmons
121 West Loop
Tacoma, WA 00000
phone 555-0404

For _Sharon Parker_   Date _1-21_

Address _____

℞

Dopamine 400mg added
to 500ml of NS
Stock: Dopamine HCl
Injection 80mg/ml

_____   _____
SUBSTITUTION PERMITTED   DISPENSE AS WRITTEN
MeK-3 REFILL _____ TIMES   DEA No. _____   MO

FIGURE 14-16

Let's first look at all of the information provided to determine which we will use in solving the problem:

✓   400 mg—*the dose*

✗   500 mL—*the quantity to dispense*

✓   dopamine HCl injection 80mg/mL—*the drug name and strength*

To solve this problem, we must determine how many milliliters of the stock dopamine to add to the normal saline IV solution bag. We must set up a ratio/proportion.

$$\frac{80 \text{ mg}}{1 \text{ mL}} = \frac{400 \text{ mg}}{X \text{ mL}}$$

Cross-multiply and then set up the equation to solve for X.

$1 \cdot 400 = 400$ and $80 \cdot X = 80X$

$400 = 80X$

Now divide both sides by 80 to solve for X.

$$\frac{400}{80} = \frac{80X}{80}$$

$X = 5$

So, we must add 5 mL of the stock dopamine HCl injection to the IV solution.

PRACTICE Problems 14.3 Calculating the Quantity of Ingredient

1. Z-Pak®s contain 6 tablets of azithromycin 250 mg, which are taken over the course of five days. How many total mg of active ingredient are contained in a Z-Pak®?

2. How many mcg of Fentanyl® would be contained in 1.5 mL (see Figure 14-17)?

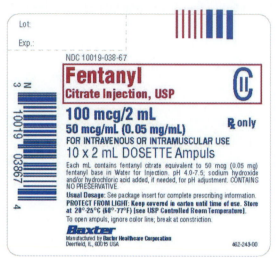

FIGURE 14-17 Drug label for Fentanyl®.
(Courtesy of Baxter Health Care Corporation.)

3. How many milligrams of acetaminophen are contained in 2 Lortab® 2.5 tablets (2.5 mg hydrocodone/500 mg acetaminophen)?

4. How many milligrams of dexamethasone are contained in the stock bottle (500 mL) shown in Figure 14-18?

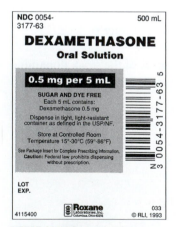

FIGURE 14-18 Drug label for dexamethasone oral solution.
(© Copyright Boehringer Ingelheim Roxane, Inc. and/or affiliated companies 2009. All Rights Reserved.)

5. How many mg of hydrocortisone are found in 1 tbsp. of Cortef® 10 mg/5 mL?

Calculating the Correct Days Supply

Accurate calculation of the number of days a prescription should last, or **days supply**, is important, especially when billing through a third-party insurance provider. If an incorrect days supply is entered, the original prescription could be denied, the co-pay may be miscalculated, or refill coverage could be affected. In this section, you will learn how to calculate the correct days supply.

days supply the expected duration for a prescription being dispensed; how long the amount of medication dispensed will last if taken as directed.

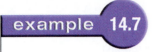
example 14.7

How many days should the prescription shown in Figure 14-19 last?

Dr. Barbara Clemmons
121 West Loop
Tacoma, WA 00000
phone 555-0404

For _Sharon Parker_   Date _1-21_

Address _____

℞

Pamelor® 75 mg
ĭ po BID
Disp. # 50

_____   _____
SUBSTITUTION PERMITTED   DISPENSE AS WRITTEN
MeK-3 REFILL _3_ TIMES   DEA No. _____   MO

FIGURE 14-19

Let's determine what parts of the information provided we will need to solve the problem.

✓   1 po—*the dose*

✓ BID—*the frequency*

✓   50—*the quantity to dispense*

✗ Pamelor® 75 mg—*the drug name and strength*

✗ 100 capsules—*the quantity of the stock bottle*

To calculate the appropriate days supply, use the following formula:

$$\text{Days supply} = \frac{\text{qty. dispensed}}{\text{dose} \cdot \text{frequency}}$$

Using the information provided, set up the formula as follows.

$$X = \frac{50 \text{ (qty. dispensed)}}{1 \times 2 \text{ (dose} \times \text{frequency)}}$$

This becomes

$$X = \frac{50}{2} \text{ or } X = 25$$

So, this prescription should last for 25 days.

---

example 14.8

How many days should the prescription shown in Figure 14-20 last?

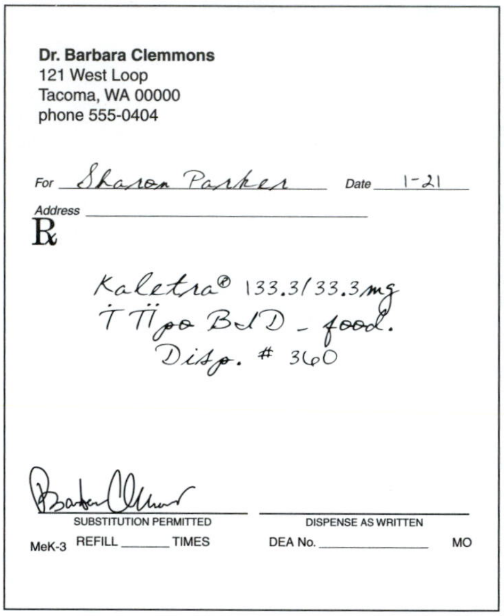

Dr. Barbara Clemmons
121 West Loop
Tacoma, WA 00000
phone 555-0404

For _Sharon Parker_   Date _1-21_

Address _____

℞

Kaletra® 133.3/33.3 mg
ī Tī po BID - food.
Disp. # 360

(signature)
SUBSTITUTION PERMITTED   DISPENSE AS WRITTEN

MeK-3 REFILL _____ TIMES   DEA No. _____ MO

FIGURE 14-20

Let's determine what parts of the information provided we will need to solve the problem.

✓   1–2 po—*the dose*

✓ BID—*the frequency*

✓   360—*the quantity to dispense*

✗ Kaletra® 133.3/33.3 mg—*the drug name and strength*

To calculate the appropriate days supply, use the following formula:

$$\text{Days supply} = \frac{\text{qty. dispensed}}{\text{dose} \times \text{frequency}}$$

Using the information provided, set up the formula as follows.

$$X = \frac{360 \text{ (qty. dispensed)}}{2 \cdot 2 \text{ (dose} \cdot \text{frequency)}}$$

This becomes

$$X = \frac{360}{4} \text{ or } X = 90$$

So, this prescription should last for 3 months, or 90 days.

PRACTICE Problems 14.4 Calculating the Correct Days Supply

1. How many days will the prescription shown in Figure 14-21 last?

```
Dr. Barbara Clemmons
121 West Loop
Tacoma, WA 00000
phone 555-0404


For  Sharon Parker        Date  1-21
Address _____
℞

        Diabinese® 100mg
          ī po ğ AM
        Disp. # 45




  Barbara Clemmons
  SUBSTITUTION PERMITTED        DISPENSE AS WRITTEN
MeK-3  REFILL _____ TIMES    DEA No. _____  MO
```

FIGURE 14-21

2. How many days will a 150 mL bottle of Ceclor® 125 mg/5 mL last, if the patient is to take 2 teaspoonfuls 3 times daily? (See Figure 14-22.)

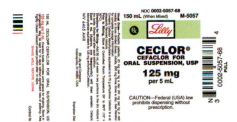

FIGURE 14-22 Drug label for Ceclor®.
(Courtesy of Eli Lilly and Company.)

3. How many days will the prescription shown in Figure 14-23 last?

```
Dr. Barbara Clemmons
121 West Loop
Tacoma, WA 00000
phone 555-0404


For  Sharon Parker        Date  1-21
Address _____
℞

        Valium® 5mg
          ī po BID
        Disp. # 60




  Barbara Clemmons
  SUBSTITUTION PERMITTED        DISPENSE AS WRITTEN
MeK-3  REFILL _____ TIMES    DEA No. _____  MO
```

FIGURE 14-23

4. How many days should 10 tablets of Cialis® 5 mg last, if the prescription directs the patient to use a maximum of one tablet q 3 days?

5. How many days will the prescription shown in Figure 14-24 last?

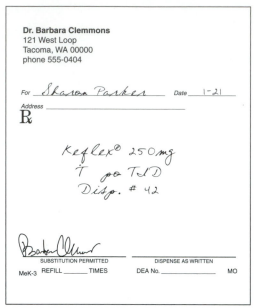

Dr. Barbara Clemmons
121 West Loop
Tacoma, WA 00000
phone 555-0404

For _Sharon Parker_   Date _1-21_

Address _____

℞

Keflex® 250mg
ī̄ po TID
Disp. # 42

SUBSTITUTION PERMITTED   DISPENSE AS WRITTEN

MeK-3   REFILL _____ TIMES   DEA No. _____   MO

FIGURE 14-24

Solving Multiple Dosage Calculations

In practical application, pharmacy technicians most often need to perform a combination of the dosage calculations previously covered to prepare and fill a prescription. In this section, you will practice solving multiple dosage calculations for an individual prescription. The calculations required are those we have already reviewed.

PRACTICE Problems 14.5 Solving Multiple Dosage Calculations

1.

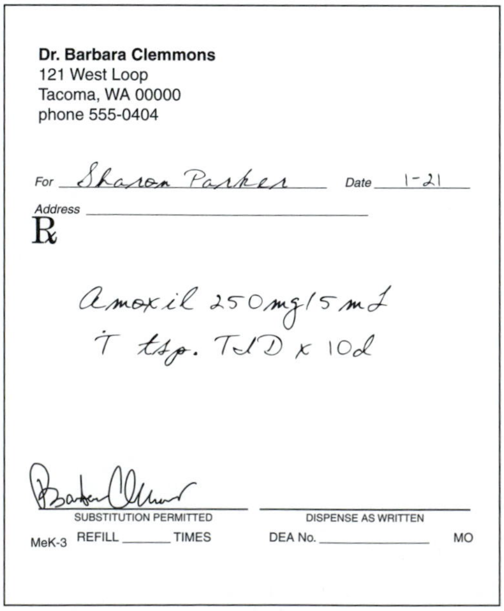

Dr. Barbara Clemmons
121 West Loop
Tacoma, WA 00000
phone 555-0404

For _Sharon Parker_   Date _1-21_

Address _____

℞

Amoxil 250mg/5mL
ī̄ tsp. TID x 10d

SUBSTITUTION PERMITTED   DISPENSE AS WRITTEN

MeK-3   REFILL _____ TIMES   DEA No. _____   MO

FIGURE 14-25

a. What is the appropriate quantity to dispense?

b. How many total doses are to be dispensed?

c. What is the total amount of amoxicillin, in mg, to be dispensed?

d. How many days should this prescription last?

2.

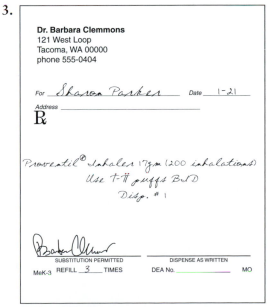

Dr. Barbara Clemmons
121 West Loop
Tacoma, WA 00000
phone 555-0404

For _Sharon Parker_ Date _1-21_

Address _____

℞

Dexamethasone Oral Soln. 0.5 mg/5 ml
Give 0.25 mg QOD
Disp. # 1 bottle

_____ _____
SUBSTITUTION PERMITTED   DISPENSE AS WRITTEN
MeK-3 REFILL _____ TIMES   DEA No. _____ MO

FIGURE 14-26

a. What is the appropriate quantity to dispense?

b. How many total doses are to be dispensed?

c. What is the total amount of dexamethasone, in mg, to be dispensed?

d. How many days should this prescription last?

3.

Dr. Barbara Clemmons
121 West Loop
Tacoma, WA 00000
phone 555-0404

For _Sharon Parker_ Date _1-21_

Address _____

℞

Proventil® Inhaler 17gm (200 inhalations)
Use I-II puffs BID
Disp. # 1

_____ _____
SUBSTITUTION PERMITTED   DISPENSE AS WRITTEN
MeK-3 REFILL _3_ TIMES   DEA No. _____ MO

FIGURE 14-27

a. What is the appropriate quantity to dispense?

b. How many total doses are to be dispensed?

c. What is the total amount of albuterol, in mg, per inhalation?

d. How many days should this prescription last?

4.

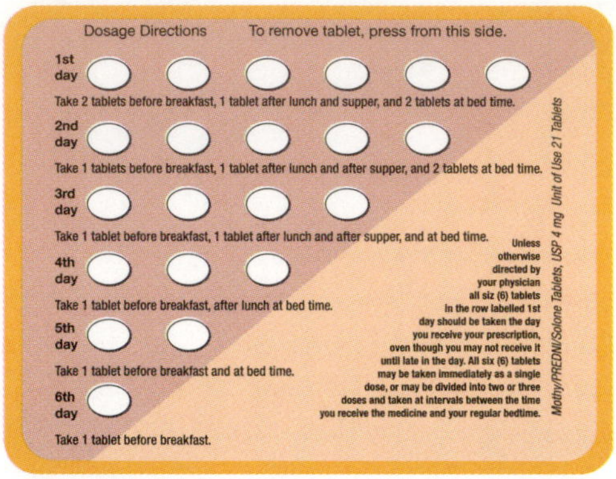

Dosage Directions   To remove tablet, press from this side.

1st day
Take 2 tablets before breakfast, 1 tablet after lunch and supper, and 2 tablets at bed time.

2nd day
Take 1 tablets before breakfast, 1 tablet after lunch and after supper, and 2 tablets at bed time.

3rd day
Take 1 tablet before breakfast, 1 tablet after lunch and after supper, and at bed time.

4th day
Take 1 tablet before breakfast, after lunch at bed time.

5th day
Take 1 tablet before breakfast and at bed time.

6th day
Take 1 tablet before breakfast.

Unless otherwise directed by your physician all six (6) tablets in the row labelled 1st day should be taken the day you receive your prescription, even though you may not receive it until late in the day. All six (6) tablets may be taken immediately as a single dose, or may be divided into two or three doses and taken at intervals between the time you receive the medicine and your regular bedtime.

Methyl PREDNI/Solone Tablets, USP 4 mg Unit of Use 21 Tablets

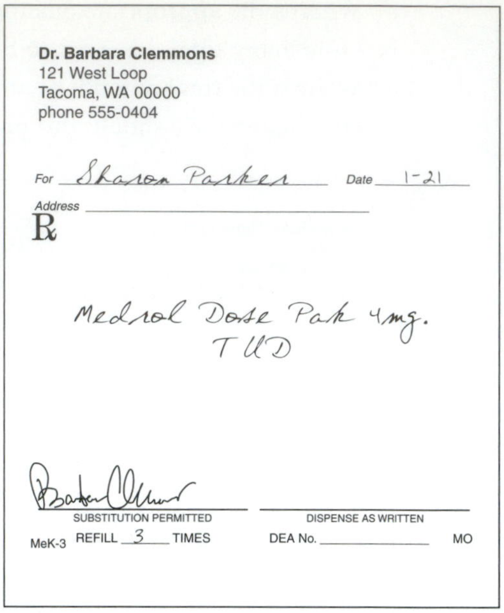

Dr. Barbara Clemmons
121 West Loop
Tacoma, WA 00000
phone 555-0404

For _Sharon Parker_   Date _1-21_

Address _____

Rx

Medrol Dose Pak 4mg.
TUD

SUBSTITUTION PERMITTED   DISPENSE AS WRITTEN

MeK-3   REFILL _3_ TIMES   DEA No. _____   MO

FIGURE 14-28

a. What is the appropriate quantity to dispense?
b. How many total doses are to be dispensed?
c. What is the total amount of methylprednisolone, in mg, to be dispensed in the pack?
d. How many days should this prescription last?

5.

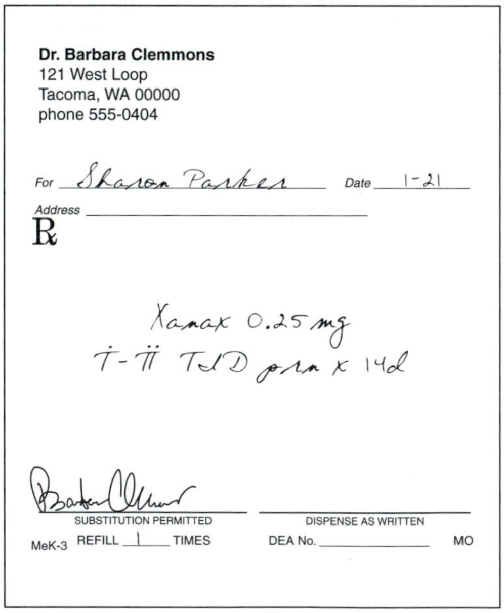

Dr. Barbara Clemmons
121 West Loop
Tacoma, WA 00000
phone 555-0404

For _Sharon Parker_   Date _1-21_

Address _____

Rx

Xanax 0.25 mg
T-II TUD prn x 14d

SUBSTITUTION PERMITTED   DISPENSE AS WRITTEN

MeK-3   REFILL _1_ TIMES   DEA No. _____   MO

FIGURE 14-29

a. What is the appropriate quantity to dispense?
b. What is the maximum number of doses available if 60 tablets are dispensed?
c. What is the maximum amount of alprazolam, in mg, to be taken daily?
d. How many days could this prescription last, if 60 tablets are dispensed?

FORMULA	Pediatric Dosing

FIGURE 14-30 Pediatric dosing.

Fried's Rule

$$\text{Child's dosage} = \frac{\text{Age in months}}{150} \times \text{Adult dosage}$$

Young's Rule

$$\text{Child's dosage} = \frac{\text{Age of child in years}}{\text{Age of child in years} + 12} \times \text{Adult dosage}$$

Clark's Rule

$$\text{Child's dosage} = \frac{\text{Child's weight in pounds}}{150} \times \text{Adult dosage}$$

Calculating Pediatric Dosages

Pediatric patients (a group that includes both infants and children) require special dosing that is adjusted for their age and body weight (Figure 14-30). A number of formulas have been used throughout the years to determine the best dosage for pediatric patients; the most common are reviewed in this section. Chapter 32 reviews additional special considerations concerning pediatric patients.

Calculating Pediatric Dosages Using Fried's Rule

Fried's Rule is a formula used in calculating pediatric dosages based on the child's age, stated in months.

Fried's Rule formula for solving pediatric dosage calculations based on the patient's age in months.

example 14.9

An infant, 15 months old and weighing 20 pounds, needs streptomycin sulfate, which is usually administered to adults as 1 gm (1,000 mg) in a daily IM injection. What is the appropriate dosage for the infant?

To calculate the pediatric dosage based on a child's age in months, simply use the formula for Fried's Rule. Using the information provided, set up the calculation as follows:

$$\text{Pediatric dose} = \frac{15 \text{ (age in months)}}{150} \times 1,000 \text{ mg (adult dose)}$$

$$\text{Pediatric dose} = \frac{15}{150} \times 1,000$$

$$\text{Pediatric dose} = 0.1 \times 1,000$$

$$\text{Pediatric dose} = 100 \text{ mg}$$

So, according to Fried's Rule, the pediatric dosage appropriate for a 15-month-old would be 100 mg.

PRACTICE Problems 14.6 Calculating Pediatric Dosages
Using Fried's Rule

1. A 24-month-old child needs acetaminophen; the normal adult dose is 650 mg. What is the appropriate dosage for the child?

2. An 18-month-old needs amikacin sulfate; the normal adult dose is 250 mg. What is the appropriate dosage for the child?

3. A child who is 30 months old needs erythromycin; the normal adult dose is 250 mg QID. What is the appropriate dosage for the child?

Calculating Pediatric Dosages Using Young's Rule

Young's Rule formula for solving pediatric dosage calculations based on the patient's age in years.

Young's Rule is another formula used in calculating pediatric dosages; it too is based on age. The difference between Young's Rule and Fried's Rule is that Young's Rule uses a formula based on the age expressed in years rather than months.

example 14.10

Let's reexamine Example 14.9 in light of Young's Rule, which uses the child's age in years. The age of a 15-month-old could be expressed as 1.25 years, since the child has lived for 12 months (1 year) + 3 months ($\frac{1}{4}$ or 0.25 of a year).

Using an age of 1.25 years and the information provided in Example 14.9, set up the calculation, using Young's Rule, as follows:

$$\text{Pediatric dose} = \frac{1.25 \text{ (age in years)}}{13.25 \text{ (age of child} + 12)} \times 1{,}000 \text{ mg (adult dose)}$$

$$\text{Pediatric dose} = \frac{1.25}{13.25} \times 1{,}000$$

$$\text{Pediatric dose} = 0.094 \times 1{,}000$$

$$\text{Pediatric dose} = 94 \text{ mg}$$

So, according to Young's Rule, the pediatric dosage appropriate for a 15-month-old would be 94 mg.

PRACTICE Problems 14.7 Calculating Pediatric Dosages
Using Young's Rule

1. A 2-year-old child is prescribed amoxicillin; the normal adult dose is 500 mg. What is the appropriate dosage for the child?

2. A 7-year-old needs propylthiouracil; the normal adult daily dose is 150 mg. What is the appropriate dosage for the child?

3. A child who is 10 years old is prescribed Tavist® syrup; the normal adult dose is 1.34 mg BID. What is the appropriate dosage for the child?

Calculating Pediatric Dosages Using Clark's Rule

Clark's Rule formula for solving pediatric dosage calculations based on the patient's weight in pounds.

Clark's Rule is yet another method for calculating a pediatric dosage. This formula is based on the patient's weight expressed in pounds.

example 14.11

Let's reexamine Example 14.9 in light of Clark's Rule, which uses the child's weight in pounds.

Using a weight of 20 pounds and the information provided in Example 14.9, set up the calculation using Young's Rule as follows:

$$\text{Pediatric dose} = \frac{20 \text{ (weight in pounds)}}{150} \times 1{,}000 \text{ mg (adult dose)}$$

$$\text{Pediatric dose} = \frac{20}{150} \times 1{,}000$$

$$\text{Pediatric dose} = 0.133 \times 1{,}000$$

$$\text{Pediatric dose} = 133 \text{ mg}$$

So, according to Clark's Rule, the pediatric dosage appropriate for a 15-month-old who weights 20 pounds would be 133 mg.

PRACTICE Problems 14.8 Calculating Pediatric Dosages Using Clark's Rule

1. A child weighing 85 pounds is prescribed hydrochlorothiazide; the normal adult dose is 50 mg. What is the appropriate dosage for the child?

2. A child weighing 70 pounds is prescribed quinine sulfate; the normal adult dose is 325 mg TID. What is the appropriate dosage for the child?

3. A child weighing 112 pounds is prescribed Kaletra®, a protease inhibitor combination therapy; the normal adult dose is 400 mg lopinavir/100 mg ritonavir. What is the appropriate dosage for the child?

Converting Weight from Pounds to Kilograms

Although it is not technically a dosage calculation, the conversion of a patient's weight from pounds to kilograms is a calculation needed when performing dosage calculations based on mg/kg, which is discussed in the next section.

example 14.12

If an infant weighs 20 pounds, what is her weight in kg?

Using the weight conversion formula, you divide the patient's weight, which in this case is 20 pounds, by 2.2 to convert the weight from pounds to kilograms.

$$20 \div 2.2 = 9.09$$

So, the infant weighs 9.09 kg.

PRACTICE Problems 14.9 Converting Weight

Convert the following.

1. 115 pounds = _____ kg

2. 18 kg = _____ pounds

3. 74 pounds = _____ kg

4. 50 kg = _____ pounds

5. 41 kg = _____ pounds

6. 60 pounds = _____ kg

7. 24 kg = _____ pounds

8. 100 pounds = _____ kg

Calculating Dosages Using mg/kg/day

mg/kg/day formula for solving dosage calculations based on the patient's weight in kilograms.

The most precise, and preferred, method of calculating dosages is based on the number of milligrams suggested per kilogram per day, or **mg/kg/day**. This method is also the most accurate and preferred method when calculating pediatric dosages.

example 14.13

Using the infant from Examples 14.9–14.11, determine the pediatric dosage if it is recommended to administer 20 mg/kg/day (maximum of 1 g) of streptomycin sulfate to this infant.

We have already calculated this infant's weight in kg as 9.09 kg, so now we will multiply the recommended number of milligrams by her weight in kilograms to calculate the appropriate daily pediatric dosage.

20 mg × 9.09 kg × 1 day = Pediatric daily dosage

20 × 9.09 × 1 = Pediatric daily dosage

181.8 = Pediatric daily dosage

So, according to the mg/kg/day formula, the patient should be given 181.8 mg of streptomycin sulfate as a daily IM injection.

PRACTICE Problems 14.10 Calculating Dosages Using mg/kg/day

1. A dose of 4 mg/kg/day of Plaquenil® can be recommended for certain children suffering from lupus. What would be the appropriate dosage for a patient who weighs 47 kg?

2. For children, the daily dose of Omnicef® is 14 mg/kg, up to a maximum dose of 600 mg/day. What is the appropriate daily dosage for a patient who weighs 98 pounds?

3. The recommended dosage of fluconazole for oropharyngeal candidiasis is 6 mg/kg on day one, followed by 3 mg/kg/day thereafter. What are the appropriate dosages for a child weighing 30 kg?

4. A child who weighs 76 pounds is prescribed the antibiotic cefaclor. It is recommended that children receive 20 mg/kg/day in divided doses every 8 hours. How many mg should this child take per dose?

5. Acute lymphatic leukemia in children can respond well to methotrexate given 2.5 mg/kg every 14 days by IV. What would be the appropriate dosage of methotrexate to administer biweekly to a child weighing 110 pounds?

PROFILES IN PRACTICE

David is a pharmacy technician who works at a chain drugstore pharmacy. Recently he filled a prescription for a patient that contained 60 tablets, with directions to take 1–2 tablets twice daily. David entered the prescription as a 30-day supply. After 2 weeks, the patient requested a refill and it is being denied by the insurance company.

- What mistake did David make?
- What steps can he take to resolve the problem?

SUMMARY

Dosage calculations are varied, and more than likely will be the pharmacy calculations you perform most often. Dosage calculations include determining the number of doses, dispensing quantities, and amount of active ingredients required, for both adult and pediatric patients.

CHAPTER REVIEW QUESTIONS

1. How many 1 tsp. doses are in 1 qt. of lactulose solution, USP 10 g/15 mL?

   a. 32 doses
   b. 64 doses
   c. 128 doses
   d. 192 doses

2. How many milligrams of estradiol are delivered over 72 hours by one 0.075 mg/day patch?

   a. 0.225 mg
   b. 1.6 mg
   c. 8 mg
   d. 0.075 mg

3. You are asked to compound maldroxyl 60 mL, diphenhydramine elixir 60 mL, and viscous lidocaine 2%, qs to 200 mL. How much viscous lidocaine 2% will you need to prepare the order?

   a. 60 mL
   b. 4 mL
   c. 80 mL
   d. 200 mL

4. The recommended pediatric dose of ampicillin is 25 mg/kg/day q8h. Your patient is a 4-week-old infant who weighs 8.7 pounds. Which is the best dose for this patient?

   a. 15 mg
   b. 25 mg
   c. 33 mg
   d. 45 mg

5. How many days will 4 oz. of clemastine fumarate syrup 0.5 mg/5 mL last if the dose is $\frac{1}{2}$ tsp. daily?

   a. 24 days
   b. 48 days
   c. 30 days
   d. 60 days

6. How many grams of drug are in 480 mL of docusate sodium syrup 60 mg/15 mL?

   a. 28.8 g
   b. 1.92 g
   c. 1,920 g
   d. 2.88 g

7. How many milligrams are in a 2 mL dose of prochlorperazine injection 5 mg/mL given IM for severe nausea and vomiting?
   a. 10 mg
   b. 5 mg
   c. 2.5 mg
   d. 15 mg

8. How many milliliters of chloral hydrate syrup 500 mg/5 mL are required for a dose of 100 mg?
   a. 2.5 mL
   b. 5 mL
   c. 2 mL
   d. 1 mL

9. The recommended pediatric dose for promethazine is 0.25 mg/kg QID. What is the best dose for a 12-year-old male who weighs 95 pounds?
   a. 2.5 mg
   b. 10 mg
   c. 12.5 mg
   d. 15 mg

10. How many total grams of active ingredient are in five syringes of testosterone 4% topical gel containing 3 g of gel each?
   a. 15 g
   b. 0.6 g
   c. 2.4 g
   d. 60 g

CRITICAL THINKING QUESTIONS

1. How do dosage calculations affect the insurance billing process?

2. Explain the various methods of calculating pediatric dosages and list the preferred method.

3. List the various types of dosage calculations, along with an explanation of how to solve each type.

REFERENCES AND RESOURCES

Hegstad, LN, & Hayek, W. *Essential Drug Dosage Calculations* (4th ed.). Upper Saddle River, NJ: Pearson, 2001.

Johnston, M. *Pharmacy Calculations*. Upper Saddle River, NJ: Pearson, 2005.

Lesmeister, MB. *Math Basics for the Healthcare Professional* (2d ed.). Upper Saddle River, NJ: Pearson, 2005.

Mikolah, AA. *Drug Dosage Calculations for the Emergency Care Provider* (2d ed.). Upper Saddle River, NJ: Prentice-Hall, 2003.

Olsen, JL, Giangrasso, AP, & Shrimpton, D. *Medical Dosage Calculations* (9th ed.). Upper Saddle River, NJ: Pearson, 2008.

Concentrations and Dilutions

15 chapter

LEARNING OBJECTIVES

After completing this chapter, you should be able to:

- Calculate weight/weight concentrations.
- Calculate weight/volume concentrations.
- Calculate volume/volume concentrations.
- Calculate dilutions of stock solutions.

Introduction

Concentrations of many pharmaceutical preparations are expressed as a **percent strength.** This is an important concept. Percent strength represents how many grams of active ingredient are in 100 mL. In the case of solids such as ointments, percent strength represents the number of grams of active ingredient contained in 100 g. Percent strength can be reduced to a fraction or to a decimal, which may be useful in solving these calculations. It is best to convert any ratio strengths to percents.

concentration term for the strength of active pharmaceutical ingredient in a medication.

percent strength representation of the number of grams of active ingredient contained in 100 mL.

> ## Workplace Wisdom Equivalents
>
> Grams and milliliters are used interchangeably in concentration problems, as they are considered equivalent measures. Which you are dealing with depends on whether you are working with solids, in grams; or liquids, in milliliters.

Concentrations

Concentrations problems are classified into three categories.

% weight/weight (%w/w)
percent strength concentration of a solid active ingredient contained within a solid base.

% weight/volume (%w/v)
percent strength concentration of a solid active ingredient contained within a liquid base.

% volume/volume (%v/v)
percent strength concentration of a liquid active ingredient contained within a liquid base.

- **Weight/weight** concentrations are those in which a solid active ingredient (e.g., a powder) is mixed with a solid base (e.g., an ointment).
- **Weight/volume** concentrations are those in which a solid active ingredient (e.g., a powder) is mixed with a liquid base (e.g., a syrup).
- **Volume/volume** concentrations are those in which a liquid active ingredient is mixed with a liquid base (e.g., an emulsion).

Weight/Weight Concentrations

Calculation of weight/weight concentrations can be easily and accurately performed by following these steps:

1. Set up a proportion with the amount of active ingredient listed over the total quantity, as grams over grams.
2. Convert the proportion to a decimal (by dividing the numerator by the denominator).
3. Multiply the converted number by 100 to express the final concentration as a percentage.

example 15.1

1 g of active ingredient powder is mixed with 99 g of white petrolatum. What is the final concentration (w/w)?

Let's look at the information that has been provided and is critical to solving the calculation:

1 g	amount of active ingredient
99 g white petrolatum	amount of base
100 g*	total quantity (1 g of active + 99 g of base)

*It is important to be careful in determining the amount for the total quantity. If you do not add both the active and base quantities for the total quantity—even if they are not both listed—the calculation will be set up incorrectly from the very start!

The first step is to set up a proportion with the amount of active ingredient listed over the total quantity.

$$\frac{1 \text{ g (active)}}{100 \text{ g (total)}}$$

Next, convert the proportion to a decimal by dividing the numerator by the denominator.

$1 \text{ g} \div 100 \text{ g} = 0.01$

Now, multiply the converted number by 100 to express the final concentration as a percentage.

$0.01 \times 100 = 1\%$

So, the final weight/weight concentration is 1%.

example 15.2

12 g of active ingredient powder is in a 120 g compounded cream.

What is the concentration (w/w)?

Let's look at the information that has been provided and is critical to solving the calculation:

12 g	amount of active ingredient
not provided	amount of base
120 g*	total quantity

*In this example, we are not given the amount of base, only the amount of active ingredient and the total quantity.

First, set up a proportion with the amount of active ingredient listed over the total quantity.

$$\frac{12 \text{ g (active)}}{120 \text{ g (total)}}$$

Now, convert the proportion to a decimal by dividing the numerator by the denominator.

$12 \text{ g} \div 120 \text{ g} = 0.1$

Finally, multiply the converted number by 100 to express the final concentration as a percentage.

$0.1 \times 100 = 10\%$

Therefore, the final weight/weight concentration of the compounded cream is 10%.

example 15.3

30 g of a compounded ointment contains 105 mg of neomycin sulfate. What is the final concentration (w/w)?

Let's look at the information that has been provided and is critical to solving the calculation:

0.105 g	amount of active ingredient
not provided	amount of base
30 g	total quantity

" **Workplace Wisdom** Calculating Concentrations

For accurate concentration calculations, the proportion must be set up as grams over grams. In Example 15.3, the problem provides the amount of active ingredient in milligrams, which must first be converted to grams. "

Set up a proportion with the amount of active ingredient listed over the total quantity.

$$\frac{0.105 \text{ g (active)}}{30 \text{ g (total)}}$$

Then, convert the proportion to a decimal by dividing the numerator by the denominator.

$$0.105 \text{ g} \div 30 \text{ g} = 0.0035$$

Now, multiply the converted number by 100 to express the final concentration as a percentage.

$$0.0035 \times 100 = 0.35\%$$

The final weight/weight concentration is 0.35%.

example 15.4

If you add 3 g of salicylic acid to 97 g of an ointment base, what is the final concentration (w/w) of the product?

Let's look at the information that has been provided and is critical to solving the calculation:

3 g	amount of active ingredient
97 g	amount of base
100 g	total quantity (3 g + 97 g)

Set up a proportion with the amount of active ingredient listed over the total quantity.

$$\frac{3 \text{ g (active)}}{100 \text{ g (total)}}$$

Now, convert the proportion to a decimal by dividing the numerator by the denominator.

$$3 \text{ g} \div 100 \text{ g} = 0.03$$

Multiply the converted number by 100 to express the final concentration as a percentage.

$$0.03 \times 100 = 3\%$$

The final weight/weight concentration of the ointment is 3%.

example 15.5

How much oxiconazole nitrate powder is required to prepare the following order?

Dr. Barbara Clemmons
121 West Loop
Tacoma, WA 00000
phone 555-0404

For _Sharon Parker_   Date _1-21_

Address _____

℞

    1% Oxiconazole
    Nitrate Ointment
        Disp. 45g

_____   _____
SUBSTITUTION PERMITTED   DISPENSE AS WRITTEN

MeK-3   REFILL _____ TIMES   DEA No. _____   MO

Let's look at the information that has been provided—and find out what is missing.

not provided	amount of active
not provided	amount of base
45 g	total quantity
1%	final

In this problem, we have been given the final concentration, and we are being asked to determine the amount of active ingredient needed. Notice that, in essence, the previous examples could have been solved by using the following formula:

$$\frac{\text{g active}}{\text{g total qty.}} \times 100 = \text{final \% strength}$$

Up to this point, we have been able to solve for the final percent strength (% strength) by filling in the other amounts and solving. We will take the same approach to solving this problem; the only difference is that we will be solving for the number of grams of active ingredient.

Using the information we know and the preceding formula, let's fill in everything we can.

$$\frac{\text{X g (active)}}{\text{45 g (total)}} \times 100 = 1\%$$

To solve for X, the unknown quantity of active ingredient, we can divide both sides of the equation by 100. This will cancel it out on the left side and create a fraction on the right side.

$$\frac{\text{X g (active)}}{\text{45 g (total)}} \times \frac{\cancel{100}}{\cancel{100}} = \frac{1}{100}$$

Now we have a ratio and proportion, which can be solved by cross-multiplication and solving for X.

$$\frac{X \text{ g (active)}}{45 \text{ g (total)}} = \frac{1}{100}$$

Cross-multiply.

$$X \times 100 = 100X$$

$$1 \times 45 = 45$$

So, $100X = 45$

Now we can divide both sides by 100 to solve for X (the quantity of active ingredient needed).

$$\frac{\cancel{100}X}{\cancel{100}} = \frac{45}{100}$$

$$X = 0.45$$

So, 0.45 g or 450 mg of oxiconazole nitrate powder is needed for this order.

example 15.6

How much fluorouracil powder is in 5% Efudex® cream 25 g?

Let's look at the information that has been provided.

not provided	amount of active
not provided	amount of base
25 g	total quantity
5%	final

Again, we have been given the final concentration and we are being asked to determine the amount of active ingredient needed.

Using the information known and the formula, fill in everything you can.

$$\frac{X \text{ g (active)}}{25 \text{ g (total)}} \times 100 = 5\%$$

Divide both sides of the equation by 100 to set up a ratio and proportion that can be solved.

$$\frac{X \text{ g 1active2}}{25 \text{ g 1total2}} \times \frac{\cancel{100}}{\cancel{100}} = \frac{5}{100}$$

Now we have a ratio and proportion, which can be solved by cross-multiplication and solving for X.

$$\frac{X \text{ g (active)}}{25 \text{ g (total)}} = \frac{5}{100}$$

Cross-multiply.

$X \times 100 = 100X$

$5 \times 25 = 125$

So, $100X = 125$

Now, divide both sides by 100 to solve for X (the quantity of active ingredient needed).

$$\frac{\cancel{100}X}{\cancel{100}} = \frac{125}{100}$$

$X = 1.25$

So, 1.25 g of fluorouracil powder is contained in 25 g of 5% Efudex® cream.

PRACTICE Problems 15.1 Weight/Weight Concentrations

1. 3 g of Zovirax® ointment contains 150 mg of acyclovir. What is the concentration of this product?

2. 15 g of Tinactin® contains 0.15 g of tolnaftate powder. What is the % strength of this cream?

3. Bactroban® ointment contains 0.6 g of mupirocin per 30 g tube. What is the % strength?

4. Zonalon® cream contains 1.5 g of doxepin HCl with 28.5 g of a cream base. What is the concentration of Zonalon®?

5. To prepare a topical cream, you add 150 mg of metronidazole to 14.85 g of a cream base. What is the final % strength of the cream?

6. 6 g of azelaic acid is added to 24 g of cream base to produce Azelex® cream. What is the concentration of this product?

7. Hytone® contains 500 mg of hydrocortisone powder with 19.5 g of emollient base. What is the % strength of Hytone®?

8. How much boric acid is contained in 30 g of a 10% boric acid ointment?

9. How much sulfur is contained in 120 g of 5% Plexion SCT® cream?

10. Vaniqa® cream contains 13.9% eflornithine HCl. How many grams of active ingredient is contained in 30 grams of Vaniqa®?

Weight/Volume Concentrations

Calculation of weight/volume concentrations can be easily and accurately performed by following these steps:

1. Set up a proportion with the amount of active ingredient listed over the total quantity, as grams over milliliters.

2. Convert the proportion to a decimal (by dividing the numerator by the denominator).

3. Multiply the converted number by 100 to express the final concentration as a percentage.

example 15.7

100 g of active ingredient powder is mixed with 500 mL normal saline. What is the final concentration (w/v)?

Let's look at the information that has been provided and is critical to solving the calculation:

100 g	amount of active ingredient
500 mL normal saline	amount of base
500 mL	total quantity

Workplace Wisdom Weight/Volume Concentrations

When mixing powders with liquids, the liquid (base) quantity is considered the total quantity, because the powder will either dissolve or suspend within the base liquid.

The first step is to set up a proportion with the amount of active ingredient listed over the total quantity.

$$\frac{100 \text{ g (active)}}{500 \text{ mL (total)}}$$

Next, convert the proportion to a decimal by dividing the numerator by the denominator.

$100 \text{ g} \div 500 \text{ mL} = 0.2$

Now, multiply the converted number by 100 to express the final concentration as a percentage.

$0.2 \times 100 = 20\%$

So, the final weight/volume concentration is 20%.

example 15.8

25 g of active ingredient powder is mixed with 250 mL of distilled water. What is the final percent strength (w/v)?

Let's look at the information that has been provided and is critical to solving the calculation:

25 g	amount of active ingredient
250 mL	total quantity

First, set up a proportion with the amount of active ingredient listed over the total quantity.

$$\frac{25 \text{ g (active)}}{250 \text{ mL (total)}}$$

Next, convert the proportion to a decimal by dividing the numerator by the denominator.

25 g ÷ 250 mL = 0.1

Now, multiply the converted number by 100 to express the final concentration as a percentage.

0.1 × 100 = 10%

So, the final weight/volume percent strength is 10%.

example 15.9

9 g of sodium chloride is diluted in 1 L of sterile water for injection (SWFI). What is the final percent strength (w/v)?

Let's look at the information that has been provided and is critical to solving the calculation:

9 g   amount of active ingredient
1,000 mL*   total quantity

*Remember that the total quantity must be expressed as milliliters, so the 1 L given in the original problem statement is converted to 1,000 mL.

Set up a proportion with the amount of active ingredient listed over the total quantity.

$$\frac{9 \text{ g (active)}}{1,000 \text{ mL (total)}}$$

Next, convert the proportion to a decimal by dividing the numerator by the denominator.

9 g ÷ 1000 mL = 0.009

Now, multiply the converted number by 100 to express the final concentration as a percentage.

0.009 × 100 = 0.9%

So, the final weight/volume percent strength is 0.9%.

example 15.10

30 mL of Xylocaine® liquid contains 1.5 g of lidocaine HCl. What is the final concentration (w/v)?

Let's look at the information that has been provided and is critical to solving the calculation:

1.5 g   amount of active ingredient
30 mL   total quantity

Set up a proportion with the amount of active ingredient listed over the total quantity.

$$\frac{1.5 \text{ g (active)}}{30 \text{ mL (total)}}$$

Now, convert the proportion to a decimal by dividing the numerator by the denominator.

1.5 g ÷ 30 mL = 0.05

Finally, multiply the converted number by 100 to express the final concentration as a percentage.

0.05 × 100 = 5%

So, the final weight/volume concentration is 5%.

example 15.11

Melanex® solution contains 0.9 g of hydroquinone in every 1 oz. bottle. What is the final percent strength (w/v)?

Let's look at the information that has been provided and is critical to solving the calculation:

0.9 g   amount of active ingredient

30 mL*   total quantity

*Remember that the total quantity must be expressed as milliliters, so the 1 oz. is converted to 30 mL.

Set up a proportion with the amount of active ingredient listed over the total quantity.

$$\frac{0.9 \text{ g (active)}}{30 \text{ mL (total)}}$$

Next, convert the proportion to a decimal by dividing the numerator by the denominator.

0.9 g ÷ 30 mL = 0.03

Now, multiply the converted number by 100 to express the final concentration as a percentage.

0.03 × 100 = 3%

So, the final weight/volume percent strength is 3%.

example 15.12

Rogaine® Extra Strength is a 5% solution of minoxidil in alcohol. How much active ingredient is in a 60 mL bottle?

Let's look at the information that has been provided—and find out what is missing.

not provided   amount of active ingredient

60 mL   total quantity

5%   final strength

In this problem, we have been given the final concentration and we are being asked to determine the amount of active ingredient needed. Notice that, in essence, the previous examples could be solved by using the following formula:

$$\frac{\text{g active}}{\text{mL total qty.}} \times 100 = \text{final \% strength}$$

Using the information we know and the preceding formula, let's fill in everything we can.

$$\frac{X \text{ g (active)}}{60 \text{ mL (total)}} \times 100 = 5\%$$

To solve for X, the unknown quantity of active ingredient, we can divide both sides of the equation by 100. This will cancel it out on the left side and create a fraction on the right side.

$$\frac{X \text{ g (active)}}{60 \text{ mL (total)}} \times \frac{\cancel{100}}{\cancel{100}} = \frac{5}{100}$$

Now we have a ratio and proportion, which can be solved by cross-multiplication and solving for X.

$$\frac{X \text{ g (active)}}{60 \text{ mL (total)}} = \frac{5}{100}$$

Cross-multiply.

$$X \times 100 = 100X$$

$$60 \times 5 = 300$$

So, $100X = 300$

Now we can divide both sides by 100 to solve for x (the quantity of active ingredient needed).

$$\frac{\cancel{100}X}{\cancel{100}} = \frac{300}{100}$$

$$X = 3$$

So, a 60 mL bottle of 5% Rogaine® Extra Strength contains 3 g of minoxidil powder.

PRACTICE Problems 15.2 Weight/Volume Concentrations

1. Betagan Liquifilm® contains 25 mg of levobunolol HCl in 10 mL of solution. What is the % strength?
2. 50 g of dextrose is added to 1 L of SWFI. What is the final concentration?
3. Cleocin T® contains 10 mg of clindamycin phosphate per mL of solution. What % strength is this product?
4. Pred Forte® contains 0.15 g of prednisolone in 15 mL of opthalmic suspension. What is the concentration?
5. How much sodium chloride powder is needed to prepare 500 mL of a 0.45% NaCL solution?
6. How much phenylephrine HCl would be needed to prepare 20 mL of a 5% ophthalmic solution?
7. Sebizon® lotion contains 8.5 g sulfacetamide sodium in 85 mL. What is the final concentration of this product?
8. How much silver nitrate is needed to prepare one ounce of a 35% silver nitrate solution?
9. How much albuterol sulfate is needed to compound 120 unit-dose vials (3 mL) of 0.042% albuterol for nebulization?
10. Drysol® contains 7.5 g of aluminum chloride hexahydrate in 37.5 mL of an alcohol base. What is the final % strength of Drysol®?

Volume/Volume Concentrations

Calculation of volume/volume concentrations can be easily and accurately performed by following these steps:

1. Set up a proportion with the amount of active ingredient listed over the total quantity, as milliliters over milliliters.
2. Convert the proportion to a decimal (by dividing the numerator by the denominator).
3. Multiply the converted number by 100 to express the final concentration as a percentage.

example 15.13

10 mL of active ingredient is mixed with distilled water to total 200 mL. What is the final concentration (v/v)?

Let's look at the information that has been provided and is critical to solving the calculation:

10 mL   amount of active ingredient
200 mL   total quantity

The first step is to set up a proportion with the amount of active ingredient listed over the total quantity.

$$\frac{10 \text{ mL (active)}}{200 \text{ mL (total)}}$$

Next, convert the proportion to a decimal by dividing the numerator by the denominator.

10 mL ÷ 200 mL = 0.05

Now, multiply the converted number by 100 to express the final concentration as a percentage.

0.05 × 100 = 5%

So, the final volume/volume concentration is 5%.

example 15.14

180 mL of active ingredient is added to 820 mL of an alcohol-based solution. What is the final strength (v/v)?

Let's look at the information that has been provided and is critical to solving the calculation:

180 mL   amount of active ingredient
820 mL   amount of base
1,000 mL   total quantity

Workplace Wisdom Volume/Volume Concentrations

It is important to be careful when determining the amount for the total quantity. If you do not add both the active and base quantities for the total quantity, even if they are not both listed, the calculation will be set up incorrectly from the very start!

The first step is to set up a proportion with the amount of active ingredient listed over the total quantity.

$$\frac{180 \text{ mL (active)}}{1,000 \text{ mL (total)}}$$

Next, convert the proportion to a decimal by dividing the numerator by the denominator.

$$180 \text{ mL} \div 1000 \text{ mL} = 0.18$$

Now, multiply the converted number by 100 to express the final concentration as a percentage.

$$0.18 \times 100 = 18\%$$

So, the final volume/volume strength is 18%.

example 15.15

36 mL of bezoin tincture is combined with 84 mL of an 80% alcohol solution. What is the final strength (v/v)?

Let's look at the information that has been provided and is critical to solving the calculation:

36 mL	amount of active ingredient
84 mL	amount of base
120 mL	total quantity

Be careful: 80% is not a factor in solving this problem. It is simply describing the base product.

The first step is to set up a proportion with the amount of active ingredient listed over the total quantity.

$$\frac{36 \text{ mL (active)}}{120 \text{ mL (total)}}$$

Next, convert the proportion to a decimal by dividing the numerator by the denominator.

$$36 \text{ mL} \div 120 \text{ mL} = 0.3$$

Now, multiply the converted number by 100 to express the final concentration as a percentage.

$$0.3 \times 100 = 30\%$$

So, the final volume/volume strength is 30%.

example 15.16

How many mL of active ingredient must be added to distilled water to produce 60 mL of a 25% solution (v/v)?

Let's look at the information that has been provided—and find out what is missing.

not provided   amount of active ingredient
60 mL   total quantity
25%   final strength

In this problem, we have been given the final concentration, and we are being asked to determine the amount of active ingredient needed. Notice that, in essence, the previous examples could have been solved by using the following formula:

$$\frac{\text{mL active}}{\text{mL total qty.}} \times 100 = \text{final \% strength}$$

Using the information we know and the preceding formula, let's fill in everything we can.

$$\frac{\text{X mL (active)}}{60 \text{ mL (total)}} \times 100 = 25\%$$

To solve for X, the unknown quantity of active ingredient, we can divide both sides of the equation by 100. This will cancel it out on the left side and create a fraction on the right side.

$$\frac{\text{X mL 1active2}}{60 \text{ mL 1total2}} \times \frac{\cancel{100}}{\cancel{100}} = \frac{25}{100}$$

Now we have a ratio and proportion, which can be solved by cross-multiplication and solving for X.

$$\frac{\text{X mL (active)}}{60 \text{ mL (total)}} = \frac{25}{100}$$

Cross-multiply.

$$\text{X} \times 100 = 100\text{X}$$

$$60 \times 25 = 1500$$

So, $100\text{X} = 1500$

Now we can divide both sides by 100 to solve for X (the quantity of active ingredient needed).

$$\frac{\cancel{100}\text{X}}{\cancel{100}} = \frac{1500}{100}$$

$$\text{X} = 15$$

So, 15 mL of active ingredient is necessary to produce 60 mL of a 25% solution.

PRACTICE Problems 15.3 Volume/Volume Concentrations

1. 10 mL of alcohol combined with 90 mL of distilled water would yield what % v/v concentration?
2. 150 mL of active ingredient is combined with 350 mL of normal saline. What is the final % strength?
3. Two tablespoons of extract are mixed with 120 mL of oral suspension base. What is the final concentration of the suspension?
4. 5 mL of medicated tincture is combined with simple syrup to total 2 ounces. What is the final % strength of the product?

5. 48 mL of lidocaine is mixed with 552 mL of a suspension base. What is the final % v/v?

6. How many milliliters of active ingredient are required to be added to normal saline to produce a total of 250 mL of 15% solution?

7. How much gentian violet should be added to alcohol to produce a total of 1 L of a 10% solution?

8. How much active ingredient must be added to distilled water to produce a total of 20 mL of a 70% solution?

9. 20 mL of butyl stearate is mixed with 380 mL of alcohol. What is the final % strength?

10. 35 mL of artificial flavor concentrate is mixed with 105 mL of SWFI. What is the final concentration?

Dilutions

Stock solutions are strong (very concentrated) solutions that you can later dilute to the strength ordered or desired. The larger volume that you mix with the stock solution is called the **diluent**. You can use the following formula to calculate dilutions, where Q represents the quantity, expressed in milliliters or grams, and C represents the concentration listed as a percentage strength:

diluent a substance used to dilute another substance.

$$Q_1 \times C_1 = Q_2 \times C_2$$

The equation may also be shown this way, as a ratio and proportion:

$$\frac{Q_1}{Q_2} :: \frac{C_2}{C_1}$$

Notice that the quantities are shown on one side and the concentrations on the other. Note also that the initial values, represented by the number 1, are diagonal to each other and that the final values, represented by the number 2, are on the opposite diagonal.

Calculating dilution problems requires you to place the provided elements in the formula appropriately before solving.

Q_1 = initial quantity or volume

Q_2 = final, or desired, quantity or volume

C_1 = initial concentration expressed as a percentage (stock solution)

C_2 = final, or desired, concentration expressed as a percentage (final solution)

When solving dilutions, three of these four elements will be provided; you must place them appropriately in the formula and then solve for the unknown.

example 15.17

How much stock solution of hydrogen peroxide 12% solution will you need to make 480 mL of hydrogen peroxide 3% solution?

$Q_1 = X$

$C_1 = 12\%$

$Q_2 = 480$ mL

$C_2 = 3\%$

Use the formula by plugging in the known elements:

$X \times 12 = 480 \times 3$

$12X = 1440$

To solve for X, divide both sides by 12.

$$\frac{\cancel{12}X}{\cancel{12}} = \frac{1440}{12}$$

X = 120 mL

So, you would need 120 mL of the 12% solution to dilute to 480 mL of a 3% solution.

example 15.18

You had 60 g of a 20% coal tar solution, which you diluted to produce 100 g. What is the strength of the final product?

Q1 = 60 g

C1 = 20%

Q2 = 100 g

C2 = X

Use the formula by plugging in the known elements:

$60 \times 20 = 100 \times X$

$1200 = 100X$

To solve for X, divide both sides by 100.

$$\frac{1200}{100} = \frac{\cancel{100}X}{\cancel{100}}$$

12 = X

So, the final product is a 12% coal tar solution.

example 15.19

If you diluted 90 mL of an 8% benzocaine lotion to 6%, how much could you produce?

Q1 = 90 mL

C1 = 8%

Q2 = X

C2 = 6%

Use the formula by plugging in the known elements:

$90 \times 8 = X \times 6$

$720 = 6X$

To solve for X, divide both sides by 6.

$$\frac{720}{6} = \frac{6X}{6}$$

120 = X

So, you would be able to produce 120 mL of the diluted 6% lotion.

PRACTICE Problems 15.4 Dilutions

1. How much of a 10% solution will you need to produce 150 mL of a 6% solution?

2. How much 50% silver nitrate solution do you need to produce one ounce of a 10% silver nitrate solution?

3. How much 8% solution can you make by diluting 500 mL of a 20% solution?

4. How much 500 mcg/mL prostaglandin solution is needed to prepare 10 cc of prostaglandin 20 mcg/mL solution?

5. How much doxepin 10 mg/mL concentrate should you dilute to prepare 240 mL of doxepin 25 mg/5 mL?

6. Rx: povidone iodine 1% soaking solution 1 L. How much povidone iodine 12% solution should you dilute to prepare the order?

7. You have a stock solution of lidocaine HCl 4% solution. How much of the stock solution is needed to prepare 1 oz. of lidocaine HCl 1% nasal spray?

8. Rx: hydrochloric acid 1% solution 4 oz. You have a stock solution of hydrochloric acid 50%. How much of the stock solution is required to prepare the order?

9. You have a stock solution of hydroxycobalamin 10 mg/mL. How much of the stock solution is needed to prepare 30 mL of a hydroxycobalamin 5,000 mcg/mL solution?

10. Rx: vancomycin 50 mg/100 mL Disp: 100 mL. In stock, you have vials that contain vancomycin 50 mg/10 mL. How many milliliters of stock solution will you need to prepare this order?

PROFILES IN PRACTICE

Liz works as a pharmacy technician in a hospital inpatient pharmacy. The pharmacist asks Liz to dilute a stock solution to 25% of the original strength. Liz determines that the easiest way to do this is to take one-fourth of the volume of the original stock solution and q.s. to the original volume with SWFI.

- Does Liz obtain the desired dilution using this method?

SUMMARY

Concentrations and dilutions, which can appear overwhelming and intimidating, are in essence no more than a series of simple ratios and proportions. You will use concentrations and dilutions in a variety of pharmacy practice settings, so it is important that you master this skill.

CHAPTER REVIEW QUESTIONS

1. 50% w/w contains how many grams of active ingredient per 100 grams?
   a. 50 g
   b. 25 g
   c. 100 g
   d. 5 g

2. How many milligrams of active ingredient will you need to prepare 120 mL of a product that contains 4 mg/mL of active ingredient?
   a. 120 mg
   b. 4 mg
   c. 480 mg
   d. 400 mg

3. What is the percent strength of clemastine fumarate syrup 0.5 mg/5 mL?
   a. 0.05%
   b. 0.01%
   c. 0.025%
   d. 0.5%

4. Which of the following has the highest concentration?
   a. 4 mg/mL
   b. 4%
   c. 2 mg/mL
   d. 2%

5. What is the final volume when you dilute 10 mL of a lidocaine 6% nasal spray to a lidocaine 2% nasal spray?
   a. 10 mL
   b. 12 mL
   c. 15 mL
   d. 30 mL

6. How many milliliters of gentian violet 2% solution will you need to make 500 mL of a 0.025% solution?
   a. 6.25 mL
   b. 20 mL
   c. 50 mL
   d. 250 mL

7. What is the final strength when you dilute 25 mL of a 12% solution with 100 mL water (final volume 125 mL)?
   a. 5.0%
   b. 2.0%
   c. 2.4%
   d. 3.0%

8. What is the resulting ratio strength when you dilute 12 mL of liquid coal tar to make 240 mL of coal tar solution?
   a. 1:5
   b. 1:10
   c. 1:12
   d. 1:20

9. How many grams of thymol should you dilute to make 30 mL of a 4% thymol in alcohol topical nail solution?
   a. 0.12 g
   b. 1.2 g
   c. 4.0 g
   d. 7.5 g

10. What is the final volume when you dilute 100 mL of sorbitol 50% solution to a 20% solution?
    a. 120 mL
    b. 150 mL
    c. 250 mL
    d. 300 mL

CRITICAL THINKING QUESTIONS

1. Can a solution ever be diluted to a strength higher than the starting solution? Why or why not?

2. Why is it important to determine whether the active ingredient is contained within, or being added to, the base when calculating w/w and v/v concentrations?

3. How much normal saline (NS), would be needed to produce 1 L of 0.45% sodium chloride solution?

REFERENCES AND RESOURCES

Hegstad, LN, & Hayek, W. *Essential Drug Dosage Calculations* (4th ed.). Upper Saddle River, NJ: Pearson, 2001.

Johnston, M. *Pharmacy Calculations.* Upper Saddle River, NJ: Pearson, 2005.

Lesmeister, MB. *Math Basics for the Healthcare Professional* (2d ed.). Upper Saddle River, NJ: Pearson, 2005.

Mikolah, AA. *Drug Dosage Calculations for the Emergency Care Provider* (2d ed.). Upper Saddle River, NJ: Prentice-Hall, 2003.

Olsen, JL, Giangrasso, AP, & Shrimpton, D. *Medical Dosage Calculations* (9th ed.). Upper Saddle River, NJ: Pearson, 2008.

Alligations

16 chapter

alligation 287

After completing this chapter, you should be able to:

- Understand when to use the alligation principle for calculations.
- Calculate and solve a variety of alligation-related problems.

alligation 287

Introduction

Alligations are used when mixing two products with different percent strengths of the same active ingredient. The strength of the final product will fall between the strengths of each original product.

alligation a principle relating to the solution of questions concerning the compounding or mixing of different ingredients.

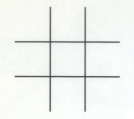

FIGURE 16-1 The alligation grid.

Solving Alligations

You can use the alligation method to determine how many parts of the same product, with different strengths, you will need to create the final strength requested. Further, you can calculate exactly how many milliliters or grams you need of each constituent (beginning) product.

The Alligation Grid

The alligation grid shown in Figure 16-1, which is also referred to as a tic-tac-toe board, is simply a tool that makes it easier to solve pharmacy alligation problems. In the following sections, you will learn what each segment of the grid represents.

INFORMATION

It is critical that you understand the following points when working alligation problems.

- Solvents and diluents, such as water, vanishing cream base, and white petrolatum, are considered to be a percent strength of zero.
- Liquids, including solutions, syrups, elixirs, and even lotions, are expressed in milliliters.
- Solids, including powders, creams, and ointments, are expressed in grams.
- The alligation formula requires that you express the strength as a percentage when setting up the problem. You must convert any ratio strength in the initial question to a percent strength.
- When writing percents or using decimals, always use a leading zero (e.g., 0.25%). This helps prevent errors in interpretation. It would be a terrible error—possibly even fatal—to dispense something in 25% strength that was really supposed to be 0.25% strength.
- 1 fl. oz. = 29.57 mL. This is commonly rounded to 30 mL.
- 1 avoirdupois oz. = 28.35 g. This measurement, used for solids, is also commonly rounded to 30 g.

---

example 16.1

Rx: Prepare 120 g of a 2% hydrocortisone ointment using a 1% ointment and a 2.5% ointment.

Let's look at the information that has been provided.

2.5%	higher strength
1 %	lower strength
2%	desired strength
120 g	desired quantity

First, draw the alligation grid.

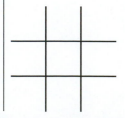

Now, fill in the alligation grid with the information provided in the problem.

- The higher strength goes in the top left box.
- The lower strength goes in the bottom left box.
- The desired strength goes in the center box.

Higher 2.5

Desired 2

Lower 1

Next, we calculate the numbers that should go into the top right and bottom right boxes.

Higher 2.5

Desired 2

Lower 1

This is done by working diagonally and taking the difference between the two numbers already in place.

Let's look at the first diagonal, which contains 2.5 and 2. The difference between these two numbers goes in the bottom right box.

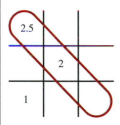

The difference between 2.5 and 2 is 0.5, so 0.5 goes in the bottom right box.

$2.5 - 2 = 0.5$

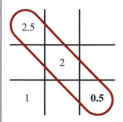

Now, we can work on the other diagonal, which contains 1 and 2. The difference between these two numbers goes into the top right box.

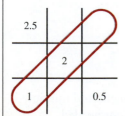

The difference between 1 and 2 is 1, so 1 goes in the top right box.

$1 - 2 = -1$

Only positive numbers can go into the alligation grid, so −1 is changed to 1.

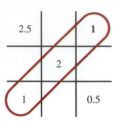

The numbers on the right-hand side of the alligation grid represent the number of parts per ingredient, when read straight across. This means that there should be 1 part of the 2.5% (higher-strength) ointment and 0.5 parts of the 1% (lower-strength) ointment to make the 2% ointment.

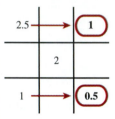

Now, by adding the numbers in the right column, we can determine the total number of parts necessary. In other words,

1 part (2.5%) + 0.5 parts (1%) = 1.5 parts total

Now that we have determined the number of parts needed for each ingredient and the total number of parts to be used, we can set these up as proportions.

$$\frac{\text{parts needed}}{\text{total parts}}$$

2.5% ointment

$$\frac{1 \text{ part}}{1.5 \text{ parts}} \text{ or } \frac{1}{1.5}$$

1% ointment

$$\frac{0.5 \text{ parts}}{1.5 \text{ parts}} \text{ or } \frac{0.5}{1.5}$$

Finally, we can take the proportion of parts needed of each ointment and multiply it by the desired quantity to determine the quantity of each ingredient needed.

2.5% ointment

$$\frac{120\text{ g}}{1.5} \times 1 = 80\text{ g}$$

1% ointment

$$\frac{120\text{ g}}{1.5} \times 0.5 = 40\text{ g}$$

So, we would combine 80 g of the 2.5% ointment and 40 g of the 1% ointment to produce 120 g of a 2% ointment.

Workplace Wisdom Positive Numbers Only

Remember that only positive numbers can be used within the alligation grid. If you are working with a negative number, remove the minus sign.

example 16.2

Rx: Prepare 90 g of triamcinolone 0.05% cream. In stock, you have 454 g each of triamcinolone 0.025% cream and triamcinolone 0.1% cream.

Let's look at the information that has been provided.

0.1%	higher strength
0.025	lower strength
0.05%	desired strength
90 g	desired quantity

First, draw the alligation grid.

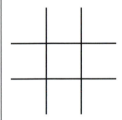

Now, fill in the alligation grid with the information provided in the problem.

- The higher strength goes in the top left box.
- The lower strength goes in the bottom left box.
- The desired strength goes in the center box.

Higher 0.1

Desired 0.05

Lower 0.025

Next, we calculate the numbers that should go into the top right and bottom right boxes.

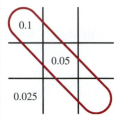

This is done by working diagonally and taking the difference between the two numbers already in place.

Let's look at the first diagonal, which contains 0.1 and 0.05. The difference between these two numbers goes in the bottom right box.

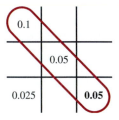

The difference between 0.1 and 0.05 is 0.05, so 0.05 goes in the bottom right box.

$$0.1 - 0.05 = 0.05$$

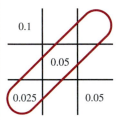

Now, we can work on the other diagonal, which contains 0.025 and 0.05. The difference between these two numbers goes in the top right box.

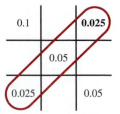

The difference between 0.025 and 0.05 is 0.025, so 0.025 goes in the top right box.

$$0.025 - 0.05 = -0.025$$

Remember, only positive numbers can go into the alligation grid, so -0.025 is changed to 0.025.

The numbers on the right-hand side of the alligation grid represent the number of parts per ingredient, when read straight across. This means that there should be 0.025 parts of the 0.1% cream and 0.05 parts of the 0.025% cream to make the 0.05% cream.

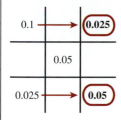

Now, by adding the numbers in the right-hand column, we can determine the total number of parts necessary. In other words,

0.025 parts (0.1%) + 0.05 parts (0.025%) = 0.075 parts total

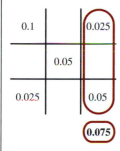

Now that we have determined the number of parts needed for each ingredient and the total number of parts to be used, we can set these up as proportions.

parts needed
─────────────
  total parts

0.1% cream

$$\frac{0.025 \text{ parts}}{0.075 \text{ parts}} \text{ or } \frac{0.025}{0.075}$$

0.025% cream

$$\frac{0.05 \text{ parts}}{0.075 \text{ parts}} \text{ or } \frac{0.05}{0.075}$$

Finally, we can take the proportion of parts needed of each cream and multiply it by the desired quantity to determine the quantity of each ingredient needed.

0.1% cream

$$\frac{90 \text{ g}}{0.075} \times 0.025 = 30 \text{ g}$$

0.025% cream

$$\frac{90 \text{ g}}{0.075} \times 0.05 = 60 \text{ g}$$

So, we would combine 30 g of the 0.1% cream and 60 g of the 0.025% cream to produce 90 g of a 0.5% cream.

example   16.3

Rx: How much of a 2.5% cream and a 0.5% cream would be required to compound 100 g of a 1% cream?

Let's look at the information that has been provided.

2.5%   higher strength
0.5%   lower strength
1%   desired strength
100 g   desired quantity

First, draw the alligation grid.

Now, fill in the alligation grid with the information provided in the problem.

- The higher strength goes in the top left box.
- The lower strength goes in the bottom left box.
- The desired strength goes in the center box.

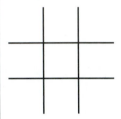

Higher 2.5

Desired 1

Lower 0.5

Next, we calculate the numbers that should go into the top right and bottom right boxes.

Higher 2.5

Desired 1

Lower 0.5

This is done by working diagonally and taking the difference between the two numbers already in place.

Let's look at the first diagonal, which contains 2.5 and 1. The difference between these two numbers goes in the bottom right box.

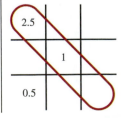

The difference between 2.5 and 1 is 1.5, so 1.5 goes in the bottom right box.

2.5 − 1 = 1.5

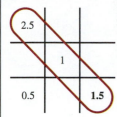

Now we can work on the other diagonal, which contains 0.5 and 1. The difference between these two numbers goes in the top right box.

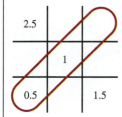

The difference between 0.5 and 1 is 0.5, so 0.5 goes in the top right box.

0.5 − 1 = −0.5

Remember, only positive numbers can go into the alligation grid, so −0.5 is changed to 0.5.

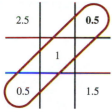

The numbers on the right-hand side of the alligation grid represent the number of parts per ingredient, when read straight across. This means that there should be 0.5 parts of the 2.5% cream and 1.5 parts of the 0.5% cream to make the 1% cream.

Now, by adding the numbers in the right-hand column, we can determine the total number of parts necessary. In other words,

0.5 parts (2.5%) + 1.5 parts (0.5%) = 2 parts total

Now that we have determined the number of parts needed for each ingredient and the total number of parts to be used, we can set these up as proportions.

$$\frac{\text{parts needed}}{\text{total parts}}$$

2.5% cream

$$\frac{0.5 \text{ parts}}{2 \text{ parts}} \text{ or } \frac{0.5}{2}$$

0.5% cream

$$\frac{1.5 \text{ parts}}{2 \text{ parts}} \text{ or } \frac{1.5}{2}$$

Finally, we can take the proportion of parts needed of each cream and multiply it by the desired quantity to determine the quantity of each ingredient needed.

2.5% cream

$$\frac{100 \text{ g}}{2} \times 0.5 = 25 \text{ g}$$

0.5% cream

$$\frac{100 \text{ g}}{2.0} \times 1.5 = 75 \text{ g}$$

So, we would combine 25 g of the 2.5% cream and 75 g of the 0.5% cream to produce 100 g of a 1% cream.

example 16.4

Rx: Prepare 500 mL of a 7.5% dextrose solution using SWFI and D10W.

Let's look at the information that has been provided.

10%	higher strength
0%	lower strength
7.5%	desired strength
500 mL	desired quantity

D10W stands for dextrose 10% in water, thus making it a 10% strength.

Remember that bases, such as SWFI, are 0% strength, because they contain no active ingredient.

Now, fill in the alligation grid with the information provided in the problem.

- The higher strength goes in the top left box.
- The lower strength goes in the bottom left box.
- The desired strength goes in the center box.

Higher 10

Desired 7.5

Lower 0

Next, we will calculate the numbers that should go into the top right and bottom right boxes. This is done by working diagonally and taking the difference between the two numbers already in place.

Let's look at the first diagonal, which contains 10 and 7.5. The difference between these two numbers goes in the bottom right box.

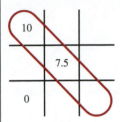

The difference between 10 and 7.5 is 2.5, so 2.5 goes in the bottom right box.

10 − 7.5 = 2.5

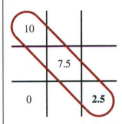

Now we can work on the other diagonal, which contains 0 and 7.5. The difference between these two numbers goes in the top right box.

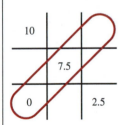

The difference between 0 and 7.5 is 7.5, so 7.5 goes in the top right box.

0 − 7.5 = −7.5

Remember, any negative number must be changed to a positive number to be used in the grid.

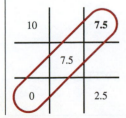

The numbers on the right-hand side of the alligation grid represent the number of parts per ingredient, when read straight across. This means that there should be 7.5 parts of the D10W and 2.5 parts of the SWFI in a 7.5% dextrose solution.

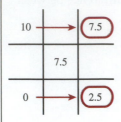

Now, by adding the numbers in the right-hand column, we can determine the total number of parts necessary. In other words,

7.5 parts (10%) + 2.5 parts (0%) = 10 parts total

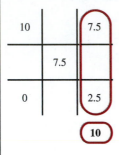

Now that we have determined the number of parts needed for each ingredient and the total number of parts to be used, we can set these up as proportions.

$$\frac{\text{parts needed}}{\text{total parts}}$$

D10W

$$\frac{7.5 \text{ parts}}{10 \text{ parts}} \quad \text{or} \quad \frac{7.5}{10}$$

SWFI

$$\frac{2.5 \text{ parts}}{10 \text{ parts}} \quad \text{or} \quad \frac{2.5}{10}$$

Finally, we can take the proportion of parts needed of each cream and multiply it by the desired quantity to determine the quantity of each ingredient needed.

D10W

$$\frac{500 \text{ mL}}{10} \times 7.5 = 375 \text{ mL}$$

SWFI

$$\frac{500 \text{ mL}}{10} \times 2.5 = 125 \text{ mL}$$

So, we would combine 375 mL of the D10W and 125 mL of the SWFI to prepare 500 mL of a 7.5% dextrose solution.

example **16.5**

Rx: Prepare 1 L of a 20% alcohol solution using a 90% alcohol and a 10% alcohol.

Let's look at the information that has been provided.

90%	higher strength
10%	lower strength
20%	desired strength
1 L (1,000 mL)	desired quantity

Now, fill in the alligation grid with the information provided in the problem.

- The higher strength goes in the top left box.
- The lower strength goes in the bottom left box.
- The desired strength goes in the center box.

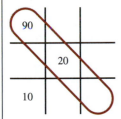

Next, we calculate the numbers that should go into the top right and bottom right boxes. This is done by working diagonally and taking the difference between the two numbers already in place.

Let's look at the first diagonal, which contains 90 and 20. The difference between these two numbers goes in the bottom right box.

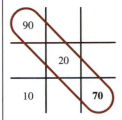

The difference between 90 and 20 is 70, so 70 goes in the bottom right box.

$$90 - 20 = 70$$

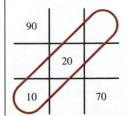

Now we can work on the other diagonal, which contains 10 and 20. The difference between these two numbers goes in the top right box.

The difference between 10 and 20 is 10, so 10 goes in the top right box.

10 − 20 = −10

Remember, any negative number must be changed to a positive number to be used in the grid.

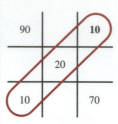

The numbers on the right-hand side of the alligation grid represent the number of parts per ingredient, when read straight across. This means that there should be 10 parts of the 90% alcohol and 70 parts of the 10% alcohol to prepare a 20% alcohol solution.

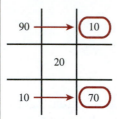

Now, by adding the numbers in the right-hand column, we can determine the total number of parts necessary. In other words,

10 parts (90%) + 70 parts (10%) = 80 parts total

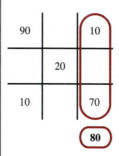

Now that we have determined the number of parts needed for each ingredient and the total number of parts to be used, we can set these up as proportions.

$$\frac{\text{parts needed}}{\text{total parts}}$$

90% alcohol

$$\frac{10 \text{ parts}}{80 \text{ parts}} \quad \text{or} \quad \frac{10}{80}$$

10% alcohol

$$\frac{70 \text{ parts}}{80 \text{ parts}} \quad \text{or} \quad \frac{70}{80}$$

Finally, we can take the proportion of parts needed of each cream and multiply it by the desired quantity to determine the quantity of each ingredient needed.

90% alcohol

$$\frac{1,000 \text{ mL}}{80} \times 10 = 125 \text{ mL}$$

10% alcohol

$$\frac{1,000 \text{ mL}}{80} \times 70 = 875 \text{ mL}$$

So, we would combine 125 mL of the 90% alcohol and 875 mL of the 10% alcohol to prepare 1 L of a 20% alcohol.

PRACTICE Problems 16.1

1. Rx: silver nitrate 0.25% solution 1% 1 L. You have one gallon of silver nitrate 1% stock solution, which you can dilute with distilled water. How many milliliters of each will you need to make the final product?

2. Rx: soaking solution 1:100 1 L. You have a 1:25 stock solution and water. How many milliliters of each will you need to prepare the order?

3. Rx: coal tar 5% ointment 120 g. You have coal tar 10% ointment and coal tar 2% ointment. How many grams of each will you use to prepare the final product?

4. You are instructed to prepare 454 g of a 15% ointment. In stock you have 5% and 30%. How much of each will you need to use to make the order?

5. Rx: Prepare 480 mL of a 1:30 solution using a 1:10 solution and a 1:50 solution. What quantities will be used of each stock solution to make the 1:30 solution?

6. You need to prepare 80 g of a 9% cream using a 20% stock cream and a cream base. How much is needed of each?

7. You are asked to prepare 1 L of a 1:200 soaking solution, using a stock 1:50 soaking solution and distilled water. How much of each will you need to use?

8. How much SWFI would you need to add to 500 mL stock normal saline (0.9% NaCl) to produce a 0.45% sodium chloride solution?

9. Rx: alcohol 30%. How many milliliters of 90% alcohol should you add to 25 mL of 10% alcohol to make 30% alcohol?

10. Rx: hydrocortisone 2% ointment. How many grams of petrolatum should you add to 30 g of hydrocortisone 2.5% ointment to reduce its strength to 2.0%? (The percent strength of petrolatum is zero.)

11. Rx: normal saline. How many milliliters of water must you add to 500 mL of a 10% stock solution of sodium chloride to make a batch of normal saline (sodium chloride 0.9% solution)?

12. Rx: ichthammol 5% ointment. How many grams of ichthammol 10% ointment should you add to 20 g of ichthammol 2% ointment to make ichthammol 5% ointment?

13. Rx: benzalkonium chloride 1:1000 solution. How many milliliters of water should you add to 50 mL of benzalkonium chloride 0.25% solution to prepare the order?

14. Rx: zinc oxide 10% ointment 45 g. How many grams of zinc oxide 20% ointment and zinc oxide 5% ointment should you mix to prepare the order?

15. Rx: aluminum acetate 1:400 solution 1 gallon. How many milliliters of Burrow's solution (aluminum acetate 5%) should you use to prepare the order?

16. Rx: histamine phosphate 1:10,000 solution 10 mL. How many milliliters of a histamine phosphate 1:10 solution do you need to prepare the order?

17. Rx: benzocaine 5% ointment 2 oz. How many grams of benzocaine 2% ointment should you mix with 22.5 g of benzocaine 10% ointment to prepare the order?

18. When using a 0.5% cream and a 2% cream to produce a 1.25% cream, how many parts of each initial ingredient are needed?

19. In what proportion would you add SWFI to D10W to produce D6W?

20. In what proportion should you add a 1:20 soaking solution and distilled water to create a 1:50 solution?

PROFILES IN PRACTICE

Nick is a pharmacy technician who works at an independent, compounding pharmacy. A dermatologist has prescribed a topical ointment in precisely 0.45%, to accommodate the patient's sensitivities. After researching the substance, Nick discovers that the lowest strength available for the medication is 2%.

- What can Nick compound the stock medication with to produce 60 g of the 0.45% ointment, and with what quantities?

SUMMARY

In certain situations, a pharmacy must use the alligation method to combine two varying strengths of a drug, or combine a drug with a base or diluent, to achieve the prescribed strength. Although these calculations can be confusing at first, once you master the alligation grid you should be able to perform these calculations easily.

CHAPTER REVIEW QUESTIONS

1. How much 20% cream should you add to 26 g of 1% cream to make a 4% cream?
   a. 6.00 g
   b. 5.20 g
   c. 4.88 g
   d. 3.00 g

2. How much 25% stock solution and distilled water will you need to make 1 L of a 1:400 solution?
   a. 10 mL of the 25% solution and 990 mL of water
   b. 100 mL of the 25% solution and 900 mL of water
   c. 990 mL of the 25% solution and 10 mL of water
   d. 900 mL of the 25% solution and 10 mL of water

3. How much of a 10% cream and a 0.5% cream will you need to prepare 120 g of a 2.5% cream?
   a. 20 g of the 10% cream and 100 g of the 0.5% cream
   b. 100 g of the 10% cream and 20 g of the 0.5% cream
   c. 25 g of the 10% cream and 95 g of the 0.5% cream
   d. 95 g of the 10% cream and 25 g of the 0.5% cream

4. How much povidone iodine 20% solution and water will you need to make 500 mL of a povidone iodine 3% rinse?
   a. 75 mL of the 20% solution and 425 mL of water
   b. 425 mL of the 20% solution and 25 mL of water
   c. 20 mL of the 20% solution and 480 mL of water
   d. 480 mL of the 20% solution and 20 mL of water

5. How much lidocaine 0.5% topical gel should you mix with lidocaine 10% topical gel to make 15 g of a lidocaine 2% topical gel?

   a. 2.4 g
   b. 5.0 g
   c. 9.5 g
   d. 12.6 g

6. How much 1:25 solution and 1:500 solution should you mix to make 1 L of a 1:250 soaking solution?

   a. 947 mL of the 1:25 solution and 53 mL of the 1:500 solution
   b. 53 mL of the 1:25 solution and 947 mL of the 1:500 solution
   c. 250 mL of the 1:25 solution and 750 of the 1:500 solution
   d. 750 mL of the 1:25 solution and 250 mL of the 1:500 solution

7. Convert 50% to a ratio strength.

   a. 1:2
   b. 1:4
   c. 1:6
   d. 1:8

8. How much NaCl 10% stock solution should you add to 100 mL of NaCl 0.45% solution to make normal saline?

   a. 1 mL
   b. 2 mL
   c. 5 mL
   d. 10 mL

9. How many grams of 0.1% cream should you mix with 12 g of 12% cream to make a 6% cream?

   a. 10.4 g
   b. 12.2 g
   c. 24 g
   d. 33 g

10. How many parts of each of a 1% product and a 3% product do you need to make a 2.5% product?

   a. 2.5 parts of the 1% product and 1 part of the 3% product
   b. 1 part of the 1% product and 2.5 parts of the 3% product
   c. 1.5 parts of the 1% product and 0.5 part of the 3% product
   d. 0.5 part of the 1% product and 1.5 parts of the 3% product

CRITICAL THINKING QUESTIONS

1. Why are bases, such as vanishing cream, considered 0% strength?

2. How can alligation problems be double-checked after solving, to ensure accuracy?

3. In what scenario might a pharmacy technician be required to perform an alligation problem, outside of an independent, compounding pharmacy?

REFERENCES AND RESOURCES

Hegstad, LN, & Hayek, W. *Essential Drug Dosage Calculations* (4th ed.). Upper Saddle River, NJ: Pearson, 2001.

Johnston, M. *Pharmacy Calculations.* Upper Saddle River, NJ: Pearson, 2005.

Lesmeister, MB. *Math Basics for the Healthcare Professional* (2d ed.). Upper Saddle River, NJ: Pearson, 2005.

Mikolah, AA. *Drug Dosage Calculations for the Emergency Care Provider* (2d ed.). Upper Saddle River, NJ: Prentice-Hall, 2003.

Olsen, JL, Giangrasso, AP, & Shrimpton, D. *Medical Dosage Calculations* (8th ed.). Upper Saddle River, NJ: Pearson, 2004.

LEARNING OBJECTIVES

After completing this chapter, you should be able to:

- Illustrate the principle of basic dimensional analysis.
- Calculate flow duration for parenteral products.
- Calculate the volume per hour for parenteral orders.
- Calculate the drug per hour for parenteral products.
- Calculate drip rates in both drops/minute and milliliters/hour.
- Calculate TPN milliequivalents.

Introduction

The preparation and administration of parenteral products, such as IVs, infusions, TPN, and chemotherapy, require the performance of specific calculations. It is common for individuals to become overwhelmed and confused when approaching complex pharmacy calculations. The truth is, however, that although many pharmacy calculations may appear to be complex, they are in actuality very simple. This chapter explains parenteral calculations using the principle of basic dimensional analysis.

Basic Dimensional Analysis

Calculations regarding sterile product and flow rates are typically viewed as among the most difficult in pharmacy practice, but each problem can be solved by using either basic dimensional analysis or ratios/proportions. We covered ratios/proportions extensively in earlier chapters of this book, so now we investigate the basics of dimensional analysis.

Before moving forward, however, let's review several fundamental math principles.

1. Any number multiplied by 1 retains the same value.

    example: $4 \times 1 = 4$
    example: $\frac{1}{2} \times 1 = \frac{1}{2}$

2. Any whole number can be expressed as a fraction by placing a 1 as the denominator.

    example: $3 = \frac{3}{1}$
    example: $18 = \frac{18}{1}$

3. Any number divided by itself equals 1.

    example: $4 \div 4 = 1$
    example: $\frac{2}{2} = 1$

The first set of examples and practice problems (Examples 17.1–17.5) in this chapter will not appear to have anything at all to do with sterile product calculations, but be patient: These early examples are laying a foundation so that you can better comprehend more "advanced" flow rate calculations and solve these problems more easily.

example 17.1 Basic Dimensional Analysis

How many hours are there in 6 days?

In this problem, we are working with days and hours. What information, or facts, do we know about days and hours?

- There are 24 hours in 1 day.

This could be written as:

- 24 hours = 1 day

- $\dfrac{1 \text{ day}}{24 \text{ hours}}$

- $\dfrac{24 \text{ hours}}{1 \text{ day}}$

Using the principle of dimensional analysis, we can use this information to solve the problem.

$$6 \text{ days} = \frac{6 \text{ days}}{1} \times \frac{24 \text{ hours}}{1 \text{ day}} = ?$$

After setting the problem up, we cancel out like units and/or numbers.

$$6 \text{ days} = \frac{6 \text{ \cancel{days}}}{1} \times \frac{24 \text{ hours}}{1 \text{ \cancel{day}}} = ?$$

Which can now be written as:

$$6 \text{ days} = 6 \times 24 = ?$$

Therefore, six days is equivalent to 144 hours.

$$6 \text{ days} = 6 \times 24 = 144$$

example 17.2   Basic Dimensional Analysis

How many minutes are in 5 hours?

In this problem we are working with minutes and hours. What information, or facts, do we know about minutes and hours?

- There are 60 minutes in 1 hour.

This could be written as:

- 1 hour = 60 minutes

- $\dfrac{1 \text{ hour}}{60 \text{ minutes}}$

- $\dfrac{60 \text{ minutes}}{1 \text{ hour}}$

Using the principle of dimensional analysis, we can use this information to solve the problem.

$$5 \text{ hours} = \frac{5 \text{ hours}}{1} \times \frac{60 \text{ minutes}}{1 \text{ hour}} = ?$$

After setting the problem up, we cancel out like units and/or numbers.

$$5 \text{ hours} = \frac{5 \text{ \cancel{hours}}}{1} \times \frac{60 \text{ minutes}}{1 \text{ \cancel{hour}}} = ?$$

Which can now be written as:

$$5 \text{ hours} = 5 \times 60 = ?$$

Therefore, 5 hours is equivalent to 300 minutes.

$$5 \text{ hours} = 5 \times 60 = 300$$

example 17.3   Basic Dimensional Analysis

45 minutes is equal to how many seconds?

We know that there are 60 seconds in every 1 minute. This could be written as:

- 1 minute = 60 seconds

- $\dfrac{1 \text{ minute}}{60 \text{ seconds}}$

- $\dfrac{60 \text{ seconds}}{1 \text{ minute}}$

Using the principle of dimensional analysis, we can use this information to solve the problem.

$$45 \text{ minutes} = \frac{45 \text{ minutes}}{1} \times \frac{60 \text{ seconds}}{1 \text{ minute}} = ?$$

After setting the problem up, we cancel out like units and/or numbers.

$$45 \text{ minutes} = \frac{45 \text{ \cancel{minutes}}}{1} \times \frac{60 \text{ seconds}}{1 \text{ \cancel{minute}}} = ?$$

Which can now be written as:

45 minutes = 45 × 60 = ?

Therefore, 45 minutes is equivalent to 2,700 seconds.

45 minutes = 45 × 60 = 2,700

---

example 17.4 Basic Dimensional Analysis

How many seconds are in 3 hours?

We know that there are 60 seconds in every 1 minute and that there are 60 minutes in every hour. Using the principle of dimensional analysis, we can use this information to solve the problem—but to solve this problem, we now have to add a third component.

$$3 \text{ hours} = \frac{3 \text{ hours}}{1} \times \frac{60 \text{ minutes}}{1 \text{ hour}} \times \frac{60 \text{ seconds}}{1 \text{ minute}} = ?$$

After setting the problem up, we cancel out like units and/or numbers.

$$3 \text{ hours} = \frac{3 \cancel{\text{ hours}}}{1} \times \frac{60 \cancel{\text{ minutes}}}{1 \cancel{\text{ hour}}} \times \frac{60 \text{ seconds}}{1 \cancel{\text{ minute}}} = ?$$

Which can now be written as:

3 hours = 3 × 60 × 60 = ?

3 hours = 3 × 60 × 60 = 10,800

Therefore, there are 10,800 seconds in 3 hours.

---

example 17.5 Basic Dimensional Analysis

How many seconds are in 4 days?

We know that there are 60 seconds in every 1 minute, 60 minutes in every hour, and 24 hours in every 1 day. Using the principle of dimensional analysis, we can use this information to solve the problem—but once again we need to add an additional component not present in previous examples.

$$4 \text{ days} = \frac{4 \text{ days}}{1} \times \frac{24 \text{ hours}}{1 \text{ day}} \times \frac{60 \text{ minutes}}{1 \text{ hour}} \times \frac{60 \text{ seconds}}{1 \text{ minute}} = ?$$

After setting the problem up, we cancel out like units and/or numbers.

$$4 \text{ days} = \frac{4 \cancel{\text{ days}}}{1} \times \frac{24 \cancel{\text{ hours}}}{1 \cancel{\text{ day}}} \times \frac{60 \cancel{\text{ minutes}}}{1 \cancel{\text{ hour}}} \times \frac{60 \text{ seconds}}{1 \cancel{\text{ minute}}} = ?$$

Which can now be written as:

4 days = 4 × 24 × 60 × 60 = ?

4 days = 4 × 24 × 60 × 60 = 345,600

Now we know: there are 345,600 seconds in 4 days.

PRACTICE Problems 17.1 Basic Dimensional Analysis

1. How many hours are in 8 days?

2. How many minutes are there in 14 hours?

3. How many minutes are in a day?

4. Ten minutes is equivalent to how many seconds?

5. How many seconds are in 50 minutes?

6. 1.5 days is equal to _____ hours.

7. There are _____ minutes in 2.1 hours.

8. How many seconds are in 8 hours?

9. One hour is equal to _____ seconds.

10. How many seconds make up a full day?

Flow Rates

flow rates a term used to describe a number of common pharmacy calculations used in the preparation of IV infusions.

Flow rates is a term used to describe a number of common pharmacy calculations used in the preparation of **IV infusions** (compounded solutions that provide fluids, specific medications, nutrients, electrolytes, and minerals to a patient). Precise calculations are required for IV infusions to ensure that the fluid and medication(s) are being delivered at the right speed, at the right strength, and for the right amount of time.

Flow Rate Duration

IV infusion a compounded solution that provides fluids, specific medications, nutrients, electrolytes, and minerals to a patient.

Flow rate duration refers to the length of time over which an IV will be administered, or how long an IV bag will last before it must be changed.

flow rate duration length of time for which an IV will be administered, or how long an IV bag will last before it must be changed.

example 17.6   Flow Rate Duration

A 1 L IV bag is being administered at a rate of 200 mL per hour. How long will this IV bag last?

Do not get overwhelmed or confused now that the problems are talking about IV bags instead of days, hours, and seconds. Just as before, we can use dimensional analysis to solve this problem. In essence, the problem being asked is: 1 L is equal to how many hours?

Again, we should start by looking at the information, or facts, that we know. We know that there are 1,000 mL in every 1 L, which could be written as:

- 1 L = 1,000 mL

- $\dfrac{1\ L}{1{,}000\ mL}$

- $\dfrac{1{,}000\ mL}{1\ L}$

We also know, according to the problem, that 200 mL are being administered per hour, which can be written as:

- 1 hr = 200 mL

- $\dfrac{1\ hr}{200\ mL}$

- $\dfrac{200\ mL}{1\ hr}$

Using the principle of dimensional analysis, we can use this information to solve the problem.

$$1 \text{ L} = \frac{1 \text{ L}}{1} \times \frac{1{,}000 \text{ mL}}{1 \text{ L}} \times \frac{1 \text{ hr}}{200 \text{ mL}} = ?$$

After setting the problem up, we cancel out like units and/or numbers.

$$1 \text{ L} = \frac{1 \cancel{\text{L}}}{1} \times \frac{1{,}000 \cancel{\text{mL}}}{1 \cancel{\text{L}}} \times \frac{1 \text{ hr}}{200 \cancel{\text{mL}}} = ?$$

Which can now be written as:

$$1 \text{ L} = \frac{1 \times 1{,}000 \times 1 \text{ hr}}{200} = ?$$

$$1 \text{ L} = \frac{1{,}000}{200} = 5 \text{ hrs.}$$

Therefore, the 1 L bag will last 5 hours.

example **17.7**   **Flow Rate Duration**

A 2 L IV is to be administered at 250 mL/hr. How long will the IV last?

Let's start by looking at the information, or facts, that we know. We know that there are 1,000 mL in every 1 L, which could be written as:

- 1 L = 1,000 mL
- $\dfrac{1 \text{ L}}{1{,}000 \text{ mL}}$
- $\dfrac{1{,}000 \text{ mL}}{1 \text{ L}}$

We also know, according to the problem, that 250 mL are being administered per hour, which can be written as:

- 1 hr = 250 mL
- $\dfrac{1 \text{ hr}}{250 \text{ mL}}$
- $\dfrac{250 \text{ mL}}{1 \text{ hr}}$

Using the principle of dimensional analysis, we can use this information to solve the problem.

$$2 \text{ L} = \frac{2 \text{ L}}{1} \times \frac{1{,}000 \text{ mL}}{1 \text{ L}} \times \frac{1 \text{ hr}}{250 \text{ mL}} = ?$$

After setting the problem up, we cancel out like units and/or numbers.

$$2 \text{ L} = \frac{2 \cancel{\text{L}}}{1} \times \frac{1{,}000 \cancel{\text{mL}}}{1 \cancel{\text{L}}} \times \frac{1 \text{ hr}}{250 \cancel{\text{mL}}} = ?$$

Which can now be written as:

$$2 \text{ L} = \frac{2 \times 1{,}000 \times 1 \text{ hr}}{250} = ?$$

$$2 \text{ L} = \frac{2{,}000}{250} = 8 \text{ hrs.}$$

Therefore, the 2 L bag will last 8 hours.

example 17.8   Flow Rate Duration

A patient is set to get a 500 mL infusion of cimetidine in lactated Ringer's 5% at 10:00 a.m. The bag is to be administered at a rate of 125 mL per hour. At what time will the infusion be complete?

This example provides us with additional information, such as the drug name, solution strength, and administration start time. As always, let's start by looking at the information that we know and that we will need to calculate the problem. We know that:

- the bag contains a total of 500 mL
- 125 mL are being administered per hour
- the infusion is scheduled to start at 10:00 a.m.

Using the principle of dimensional analysis, we can use this information to determine how long the infusion will last.

$$500 \text{ mL} = \frac{500 \text{ mL}}{1} \times \frac{1 \text{ hr}}{125 \text{ mL}} = ?$$

After setting the problem up, we cancel out like units and/or numbers.

$$500 \text{ mL} = \frac{500 \text{ \cancel{mL}}}{1} \times \frac{1 \text{ hr}}{125 \text{ \cancel{mL}}} = ?$$

Which can now be written as:

$$500 \text{ mL} = \frac{500 \times 1 \text{ hr}}{125} = ?$$

$$500 \text{ mL} = \frac{500 \times 1 \text{ hr}}{125} = 4$$

Therefore, the 500 mL bag will last 4 hours.

The question being asked, however, is what time will the infusion be completed?

To answer this, simply take the start time (10:00 a.m.) and add the length of duration (4 hours).

10:00 a.m. + 4 hours = 14:00 hours, or 2:00 p.m.

example 17.9   Flow Rate Duration

Three 1 L IV bags are to be infused at a rate of 150 mL/hour. How long will these three bags last?

Let's start by looking at the information, or facts, that we know. We know that:

- there are 3 IV bags to be administered
- 1 IV bag contains 1 L
- there are 1,000 mL in every 1 L
- 150 mL are being administered per hour

Using the principle of dimensional analysis, we can use this information to solve the problem.

$$3 \text{ bags} = \frac{3 \text{ bags}}{1} \times \frac{1 \text{ L}}{1 \text{ bag}} \times \frac{1{,}000 \text{ mL}}{1 \text{ L}} \times \frac{1 \text{ hr}}{150 \text{ mL}} = ?$$

After setting the problem up, we cancel out like units and/or numbers.

$$3 \text{ bags} = \frac{3 \text{ bags}}{1} \times \frac{1 \text{ L}}{1 \text{ bag}} \times \frac{1,000 \text{ mL}}{1 \text{ L}} \times \frac{1 \text{ hr}}{150 \text{ mL}} = ?$$

Which can now be written as:

$$3 \text{ bags} = \frac{3 \times 1 \times 1,000 \times 1 \text{ hr}}{150} = ?$$

$$3 \text{ bags} = \frac{3 \times 1 \times 1,000 \times 1 \text{ hr}}{150} = 20$$

Therefore, the 3 bags will last 20 hours.

---

example **17.10** **Flow Rate Duration**

Two 2 L IV bags containing heparin sodium and NS are set for administration at a rate of 250 mL per hour at 7:00 a.m. When will both bags be completely administered?

Let's start by looking at the information, or facts, that we know. We know that:

- 1 IV bag contains 2 L
- there are 1,000 mL in every 1 L
- 250 mL are being administered per hour

Using the principle of dimensional analysis, we can use this information to solve the problem.

$$2 \text{ bags} = \frac{2 \text{ bags}}{1} \times \frac{2 \text{ L}}{1 \text{ bag}} \times \frac{1,000 \text{ mL}}{1 \text{ L}} \times \frac{1 \text{ hr}}{250 \text{ mL}} = ?$$

After setting the problem up, we cancel out like units and/or numbers.

$$2 \text{ bags} = \frac{2 \text{ bags}}{1} \times \frac{2 \text{ L}}{1 \text{ bag}} \times \frac{1,000 \text{ mL}}{1 \text{ L}} \times \frac{1 \text{ hr}}{250 \text{ mL}} = ?$$

Which can now be written as:

$$2 \text{ bags} = \frac{2 \times 2 \times 1,000 \times 1 \text{ hr}}{250} = ?$$

$$2 \text{ bags} = \frac{2 \times 2 \times 1,000 \times 1 \text{ hr}}{250} = 16$$

Therefore, the 2 bags will last 16 hours.

The question being asked, however, is what time will the infusion be completed?

To answer this, simply take the start time (7:00 a.m.) and add the length of duration (16 hours).

7:00 a.m. + 16 hours = 23:00 hours, or 11:00 p.m.

PRACTICE Problems 17.2 Flow Rate Duration

1. A 250 mL bag is to be administered at 100 mL per hour. How long will the IV bag last?

2. A 1 L IV is running at 250 mL/hr. How long will the infusion last?

3. 500 mL of NS is being infused at 150 mL per hour. What will be the duration of the infusion?

4. 500 mg cefazolin in 100 mL D5W is being administered at 200 mL/hr. How long will the IV last?

5. A 500 mL bag with Diamox® is being infused at 250 mL per hour. How long will it take to infuse the entire bag?

6. 1 L is being infused at a rate of 200 mL/hr. If the infusion began at 8:15 a.m., when will it be finished?

7. Two 1 L bags are being infused at 250 mL/hr. How long will both bags last?

8. 750 mL of NS is set to be administered at 150 mL per hour, starting at 11:00 a.m. At what time will the infusion be finished?

9. Two 1 L IV bags with ascorbic acid are being administered 200 mL/hr. How long will it take to infuse both bags?

10. A 250 mL bag with ranitidine is being administered at the maximum rate of 10.7 mL per hour. How long will the bag last?

Volume per Hour

volume per hour (mL/hr) the amount of fluid, or solution, that will be administered to the patient intravenously per hour.

Volume per hour, or **mL/hr,** refers to the amount of fluid, or solution, that will be administered to the patient intravenously per hour.

example 17.11   Volume per Hour

A patient is to receive 750 mL infused over 3 hours. What is the rate of infusion in mL per hour?

Unlike the previous IV flow rate problems, solving volume per hour is easily done by setting up a ratio and proportion and then solving for the unknown, as illustrated here.

$$\frac{\text{Total mL}}{\text{Total hrs}} = \frac{X}{1 \text{ hr}}$$

Using the information provided in the problem, set up a ratio and proportion.

$$\frac{750 \text{ mL}}{3 \text{ hrs}} = \frac{X}{1 \text{ hr}}$$

Now we must cross-multiply.

$$3 \times X = 750 \times 1$$

$$3X = 750$$

Using basic algebra principles, isolate the unknown (X) to solve. In this example, we must divide both sides of the equation by 3 to isolate X.

$$\frac{3X}{3} = \frac{750}{3}$$
$$X = 250$$

This infusion will be administered at 250 mL per hour.

example 17.12 Volume per Hour

A 250 mL IV, containing 1 mg of Isuprel®, is to be given over 100 minutes. What is the rate of infusion in mL per hour?

Using the information provided in the problem, set up a ratio and proportion. Since the administration time is given in minutes, we can substitute 60 minutes for the 1 hr. beneath the unknown (X).

$$\frac{250 \text{ mL}}{100 \text{ min}} = \frac{X}{60 \text{ min}}$$

Next, cross-multiply.

$100 \times X = 250 \times 60$

$100X = 15,000$

Now, solve for X.

$$\frac{\cancel{100}X}{\cancel{100}} = \frac{15,000}{100}$$

So, X = 150

This infusion will be administered at 150 mL per hour (60 minutes).

example 17.13 Volume per Hour

500 mL of D5W containing 1 g of lidocaine hydrochloride is to be given over 250 minutes. What is the infusion rate in mL per hour?

First, set up the ratio and proportion.

$$\frac{500 \text{ mL}}{250 \text{ min}} = \frac{X}{60 \text{ min}}$$

Next, cross-multiply.

$250 \times X = 500 \times 60$

$250X = 30,000$

Now, solve for X.

$$\frac{\cancel{250}X}{\cancel{250}} = \frac{30,000}{250}$$

X = 120

This infusion will be administered at 120 mL per hour (60 minutes).

example 17.14 Volume per Hour

A 250 mL IV is to be administered over 50 minutes. What is the infusion rate in mL/hr?

First, set up the ratio and proportion.

$$\frac{250 \text{ mL}}{50 \text{ min}} = \frac{X}{60 \text{ min}}$$

Next, cross-multiply.

$50 \times X = 250 \times 60$

$50X = 15,000$

Now, solve for X.

$$\frac{\cancel{50}X}{\cancel{50}} = \frac{15,000}{50}$$

$X = 300$

This infusion will be administered at 300 mL per hour (60 minutes).

Notice that the actual IV is being administered in less than an hour, so the rate per hour should logically contain more volume than the actual IV.

example 17.15 Volume per Hour

1,000 mL NS containing 50 mg nitroprusside sodium is to be administered over 50 minutes. What is the infusion rate in mL/hr?

First, set up the ratio and proportion.

$$\frac{1,000 \text{ mL}}{50 \text{ min}} = \frac{X}{60 \text{ min}}$$

Next, cross-multiply.

$50 \times X = 1,000 \times 60$

$50X = 60,000$

Now, solve for X.

$$\frac{\cancel{50}X}{\cancel{50}} = \frac{60,000}{50}$$

$X = 1,200$

This infusion will be administered at 1,200 mL, or 1.2 L, per hour (60 minutes).

PRACTICE Problems 17.3 Volume per Hour

1. 1 L is being infused over 6 hours. What is the rate of infusion in mL per hour?

2. 500 mL is being administered over 4 hours. What is the administration rate per hour?

3. 2 L is to be given via IV over 8 hours. What is the rate of infusion per hour?

4. 480 mL of D5W containing dobutamine is being given over 8 hours. What is the administration rate per hour?

5. 1 g of Gemzar® in 25 mL NS is to be administered over 30 minutes. What is the rate of infusion in mL per hour?

6. 100 mL is being infused over 30 minutes. What is the rate of infusion in mL per hour?

7. 250 mL is being given over 100 minutes. What is the administration rate per hour?

8. 500 mL NS is being administered over 6 hours. What is the rate in mL per hour?

9. 50 mL SWFI containing folic acid is to be infused over 30 minutes. What is the infusion rate per hour?

10. 100 mL Iveegam® is infused over 100 minutes. What is the rate of infusion per hour?

Drug per Hour

Drug per hour, or **mg/hr**, refers to the dosage, or amount of medication in milligrams, that will be administered per hour of infusion.

drug per hour (mg/hr) the dosage, or amount of medication in milligrams, that will be administered per hour of infusion.

example 17.16 Drug per Hour

100 mg of medication is to be administered in 500 mL of LR (lactated Ringer's) over 2 hours. How much drug will be administered per hour?

Like solving volume per hour, calculating the amount of medication administered per hour is easily done by setting up a ratio and proportion and then solving for the unknown, as illustrated here.

$$\frac{\text{Total mg}}{\text{Total hrs}} = \frac{X}{1 \text{ hr}}$$

Using the information provided in the problem, set up a ratio and proportion.

$$\frac{100 \text{ mg}}{2 \text{ hrs}} = \frac{X}{1 \text{ hr}}$$

Now we must cross-multiply.

$2 \times X = 100 \times 1$

$2X = 100$

Using basic algebra principles, isolate the unknown (X) to solve. In this example, we must divide both sides of the equation by 2 to isolate X.

$$\frac{2X}{2} = \frac{100}{2}$$

$X = 50$

This infusion will provide 50 mg per hour.

example 17.17 Drug per Hour

600 mg of fluorouracil is to be administered by continuous infusion over 24 hours. How much drug will be administered per hour?

Using the information provided in the problem, set up a ratio and proportion.

$$\frac{600 \text{ mg}}{24 \text{ hrs}} = \frac{X}{1 \text{ hr}}$$

Now cross-multiply.

$24 \times X = 600 \times 1$

$24X = 600$

Using basic algebra principles, isolate the unknown (X) to solve. In this example, we must divide both sides of the equation by 24 to isolate X.

$$\frac{24X}{24} = \frac{600}{24}$$

$X = 25$

This infusion will provide 25 mg per hour.

example 17.18 Drug per Hour

200 mg of Vibramycin IV® is diluted in 400 mL LR to be administered over 4 hours. How much drug will be administered per hour?

First, set up a ratio and proportion.

$$\frac{200 \text{ mg}}{4 \text{ hrs}} = \frac{X}{1 \text{ hr}}$$

Next, cross-multiply.

$4 \times X = 200 \times 1$

$4X = 200$

Now solve for X.

$$\frac{4X}{4} = \frac{200}{4}$$

$X = 50$

This infusion will provide 50 mg per hour.

example 17.19 Drug per Hour

125 mg of Cardizem® is being infused in 125 mL over 12.5 hours. How much drug will be administered per hour?

First, set up a ratio and proportion.

$$\frac{125 \text{ mg}}{12.5 \text{ hrs}} = \frac{X}{1 \text{ hr}}$$

Next, cross-multiply.

$12.5 \times X = 125 \times 1$

$12.5X = 125$

Now solve for X.

$$\frac{12.5X}{12.5} = \frac{125}{12.5}$$

$X = 10$

This infusion will provide 10 mg per hour.

example 17.20 Drug per Hour

5 million units of Penicillin G Aqueous® are being delivered in 1 L of D5W over 12 hours. How much drug will be administered per hour?

First, set up a ratio and proportion.

$$\frac{5,000,000 \text{ units}}{12 \text{ hrs}} = \frac{X}{1 \text{ hr}}$$

Next, cross-multiply.

$12 \times X = 5,000,000 \times 1$

$12X = 5,000,000$

Now solve for X.

$$\frac{\cancel{12}X}{\cancel{12}} = \frac{5,000,000}{12}$$

$X = 416,666.67$

Therefore, this infusion will provide 416,667 units per hour.

PRACTICE Problems 17.4 Drug per Hour

1. 250 mg of medication in 1 L is administered over 5 hours. How much drug will be administered per hour?

2. 800 mg of medication in 2 L is to be infused over 4 hours. How much drug will be administered per hour?

3. 500 mg of medication in 500 mL is to be given over 4 hours. How much drug will be administered per hour?

4. 250 mL Plasmanate®, which contains 25 g of plasma protein, is to be administered over 250 minutes. How much drug will be administered per hour?

5. 500 mg of nafcillin sodium in 150 mL is to be infused over 30 minutes. How much drug will be administered per hour?

6. A 100 mL bag contains 75 mg of medication to be given over 30 minutes. How much drug will be administered per hour?

7. 25 mcg of medication in 250 mL is to be infused over 2 hours. How much drug will be administered per hour?

8. 250,000 units of medication in 1 L is administered over 8 hours. How much drug will be administered per hour?

9. 100 mg teniposide in 500 mL is given over 45 minutes. How much drug will be administered per hour?

10. 75 mg of Demadex® in D5W is to be administered over 24 hours. How much drug will be administered per hour?

Drop Factors

When preparing sterile products, pharmacy personnel are often responsible for calculating the rate of IV administration, expressed as **drops per minute (gtts/min)**. Literally, this drip rate will determine how the IV pump is calibrated and the volume of medication to be administered each minute.

drops per minute (gtts/min) the volume of medication to be administered each minute.

Various IV administration sets release specific drops per milliliter. Microdrip sets are calibrated to deliver 60 drops per mL, whereas macrodrip sets might be calibrated to deliver 10, 15, or 20 drops per mL. The larger the number of drops per milliliter, the smaller the drops will be—because, of course, one milliliter is one milliliter.

In pharmacy, you will work with four common IV drip rates: 10 gtts/mL, 15 gtts/mL, 20 gtts/mL, and 60 gtts/mL. Drip rates can be expressed by their **drop factor**, which is just a simpler way of stating a drip rate (see Table 17-1).

drop factor an abbreviated form referring to a specific drip rate.

FIGURE 17-1 Illustration of drip sets.

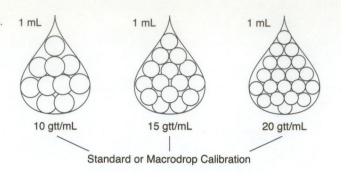

10 gtt/mL   15 gtt/mL   20 gtt/mL   60 gtt/mL

Standard or Macrodrop Calibration   Microdrop Calibration

Table 17-1 Drip Rates Expressed by Drop Factor

DROP FACTOR	DRIP RATE
60	60 gtts/mL
20	20 gtts/mL
15	15 gtts/mL
10	10 gtts/mL

" Workplace Wisdom Always Assume 60 gtts/mL

The most commonly used drip rate is the **microdrip**, 60 gtts/mL. Therefore, if a problem does not indicate a specific drip rate or drop factor, you should always assume 60 gtts/mL. **"**

microdrip the most commonly used drip rate; 60 gtts/mL.

example 17.21 Drip Rates

A 1 L bag of D5W is to be administered at a drop factor of 60 over 6 hours. What is the flow rate in gtts/min?

Let's start by looking at the information, or facts, that we know. We know that:

- 1 IV bag contains 1 L
- there are 1,000 mL in every 1 L
- the drop factor is 60, so there are 60 gtts/mL
- the duration of administration is 6 hours
- there are 60 minutes in 1 hour

Using the principle of dimensional analysis, we can use this information to solve the problem.

$$1 \text{ bag} = \frac{1,000 \text{ mL}}{6 \text{ hrs}} \times \frac{60 \text{ gtts}}{1 \text{ mL}} \times \frac{1 \text{ hr}}{60 \text{ min}} = ?$$

After setting the problem up, we cancel out like units and/or numbers.

$$1 \text{ bag} = \frac{1,000 \text{ mL}}{6 \text{ hrs}} \times \frac{60 \text{ gtts}}{1 \text{ mL}} \times \frac{1 \text{ hr}}{60 \text{ min}} = ?$$

Which can now be written as:

$$1 \text{ bag} = \frac{1,000 \times 1 \text{ gtts}}{6 \text{ min}} = ?$$

$$1 \text{ bag} = \frac{1,000 \times 1 \text{ gtts}}{6 \text{ min}} = 166.66$$

So, the infusion rate is 167 gtts/min.

example 17.22 Drip Rates

500 mL is to be administered to a patient over 5 hours, using a drop factor of 15. What is the flow rate in gtts/min?

Let's start by looking at the information, or facts, that we know. We know that:

- 1 IV bag contains 500 mL
- the drop factor is 15, so there are 15 gtts/mL
- the duration of administration is 5 hours
- there are 60 minutes in 1 hour

Using the principle of dimensional analysis, we can use this information to solve the problem.

$$1 \text{ bag} = \frac{500 \text{ mL}}{5 \text{ hrs}} \times \frac{15 \text{ gtts}}{1 \text{ mL}} \times \frac{1 \text{ hr}}{60 \text{ min}} = ?$$

After setting the problem up, we cancel out like units and/or numbers.

$$1 \text{ bag} = \frac{500 \text{ mL}}{5 \text{ hrs}} \times \frac{15 \text{ gtts}}{1 \text{ mL}} \times \frac{1 \text{ hr}}{60 \text{ min}} = ?$$

Which can now be written as:

$$1 \text{ bag} = \frac{500 \times 15 \text{ gtts}}{300 \text{ min}} = ?$$

$$1 \text{ bag} = \frac{7,500 \text{ gtts}}{300 \text{ min}} = 25$$

So, the infusion rate is 25 gtts/min.

example 17.23 Drip Rates

Rx: Vancomycin® 250 mg/250 mL Disp. 500 mg over 3 hours q8hr. What is the flow rate in gtts/min?

Let's start by looking at the information, or facts, that we know. We know that:

- 1 IV bag contains 500 mL
- the drop factor is not stated, so we must assume 60 gtts/mL
- the duration of administration is 3 hours
- there are 60 minutes in 1 hour

Notice that the additional information provided is not necessary in solving this problem.

Using the principle of dimensional analysis, we can use this information to solve the problem.

$$1 \text{ bag} = \frac{500 \text{ mL}}{3 \text{ hrs}} \times \frac{60 \text{ gtts}}{1 \text{ mL}} \times \frac{1 \text{ hr}}{60 \text{ min}} = ?$$

After setting the problem up, we cancel out like units and/or numbers.

$$1 \text{ bag} = \frac{500 \text{ mL}}{3 \text{ hrs}} \times \frac{60 \text{ gtts}}{1 \text{ mL}} \times \frac{1 \text{ hr}}{60 \text{ min}} = ?$$

Which can now be written as:

$$1 \text{ bag} = \frac{500 \times 1 \text{ gtts}}{3 \text{ min}} = ?$$

$$1 \text{ bag} = \frac{500 \text{ gtts}}{3 \text{ min}} = 166.66$$

So, the infusion rate is 167 gtts/min.

---

example 17.24 Drip Rates

A 100 mL bag containing 1 g of Zanosar® is to be infused, with a drop factor of 15, over 1 hour. What is the flow rate in gtts/min?

We know that:

- 1 IV bag contains 100 mL
- the drop factor is 15, so there are 15 gtts/mL
- the duration of administration is 1 hour
- there are 60 minutes in 1 hour

Using the principle of dimensional analysis, we can use this information to solve the problem.

$$1 \text{ bag} = \frac{100 \text{ mL}}{1 \text{ hr}} \times \frac{15 \text{ gtts}}{1 \text{ mL}} \times \frac{1 \text{ hr}}{60 \text{ min}} = ?$$

After setting the problem up, we cancel out like units and/or numbers.

$$1 \text{ bag} = \frac{100 \text{ m\cancel{L}}}{1 \text{ \cancel{hr}}} \times \frac{15 \text{ gtts}}{1 \text{ m\cancel{L}}} \times \frac{1 \text{ \cancel{hr}}}{60 \text{ min}} = ?$$

Which can now be written as:

$$1 \text{ bag} = \frac{100 \times 15 \text{ gtts}}{60 \text{ min}} = ?$$

$$1 \text{ bag} = \frac{1,500 \text{ gtts}}{60 \text{ min}} = 25$$

So, the infusion rate is 25 gtts/min.

---

example 17.25 Drip Rates

Rx: 2 g Mandol® in 1 L of D10W over 4 hours TID. What is the flow rate in gtts/min?

Let's start by looking at the information, or facts, that we know. We know that:

- 1 IV bag contains 1,000 mL (1 L)
- the drop factor is not stated, so we must assume 60 gtts/mL
- the duration of administration is 4 hours
- there are 60 minutes in 1 hour

Notice that the additional information provided is not necessary in solving this problem.

Using the principle of dimensional analysis, we can use this information to solve the problem.

$$1 \text{ bag} = \frac{1,000 \text{ mL}}{4 \text{ hrs}} \times \frac{60 \text{ gtts}}{1 \text{ mL}} \times \frac{1 \text{ hr}}{60 \text{ min}} = ?$$

After setting the problem up, we cancel out like units and/or numbers.

$$1 \text{ bag} = \frac{1,000 \text{ mL}}{4 \text{ hrs}} \times \frac{60 \text{ gtts}}{1 \text{ mL}} \times \frac{1 \text{ hr}}{60 \text{ min}} = ?$$

Which can now be written as:

$$1 \text{ bag} = \frac{1,000 \times 1 \text{ gtts}}{4 \text{ min}} = ?$$

$$1 \text{ bag} = \frac{1,000 \times 1 \text{ gtts}}{4 \text{ min}} = 250$$

So, the infusion rate is 250 gtts/min.

PRACTICE Problems 17.5 Drip Rates

1. Rx: Claforan (cefotaxime) 500 mg/50 mL IV over 30 minutes. What is the flow rate in gtts/min?

2. Rx: ampicillin 0.5 g/100 mL 50 mg/kg/day q8h over 90 min. The patient weighs 30 kg. What is the flow rate in mL/hr?

3. Rx: penicillin G potassium 20,000,000 units/L over 24 hours. What is the flow rate in mL/hr?

4. Rx: dexamethasone sodium phosphate 0.25 mg/kg/dose q8h over 15 minutes. The patient weighs 14 lb. You have a stock vial containing 4 mg/mL in a 10 mL vial; the IV bag holds 50 mL and the IV administration set delivers 30 gtts/mL. What is the flow rate in gtts/min?

5. Rx: Ringer's Solution 500 mL over 8 hours. What is the flow rate in mL/hr?

6. Rx: D5W 1.44 L over 24 hours. What is the flow rate in gtts/min?

7. Rx: electrolyte solution 500 mL over 250 minutes. What is the flow rate in mL/hr?

8. Rx: antibiotic 250 mL over 2 hr. The IV administration set delivers 15 gtts/mL. What is the flow rate in gtts/min?

9. Rx: Rocephin 2 g/100 mL over 1 hour. The IV administration set delivers 30 gtts/mL. What is the flow rate in mL/hr?

10. Rx: insulin 100 units/250 mL over 2.5 hours. The IV administration set delivers 30 gtts/mL. What is the flow rate in gtts/min?

TPN Milliequivalents

Total parenteral nutrition, also called **TPN**, is a solution made to supply many of the body's basic nutritional needs. It also contains necessary fluids, vitamins, and lipids. In essence, it is everything needed to sustain a human body nutritionally.

total parenteral nutrition (TPN) a solution made to supply many of the body's basic nutritional needs via parenteral cadministration.

Electrolyte Solutions

Electrolytes in solution conduct electricity. When electrolytes are dissolved in water, they split into charged particles known as *ions*, which carry an electric charge. Electrolytes are important in maintaining acid-base balance in body fluids, controlling body water volume, and regulating metabolism.

Electrolytes are commonly added to TPN solutions according to the needs of the patient as indicated by the physician on the order. *Parenteral* indicates that the solution is delivered into the bloodstream via IV infusion.

Milliequivalents are used to express the concentration of electrolytes in solution. Solutions can be isotonic, hypertonic, or hypotonic, depending on their concentration as it relates to the osmotic pressure of human red blood cells. Solutions, therefore, are classified as one of the three following, depending upon the tonicity:

isotonic solutions solutions that have an osmotic pressure equal to that of cell contents.

hypertonic solutions solutions that have greater osmotic pressure than cell contents. Hypertonic solutions cause cells to dehydrate and shrink.

hypotonic solutions solutions that have a lower osmotic pressure than cell contents. Hypotonic solutions cause cells to take on water and expand.

Isotonic solutions: Solutions that have an osmotic pressure equal to that of cell contents. Normal saline (sodium chloride 0.9% solution), is considered isotonic with human red blood cells.

Hypertonic solutions: Solutions that have greater osmotic pressure than cell contents. Hypertonic solutions cause cells to dehydrate and shrink.

Hypotonic solutions: Solutions that have a lower osmotic pressure than cell contents. Hypotonic solutions cause cells to take on water and expand.

After receiving a TPN order, the pharmacy technician must determine how many milliliters will be extracted from the stock vial and injected into the TPN bag. Each item is extracted from the stock vial and injected into the TPN bag separately; that is, only one item is added at a time. TPNs are prepared in the clean room using aseptic technique.

Workplace Wisdom TPN Automixers

Most health-system pharmacies now use automated machines called *automixers* to prepare TPN orders. The user need only enter the Rx order. These machines are connected to common stock solutions and automatically perform the necessary calculations and fluid draws. However, pharmacy technicians are still required to be proficient in performing these calculations.

example 17.26 TPN Milliequivalents

Electrolyte	Stock Vial	Rx Order	Volume Required
NaCl	4 mEq/mL	60 mEq	X

To calculate the volume required for electrolyte milliequivalents, you could set up a proportion and solve for X; you could set up a basic algebraic equation; or, most easily, you can divide the ordered amount of milliequivalents by the stock vial concentration, as long as the concentration is stated as X mEq per 1 mL.

$60 \div 4 = 15$

So, you need to add 15 mL of the stock NaCl to the TPN.

example 17.27 TPN Milliequivalents

Electrolyte	Stock Vial	Rx Order	Volume Required
K acetate	2 mEq/mL	20 mEq	X

Again, because the stock concentration is listed as "per 1 mL," it is not necessary to set up a proportion or equation. Simply divide the quantity ordered by the stock concentration.

$20 \div 2 = 10$

10 mL of K acetate 2 mEq/mL must be added to the TPN.

PRACTICE Problems 17.6 Milliequivalents

Electrolyte	Stock Vial	Rx Order	Volume Required
Na phosphate	4 mEq/mL	34 mEq	X
MgSO$_4$	4mEq/mL	30 mEq	X
Na acetate	2 mEq/mL	10 mEq	X
KCl	2 mEq/mL	40 mEq	X
Ca gluconate	0.465 mEq/mL	20 mEq	X

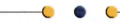

PROFILES IN PRACTICE

Juan is a pharmacy technician who works at an infusion clinic pharmacy. When preparing a TPN, Juan makes a mistake and withdraws the "strengths" of the electrolytes listed, rather than the calculated volumes needed.

• The error is caught by the pharmacist, but what would have been the consequences had this error gone unchecked?

SUMMARY

Often described as the most difficult and challenging calculations used in pharmacy, parenteral calculations, drip rates, and TPN milliequivalents are all solved with basic, fundamental mathematics. If you properly use proportions, cross-multiplication, and dimensional analysis, you will be able to perform virtually all parenteral calculations that are done by pharmacy technicians.

CHAPTER REVIEW QUESTIONS

1. You have a stock vial of cefotaxime 500 mg/10 mL. The dose is 2 g over 30 minutes. How many mg/min will the patient receive?
   a. 17 mg/min
   b. 27 mg/min
   c. 47 mg/min
   d. 67 mg/min

2. You have a stock vial of cefotaxime 500 mg/10 mL. The dose is 2 g over 30 minutes. What is the flow rate in mL/hr?
   a. 40 mL/hr
   b. 60 mL/hr
   c. 80 mL/hr
   d. 100 mL/hr

3. You have a stock vial of cefotaxime 500 mg/10 mL. The dose is 2 g over 30 minutes. What is the flow rate in gtts/min if the administration set is calibrated to 20 gtts/mL?

   a. 27 gtts/min
   b. 67 gtts/min
   c. 80 gtts/min
   d. 87 gtts/min

4. What is the flow rate, in gtts/min, for a 1 L TPN over 12 hours if the IV administration set is calibrated to deliver 30 gtts/mL?

   a. 42 gtts/min
   b. 30 gtts/min
   c. 12 gtts/min
   d. 60 gtts/min

5. What is the flow rate in gtts/min for 50 mL of an antibiotic administered over 60 minutes?

   a. 30 gtts/min
   b. 50 gtts/min
   c. 60 gtts/min
   d. 83 gtts/min

6. You have an order for cefuroxime 1.5 g/50 mL with a maximum dose of 1.5 g q8h. The patient weighs 200 pounds. What is the flow rate in gtts/min if his dose is administered over 90 minutes?

   a. 90 gtts/min
   b. 50 gtts/min
   c. 40 gtts/min
   d. 33 gtts/min

7. You have a stock vial of product 30 mg/mL. How many milliliters will you need to prepare an IV infusion containing a dose of 150 mg/50 mL?

   a. 5 mL
   b. 10 mL
   c. 20 mL
   d. 30 mL

8. You have a stock vial of sodium bicarbonate 0.5 mEq/mL. How many milliliters do you need to provide 80 mEq?

   a. 40 mL
   b. 80 mL
   c. 120 mL
   d. 160 mL

9. You have a stock vial of magnesium sulfate 4 mEq/mL. How many milliliters do you need to provide 24 mEq?

   a. 4 mL
   b. 6 mL
   c. 8 mL
   d. 12 mL

10. You have a stock vial of calcium gluconate injection 4.65 mEq/10 mL. How many milliliters do you need to provide 70 mEq?

    a. 70 mL
    b. 120 mL
    c. 150 mL
    d. 325 mL

CRITICAL THINKING QUESTIONS

1. In what ways are calculations using milliequivalents similar to ratio-and-proportion calculations?

2. Why does pharmacy assume a drop factor of 60 unless notified otherwise?

3. What impact can miscalculated flow rates have on the nursing staff, and ultimately the patient?

REFERENCES AND RESOURCES

Hegstad, LN, & Hayek, W. *Essential Drug Dosage Calculations* (4th ed.). Upper Saddle River, NJ: Pearson, 2001.

Johnston, M. *Pharmacy Calculations.* Upper Saddle River, NJ: Pearson, 2005.

Lesmeister, MB. *Math Basics for the Healthcare Professional* (2d ed.). Upper Saddle River, NJ: Pearson, 2005.

Mikolah, AA. *Drug Dosage Calculations for the Emergency Care Provider* (2d ed.). Upper Saddle River, NJ: Prentice-Hall, 2003.

Olsen, JL, Giangrasso, AP, & Shrimpton, D. *Medical Dosage Calculations* (8th ed.). Upper Saddle River, NJ: Pearson, 2004.

Pharmacology

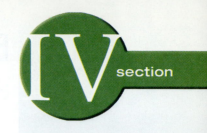

IV
section

18 Dosage Formulations and Administration

LEARNING OBJECTIVES

After completing this chapter, you should be able to:

- Explain drug nomenclature.
- Define medication error.
- List and explain the rights of medication administration.
- Identify various dosage formulations.
- Identify the advantages and disadvantages of solid and liquid medication dosage formulations.
- Explain the differences between solutions, emulsions, and suspensions.
- Explain the difference between ointments and creams.
- Identify the various routes of administration and give examples of each.
- Give examples of common medications for various routes of administration.
- Identify the advantages and disadvantages of each route of administration.
- Identify the parenteral routes of administration.
- Explain the difference between transdermal and topical routes of administration.
- Explain the difference between sublingual and buccal routes of administration.
- Identify the abbreviations for the common routes of administration and dosage formulations.

Introduction

Technological advances over the last century have vastly changed the way the world lives and have given us a wider variety of choices in our daily lives. Pharmacy is no longer restricted to using plants and animals as the basis of new medications, and advances have enabled the pharmaceutical industry to produce more new medications, in a greater variety of forms, than ever before. However, with the higher number of new medications available, more medication errors are likely to occur. How does one identify and differentiate all these new medications, and how does pharmacy prevent medication errors? This chapter discusses the different sources from which medications are derived, how medications are named, and how the pharmacy technician can play a vital role in reducing medication errors. Various dosage formulations and routes of administration, as well as common medications in each of the categories, are also introduced.

Sources of Drugs

Although most people are familiar with the trade or brand names of the medications they take, they may be unfamiliar with the various names used to identify the same drug products, or the fact that their medications are derived from many different sources, including plants and animals. Drugs are derived from a variety of sources that can be categorized into three classifications: natural, synthetic, and genetically engineered. This section briefly discusses each source.

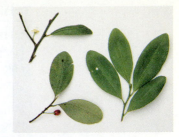

FIGURE 18-1 Coca plant (*Erythroxylum coca*).

Natural Drug Sources

Natural drugs are substances that occur in nature (naturally occurring). These include substances that are derived or extracted from plants, animals, and minerals. Examples of natural drugs include:

- acetylsalicylic acid (aspirin)—analgesic derived from white willow bark.
- bovine insulin—derived from cattle.
- cocaine—local anesthetic derived from the coca plant (see Figure 18-1).
- codeine, morphine—analgesics derived from the opium poppy plant (see Figure 18-2).
- digoxin—cardiac glycoside derived from the foxglove plant (see Figure 18-3).
- ferrous sulfate (iron)—used to treat iron deficiencies.
- gold—used to treat arthritis.
- human growth hormone—derived from the pituitary gland.
- porcine insulin—derived from pigs.
- vincristine, vinblastine—anticancer drugs derived from the periwinkle plant (see Figure 18-4).

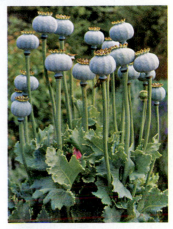

FIGURE 18-2 Opium poppy (*Papaver somniferum*).

Synthetic Drug Sources

Synthetic drugs are produced in the laboratory and are not naturally occurring. A drug is **semi-synthetic** if it is a naturally occuring substance that has been chemically altered. A drug is considered to be **synthesized** if it is made in a laboratory to imitate a drug that is naturally occurring. In pharmacy practice, it is common for any drug that does not occur in nature and is produced in the laboratory to be called *synthetic*. Examples of synthetic drugs include:

- Adrenalin—synthesized epinephrine for the treatment of hypersensitivity and asthmatic attacks.
- amoxicillin, ampicillin, piperacillin—semi-synthetic penicillins used to treat infection.
- barbiturates—synthetic central nervous system depressants.
- OxyContin®—synthetic opiate used for pain management.

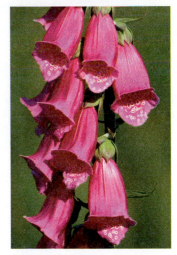

FIGURE 18-3 Foxglove (*Digitalis purpurea*).

Genetically Engineered Drug Sources

Genetically engineered drugs are synthetic drugs produced by means of recombinant DNA or monoclonal antibodies (MAbs). When manufacturers use *recombinant DNA*, they combine two different DNA strands to produce a new strand of DNA (deoxyribonucleic acid) or rDNA. Monoclonal antibodies are hybrid cells created in the laboratory from animals. These new cells can be used to treat tumors and diagnose various conditions. Examples of rDNA and MAb drugs include:

- human insulin—created by rDNA to treat diabetes.
- recombinant hepatitis B vaccine—created by rDNA to vaccinate against hepatitis B.
- Rituxan®, Zevalin®, Erbitux®, Avastin®—MAbs used in the treatment of various cancers.

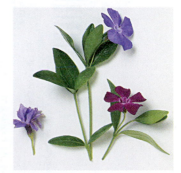

FIGURE 18-4 Periwinkle (*Vinca minor*).

Table 18-1   Drug Nomenclature Examples

CHEMICAL NAME	GENERIC NAME	TRADE NAME(S)
(±)- 2- (p- isobutylphenyl) propionic acid	ibuprofen	Motrin®, Advil®
4'-hydroxyacetanilide	acetaminophen	Tylenol®
4-thia-1-azabicyclo[3.2.0]-heptane-2-carboxylic acid, 3,3-dimethyl-7-oxo-6-[(phenoxyacetyl)amino]-, monopotassium salt, [2S-(2a,5a,6b)]-	penicillin VK	Veetids®

synthetic drugs that are not naturally occurring; produced in a laboratory.

semi-synthetic a naturally occurring compound that has been chemically altered.

synthesized produced in a laboratory to imitate a naturally occurring compound.

nomenclature set of names; way of naming.

Drug Nomenclature

The three classifications of drug **nomenclature** are the chemical name, the generic name, and the brand or trade name. All drug products have a chemical name and a generic name, but not all drugs have a trade name. Understanding drug nomenclature is very important for a pharmacy technician.

Chemical Name

The *chemical name* of a drug product reflects the chemical structure of the compound. The chemical name is often complicated, extremely lengthy, and difficult to remember and pronounce (see Table 18-1). Each drug is named according to the strict nomenclature guidelines of the International Union of Pure and Applied Chemistry (IUPAC), an organization the main purpose of which is to advance worldwide aspects of the chemical sciences. The chemical names of drugs are used primarily in chemistry and pharmaceutical research; they are not commonly used in daily pharmacy practice.

Generic Name

The *generic name* of a drug is a convenient and concise name used by the public to identify the active ingredient in the drug. The generic name is assigned to the drug by the manufacturer in collaboration with the Food and Drug Administration (FDA). A generic drug name is usually not capitalized, and may be used by anyone because it is not restricted by copyright or trademark. It is also the name used in the *United States Pharmacopoeia* (USP) and the *United States Pharmacopoeia National Formulary* (USP-NF). The USP is the official standards-setting authority for prescription and over-the-counter drugs; the USP-NF is the publication containing the official standards. Identical substances always use the same generic name; that is, a substance never has more than one generic drug name assigned to it. The generic name is also known as the *nonproprietary name* (see Figure 18-5).

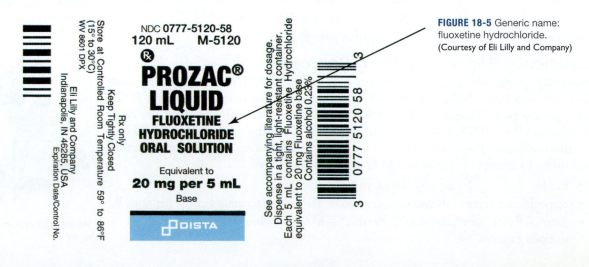

FIGURE 18-5 Generic name: fluoxetine hydrochloride. (Courtesy of Eli Lilly and Company)

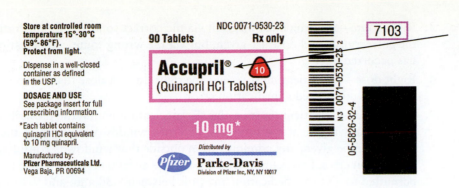

Store at controlled room
temperature 15°-30°C
(59°-86°F).
Protect from light.

Dispense in a well-closed
container as defined
in the USP.

DOSAGE AND USE
See package insert for full
prescribing information.

*Each tablet contains
quinapril HCl equivalent
to 10 mg quinapril.

Manufactured by:
Pfizer Pharmaceuticals Ltd.
Vega Baja, PR 00694

NDC 0071-0530-23
90 Tablets   **Rx only**

7103

Accupril® 10
(Quinapril HCl Tablets)

10 mg*

Distributed by
Pfizer **Parke-Davis**
Division of Pfizer Inc, NY, NY 10017

N3 0071-0530-23 2
05-5826-32-4

FIGURE 18-6 Trade name: Accupril®. (Reg. Trademark of Pfizer, Inc. Reproduced with permission)

In efforts to contain escalating drug costs, many insurance companies and **health maintenance organizations (HMOs)** will pay the pharmacy only for generic medications, according to their **formularies**. Additionally, many pharmacies stock their shelves alphabetically by generic name.

health maintenance organization (HMO) a type of healthcare/insurance plan.

formulary a listing of drugs approved for use or for reimbursement.

Trade or Brand Name

The *trade* or *brand name* of a drug is registered or trademarked by a specific producer or manufacturer to identify its particular drug. Because a trade name is trademarked, it cannot be used by other manufacturers. Trade names are normally capitalized, and a single generic drug, such as ibuprofen, may be produced, marketed, and sold under more than one trade name. The trade or brand name may also be referred to as the *proprietary name* (see Figure 18-6). Table 18-1 lists some examples of drug nomenclature.

Medication Errors

Medication errors are a very serious problem in the medical field and, unfortunately, happen quite frequently. For example, suppose that a pharmacy has a 1 percent prescription error rate. In most professions, this would be considered a very low number and would be acceptable. However, if the pharmacy fills 10,000 prescriptions per year, it would make 100 prescription errors. Although this may seem like a small number of errors, any error can be quite serious and even deadly; thus, *any* error in pharmacy should be considered unacceptable. This section discusses why it is important for a pharmacy technician to know and be able to identify the different types of medication errors, and to learn how to avoid them.

The National Coordinating Council for Medication Error Reporting and Prevention defines a *medication error* as "any preventable event that may cause or lead to inappropriate medication use or patient harm while the medication is in the control of the health care professional, patient, or consumer. Such events may be related to professional practice, health care products, procedures, and systems, including prescribing; order communication; product labeling, packaging, and nomenclature; compounding; dispensing; distribution; administration; education; monitoring; and use." Medication errors can occur at any point in the medication distribution process, from the moment the prescription is written until the medication is ultimately administered to the patient. However, although everyone involved in the process must take precautions to detect and prevent medication errors, the majority of responsibility and blame seems—perhaps too often—to fall on pharmacy staff.

The Five Rights of Medication Administration

Let's review the Five Rights of medication administration presented earlier in Chapter 3, as they can greatly decrease the occurrence of medication errors. The Five Rights are:

1. Right patient—the drug must always go to the correct patient.
2. Right drug—the right drug must always be chosen.

3. Right route—the drug must be given via the correct route of administration. If the correct drug and dose are given, but via the wrong route, a medication error has occurred.

4. Right dose—the patient must receive the right dose. A dose that is too high or too low is considered a medication error.

5. Right time—the patient must receive the medication within the prescribed time frame. Many inpatient institutions have a time window within which the medication can be given; any administration outside that window is considered a medication error. For example, if a dose is due at 9:00 a.m., the nurse may be permitted to give the medication any time between 8:30 a.m. and 9:30 a.m. Medication given outside the set parameters is considered a medication error.

There are two new, additional "rights" of medication administration outside of the five traditional rights. The first is the *right technique*. The correct technique must be used when preparing the drug (e.g., IV products must be made in sterile environments). The second is the *right documentation*. Correct documentation must be done (whether by doctor, nurse, pharmacy, etc.), or a medication error has occurred.

Types of Medication Errors

The American Hospital Association lists the following as some common types of medication errors:

- Incomplete patient information, such as not knowing about patients' allergies, other medicines they are taking, previous diagnoses, and lab results.
- Unavailable drug information, such as lack of up-to-date clinical warnings.
- Miscommunication of drug orders, which can be caused by poor handwriting, confusion between drugs with similar names, misuse of zeroes and decimal points, confusion of metric and other dosing units, and inappropriate abbreviations.
- Lack of appropriate labeling as a drug is prepared and repackaged into smaller units.
- Environmental factors, such as lighting, heat, noise, and interruptions that can distract health professionals from their medical tasks.

Dosage Formulations

dosage form the actual form of the drug (tablet, capsule, suppository, solution, etc.); also called *dosage formulation*.

Medications are available in various **dosage forms**; the term refers to how the medication is prepared for administration to the patient. The two primary dosage preparations are liquid and solid. As you learned in Chapter 10, common dosage forms include tablets, solutions, suspensions, inhalants, creams, and ointments. A single medication may be available in multiple dosage forms to allow use for various disease states, patient age ranges, and desired results.

Solid Dosage Forms

Medications are most widely available as solid dosage forms (see Figure 18-7). These may be administered by different routes, such as orally, rectally, vaginally, or topically.

A physician must review many factors when deciding if a solid dosage form is an appropriate choice for the patient. Solid medications have several advantages over other forms of medication, including:

- Patients are able to self-administer solid medications more easily.
- Solid medications usually have a longer shelf life before reaching the expiration date.
- Solid medications are easier to package, distribute, ship, and store.
- Dosing is more accurate with solid dosage forms, because the medication is already in a distinctive unit/measure.

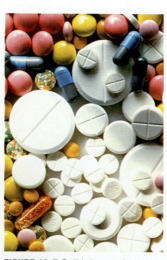

FIGURE 18-7 Solid dosage forms.

- Solid medications usually have little or no taste, whereas liquid medications often taste bad.
- Solid dosage forms have been created to release the medication over a longer period of time in the patient's body, as in extended-release medications. This allows the patient to take fewer doses while still getting the desired effects.

Solid medications also have several disadvantages:

- Some patients may have difficulty swallowing large tablets or capsules.
- Solid medications are not an appropriate choice for patients who are unconscious or are using nasal/mouth breathing tubes for ventilation.
- Solid medications take longer to be absorbed, broken down, and distributed in the body. The stomach has to metabolize the medication before it can take effect.
- Solid medications are not fast enough for immediate-action treatments. When immediate-action treatments are required, liquids or injectable medications are more appropriate.

Tablets

Tablets are solid medications that are compacted into small, formed shapes. They are usually taken by mouth (oral administration). Tablets consist of several components that work together to ensure that the tablet is easy to swallow, has flavorings or sweeteners for improved taste, is properly digested in the body, and releases the drug at the proper time to produce the desired effect. All of the ingredients in a medication except the active drug(s) are called *inactive*, or *inert*, *ingredients*.

Tablets are classified by the way they are made. The two most common tablet classifications are molded and compressed. *Molded* tablets are made by using a mold and wet materials. *Compressed* tablets are formed by die-punching compressed, powdered, crystalline, or granular substances into a uniform shape. One characteristic of a compressed tablet is the film, sugar coating, or enteric coating on the outside of the tablet, commonly used to mask a bad taste or foul smell and protect the tablet from the air and humidity. The film coating is also used to make the tablet smooth and easier to swallow. Enteric coating is used to keep the tablet from being dissolved in the stomach by the gastric acids and to protect the lining of the gastrointestinal tract and stomach from irritation by the drug. Medications that are to be released in the body over a period of time are made with enteric coatings.

The five common types of tablets are chewable, effervescent, sublingual, buccal, and vaginal. The following briefly describes each type and its unique characteristics and uses.

Chewable Tablets

Chewable tablets are tablets that should be chewed, instead of swallowed whole, to achieve the desired results. Chewable tablets are most commonly used for pediatric medications, because small children have a difficult time swallowing tablets. Most chewable tablets include sweeteners and flavorings to mask bad tastes and make the medication easier to take. Some adult medications are also chewable, such as antacids and aspirin.

Effervescent Tablets

Effervescent tablets are dissolved into a liquid before administration. These tablets contain special ingredients that release the active chemical ingredient by reacting with the liquid; this is what causes the bubbling and fizzing when an effervescent tablet is placed in liquid. Effervescent tablets have the advantage of being completely dissolved in the liquid before the patient takes the medication. This allows for quicker absorption in the body than a solid tablet.

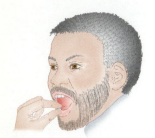

FIGURE 18-8 Sublingual tablet and route.

Sublingual Tablets

Sublingual tablets are disintegrated and absorbed when the tablet is placed sublingually; that is, under the tongue (see Figure 18-8). The ingredients in these tablets are absorbed through the lining of the mouth into the bloodstream; thus, sublingual tablets are useful for medications that are destroyed by stomach acid or poorly absorbed through the GI tract.

Buccal Tablets

Buccal tablets are similar to sublingual, except that they are disintegrated in the buccal pouch of the mouth, located between the gums and the cheek, and absorbed into the bloodstream through the lining of the cheek.

Vaginal Tablets

Vaginal tablets are solid dosage forms that are administered into the vagina and are dissolved and absorbed through the mucous lining of the vagina. Vaginal tablets are useful if immediate treatment and medication are needed within the walls of the vagina.

Capsules

Capsules are solid medication forms in which the active and inactive ingredients of a drug are contained in a shell. The most common shell is composed of gelatin, which is made of protein from animals. The smooth surface of the gelatin shells allows easier swallowing. Gelatin shells may be either soft or hard.

Soft Gelatin Shells

Soft gelatin shells have had ingredients added to the shell to give it a soft, elastic consistency. This allows the capsule to be flexible during administration. The two halves of a soft capsule are sealed together and cannot be broken apart. The shape of soft capsules can vary from round to oblong (see Figure 18-9). They are filled with powdered, pasty, or liquid medications. The soft gelatin capsule dissolves once in the body, allowing the medication to be absorbed and distributed to the body tissues.

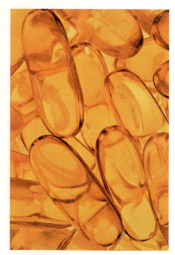

FIGURE 18-9 Soft gelatin shell capsules.

Hard Gelatin Shells

Hard gelatin capsules are characterized by two oblong halves joined together (see Figure 18-10). These capsules are only filled with powdered medications, never liquid, as liquid would dissolve the capsule shells. Hard gelatin capsules are most often intended for oral administration, and such capsules should be swallowed whole. However, an advantage of a hard gelatin capsule is that it can be opened and its contents sprinkled over a food substance or into water before administration. This is helpful for patients who are not able to swallow a whole capsule. The ingredients will be dissolved more quickly outside the gelatin shell.

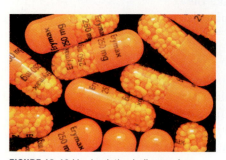

Lozenges

Also called *pastilles* or *troches*, *lozenges* are a hard, disk-shaped solid dosage form that contain a sugar base. Lozenges are used to deliver a variety of local therapeutic effects to the patient's mouth and throat, including antiseptic, analgesic, anesthetic, antibiotic, decongestant, astringent, and antitussive effects. The lozenge remains in the patient's mouth until it has completely dissolved and all the medication has been released.

FIGURE 18-10 Hard gelatin shell capsules.

Ointments

Ointments are semisolid dosage forms composed of solid and liquid medications. Ointments are applied externally to the skin or mucous membranes and are used to deliver medication to the skin, lubricate the skin, or protect the skin. Ointments may or may not contain a medication. They are categorized into the following types: oleaginous, water-soluble, anhydrous, and emulsions. The choice of an ointment depends on the specific characteristics and desired results. Certain medications are more effective in a water-based ointment than in a heavy, greasy base.

Oleaginous Ointments

Oleaginous ointments are **emollients** used to soothe and cool the skin or mucous membrane. Their primary function is to protect the surface from the air. An advantage of an oleaginous ointment is that it is **hydrophobic** and not easily washed off. These ointments keep moisture from leaving the skin and therefore are commonly used as lubricants. They can remain on the skin for a long period of time. One disadvantage of oleaginous ointments is their greasy feel.

oleaginous containing oil; having oil-like properties.

emollient softening and soothing to the skin.

hydrophobic repels water.

Water-Soluble Ointments

Water-soluble ointments have characteristics that are the opposite of those of oleaginous ointments. They are nongreasy to the touch and easily wash off with water. These types of ointments usually do not contain fats or water. Water-soluble ointment bases can be mixed with a nonaqueous or solid medication.

Anhydrous Ointments

Anhydrous ointments are emollients similar to oleaginous ointments. The major difference between the two is that anhydrous ointments absorb water instead of repelling it, because anhydrous ointments contain no water. A main function is to soften and moisturize the skin, but not to the same degree as ointments with an oleaginous base. As it absorbs water, the anhydrous ointment turns into a water-in-oil emulsion.

anhydrous without water.

emulsion liquid mixture of water and oil.

occlusive closing or blocking; refers to a substance that closes or covers a wound and keeps the air from reaching the wound.

Emulsions

Emulsions are emollient bases that are comprised of water and oil. The two types of emulsions are oil-in-water and water-in-oil. The water-in-oil bases are heavy, greasy, emollient, and **occlusive**. The oil-in-water bases are the opposite: water-washable, nongreasy, and nonocclusive.

aqueous containing water.

Creams

Creams are semisolid preparations that may or may not contain medication and are composed of an oil-in-water base or a water-in-oil base. They are lighter than ointments and can be applied to the skin more easily. Creams function to soothe, cool, dry, and protect the skin. Creams are usually preferred over ointments because they are easier to apply and wash off the skin.

Liquid Dosage Forms

The most common liquid dosage forms are syrups, solutions, emulsions, and suspensions (see Figure 18-11). The fluid medium is also called the *vehicle* or *delivery system* and is considered to carry the active ingredient or medication. The vehicle may be **aqueous** (water), or the liquid used may be oil or alcohol. The medication may be dissolved in the vehicle or may remain as a fine solid particle suspended in the fluid. The consistency of the liquid can be as thin as water or as thick as a syrup.

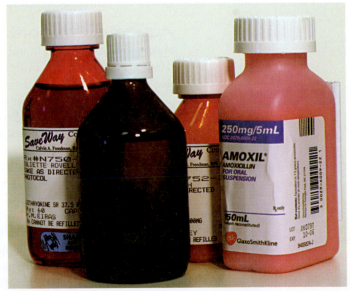

FIGURE 18-11 Liquid dosage forms.

Liquids have several advantages over other dosage forms, including:

- Patients who have difficulty swallowing solid dosage forms such as tablets can better tolerate liquid dosage forms.
- Liquid medications are absorbed faster in the body than solid dosage forms because the active ingredient has already begun to break down and can readily be absorbed in the bloodstream. Solid dosage forms must be dissolved and broken down in the body before absorption of the active medication can take place.
- Liquid forms provide much more flexibility for achieving the proper dosage of the medication.

Liquids also have several disadvantages compared to other dosage forms, including:

- Liquids often have a shorter life before expiration than other dosage forms.
- Liquids may have a bad taste, as the medication is already dissolved and this dosage form cannot provide a protective coating like a tablet or capsule. This may make compliance especially difficult for children who do not like the taste of the medication. Sweeteners and flavorings are often used to make liquid medications tolerable for the patient. (Solid medications such as tablets and capsules are often coated to diminish contact with the taste receptors before they are swallowed.)
- Liquids may be more difficult to administer for some patients; thick liquids can be hard to pour, and patients often spill liquids.
- Liquids may promote dosage errors, as some patients may not measure a liquid correctly.
- Liquids usually have special storage requirements that must be maintained for the medication to work properly. For example, if refrigeration is needed, patient travel and compliance may be difficult.

Solutions

Solutions are a dosage form in which the medication is completely dissolved and evenly distributed in a **homogenous** mixture. The molecules of the solid, liquid, or gas medications are equally distributed among the molecules of the liquid vehicle. Solutions are usually absorbed quickly, because the medication is already completely dissolved; this allows the medication to take effect faster. This may be the greatest advantage of solution dosage forms. There are several subcategories of solutions, based on characteristics of the vehicle in which the medication is dissolved.

homogenous having all the same qualities within a group.

Aqueous Solutions

Aqueous solutions are liquid mixtures that use purified or sterile water as the vehicle. They are available for oral, topical, or parenteral administration. Aqueous solutions are available as douches, irrigating solutions, enemas, gargles, washes, and sprays.

Douches are directed into a body cavity or against a part of the body to clean and disinfect. These can be used to remove debris from the eyes, nose, throat, or vagina.

Irrigating solutions are also used to cleanse parts of the body, such as the eyes, urinary bladder, abraded skin, or open wounds. These types of solutions contain antibiotics and antimicrobial medications to rid the site of infection. Irrigating solutions are often used over a larger part of the body, and in surgical procedures, to clear blood and debris.

Enemas are aqueous solutions administered rectally to empty the bowel or treat infections and diseases of the lower gastrointestinal tract. Enemas are also often used to relieve constipation and to cleanse the bowel before a surgical procedure.

Gargles and *washes* are used to cleanse and treat diseases of the mouth and throat. Gargles are swished in the patient's mouth and then spit out. Washes are used more often for cosmetic and disinfecting purposes in the mouth. Like gargles, washes are used in the mouth and not swallowed.

Viscous Aqueous Solutions

Viscous aqueous solutions also use purified or sterile water as the liquid vehicle. These liquid preparations are thick, sticky, sweet solutions that may be either liquid or semi-solid preparations. Viscous aqueous solutions include syrups, jellies, and mucilages.

Syrups are concentrated mixtures of sugar and water, and may be medicated or nonmedicated. Syrups are distinguished from other solutions by the high concentration of sugar contained in the mixture. In addition to the active ingredient, syrups may also contain flavorings or sweeteners that have no medicinal value. Nonmedicated syrups may be used as a vehicle for unpleasant-tasting medications. The biggest advantage of a syrup is its ability to cover up the bad taste of a medication; because it is so thick, only a small portion of the medication comes in contact with the taste receptors in the mouth. The thicker consistency of a syrup can also have a soothing effect on irritated or infected tissues of the mouth and throat. The most common use of syrups is in pediatric and adult cough and cold syrups.

Jellies are semisolid preparations that contain water. They are most often used as lubricants for surgical gloves, vaginal contraceptive agents, and rectal thermometers. Jellies can be used as lubricants to aid in the insertion and removal of diagnostic probes into orifices or to reduce friction during an ultrasound procedure.

Mucilages are much thicker, viscous, adhesive liquids that contain water and the thick components of vegetable matter. They are useful to prevent insoluble, solid medication particles from settling at the bottom of the liquid.

viscous thick; almost jelly-like.

Nonaqueous Solutions

Nonaqueous solutions use dissolving agents other than water, although the vehicle may be combined with water. Vehicles commonly used in nonaqueous solvents include alcohol, glycerin, and propylene glycol. The solutions that use only alcohol as the dissolving agent are called *alcoholic* solutions.

Hydro-Alcoholic Solutions

Hydro-alcoholic solutions are nonaqueous solutions, but differ from pure aqueous solutions in that they contain alcohol in addition to water to act as the vehicle or dissolving agent. The most common example of a hydro-alcoholic solution is an elixir.

Elixirs are liquid preparations that contain flavored water and alcohol mixtures intended for oral administration. They are clear, sweet solutions that may or may not contain medication. The amount of alcohol in the mixture will vary, depending on the ability of the other ingredients to dissolve easily in pure water. Many drugs dissolve more easily in a water-and-alcohol mixture than in water alone. The range of alcohol contents in one solution may vary from 2 percent to 30 percent.

Alcohol, the greatest advantage of an elixir, may also be its greatest disadvantage. Many patients are not able to consume alcohol, and it may have undesired side effects or interactions with other medications currently being taken. Patients, especially pediatric and elderly, should pay attention to the ingredient contents in elixirs. These populations can be extra-sensitive to even the smallest alcohol content. Medicated elixirs are often given to patients who have a difficult time swallowing tablets or capsules.

Two examples of commonly prescribed medicated elixirs are phenobarbital and digoxin. Elixirs can also be used as sweeteners or flavoring agents. **Aromatic** elixirs are nonmedicated and are used as vehicles to mask the unpleasant taste of a medication.

aromatic having a strong or fragrant smell (aroma).

Alcoholic Solutions

Alcoholic solutions contain only alcohol as the dissolving agent and have no water. The most common alcohols used in preparing alcoholic solutions are ethyl and ethanol alcohols. Examples of alcoholic solutions include collodions, spirits, and glycerite solutions.

Collodions are alcoholic solutions that contain pyroxylin (which is found in cotton fibers) dissolved in either ethanol or ethyl alcohol. When this liquid preparation is applied to the skin, the alcohol evaporates, leaving only a thin film covering of the pyroxylin. An added advantage of a collodion is that it can carry an added medication. These preparations are used to treat and dissolve corns or warts. A more common example of a collodion is the Band-Aid® liquid bandage, which applies a medication and a thin covering to prevent infection.

Spirits are liquid solutions that may be either alcoholic or hydro-alcoholic. Spirits contain **volatile** and aromatic substances. Alcohol dissolves these substances more easily than water, allowing a greater concentration of these materials. Spirits may be administered internally or inhaled. Spirits are also known for their flavoring ability, such as peppermint spirits. Other spirits, known as aromatic ammonia spirits or smelling salts, may be inhaled through the nose. If spirits contain water in addition to alcohol, they are identified as hydro-alcoholic solutions.

Glycerite solutions are nonaqueous solutions that contain a medication dissolved in glycerin. Glycerin is a sweet, oily fluid made from fat and oils. Glycerin is considered a flexible vehicle. It can be used alone or in any combination with water or alcohol. Glycerin is often used as a solvent for medications that do not easily dissolve in water or alcohol alone. Usually, a medication is dissolved in the glycerin, which is then further mixed into a water or alcohol vehicle. Glycerite solutions are often viscous and have the thick consistency of a jelly. Glycerite solutions are rarely used today.

volatile evaporates rapidly.

Inhalants

Inhalants are medications that contain a fine powder or solution delivered through a mist into the mouth or nose. The medication immediately enters the respiratory tract for absorption. The most common inhalant medications are inhalers used to treat asthma. Allergy nasal sprays may also be delivered as an inhalant through the nose.

Liniments

Liniments are medications that are applied to the skin with friction and rubbing. They can be solutions, suspensions, or emulsions and are used to relieve minor cuts, scrapes, burns, aches, and pains. Most contain a medication that produces a mild irritation or reddening of the skin when applied. This irritation then produces a counterirritation, or mild inflammation, of the skin. This counterirritation relieves the inflammation of a deeper structure such as tissues or muscles. Ben-Gay® is the most commonly used over-the-counter liniment today.

INFORMATION

Liniments are prepared with alcohol or acetone, contain other irritants such as capsaicin, and should not be applied to bruised or broken skin, as pain and irritation would occur.

Emulsions

Emulsions are liquid mixtures of water and oil, which normally do not mix. One liquid is broken down into smaller elements and evenly distributed throughout the other liquid. The liquid that was broken down into small elements is called the *internal phase*; the other liquid is the *external phase*. The external phase may also be referred to as the *continuous phase*, because it remains a liquid substance.

Emulsions are named for the emulsifying agent that is used with the two phases. The emulsifying agent is added to the liquid mixture to prevent the internal phase from fusing together and separating from the external phase. If an emulsifying agent is not used, the two liquids will eventually separate and create two distinct layers. This is commonly seen in a bottle of oil and vinegar salad dressing. Before you shake the bottle, you can see the individual layers of oil and vinegar that have settled and separated. Once shaken, the two layers are mixed together again. This is an example of what happens when an emulsifying agent is not added to a liquid mixture.

Water-in-oil emulsions are liquid mixtures of water droplets distributed throughout an oil substance. These mixtures are commonly used on unbroken skin wounds.

Water-in-oil emulsions spread out more evenly than oil-in-water emulsions, because the skin's natural oils mix well with the external oil phase in the emulsion. The oils also soften the skin better by adding moisture and remaining on the skin when washed with water. These emulsions are often avoided, though, because they easily stain clothing and have a greasy texture.

Oil-in-water emulsions contain small oil globules dispersed throughout water. These mixtures are commonly used as oral medications. The undesirably oily medications are broken into small particles and dispersed in a sweetened, flavored aqueous vehicle. These small particles can then be swallowed without contacting the taste buds. The small size of the particles increases absorption in the stomach and bloodstream. Oil-in-water emulsions are lighter and nongreasy. For these reasons, they are the first choice for application to a hairy part of the body. The two common types of oil-in-water emulsions are mineral oil and castor oil.

Comparison of Water-in-Oil and Oil-in-Water Emulsions

Each type of emulsion has several advantages and disadvantages. Several factors will drive the choice of the proper emulsion. For irritated skin, the medication is better tolerated if applied to the skin as small particles in the internal phase. The external phase keeps these particles from direct contact with the irritation. The rule of thumb is:

- Medications that dissolve more easily in water are applied as water-in-oil emulsions.
- Medications that dissolve more easily in oil are applied as oil-in-water emulsions.

Suspensions

Suspensions contain very fine solid particles mixed with a gas, liquid, or solid preparation. Most suspensions are solid particles dispersed in a liquid. A suspension is often used when a solid medication form is not appropriate for a particular patient. Because the solid particles in the suspension are very small, the breakdown and absorption process is much quicker than with tablets or capsules. The medication reaches the bloodstream much sooner than it would if a solid medication form were used.

The key difference between a solution and a suspension is that a suspension must be shaken well before use, to redistribute any of the solid particles that have settled in the liquid mixture. Suspensions are usually intended for oral ingestion in cases where a large amount of medication is needed. Suspensions are also available for administration by other routes, including ophthalmic, parenteral, otic, and rectal. Suspensions for oral use are combined with water, although other suspensions may use oil as the vehicle or dissolving agent.

Magmas and Milks

Magmas and *milks* are suspensions of undissolved medications in water. They are very thick, viscous liquids. These suspensions are intended only for oral use and must be shaken thoroughly before use. Milk of Magnesia® is the most common example of a magma suspension.

Lotions

Lotions are suspensions for external use only. They are made up of a powdered medication in a liquid mixture. Lotions are used to soothe, cool, dry, and protect irritated skin and wounds. Lotions can function as disinfectants, protectants, moisturizers, and anti-inflammatories. Lotions have an advantage over other external medications in that they can easily be applied over large areas of the skin. They do not leave an oily or greasy feel on the skin after application. The most common over-the-counter example of a lotion is Calamine® lotion.

Gels

Gels are suspensions similar to magmas and milks, but the solid particles in gels are much smaller. Gels can be used for oral or topical administration. Over-the-counter antacids are common examples of gel suspensions.

Extractives

Extractives are liquid mixtures made from concentrated active ingredients derived from plants or animals. The drug is withdrawn by soaking the dried tissue in a solvent. After the liquid is evaporated, the only thing remaining is the active, or crude, drug ingredient. Some examples of extractives are tinctures, extracts, and fluidextracts. The various types of extractives are distinguished by the potency of their active ingredient.

Tinctures are extractive alcoholic or hydro-alcoholic solutions. The potency of each mixture is adjusted so that each milliliter of tincture contains the exact same potency of 100 mg of crude ingredient. Iodine and paregoric tinctures are two common examples of this type of extractive.

Fluidextracts are more potent than tinctures, as each milliliter of fluidextract contains 1,000 mg of the crude drug.

Extracts are very similar to tinctures and fluidextracts, except for potency. The potency of the crude drug in extracts is two to six times stronger than in the others. Common examples of extracts are vanilla, peppermint, and almond extracts used for cooking.

Powders

Powders are a solid preparation in which fine, uniform particles of active and inactive ingredients are ground up. Powders are usually manufactured and packaged as large supplies for bulk compounding. They may be applied internally or externally. Internal administration is done after the powder mixture has been dissolved in a liquid. External powders can be applied directly to the skin to be absorbed into the bloodstream. External powders are also referred to as *dusting powders*. Commonly used internal powders are potassium supplements, which must be dissolved in water or juice for administration. Mycostatin® powder is an external powder used to treat fungal infections on the skin.

Powders packaged in bulk supply are difficult to measure accurately. This accuracy is achieved at the individual dose level by packaging the powder in a *powder paper*, a small piece of paper that measures out exactly one dose. BC Powder® comes packaged in powder papers, each one equivalent to one dose.

Granules

Granules are made from powders that are wetted and then dried. Once completely dried, the powder is ground into coarse, nonuniform particles. Granules are commonly used in pediatric antibiotic suspensions. Distilled water is added to the package of granules, and the suspension is shaken until the solid particles dissolve completely in the liquid.

Aerosols

Aerosols are very fine liquid or solid particles mixed in a vehicle. The aerosol mixture is packed with gas and pressure to be administered via the respiratory tract or applied topically. When used properly, the gaseous pressure forces the liquid or solid particles out of the inhaler. Internal aerosols are contained in inhalers and can be used in the nose or mouth. The inhaler forces the medication directly into the lungs and respiratory system so it can immediately provide relief. External aerosols are usually applied topically. Common external aerosols are Tinactin® and Bactine® sprays. One advantage of external aerosols is their ability to be used in hard-to-reach areas or on severely irritated areas of the skin. Aerosols do not cause as much irritation to the wound as other topical treatments, such as ointments or creams.

The need for a variety of alternative dosage forms is not exclusive to humans. Animals need variety, too! Think of trying to give a cat a capsule by mouth—depending on the cat's mood, it is probably not going to happen. Specialty pharmacies can, however, compound the prescribed medication into a transdermal gel that the owner can simply rub onto the back of the feline's ear. There are also other alternative dosage forms, not discussed in this chapter, that may be used for animals. For example, sometimes it is necessary to use a fish or a mouse as the dosage form or vehicle for patients such as dolphins and snakes.

Extended-Release Dosage Forms

Some medications are made to be released in the body over a period of time, rather than all at once. Referred to as extended-release (ER), long-acting (LA), sustained-release (SR), time-release (TR), or controlled-release (CR), these medications dissolve in the body, but allow only a portion of the active ingredient to be absorbed into the bloodstream at a time. Extended-release medications are most commonly available in tablets and capsules. There are also a few liquid preparations that are made to slowly release over a period of time. Extended-release medications are available for many common illnesses, such as hypertension, diabetes, depression, bacterial infections, and pain. The following characteristics are considered when selecting an extended-release medication:

- The same amount of medication is released into the bloodstream over a slow, consistent period.
- There is added convenience for patients, as they will take fewer doses per day to achieve the same (or better) results than they would have to take of an immediate-action medication. Most extended-release medications are taken q12h or q24h.
- Patient compliance increases when there are fewer doses and pills to take per day.
- Costs are often lower, as the patient does not need as many pills or doses. Lower prescription costs also help increase patient compliance.
- Adverse reactions and side effects are reduced, because the medication is introduced into the body slowly.

Extended-release medications are made possible by advanced technologies. Gelatin capsules can be made to contain very small beads of medication. The stomach immediately dissolves the gelatin capsule, exposing the beads for absorption. The beads of medication are then dissolved and absorbed over a period of time. Many cold and allergy medications are made in this fashion to provide relief for 6 to 12 hours after taking one dose. Some extended-release medications are made with two layers. One layer is dissolved and absorbed immediately, while the other one dissolves gradually over time.

Another method of making extended-release medications is to embed the medication in a plastic or wax matrix. As the medication is released from the matrix, it is dissolved and absorbed in the body. The matrix itself does not dissolve, but is excreted from the body as waste. A more advanced technology uses an osmotic pump to deliver the medication over a period of time. The system consists of a membrane surrounding the medication. Through the process of osmosis, and depending on the concentration, medication is diffused out to the body. Medication is pushed from the membrane to the body with the entrance and exit of water. Examples of extended-release medication are Procardia XL® and Cardizem CD®.

Routes of Administration

Medications are delivered to a patient by a variety of routes of administration. The **route of administration (ROA)** is simply the method by which a medication is introduced into the body for absorption and distribution (see Figure 18-12). The route of administration can vary from patient to patient and depends on the effect desired from

route of administration how a drug is introduced into or on the body.

ROUTES

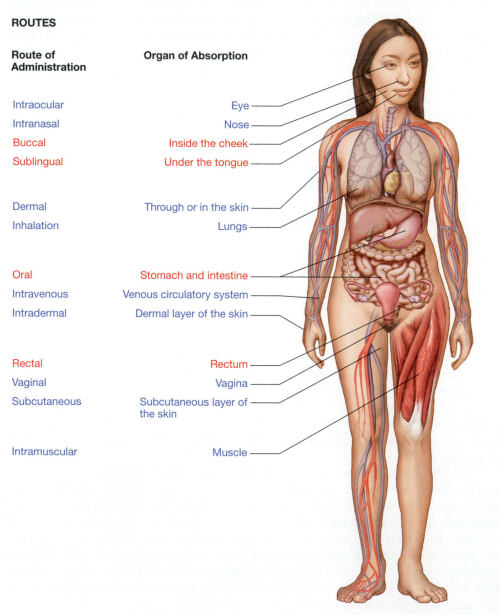

Route of Administration	Organ of Absorption
Intraocular	Eye
Intranasal	Nose
Buccal	Inside the cheek
Sublingual	Under the tongue
Dermal	Through or in the skin
Inhalation	Lungs
Oral	Stomach and intestine
Intravenous	Venous circulatory system
Intradermal	Dermal layer of the skin
Rectal	Rectum
Vaginal	Vagina
Subcutaneous	Subcutaneous layer of the skin
Intramuscular	Muscle

FIGURE 18-12 Various routes of administration.

the administered medication. Several factors are considered when determining the ROA, including:

- Patient's age. Younger and older patients may have difficulty swallowing medications.
- Patient's physical state. Consciousness versus an unconscious state may determine the best route.
- Patient's medical condition. Oral medications may not be appropriate for patients with stomach or gastrointestinal complications.
- Time to achieve results. Injections or IV routes will achieve results much faster than other routes.
- Side effects. Possible side effects should be considered when choosing a ROA.

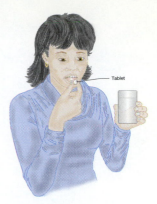

FIGURE 18-13 The oral route of administration.

Oral

The most common and uncomplicated route of administration is by mouth (see Figure 18-13). The abbreviation for the oral route of administration, PO, is derived from the Latin *per os* (by mouth). Capsules, tablets, caplets, liquids, and emulsions are some of the medication dosage formulations that may be taken orally. Most medications are available both orally and by another route. For example, one patient may be treated with an oral tablet or suspension, whereas another patient needs an injection of the same medication for immediate treatment. Most tablets, capsules, and liquids are given via the oral route of administration.

Advantages of oral medications over other routes of administration include:

- Oral medications are safer, more convenient, and easier to store.
- They may be more readily available in pharmacies. Injections may have to be special-ordered by the physician or pharmacy.
- They are generally less expensive than other available routes.
- Many are available in both immediate-release or extended-release dosage forms.
- They are easier to self-administer and generally do not require additional administration supplies.

The disadvantages of oral medications usually lead physicians and patients to choose another route by which to administer the medication in specific instances. These disadvantages include:

- Oral medications may not be appropriate for children or elderly patients.
- They may be difficult to swallow for patients who are unconscious, ventilated, or having digestion problems.
- They must be broken down and absorbed before they can be distributed throughout the body. For this reason, oral medications take longer to provide effects and relief.

Transdermal

Transdermal medications are delivered across or through the skin for systemic effects. Also known as *percutaneous*, the transdermal route generally uses a patch applied to the skin, where it delivers medication to the bloodstream. In contrast to transdermal medications, topical ointments and creams generally do not deliver medication into the bloodstream; instead, these medications are used for external treatments and protection. However, a few transdermal ointments and cream medications exist. The most common transdermal ointment is nitroglycerin ointment for the relief of cardiac chest pain.

Transdermal patches consist of an adhesive vehicle applied to the skin; the medication is released into the bloodstream over a period of time. Patches are easy to store, convenient to use, and can remain on the body for a long time. Depending on the medication, patches may be used for one day or up to a week at a time. Wearing a transdermal patch is considered more convenient than taking a tablet on a daily basis.

Two types of patches are used to deliver transdermal medications. One patch controls the rate of delivery to the skin and bloodstream; the other patch is designed so that the skin controls the rate of delivery. In the patch that controls the delivery, a special membrane that is in direct contact with the skin delivers the medication from a drug reservoir. When the skin is used to control the rate of delivery, the drug is moved from the patch into the blood. The difference between these two routes is the relatively quick delivery of a large amount of medication all at once via the second route.

Workplace Wisdom Transdermal Patches

In most cases, patients should rotate the spots where transdermal patches are applied, to avoid skin irritation. Additionally, to avoid pulling hair out during removal, patches should not be applied to hairy skin areas.

Transdermal patches are becoming more readily available and widely accepted by patients. There are patches available for several different types of medications and uses. Examples of transdermal patches available include those for hormone therapy (Climara®, Estraderm®), narcotic analgesics (Duragesic®), birth control (Ortho Evra®), cardiac problems (nitroglycerin, Catapress®), motion sickness (Transderm Scōp®), and smoking cessation (Nicoderm®).

Inhalation

When the inhalation route of administration is used, the medication is inhaled through the mouth and directly absorbed into the lungs. This is effective for lung conditions when immediate relief is needed. The most common condition for which inhalation is used is asthma; the medication is administered through an inhaler inserted into the mouth. Gases then force the medication particles into the mouth and down to the lungs. With other respiratory conditions, such as infections and congestion, inhalers may be used to help open the lungs and bronchioles if the airways are temporarily constricted. Common examples of medications administered through inhalation include albuterol (Proventil®/Ventolin®), Advair Diskus®, and over-the-counter Primatene Mist®.

Nasal

Medications can be inhaled through the nose and absorbed into the bloodstream or sprayed into the nose for local effects. Like inhalation by mouth, the nasal route of administration provides immediate relief for conditions such as nasal allergies and congestion. A nasal inhaler is used by holding it to the nostrils and inhaling through the nose; liquid medications are more commonly sprayed into the nose.

There may be additional conditions for which a nasally administered medication is more effective. One example is a narcotic analgesic, Stadol®. When administered nasally, this medication reaches the bloodstream more quickly than through the traditional oral route of administration. Common medications available for nasal administration include Flonase®, Rhinocort®, and Stadol®.

Parenteral

The second most commonly used route of administration is injection (see Figure 18-14). *Parenteral* is the route by which medication does not pass through the gastrointestinal system for absorption and distribution. The most common parenteral routes are:

1. intradermal
2. subcutaneous
3. intramuscular
4. intravenous

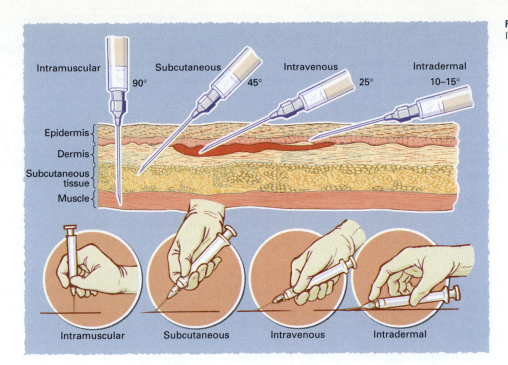

FIGURE 18-14 ID, SC, IM, and
IV routes of administration.

Medications that are delivered by the parenteral routes have several advantages over the oral route of administration:

- Quicker absorption and distribution.
- Convenience for those who cannot take oral medications.
- Varied rate of delivery (from a couple of seconds to several hours).

Care must be taken to ascertain that the dosages given parenterally are correct, because the action is usually immediate and there is no way to reverse the amount of drug administered. For many medications, there are also few or no ways to reverse any adverse effects. Adverse effects can occur when a dose given is too high, or when a dose given is too low.

Parenteral administration of medications is also very invasive. For this reason, some patients are uneasy with these routes and prefer oral medications. Injections can be very painful for children and the elderly. They also create an opportunity for bacteria and infection to enter the body. The common dosage forms of medications given by the parenteral route include suspensions, solutions, and emulsions.

Intradermal

The intradermal (ID) route injects medications into the top layers of the skin. These injections are not as invasive or as deep as those done by the subcutaneous route. The intradermal route is used to complete skin testing for allergies and some diseases, such as tuberculosis.

Subcutaneous

The subcutaneous (SC) route of administration is one of the most utilized of parenteral routes. The medication is injected into the tissue immediately under the skin and is then absorbed in the bloodstream and distributed to the body as needed. The subcutaneous route delivers the medication at a slower rate than intramuscular or intravenous routes. The ability for patients to self-administer SC injections is a great advantage. In addition, because the medication is not being delivered too far into the body, a smaller needle can be used, which is less painful and invasive than IM or IV. One disadvantage is a limitation on the volume of the drug that can be injected under the skin: the volume limit for the SC route is 3 mL.

Intramuscular

With the intramuscular (IM) route of administration, medications are injected directly into large muscle masses, such as upper arms, thighs, or buttocks, and then absorbed from the muscle into the bloodstream. Dosage forms administered intramuscularly include solutions and suspensions. IM medications are not as quick to work as medications delivered intravenously.

As with the IV route of administration, the intramuscular rate of delivery can vary from seconds to minutes, and there is little chance for reversal of a medication injected directly into the muscle. Another disadvantage of this route is that the injection is usually painful and can cause irritation.

Intravenous

The most common parenteral route is the intravenous route (IV). A medication administered IV is injected or administered directly into a vein. The medication can be a solution or suspension.

Intravenous medications can be administered at different rates of delivery. A *bolus* is a larger volume of solution administered at one time for immediate effect. A *continuous infusion* is the administration of a solution over a continued or long period of time. For an *intravenous push* (IVP), a medication is administered directly into the vein with a syringe.

Workplace Wisdom Needles

Determining the gauge and length of a needle is important when preparing medications for injection. Here are some industry guidelines. For IV injections, use a 1-inch or 1.5-inch needle with a gauge of 16 to 20. For IM injections, again use a 1-inch or 1.5-inch needle, but with a gauge of 19 to 22. SC injections are usually given with a $\frac{3}{8}$-inch to 1-inch needle with a gauge of 24 to 27.

Other Parenteral Routes

There are several other parenteral routes of administration. These include:

- Implant: a temporary or permanent medical device inserted into the body that slowly releases medication. Implants are often used to treat chronic diseases such as cancer or diabetes. Insulin pumps may be implanted in the body to deliver small amounts of insulin as needed. Norplant®, a hormone medication, is placed in an implant inserted under the skin in the arm. The implant slowly releases the hormones over a five-year period. At the end of the five years, the implant is removed, and another one is inserted, if desired.

- Intra-arterial: injects medication directly into the arteries. This route reduces the risk of adverse reactions and side effects to other parts of the body. There is, however, a greater risk of toxicity if the wrong dosage is administered. Chemotherapy drugs used to fight cancer are commonly administered this way.

- Intra-articular: injects medication directly within the joints, most commonly the elbow and knee. Treatment of arthritis often calls for the intra-articular route of administration. Medications such as Enbrel® and other steroids are used to relieve severe inflammation around the joint.

- Intracardiac: injects medication directly to the heart. This route is very invasive and used only in cardiac emergencies, as the medication is injected into the heart muscle itself. This route also poses the risk of rupturing the heart; therefore, it is not recommended except as a last resort.

- Intraperitoneal: injects medication directly into the abdominal or peritoneal cavity. The common use for this route is to administer antibiotics to treat infections inside the peritoneal cavity.

- Intrapleural: injects medication into the sac (pleura) surrounding the lungs to reduce inflammation and scarring of the tissues lining the sacs and to prevent excessive fluid buildup in the pleura.

- Intrathecal: injects medications into the cerebrospinal fluid surrounding the spinal cord. This too is a very invasive and possibly dangerous procedure. It is used to treat infections or cancers of the central nervous system.
- Intraventricular: one of the most invasive parenteral routes; injects antibiotics or chemotherapy agents into the brain cavities, or *ventricles*.
- Intravesicular: injects medications directly into the urinary bladder; used to treat urinary bladder infections as well as bladder cancer.
- Intravitreal: injects medication directly into the vitreous body of the eye. Most medications do not reach the eye from the bloodstream, so for severe infections of the eye, this route is preferred because the antibiotic goes directly into the eye. Because this route is highly invasive, it is usually used only for severe diseases that are significantly reducing a patient's sight.

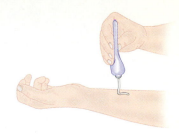

FIGURE 18-15 Topical route: Applying an ointment.

Topical

Medications that are administered externally to the skin are referred to as *topicals*. Topical medications are applied to the surface of the skin and absorbed into the mucous membrane (see Figure 18-15). The mucous membrane usually prevents the medication particles from being absorbed into the bloodstream. Dosage forms that are administered topically include ointments, creams, lotions, and emulsions. Because the medications do not enter the bloodstream, these dosage forms can be made with a higher concentration than those that do. The topical ROA is used to treat simple external skin rashes or slightly deeper-layer skin infections.

Rectal

With the *rectal* route of administration, medication is applied through the rectum. Medications administered rectally may be solids, liquids, semisolids, or aerosols. Common dosage forms include suppositories, enemas, and aerosol foams. Medications adminstered via the rectal route are used for either their local or systemic effects. For local effects, such as constipation or pain/itching, the medication is not absorbed into the bloodstream. However, for systemic effects, the medication is absorbed into the lower gastrointestinal tract or the bloodstream, for treatment of conditions such as nausea and vomiting or fever. Rectally administered medications are often used for children when an oral medication is not appropriate. Patients may also prefer a rectally administered medication when they cannot tolerate or cannot swallow an oral form of the medication. For example, rectal suppositories are commonly used to treat severe nausea and vomiting when the patient is not able to keep the solid medication down. Elderly patients who have difficulty swallowing tablets may also prefer rectally administered medications. Some common examples of medications administered rectally include Phenergan® suppositories, Fleet® enemas, and Proctofoam®.

Vaginal

With the *vaginal* route of administration, medications are inserted into the vagina for absorption and distribution. Types of dosage forms that can be administered vaginally include solutions, suppositories, tablets, and topical creams or ointments. The most common use for these medications is to treat vaginal infections. However, some medications can be administered through the vagina to deliver medication to the bloodstream to treat systemic conditions. Common examples of vaginally administered medications are Terazol®, Mycostatin® tablets, AVC® vaginal suppositories, and Massengill® douches.

Ophthalmic

Medications that are administered through the eye use the *ophthalmic* route. These medications can be solutions, ointments, suspensions, or gels. Ophthalmic medications are used to directly treat conditions of the eye such as allergies, infections, conjunctivitis, inflammation, or glaucoma. This direct route has the advantage of providing quicker relief than an oral medication that has to be absorbed and distributed throughout the entire body. Medications such as Visine® eyedrops immediately relieve the itchiness, redness, and swelling caused by allergies. Ophthalmic medications are also generally very easy to self-administer, and are convenient and easy to store. Common examples of medications delivered through the ophthalmic route include Visine®, Xalatan®, and antibiotic drops.

Otic

Medications that are administered in the ear are said to use the *otic* route of administration. These medications are delivered into the ear canal to treat infections, inflammation, and severe wax buildup. Common dosage forms administered through the otic route are solutions and suspensions. These medications are directly absorbed in the ear canal to provide immediate relief.

SUMMARY

This chapter reviewed the variety of sources from which drugs can be derived, drug nomenclature, common dosage forms, and routes of administration. Most medications come in multiple dosage forms and can be delivered by multiple routes. It is important to dispense the proper dosage form of medication; otherwise, a patient may not be able to take the medication as the physician instructed. This is a medication error.

Diligence regarding the parenteral routes of administration can be crucial to a patient. If the wrong injection route is used, toxicity can result, and usually very little can be done to reverse the effects of the injection. It is also very important to administer the correct dose of the medication. Too much or too little can be harmful to the patient.

One responsibility of a pharmacy technician is to work with the pharmacist to prepare and dispense medications to patients. The technician must understand drug names as well as the meaning and use of each dosage form and route. Although most dosage forms are commonly administered by one particular route, you cannot make assumptions about the route that is to be used. Many dosage forms may be administered via several different routes. For example, a tablet is commonly administered orally, but it could be administered vaginally as well. Liquid medications can also be administered in a variety of ways. If the prescription order is not clear as to the dosage form and route, the pharmacy staff and medical staff must work together to determine what is best for the patient and to avoid medication errors.

CHAPTER REVIEW QUESTIONS

1. It is possible for a drug to have more than one _____ name.
   a. generic
   b. chemical
   c. nonproprietary
   d. brand

2. A drug that occurs naturally but is chemically altered in the lab is considered to be:
   a. synthetic.
   b. semi-synthetic.
   c. natural.
   d. synthesized.

3. Which of the following is not a liquid dosage form?
   a. suspension
   b. emulsion
   c. cream
   d. enema

4. All of the following are common routes of administration for tablets except:
   a. buccal.
   b. vaginal.
   c. sublingual.
   d. rectal.

5. Which of the following statements is true?
   a. Ointments are a semisolid dosage form that are composed of a solid and a liquid medication.
   b. Creams are a semisolid dosage form that may or may not contain medication.
   c. Ointments are usually greasier and oilier than creams.
   d. All of the preceding statements are true.

6. Which of the following is a false statement?
   a. An IVP is injected directly into the vein.
   b. A drug administered IM is injected directly into muscle.

c. A drug administered ID is injected into the sub-cutaneous tissue.

d. All of the preceding statements are false.

7. An extended-release tablet:

a. will not cause drowsiness.

b. is administered at less frequent intervals than other tablets.

c. exits the body quickly after absorption.

d. all of the above.

8. A medication given by the parenteral route of administration:

a. passes through the skin to aid absorption.

b. requires several hours to be absorbed.

c. can be easily removed from the body after administration.

d. bypasses the GI system for absorption.

9. Which of the following drug names is not commonly used in daily pharmacy practice?

a. generic

b. trade

c. chemical

d. nonproprietary

10. Another term for a generic drug is:

a. trade drug.

b. proprietary drug.

c. chemical drug.

d. nonproprietary drug.

11. Which of the following should be considered when choosing the appropriate route of administration?

a. age

b. physical state

c. medical conditions

d. all of the above

12. Which of the following is not a suspension?

a. magma

b. elixir

c. gel

d. lotion

CRITICAL THINKING QUESTIONS

1. Explain why a prescriber might choose an extended-release dosage form over a traditional dosage form, and what impact that choice has on the patient.

2. Why is the oral route of administration safer, less complicated, and more convenient than the parenteral route? Why might the parenteral route be a better choice than the oral route?

WEB CHALLENGE

1. Go to http://www.fda.gov/cder/dsm/DRG/drg00301.htm to see other parenteral routes of administration not discussed in this chapter. List at least five of them and how they are administered.

REFERENCES AND RESOURCES

Adams, MP, Josephson, DL, & and Holland, LN Jr. *Pharmacology for Nurses—A Pathophysiologic Approach.* Upper Saddle River, NJ: Pearson Education, 2008.

American Medical Association. *Know Your Drugs and Medications.* New York: Reader's Digest Association, 1991.

American Pharmacist Association. *The Pharmacy Technician* (2d ed.). Englewood, CO: Morton Publishing, 2004.

Andreoli, T, Carpenter, C, Bennett, C, & Plum, F. *Essentials of Medicine* (4th ed.). Philadelphia: W.B. Saunders, 1997.

Ansel, HC. *Introduction to Pharmaceutical Dosage Forms.* Philadelphia: Lea & Febiger, 1995.

Ballington, DA, & Anderson, R. *Pharmacy Practice for Technicians* (3d ed.). St. Paul, MN: Paradigm Publishing, 2007.

"The Basics of Recombinant DNA" (accessed July 5, 2007): http://www.rpi.edu/dept/chem-eng/Biotech-Environ/Projects00/rdna/rdna.htm

Berkow, R. *The Merck Manual* (16th ed.). Rahway, NJ: Merck Research Laboratories, 1992.

"Drug Nomenclature" (accessed July 7, 2007): http://perth.uwlax.edu/faculty/gushiken/rth355-002/drugnomenclature.htm

Hillery, AM, et al., eds. *Drug Delivery and Targeting: For Pharmacists and Pharmaceutical Scientists.* New York: Taylor & Francis, 2001.

Hitner, H, & Nagle, B. *Basic Pharmacology* (4th ed.). New York: Glencoe/McGraw-Hill, 1999.

Holland, N, & Adams, MP. *Core Concepts in Pharmacology.* Upper Saddle River, NJ: Pearson Education, 2007.

Lambert, A. *Advanced Pharmacy Practice for Technicians.* Clifton Park, NY: Thomson Delmar Learning, 2002.

"Medication Errors" (accessed July 3, 2007): http://www.fda.gov/cder/drug/MedErrors/default.htm

O'Neil, M, et al., eds. *Merck Index: An Encyclopedia of Chemicals, Drugs, & Biologicals* (13th ed.). New York: John Wiley & Sons, 2001.

"Synthetic Drugs" (accessed July 5, 2007): http://www.ccsu.edu/counseling/New/marijuana/synthetic_drugs.htm

Taylor, L. "Plant Based Drugs and Medicines": Retrieved March 31, 2008 from http://www.rain-tree.com/plantdrugs.htm

The Body and Drugs

LEARNING OBJECTIVES

After completing this chapter, you should be able to:

- Explain the differences between pharmacodynamics and pharmacokinetics.
- Understand the ways in which cell receptors react to drugs.
- Describe mechanism of action and identify and understand its key factor.
- Explain how drugs are absorbed, distributed, metabolized, and cleared by the body.
- Explain the difference between fat-soluble and water-soluble drugs and give examples of each.
- Identify and explain the effect of bioavailability and its relationship to drug effectiveness.
- Understand addiction and addictive behavior.
- Describe the role of the pharmacy technician in identifying drug-abusing patients.
- List and identify some drugs that interact with alcohol.

Introduction

Pharmacists rely on competent pharmacy technicians to know more than how to count, pour, and prepare medications. Although the pharmacist is responsible for using his or her specialized knowledge to provide pharmaceutical care to patients, technicians too must understand the basics of pharmacology. *Pharmacology* can be defined as the study of drugs, including their composition, uses, application, and effects.

This chapter introduces some basic concepts of pharmacology, including pharmacodynamics and pharmacokinetics. You will learn how the body absorbs, distributes, transforms, and eliminates medications. You will also review the effects of drug and chemical abuse.

Pharmacodynamics

Most drugs affect the cells in the body by interacting with specific drug **receptors**. One way to think about this process is to use a lock-and-key analogy. Consider each cell in the body as having locks (the receptors), each of which requires a specific key that can lock or unlock it to produce an effect. Specific drugs "unlock" certain receptors in the body. In other words, drugs are developed to interact with certain unique receptors to produce a certain effect on the body. Ideally, this effect can be measured. The study of how drugs produce their effects on the desired cells and how a drug is processed by the body is called **pharmacodynamics**.

Receptor Complex

A receptor (again, think of it as a lock requiring a key) on a cell interacts with a specific drug because the drug "fits" the specific structure of the receptor. The drug often is designed to have a structure that is the same as or similar to that of the cells intended to be affected. Once the "key" is "turned," the chemical structure of the drug is permitted into the cell, where it can exert its effect on the particular function of the cell (see Figure 19-1).

As an example, let's look at a class of drugs that can reduce allergy symptoms. *Histamine* is a chemical released by certain cells; it is responsible for the common symptoms of allergic reactions, like burning, itchy eyes and a runny nose. Drugs called *antihistamines* interact or bind with histamine receptors on cells, effectively turning them off and thus reducing the action of histamine. The result is a reduction of the allergic symptoms.

Drugs have specific shapes and structures that match up with the shapes of the receptors on specific cells. In many instances, because of its characteristics, a drug can interact with more than one cell receptor. A classic example is diphenhydramine, which reacts with both histamine receptors and receptors in the nervous system. The interaction with the nervous system causes the main side effect of diphenhydramine, drowsiness.

Site of Action

When first developing a pharmaceutical agent, the scientists researching it usually do not merely stumble upon a receptor (although that can happen). More commonly, they create a new drug based on the knowledge that there is a specific **site of action** for each class of drug.

receptor molecular structure located on the surface of the cell that binds with a particular chemical or chemicals. When a chemical binds with a receptor, the receptor is stimulated to either produce or inhibit a specific action.

pharmacodynamics the study of the biochemical and physiologic effects of drugs and their mechanisms of action.

site of action the location where a drug will exert its effect.

FIGURE 19-1 Receptor site.

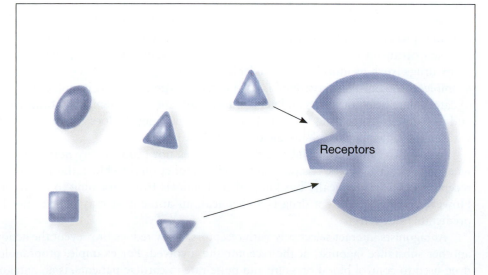

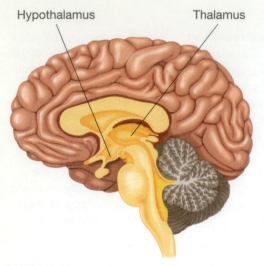

Hypothalamus   Thalamus

FIGURE 19-2 The hypothalamus.

It is true that the specific site of action of some drugs is unknown. However, the FDA requires the companies that manufacture drugs to prove two things: that the drug works (is effective), and that it is safe. If the manufacturer can prove efficacy and safety, it need not always describe or specify the site of action.

Chemistry is a science and sometimes an art as well. Aspirin is a classic example of knowing where a specific drug exerts its effects. There are specific sites located in an area of the brain called the *hypothalamus,* which is, among other things, the body's temperature regulator (see Figure 19-2). By matching some of the sites (receptors) on the cells of the hypothalamus, aspirin causes it to reduce the body's temperature.

Mechanism of Action

The term *mechanism of action* refers to how a drug works and produces its desirable (and sometimes undesirable) effects. For example, when a patient undergoes anesthesia for surgery, the drugs used for pain reduction interrupt the pathway between the central nervous system and the peripheral nervous system so that the person is no longer capable of sensing pain. Without this mechanism of action, patients who undergo massive surgical procedures would go into shock.

Receptor Site

The *receptor site* is the location where the drug (chemical) binds to the cell. Once the drug develops a bond with a body cell (at the receptor site), specific molecular changes can occur. For example, when opioids (narcotics) are used, they bind to cells and cause the changes to occur within the cell itself; the cellular changes reduce the amount of perceived pain. The pain still exists—in surgery, for example, cells are necessarily damaged in some areas—but the brain does not perceive the pain, because specific qualities of the cells that normally send pain signals are turned off. (Recall the analogy of the key that turns a lock, which in turn produces a specific response.)

The known receptors are so numerous that it would be difficult to describe every one of them. New receptors are always being discovered; hence, the market for new, more powerful, and more specific drugs is enormous.

Agonists and Antagonists

agonist a type of drug that activates the receptor to produce a predicted action.

An **agonist** is a specific type of drug that produces a certain, predicted action when it binds to the correct receptor (that is, to the receptor for which it was designed). In this situation, the drug is doing exactly what it has been designed to do, although there may or may not be side effects as well (both predicted and unpredicted). Agonists bind with cells and produce cellular responses resulting in a therapeutic effect. Many hormones and neurotransmitters (such as acetylcholine, histamine, and norepinephrine) and many drugs (such as morphine, phenylephrine, and isoproterenol) act as agonists. For example, the agonist isoproterenol is used to treat asthma because it mimics the effects of catecholamines (hormones and neurotransmitters such as adrenaline, noradrenaline, and dopamine) in relaxing bronchial muscles in the lung. It does this by interacting with one specific class of adrenergic receptor.

antagonist a type of drug that prevents receptor activation.

In contrast, an **antagonist** is a drug that does not produce any noticeable effect when it binds to a specific receptor on the cell. Its function is to block the action of that receptor, often by physically blocking other chemicals from attaching to the receptor. However, again, because a drug is a chemical, an antagonist may or may not have predictable side effects.

Antagonists interact selectively with receptors. They reduce or prevent the action of another substance (agonist) at the receptor site involved. For example, propranolol, a drug used to control blood pressure and pulse rate in cardiac patients, is an antagonist of a class of adrenergic receptors that control blood pressure and heartbeat rate.

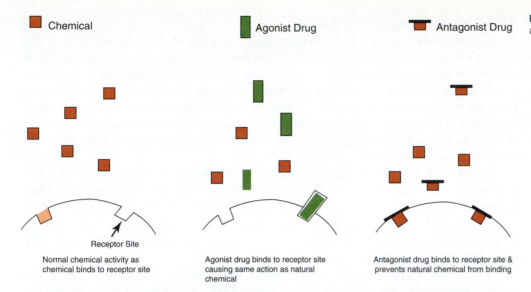

■ Chemical   ■ Agonist Drug   ⊤ Antagonist Drug

FIGURE 19-3 Example of agonistic and antagonistic drug action.

Receptor Site

Normal chemical activity as chemical binds to receptor site

Agonist drug binds to receptor site causing same action as natural chemical

Antagonist drug binds to receptor site & prevents natural chemical from binding

Agonists have two main properties. The first is *affinity*, the ability of the agonist to actually bind to the cell receptor structure. (Again, if you think about this as a lock and a key, it will make more sense.) The other property is the *efficacy* of the agonist, or the ability of the drug to impose on the cell and cellular structure and change the way the cell behaves. In essence, if the drug is an agonist, and it does what it is designed and intended to do, it is considered *efficacious*.

There are useful aspects of both kinds of drugs (see Figure 19-3). Just because an antagonist does not produce a noticeable effect, one cannot conclude that the drug is not useful. Remember that the function of an antagonist is to prevent action of another substance, rather than to produce its own effect. Antagonists have important uses; otherwise, such drugs would not exist.

Even though antagonists bind to certain receptors without producing any noticeable action, an antagonist drug could be advantageous to the life of the cell as well as the life of the organism. Think about a person who has used the wrong drug, or (a more typical example) a patient who is brought into the emergency room because he has overdosed on one of the morphine-derivative drugs. Emergency-room staff can administer a classic antagonist, called *naloxone*, which binds to the exact sites where the illicit drug attaches; the result is a prompt reversal of what would otherwise be a life-threatening situation.

There are thousands of other reasons for using antagonists as pharmacological agents, and just as many ways in which they are used. As a pharmacy technician, will you be able to identify the agonists and the antagonists? Well, maybe if you are a chemistry buff, but knowing all of them is not a specific requirement for the technician job. Knowing that they exist, how they work, and how to identify them is far more important.

Remember the **target cell**. This term actually refers to a large number of cells, all of which are similar to each other. Target cells include the nerve cells and cells that are involved with the heart or with the vascular system, especially with respect to circulation and blood pressure. These and many others make up what chemists and pharmacologists think of as target cells—the cells and receptors that become involved when a specific medication is used.

target cell general term referring to a large number of cells, all of which are similar, on which a particular drug is intended to act.

The Dose-Response Curve

A relatively simple principle of pharmacology and pharmacodynamics is that the patient's response is directly related to the amount of the drug administered. If the dose-response relationship were plotted on a chart, you would see a curve that graphically depicts this relationship, as shown in Figure 19-4. As simple as this basic principle might seem, it is probably one of the most important aspects of pharmacology you will encounter as a technician. With respect to this curve, a *dose* is defined as the specific amount of the drug required to achieve a desired effect, which is referred to as the *response to the drug*.

If you think about how a graph might represent the way a drug reacts with a cell (and with all cells that are similar to the target cell), you can easily grasp the idea that, in time, a maximal response will be attained (see Figure 19-4). After that point, adding more of the same drug will be of no benefit. That does *not* mean, however, that adding more drug will not cause harm; in fact, in most such cases, harm *does* occur, especially when people abuse drugs.

The point on the graph that represents the maximal response is called the *ceiling*. Beyond that point, drugs often become toxic, especially to the liver and the kidneys. Knowing that there are drugs that do not have a ceiling is important in pharmacodynamics; this is where your knowledge about what you do in the facility where you are employed counts the most. The pharmacy technician is slowly and quite effectively moving from being just a cashier to being an expert about certain classes of drugs.

Although you probably will not learn the mechanisms of action of drugs at the chemical level, your knowing how the drugs work generally, and why specific chemicals can be dangerous, can be an asset to the pharmacist for whom you work. It is really that simple—but it is not necessarily easy. Because the science of medicine is always producing new results, your job will always be changing, and there will always be new things to learn.

Potency

In pharmacology, the word *potency* means exactly what it does in general usage. It is a measurement of the strength of a drug that is required to produce a specific effect on the body.

ED50

ED50 is a measurement of the specific amount of a drug that will achieve 50% of the maximal response. This is an important concept, because it is used to measure the full potency of some drugs without having to achieve such a level.

FIGURE 19-4 The dose-response curve.

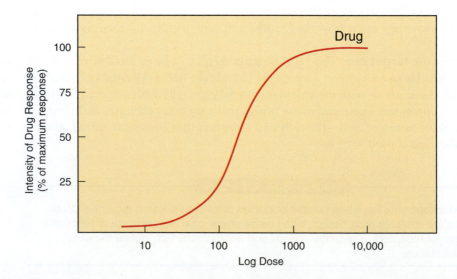

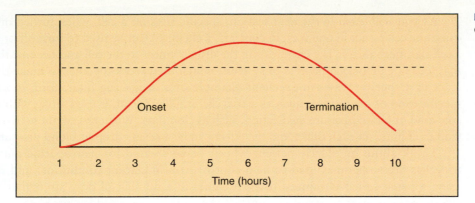

FIGURE 19-5 The time-response curve.

Half-Life

Half-life, written $T_{\frac{1}{2}}$, is the time required for plasma serum concentration levels of an absorbed and distributed drug to decrease by one-half. Once the drug is at a serum concentration of less than 3 percent, it is considered to have been removed from the body. Half-life is applicable to those drugs that follow through with the first bypass of elimination, which means that they go through the liver as well as the gastrointestinal (GI) tract. The half-life of a drug determines how many times a day a drug is dosed. Patients on drugs with longer half-lives, such as digoxin or coumadin, take fewer doses per day. In contrast, drugs with shorter half-lives, such as ibuprofen and acetaminophen, must be taken more frequently to maintain therapeutic serum levels.

half-life the time required for serum concentration levels of an absorbed and distributed drug to decrease by one-half.

Time-Response Curve

The time-response curve provides a means to determine the length of time for which a specific drug will continue to have the same degree of effect. The effect may be on a class of cells, an organ, or the entire body, depending on the relationship between the body, the drug, and what is being treated. Ideally, when no other drugs (or foods) have an adverse effect on a drug, the time-response curve will be a bell curve, showing a specific onset of action (which can be measured), the entire duration of action, and the termination of action (see Figure 19-5).

Pharmacodynamic Mechanisms

Much is known about the interactions between the many different drugs that can be taken into the human body. These pharmacologic drug interactions are an important aspect of pharmacology. If discovered by the pharmacy technician, any potential interactions should be brought to the attention of the pharmacist on duty.

Many of the problems related to **drug-drug interactions** occur when an antagonistic drug is added to one that is not, or an antagonistic drug is added to a number of other antagonistic drugs. This duplication of action can start a process by which a drug is either able to compete for specific sites on cells or to prevent other chemicals from binding on other cells.

drug-drug interaction an interaction between two or more drugs administered to a patient, resulting in either an increase or a decrease in the therapeutic effects of one or more of the drugs, or an adverse effect.

PROFILES IN PRACTICE

Juanita is a pharmacy technician who works in a neighborhood retail pharmacy. Mrs. Jones comes in to pick up her prescriptions. When ringing up the order, Juanita notices that Mrs. Jones has a prescription for warfarin and is also purchasing aspirin. Juanita knows that a serious drug interaction occurs between warfarin and aspirin. _____

• What should Juanita do?

As you will learn in the next section, specific sites on a cell, when turned on, will cause the cell to act in one way; in contrast, a chemical can be used to turn off or block a cellular mechanism. The chemicals in the drug connect to the cell and become the key that locks or unlocks a process of systems, which then work together to make the cell react in a specific way. An excellent example of a drug-drug interaction is when a specific kind of medication, such as a tricyclic antidepressant, is used along with a specific kind of blood pressure medication, such as clonidine. When mixed, these two drugs tend to counteract each other, and the effect can be a severe drop in blood pressure.

Think about an elderly patient who is being treated for neuropathic pain (the tricyclics are sometimes used to help control pain in certain conditions) and is also using a patch called Catapress® (which comes in a number of dose strengths). If the elderly patient were to stand up quickly, she could have a sudden problem with her blood pressure because this combination of medications can cause *postural* **hypotension**. If a patient's profile changes, and you notice that a healthcare provider (such as a pain management physician) has added a tricyclic antidepressant without realizing that the patient is also on clonidine, your job is to alert the pharmacist, to ensure that the physician is notified of the potential problem.

hypotension abnormally low blood pressure.

" Workplace Wisdom Medication Experts

Physicians are not necessarily medication experts. The medication expert is the pharmacist. The pharmacy has knowledge of all of the medications that a patient is taking, via the patient's profile. Therefore, it is important that, as a competent pharmacy technician, you alert the pharmacist whenever you suspect a problem (drug interactions, therapeutic duplication, etc.). With your help, the pharmacist can ensure that the patient receives the best, safest, and most effective drug regimen available. "

Keep in mind the following specific, and important, issues about drug-drug interactions:

- *Time.* The time needed for a drug to take effect is important. Some drugs take effect immediately, whereas other drugs take a much longer time to act. This depends, of course, on the kind of drug, how it is absorbed, and the dosage form or packaging (which also affects absorption). Some drugs, because of the way they are constituted, take a long time to become fully effective—sometimes weeks or even longer. Just because a patient has recently begun taking a new drug does not mean that the effect will be immediate. Some drugs must first be processed through the liver. Some drugs even build up **metabolites** that will not have an immediate effect on the body. Therefore, the patient could be on the way home, on the way to a supermarket, or on vacation when the individual effects of the two drugs finally merge. The result can be very dangerous, particularly if the patient is driving at the time.

metabolite any substance produced by the metabolic process.

- *Drug testing.* In many instances, drug-testing procedures are performed on healthy people. There may be significant differences in the effects of drugs in real patients, however. Suppose that a patient is taking an antibiotic; one of a number of drugs used to control acid secretion in the stomach (the H_2 blockers); and warfarin, the chief drug used to keep blood from coagulating (clotting). This patient then undergoes a heart valve transplant. The danger of using an antibiotic, such as erythromycin, along with warfarin might not have shown up in drug studies; however, in the clinical world—that is, in real life—there have been many instances in which the combination of these two drugs has caused severe problems, such as an increase in prothrombin time, which measures how well the drug warfarin is working.

Pharmacokinetics

pharmacokinetics the study of the time course of a drug and its metabolites in the body following drug administration.

Pharmacology is a very broad topic, and there are many books that explain the ways in which drugs are absorbed, used, and excreted by the body. Many readers, however, are scared off when they encounter words such as **pharmacokinetics**. A broad definition of the term is "the study of the time course of a drug and its metabolites in the body following drug administration by any route."

In simple terms, *pharmacokinetics* is the study of how the body handles drugs (whether they are administered orally, by way of IV, or any other means), how drugs are changed from their original form into something that the body can use (typically by way of the liver or other organs), and how drugs are eliminated from the body. This section focuses on medications once they are inside the body, rather than their presentation (dosage form) or the particulars of administration.

Plasma Concentration

Suppose that a patient takes a pill, or a nurse injects a patient with a medication. These are two different methods of intake, and the drugs administered follow two different pathways, but both drugs end up being absorbed into the body. After absorption is complete, the bloodstream becomes the vehicle that actually delivers the drug to the parts of the body requiring treatment. One factor that determines the amount of the drug needed to do any good (have any effect in the body) is the affinity of the drug to be bound to proteins that are available in the bloodstream.

The level and concentration of a specific drug in the patient's body can be measured through certain tests done in a laboratory setting. The tests actually involve a combination of the measurement of the drug that is bound to the cells of the body and the amount of the drug that is not bound to cells in the body (in this case, blood cells). This is a simplified version of what happens, but the entire concept of plasma concentration (Cp) is well beyond the scope of this text, and it has very little to do with the real clinical picture. Knowing that there is a way to measure the amount of a specific drug in a person's body also has little to do with pharmacy practice. So, in this section we present only a "bare-bones" overview of drug absorption, distribution, **metabolism**, and **excretion**, in discussing how drugs do the jobs for which they are designed.

Drug Absorption

Drug **absorption** refers to how a drug enters the body. In order for a drug, such as a pill taken by mouth, to enter the body, it must first be swallowed. Then a process begins by which the drug eventually enters the body's fluids, mainly the bloodstream. For example, a drug contained in a pill passes into the bloodstream by getting through specific membranes, such as the membranes inside the stomach and the intestines. Absorption depends largely on the type of drug, how it is designed, and the condition it is intended to treat; these are all reasons why a prescriber uses a particular drug or type of drug. Liquids are more readily absorbed than tablets or capsules, because they are already broken down to some extent.

Cell membranes are special linings that make up the cell wall; each membrane contains both lipids (fats) and proteins. This semipermeable barrier permits the entrance of some materials and the exit of others.

Some drugs actually bind to cell membranes. One such drug is Metamucil©, which binds to the walls of the stomach and acts to increase stool bulk. Thus, Metamucil is not absorbed by the body in any way.

Intravenous and intra-arterial injections bypass the absorption process, as the drugs are entered directly into the bloodstream. With this type of administration, results are usually much quicker than with any other method. However, with other routes of administration, it takes a certain length of time before the drugs start to act on the body.

Absorption of a drug does not always occur by way of the stomach and bloodstream. Inhaled medications, for example, enter through the mouth and go to the lungs. The mucous membranes of the alveoli absorb the medication and send it into the capillaries and then to the bloodstream. Medications administered rectally or vaginally have a very slow release rate, as the medications dissolve and are absorbed gradually through the rectal or vaginal mucous membranes (such drugs are actually considered to be applied topically).

metabolism the process of transforming drugs in the body; also known as *biotransformation.*

excretion the process by which drugs are eliminated from the body.

absorption the process by which a drug is moved from the site of administration into the bloodstream.

Topical medications (with the exception of transdermal patches) are not necessarily absorbed through the skin into the bloodstream; some display only a topical effect. An example is hydrocortisone cream used for inflammatory skin conditions. The transdermal patch, in contrast, enhances penetration through the skin by reducing the particle size of the medication.

Drug Distribution

distribution the process by which an absorbed drug is moved from the bloodstream to body tissues or receptors.

Drug **distribution** refers to the movement of an absorbed drug from the bloodstream into body tissues. Once a drug is absorbed, it is then distributed throughout the body by way of the circulatory system. Some of the drug binds to plasma proteins. Other drug molecules that do not bind to plasma proteins float through the bloodstream and may interact with various receptors, producing a therapeutic effect. Plasma proteins, such as albumin, do not provide any therapeutic effect in and of themselves.

Membrane Transport Mechanisms

All cells in the human body have specialized transport mechanisms (recall the earlier discussion of cell membranes) by which all materials, including pharmaceuticals, are moved into and out of the cells; normally, drugs must pass into cells in order to perform their functions. The types of transport include filtration, passive transport, and active transport. The type of transport merely describes the ways in which a drug gets from the outside of a cell into the cell proper.

It is important, at least for academic purposes, to understand how these mechanisms work. Following are more specific definitions of each of the mechanisms.

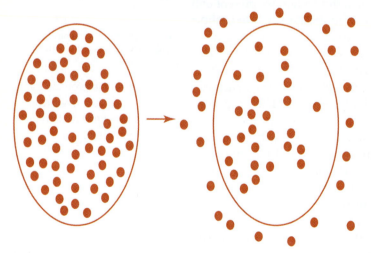

Passive Diffusion

Passive diffusion is another term for *passive transport* across a cell membrane. The force that permits a substance to be transported from outside the cell into the cell depends largely on the concentration differences between the two environments (outside the cell and inside the cell). If an equilibrium state does not exist between the two environments, the specific differences between two *gradients* will enable certain substances to pass through the membranes—that is, the drug molecules move from an area of high concentration into an area of low concentration (see Figure 19-6).

FIGURE 19-6 In passive diffusion, molecules cross to the outside of the cell membrane into an area with a lower concentration of molecules.

Facilitated Diffusion

In *facilitated diffusion*, a carrier protein permits specific molecules, such as glucose (sugar), to pass through certain parts of the cells. This is far different from the preceding process, in that it does not require the expenditure of energy. This is an important consideration with some drugs because of the rate at which the drug or other substance is permitted to pass through a membrane; there must be enough of the carrier or facilitator protein to allow the process to occur.

Active Transport

Active transport is a special kind of transportation system between the two environments (intracellular and extracellular). This process costs the cells energy; it uses the fact that certain substances are permitted to accumulate outside the cells (see Figure 19-7). After a time, the accumulation of these substances generates a special sort of concentration gradient that, in time, will permit the transportation of a substance from outside the cell into the cell.

Pinocytosis

In the form of transportation called *pinocytosis*, the cell actually engulfs the substance and, in doing so, permits the substance to enter the cell. This process also requires a degree of energy expenditure by the cell.

Bioavailability

The transport mechanisms just discussed enable drugs to become available to the body. Each drug has its own qualities and characteristics that take advantage of the specific body mechanisms for absorption; drug researchers and designers consider these aspects when shaping what a drug does, and prescribers consider these factors when prescribing specific drugs. However, there are other specific factors that also determine how well or how fast a drug becomes available to the body, such as *gastric emptying*—the ability of the stomach to permit the passage of materials from the stomach to the small intestine. (Most drugs and foods are absorbed at a much faster rate in the small intestine than in the stomach. One exception to this rule is alcohol.) So, there is a great deal more involved in the transport of a drug into the body than just swallowing a pill and expecting it to work. For various reasons, the **bioavailability** of drugs is time-restricted—some drugs require immediate access to the body's cells to become effective, whereas other drugs can survive the longer time it takes them to become available to the body.

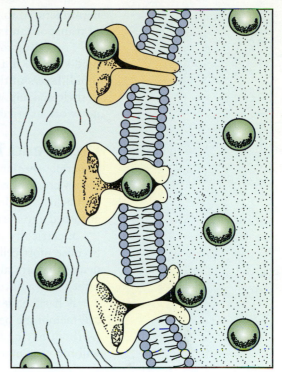

FIGURE 19-7 Active transport.

bioavailability the degree to which a drug becomes available to body tissue(s) after administration.

The Quality of Drugs—Solubility

Getting back to the cell membrane and its structure, and how drugs enter the cells themselves, recall that a cell membrane has both a protein and a lipid component. That characteristic largely determines how fast a drug can make it into the cell to perform its designated function. In general, the more lipid-soluble a drug is, the faster the drug will be absorbed into a cell. As you continue with your studies as a pharmacy technician and start to really understand the makeup of different drugs (whether they are fat-soluble or water-soluble, for example), you will better understand how quickly different drugs become available to the body. But how does this help you clinically?

Suppose, for example, that a patient has a question about how fast a specific drug works. Even if you do not have a lot of knowledge of specific drug chemistry, in time you will be able to tell from their chemical makeup which drugs are lipid-soluble (meaning that they are composed of *buffers* that are lipids) and which drugs are more water-soluble. The *Physician's Desk Reference* defines drugs in terms of their chemical structure, but some medical professionals describe a drug in terms of its makeup—for example, whether the drug is lipid-soluble, water-soluble, or both. This will help you determine whether one drug will take effect at a faster rate than another drug or a different kind of drug. This applies to most over-the-counter drugs as well; the labels will tell you about the basic chemical makeup, and you need not be a chemistry major to understand and use some of these concepts.

By and large (with the exception of highly soluble general anesthetics used during surgery), drugs are both water-soluble and only partially soluble—and there are reasons for that. First, the human body is made up mostly of water; hence, water-soluble drugs are more liable to be absorbed well and have good bioavailability. Second, except for medications used in emergencies, drugs do not have to work immediately; hence, the partial solubility of most drugs is not problematic. Because of the different cellular transport mechanisms, there are specific reasons for drugs to be both water- and lipid-soluble. Because we know a good deal about the cell membrane, drugs are manufactured to handle both the process of absorption into the body and the process of transport and use at the cellular level.

For a drug to be absorbed via the gastrointestinal tract, it must be both water- and lipid-soluble. If a drug contains too much water, it cannot pass through the very fatty (lipid) layers of the GI tract. In contrast, absorption of drugs that have too much lipid in their makeup will be delayed. (This is why some medications, such as Dilantin®, do not work as effectively in some people as in others.)

Drugs and Their Ionization

Generally speaking, chemicals that are *ionized* (positively or negatively charged) do not readily cross the cell membrane barrier. In constrast, the un-ionized form of the chemical—chemicals that do not carry a positive or negative electrical charge—are more readily absorbed into the cell.

Electrically charged molecules cannot readily cross the barrier of a cell wall because most cell walls are composed of proteins and lipids (as well as other components) that are also electrically charged. Therefore, like two magnets placed with the same poles adjacent to one another, these molecules repel each other.

A basic understanding of cell characteristics and the transport of chemicals across cell membrane barriers will make you better able to comprehend the makeup of drugs (without having to go through a lot of physiology and chemistry courses). Thus, you will function more effectively and be more valuable as a pharmacy technician.

Drug Distribution and Metabolism

You now know some of the basics about how drugs enter the human body. But what happens to medications once they are absorbed? With few exceptions, most medications must undergo a number of changes in the body to become effective. It is not quite as simple as most people think—their ability to take that pill this morning and have it work is the result of many, many years of research and development. The people who work behind the scenes in the pharmaceutical companies are responsible for ensuring that the medications work and are safe.

The Path

For a medication to become absorbed into the body, it must first undergo what is called the *first-pass process*, which is completed in the liver. This process applies only to medications taken orally, not those that are administered through other routes; these latter medications are manufactured in such a way that the body can more readily use them (see Figure 19-8).

After someone takes a pill, it goes through the many different processes that ultimately lead to its entering the bloodstream. From that point, the medication is delivered to the various organs in the body. There are several factors involved in the transportation of the drug by the blood to the tissues in the body, and these are discussed next.

Plasma-Binding Protein

Several large proteins are responsible for delivering many substances from the intestines, through the blood, and then to the tissues of the body. These proteins are albumin and the several different types of globulins. They have many different functions and capabilities, including the ability to transport chemicals through the blood. Some drugs are transported after undergoing a process called *protein binding*, in which they are attracted to and physically or chemically attached to these proteins; other drugs float freely through the blood.

The chemicals that are not bound to plasma proteins work their specific pharmacologic effects on the target organs (such as a sore, inflamed throat treated by an antibiotic). Some drugs are highly bound to the proteins, but a good majority of them

FIGURE 19-8 The path.

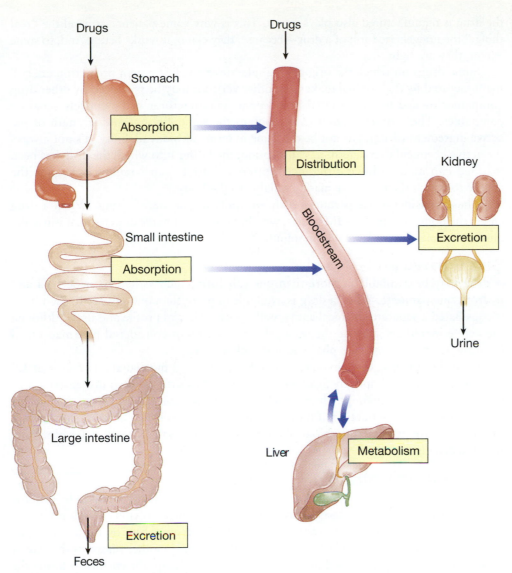

are unbound. It is the free-floating part of the drug that will make the difference. After a drug uses all available protein-binding sites, the amount of chemical available for use can be determined by measuring the portion of the drug that remains unbound. Two issues determine the degree to which a drug becomes bound to a protein site (for example, to cells in the bloodstream): (1) the binding affinity for the drug and (2) the number of available sites on the cells. As long as the volume of the drug is adequate, the amount of unbound drug will remain sufficient to get the job done.

Many equations and laws govern the pharmacokinetics of drugs, and a pharmacological chemist can tell you exactly how all of this works. Although you do not need an extensive knowledge of these laws and equations, it is helpful to understand, for example, why some drugs should be taken with food, some drugs should not be taken with milk, and some drugs should be taken only on an empty stomach. The point is to get a dosage where as much of that drug as is necessary to do the job remains unbound to plasma proteins.

Absorption

The absorption of a drug governs the bioavailability of that drug—that is, the amount of drug that is available for use. Several factors influence absorption. As mentioned previously, a drug must be both lipid- (fat) and water-soluble to enter the body through the gastrointestinal tract. There is more to it than just what gets through the gut, however; how the drug is manufactured also plays a part. This is why some patients demand the "real thing," the nongeneric form of a drug—because, they claim, it works better. And, to some extent, they are right.

Some drugs on which the original manufacturer has lost patent protection are still manufactured by the original maker, but other versions may be produced by other drug companies owned by the original brand-name manufacturer or by entirely separate companies. These other versions may contain the same amount and strength of the active ingredient (drug), but not be the same in terms of bioavailability. It's not always the active chemical that determines absorption; the buffer into which the drug has been instilled can make a huge difference. Different buffers can completely change the degree to which the drugs are made available to the body.

These considerations pertain mostly to orally administered drugs. When a drug enters the body via the IV or IM routes, whether it is brand name or generic, it is usually almost completely available within minutes.

Salt Forms

A drug may be available in more than one salt form, such as hydroxyzine HCl and hydroxyzine pamoate. When a drug is available in more than one salt form, each form is considered a separate chemical entity, with its own clinical profile and uses. Although the active ingredient may be the same, the drugs are not considered pharmaceutical equivalents. Instead, they are pharmaceutical alternatives.

Consider the drug theophylline, which, by itself, has a bioavailability factor of 1.0 (meaning that it is completely available). However, this drug is often dispensed not as theophylline, but as aminophylline, which is only 80 percent theophylline—it contains only 80 percent of the fraction of the drug salt, or *ester,* that is the "parent" compound. The ratio of the two factors, bioavailability (F) and the salt (S), will determine how well the drug is absorbed.

Rate of Administration

The rate at which a drug is administered is not measured by the time it takes to swallow a pill, but by a formula that uses the two fractions identified previously with respect to the dosing interval. Certain drugs are designed to be taken every four hours, for example, for many reasons, one of which is the half-life of the drug; another reason is the rate at which the drug can be absorbed over a given period. This helps the chemists (during the research and development process) as they determine the average rate of administration, to ensure that there is a certain amount of the drug in the system at all times.

Volume of Distribution

Theoretically, if you consider the body as a single entity, you can assume that there is a specific amount of the drug in the body at any given time. This is not always true, however, because of many factors, including the different chemicals in the bloodstream, the bioavailability of the drug, the initial plasma concentration, and the amount of drug that is freely available at any given time. The actual volume of distribution, therefore, is determined by a number of factors, including the *loading dose,* which is often higher than the patient will take on a regular basis. This is the difference between an initial loading dose and the subsequent *maintenance dose.*

═══════════════════ ◄ **INFORMATION** ► ═══════════════════

Most of the time a pharmacist considers a drug as being taken into one compartment or entity: the entire body. However, within the body the drug is actually in two compartments: (1) part of the drug is in the blood and in organs that have a relatively high rate of blood flow, such as the heart; (2) part of the drug is in the other, minute tissues of the body. (At a certain point, there will be an equilibrium; clinically speaking, though, this concept is not relevant to you or the pharmacist unless you are working in an environment where there is compounding of drugs.)

Clearance

The **clearance** of a drug—its elimination from the body—is determined by a number of factors. When a manufacturer develops a new drug, one of the questions it must answer is how the drug will be cleared (eliminated) from the body, and how fast. Ideally, a drug would be eliminated at the same rate at which it is absorbed, yielding a "steady state" level of the drug in the body at all times. However, because of the varied absorption and availability in the various bodily tissues (remember the two-compartment model), this is not always the case.

The rate of distribution, the rate of absorption, and the rate of elimination must all be balanced to ensure that the body has enough of the drug at all times, and not too much of the drug at any time. This is particularly important with antibiotics, antihypertensives, and drugs that treat cancer, because many of these drugs can be toxic. Ignoring the time it takes a drug to be removed from the body can allow a toxic buildup of drug, with deadly effects. Through a calculation, a *maintenance dose* is determined, which tells the physician a number of things about the drug. The amount to be given over a period of time is important, as is your duty to tell the patient, for example, to "Make sure that you take one of these pills every six hours" or, "Don't take more than four pills in 24 hours."

clearance the time it takes a drug to be eliminated from the body.

Addiction

The term *drug abuse* is subject to a great deal of interpretation, and is so broad as to have very little meaning outside of a specific context. In most contexts, the term carries many negative societal connotations, whether it is used in reference to pharmaceutical medications or the agents commonly called *street drugs*. Although using OxyContin®, for example, is quite different from using cocaine, the two drugs might have the same potential for abuse, depending on the user and the prescriber.

There are specific reasons for the variety of definitions, as the term *drug abuse* is actually an overly broad term applied to a large array of problems, including addiction, dependency, and even the occasional use of certain drugs. Although these problems might all present in the same way, in terms of how the patient or user acts, it is important to understand the differences between dependency and addiction, as they involve two clearly different mechanisms and have different consequences.

According to the National Institute for Drug Abuse, approximately 48 million people (aged 12 and over) have used prescription drugs for nonmedical reasons. This is almost 20 percent of the U.S. population.

Characteristics of Addiction

Addiction is a disease and should not be thought of in the same way as chemical dependency. *Addiction* is defined as both a psychological and a physiological dependency. For a drug or a chemical to be addictive, specific withdrawal symptoms must arise following an abrupt change in the practice of use. Specific signs of addiction, typically seen in persons addicted to a specific substance, include:

- **An absorbing focus**—all addictions consume some time, thought, and energy.
- **Increasing tolerance**—to achieve the same effect as when the person first started using the agent, he or she must ingest more of the chemical over time; later, there is a loss of control over the use of the agent.
- **A growing denial**—typically, users become so sensitive to the thought of using the agent that they tend to deny any interest in the agent, in order to sustain their previous pattern of life.
- **Damaging consequences**—there is no such thing as a harmless addiction, whether it is an addiction to a substance or to any other thing. All addicts eventually bring some form of destruction on themselves and their families. Typically, they lose three things: employment, interest in self, and previous reputation. Addictions are enslaving and destructive dependencies on an agent such as a drug or a pharmaceutical chemical.

addiction a pattern of compulsive substance abuse characterized by a continued psychological and physiological craving or need for the substance and its effects.

tolerance when a person requires (psychologically or physiologically) larger doses of a drug to achieve the same effect.

- **Painful withdrawal**—almost always, there is a painful physical and psychological withdrawal for some time after the agent is abruptly stopped, for whatever reason. (This is sometimes also true with chemical dependency.) The addict usually has angry, uncontrollable outbursts; periods of anxiety; panic attacks; tremors; severe depression; and a sense of loss of anything good in life.

Causes of Addiction

Specific addictive street drugs, such as cocaine, heroin, and morphine, cause the release of *dopamine*, a neurotransmitting chemical in the brain. Dopamine is only one of the many different neurotransmitters in the brain that control such things as thought, actions, emotions, and other attributes. When these neurotransmitters are functioning normally, the person is also considered normal. Dopamine has been linked to some of the more common problems seen in those who are addicted. For example, a proven link exists between dopamine and other catecholamines found in the brain and in the adrenal system; imbalances can lead to hypertension and other diseases.

Each higher dose of the abused drug causes higher dopamine levels, which is why people who are addicted to drugs are also depressed. In the addict's brain, the higher doses of dopamine activate a negative feedback system that, in time, causes the nervous system to be less sensitive to the neurotransmitter. The first high, therefore, is never duplicated by subsequent doses. Drug abusers increase the dose of a drug in an attempt to achieve the same effect as they achieved previously; this repeated effort causes the disease. Finally, the addict requires such high doses that his or her body can no longer adapt. The results are sometimes fatal.

The Criteria for Addiction

Specific criteria exist to help identify if a person is addicted to a specific chemical or drug. Depending on the level of addiction, nine different items are present in varying degrees. They include:

1. The patient takes the drug (or drugs) in larger amounts than are needed to achieve the expected results. Patients taking narcotics for pain relief reach this threshold when they take more than they need to achieve pain relief and instead are seeking other effects of the medications. The patient develops a high tolerance for the drug.

2. There have been many unsuccessful attempts to quit taking the medication, accompanied by a persistent period of craving and a desire to obtain the medication, sometimes at any cost to the patient or others involved, such as family members or friends.

3. Excessive time is used in obtaining the medication; a patient, for example, uses many different healthcare providers and pharmacies to obtain a specific medication.

4. There are periods when the patient feels intoxicated (or appears to be intoxicated or acting strangely or unusually compared with previous encounters).

5. The patient thinks about giving up other things in life for the purpose of drug seeking and use.

6. The patient continues to use the drug or medication, even after he and his family have been told of the potential damage to his life or vital organs—or danger to others in his life.

7. The marked tolerance for the medication leaves a trail of information that can sometimes be determined by checking databases or talking with other providers or pharmacists.

8. The patient manifests characteristic withdrawal symptoms with any attempt to stop taking the specific drug, particularly during times when pharmacies are closed (such as holidays or weekends), or any other periods when the drug is not available.

9. The patient consistently uses the drug to prevent withdrawal symptoms.

Alcohol

Alcohol (ETOH), although legal in certain circumstances, is a depressant. One of the largest problems associated with the use of alcohol is its concomitant use with prescribed medications. Typically, a pharmaceutical label will include instructions indicating if a medication should not be used with alcohol. Because alcohol is a highly addictive substance, it is prudent and appropriate to discuss this drug and list some of the more commonly abused drugs associated with the consumption of alcohol.

Workplace Wisdom Drug-Alcohol Interactions

A complete list of drugs that can have interactions with alcohol is too long to include here. Comprehensive lists of drugs and their interactions with alcohol can be found in pharmacy references such as *Drug Facts and Comparisons.*

Alcohol, Other Drugs, and Their Effects on the Body

Alcohol and some of the more common drugs that are addictive or cause harm to the body have an immediate and altering effect on specific perceptions and emotions. After repeated use of these substances, some form of dependence often develops—symptoms are produced that are consistent with tolerance and withdrawal.

It is essential that you, as the pharmacy technician, realize that many commonly prescribed drugs can cause devastating effects when mixed with alcohol. Certainly, an auxiliary label containing such information should be placed on the vial for that particular medication, but it might also be in your best interest to personally call a patient's attention to the warning.

According to the American Society of Addiction Medicine, alcoholism is a "primary, *chronic* disease with genetic, psychosocial, and environmental factors influencing its development and manifestations." Alcoholism is a disease, pure and simple. It refers to consuming ethanol in a potentially hazardous or harmful manner. You are not responsible for the patient's problem with this disease, but you are responsible for the types of medications that are dispensed from your institution—and the list of medications that can cause problems when alcoholics take them is long. Table 19-1 lists many medications that are potentially problematic when mixed with other medications. This list should be posted somewhere in your pharmacy to ensure that patients can review what they are currently buying and what they have at home.

Immediate Effects of Alcohol

Like some of the drugs that are dispensed from any typical pharmacy, alcohol has a number of effects. Alcohol has specific mood-altering and mind-altering effects. Alcohol and some other drugs alter the levels of dopamine in the brain. As discussed earlier in this chapter, this neurotransmitter affects the degree to which synapses interact with each other. Alcohol raises the level of dopamine in the brain; according to some recent research, even the anticipation of alcohol ingestion can have an effect on dopamine levels. Drugs such as amphetamines increase the action of dopamine by blocking the molecule that normally transports it away from the specific centers of the brain where most of its activity is centered. Another neurotransmitter, serotonin, is thought to have an even more immediate effect from the use of alcohol and from use of some other drugs, particularly those currently prescribed for the treatment of depression (the serotonin secretion reuptake inhibitors, or SSRIs).

Long-Term Effects of Alcohol

Cells in the brain, like cells in other parts of the body, are subject to change, given the right conditions. Over time, drugs and alcohol can actually change the chemical composition of the brain, altering the way the cells react to each other and resulting in

Table 19-1   Medications That May Cause Problems When Mixed with Alcohol

DRUG	COMMON PROBLEMS ASSOCIATED WITH THE USE OF ALCOHOL
alprazolam, diazepam	Drowsiness, dizziness, and an increased risk of overdose
aspirin, Advil®, Tylenol®	Stomach upset, bleeding ulcers, liver damage, increased heart rate
clonazepam, phenytoin	Drowsiness, increased risk of seizures
cimetidine, nizatidine	Rapid heart rate, sudden changes in blood pressure
diphenhydramine, temazepam	Drowsiness, dizziness, an increased risk of overdose
glyburide, metformin	Rapid heart rate, sudden changes in blood pressure, convulsions, and possibly coma
griseofulvin, Flagyl®	Rapid heart rate, sudden changes in blood pressure, liver damage
herbal preparations	Increased drowsiness
hydrocodone, oxycodone	Drowsiness, dizziness, risk of overdose
isosorbide, nitroglycerine (NTG)	Rapid heartbeat, sudden changes in blood pressure
warfarin	Occasional drinking may lead to internal bleeding; heavier drinking may have the opposite effect, resulting in clots

neuroadaptation; in other words, over time the brain learns other ways to function because of the damage done to it by drugs and alcohol. For example, excessive consumption of alcohol can cause a sudden change in the amount of neurotransmitters, which can decrease the number of dopamine receptors in the brain. In time, this can have a long-term effect on the ways in which the abuser makes decisions and exercises judgment.

Neurotoxic Effect

Over the long term, chronic abuse of drugs or alcohol (or both) can affect the brain to the point that a person develops dementia (loss of memory). Long-term use of such drugs as methamphetamine and cocaine can produce such effects as altered ability to see and impaired hearing. One of the most common seen problems associated with long-term use of alcohol is a disease called Weicke-Korsakoff's syndrome, which is a type of dementia that is often accompanied by specific nutritional problems. This disease is often associated with an inability to learn new things, recall details such as people's names and addresses, or even remember a subject that was just recently mentioned.

Alcoholism

According to the American Society of Addiction Medicine, alcoholism is a "primary, *chronic* disease" characterized by the following four symptoms:

1. Craving or urge to drink; described by some as a need.
2. Loss of control; the alcoholic person is unable to stop once drinking has begun.
3. Physical dependence. The alcoholic person experiences symptoms of withdrawal, such as nausea, shakiness, sweating, and anxiety, after drinking stops.
4. Tolerance. The alcoholic person must drink greater amounts of alcohol to get the same "buzz" or "high."

Several withdrawal syndromes are observed during the first 48 hours of cessation of drinking, or alcohol withdrawal:

- seizures
- blood pressure changes
- delirium tremens (hallucinations, tremors, and shaking caused by alcohol withdrawal; may be fatal)
- dehydration
- malnutrition
- ataxia
- nystagmus
- cognitive changes

Treatment of Alcoholism

A 12-step group support program, such as Alcoholics Anonymous, in conjunction with individual therapy and counseling, are essential in alcohol addiction. Thiamine and folate are routinely used to reverse common nutritional deficiencies, and a few benzodiazepines that are used to combat anxiety may also be used for alcohol withdrawal. Benzodiazepines are sometimes used during the first few days after a person stops drinking to help him or her safely withdraw from alcohol. Extreme agitation during withdrawal may require the use of other drugs, such as barbiturates, antipsychotics, anticonvulsants, and antihypertensives. The smallest dosage necessary to manage symptoms should be given. The liver may suffer severe benzodiazepine toxicity if the patient is given a long-acting benzodiazepine for alcohol withdrawal. The antipsychotic Haldol® (haloperidol) IV and the benzodiazepine Ativan® (lorazepam) can be given together to help control delirium tremens (the DTs). However, haloperidol must be used with caution because of the risk of torsade de pointes (an uncommon type of ventricular tachycardia in which the QT interval increases markedly, causing sudden death).

Some drugs, such as ReVia® (naltrexone), can help people remain sober. The combination of counseling and naltrexone can reduce the craving for alcohol and help prevent a return to alcohol abuse and a relapse into heavy drinking, but only *after* the patient stops drinking. Naltrexone works by blocking the same receptors and areas that narcotics and alcohol block in the brain: the mu receptors, limbic system, and reticular formation. This lessens the feeling of needing to drink alcohol, so the patient can stop drinking more easily. Side effects of naltrexone include nausea, headache, constipation, dizziness, nervousness, insomnia, drowsiness, and anxiety. Recommended dose is 50 mg daily.

Antabuse® (disulfiram) discourages drinking by making patients feel nauseated and flushed and develop sudden stomach cramps, headache, and vomiting when or if they drink alcohol. This type of management of alcoholism is called *aversion therapy*.

A new drug used in the management of alcoholism to support abstinence from alcohol is Campral® (acamprosate calcium). Studies have shown that this drug reduces alcohol intake in alcohol-dependent animals. This drug does not have disulfiram-like side effects.

Table 19-2 lists some drugs commonly used to treat withdrawal symptoms.

Smoking Withdrawal and Cessation

Statistics show that almost 23.4 percent of all adult males and 18.5 percent of all adult females in the United States continue to smoke, despite all the recognition and acknowledgment that smoking is detrimental to health. Although many people find that support groups or therapy help them quit smoking, others quit cold turkey. Still

Table 19-2   Alcohol Withdrawal Treatment

BENZODIAZEPINES	INDICATIONS	USUAL ADULT DOSE
Ativan® (lorazepam)	alcohol withdrawal and DTs; short-acting	2–4 mg IV Q1 hour prn until calm
Librium® (chlordiazepoxide)	alcohol withdrawal, DTs; long-acting	25–100 mg every 1–2 hours as needed
Serax® (oxazepam)	alcohol withdrawal; short-acting	15–30 mg, 3 or 4 times daily
Valium® (diazepam)	alcohol and cocaine withdrawal; long-acting	10–20 mg every 1–3 hours for first three doses
Antipsychotics		
Haldol® (haloperidol)	extreme agitation during withdrawal	2–4 mg IV Q 1 hour prn, until calm
Miscellaneous Antialcoholic Agents (Detoxification Helpers)		
Antabuse® (disulfiram)	management of enforced sobriety	Initial dose: 500 mg po QD for 1–2 weeks Maintenance dose: 125–500 mg po QD (not to exceed 500 mg/day)
Campral® (acamprosate calcium)	maintenance of abstinence from alcohol	Dose: two 333 mg tablets (666 mg) po TID
ReVia® (naltrexone)	treatment for alcohol dependency	Dose: 50 mg po QD

others use some of the pharmaceutical agents on the market to help them curb the urge to smoke. The pharmaceutical agents available include:

Nicotine inhalers—A nicotine oral inhalation system called Nicotrol® Inhaler is available by prescription, but requires the use of four inhalers a day, totaling 2,000 puffs per day, to achieve adequate nicotine levels. This poses compliance problems. Side effects include mouth and throat irritation due to the oral delivery.

Nicotine nasal spray—Nicotrol® NS, available by prescription, requires four sprays per hour, or a maximum of 80 sprays per day. Common side effects are nasal and throat irritation and rhinorrhea.

Nicotine gum—Nicorette® (nicotine polacrilex) is available OTC in 2 mg and 4 mg strengths. The most effective dose is the use of 10 to 15 pieces of 4 mg gum per day initially; after two weeks, most patients benefit from use of the 2 mg strength. Nicotine gum should be chewed once or twice every few minutes and then placed between the cheek and the gum (buccal placement) until the next "chew." GI upset, caused by chewing the gum too quickly and swallowing nicotine with saliva, is a common side effect.

Nicotine patch—once prescription-only, Habitrol®, Nicoderm CQ®, and Nicotrol® are now available OTC. The Fagerstrom test score determines which strength of patch the patient should begin using. A score of 5 to 6 indicates that the patient should use the 21 mg nicotine patch; a score of 3 to 4 means that the 14 mg nicotine patch is appropriate for initial therapy; and a score of zero to 2 indicates initial use of the 7 mg nicotine patch. Side effects are mild skin irritation just under the patch and possible sleep disruption. The patient may be able to alleviate these problems by rotating the patch site and removing the patch at bedtime. People who use the patch should know that concomitant smoking and nicotine patch use may cause sudden cardiac death.

Workplace Wisdom Smoking—No Longer a Habit

In 2000, the American Psychiatric Association updated its stance on smoking: it is considered a mental disorder, not a habit.

Medications Used in Smoking Cessation

The immediate-release form of the antidepressant bupropion inhibits the uptake of the monoamine neurotransmitters norepinephrine and serotonin and weakly blocks the reuptake of dopamine. The sustained-release form weakly inhibits the neuronal uptake of norepinephrine, serotonin, and dopamine. It is believed that this monoamine inhibition causes the reduction in the urge to smoke. The most common side effects of bupropion include dry mouth and sleep interruptions. If depression is also present, the patient will benefit from the antidepressant effects of this drug. Note: Bupropion is sold as antidepressant Wellbutrin® XL for anxiety/GAD, Wellbutrin® for depression, and Zyban® for smoking cessation. The combined use of antidepressant, bupropion, and nicotine replacement agents appears to be the most effective treatment for nicotine dependence (nicotine withdrawal/smoking cessation). Zyban® (bupropion) should be dosed as follows: 150 mg per day for 3 days, then 150 mg twice daily for 8 to 12 weeks.

Varenicline (Chantix®) is a new smoking-cessation medication that does not contain nicotine but helps patients by reducing their urge to smoke. It targets the same receptors that nicotine does and blocks nicotine from attaching to these receptors. Chantix® is available in 0.5 mg and 1 mg tablets and is dosed as follows:

Days 1 through 3—0.5 mg po once daily
Days 4 through 7—0.5 mg po twice daily
Day 8 through end of treatment—1 mg po twice daily

Side effects include nausea and vomiting, sleep disturbances, constipation, and gas/flatulence.

Anti-anxiety agents are also used to reduce the symptoms of anxiety associated with nicotine withdrawal and smoking cessation. Benzodiazepines enhance the effects of a brain chemical called gamma aminobutyric acid (GABA). This chemical slows down nerve cell activity and decreases nerve excitement, thus causing relaxation and quieting the anxiety symptoms that accompany smoking withdrawal. Maintenance drug therapy may include Xanax® (alprazolam) and other benzodiazepines. Alprazolam may be dosed 0.25 to 0.5 mg PO bid to tid with a maximum daily dose of 4 mg.

Drug Dependency

A great deal of confusion exists, even among clinicians, about the differences between dependency and addiction. As discussed earlier in this chapter, drug addiction involves compulsive behavior coupled with psychological and physiological dependence on a drug. Drug **dependency** is different. Drug dependency is characterized by physiological dependence and tolerance to the drug. Drug dependency does not necessarily always lead to addiction.

dependency the state of being dependent.

INFORMATION

The term *addiction* applies to a person who uses a pharmacological agent compulsively; has a psychological dependence on the agent; and continues to use the chemical in spite of all indications that continued use will be physically harmful to the body. The term *addiction*, however, is often used incorrectly in our society, including references to patients of those who have licenses to practice medicine, such as physicians and other healthcare providers. Quite simply, not all patients who ask for or take pain medications are addicts. Just because someone experiences a period of withdrawal following cessation of a medication does not mean that the person is an addict. Addiction is a psychological dependence, not just a physiological dependence.

Controlled Medications

According to the United States Controlled Substances Act of 1970, each medication that has a potential for abuse is identified by a number ranging from I through V, determined by the medication's ability to influence behavior and its potential for abuse. The following considerations apply when, for example, a new medication for pain control is released into the market: the degree to which the medication has a potential for abuse; whether the substance has been determined to have a current and acceptable medical use; and whether the use of the medication, under medical supervision, is safe. Let's look at some medications generally classified for pain relief and their properties that can lead to abuse.

An *opiate* is a drug that has its origin in the opium poppy, from which such substances as cocaine and morphine are manufactured. *Opioid* is a scientific term used to describe a large number of medications and substances, including the opiates, medications made synthetically (such as methadone), and medications having properties that interfere with specific receptors in the brain that "turn off" pain in the body.

The list of opioids also includes a number of other drugs that either compete with specific receptors or antagonize other receptors in the brain. The ultimate effect for the normal user is an eradication of the problem. The abuser is actually looking for some of the side effects of these drugs, most of which, over time, can cause damage to the brain, the kidneys, and the liver, to mention a few of the important organs that keep the body alive. The federal government controls these substances for the safety and well-being of society.

Workplace Wisdom Fraudulent Prescriptions

It is the pharmacist's duty to counsel patients on the correct ways to take their medications, the effects of the medications, and drug interactions. However, as a technician, you play a vital role in helping the pharmacist prevent drug misuse and abuse. You can help prevent prescription fraud by identifying prescriptions that appear to be fake, altered, or look false. Some pharmacies have even implemented "hotlines" to alert other pharmacies in the area when prescription fraud is detected.

Without doubt, inconsistent use of the terms *addiction*, *dependency*, and *tolerance* leads to many misunderstandings among those who regulate the system for dispensing narcotics and other medications that have a potential for chemical dependence or addiction. Most of these misconceptions concern patients who are taking medications designed for pain relief and labeled as narcotics. Because of the many misunderstandings, a good number of patients suffer with untreated pain. It is true that a small percentage of patients have been identified as using such medications for reasons other than pain relief, but many pain patients suffer needlessly because of the mistaken idea that everyone who takes narcotics is an addict or will inevitably become addicted.

The Role of the Pharmacy Technician

Certainly, it is not within your jurisdiction to take prescription counseling into your own hands. However, it *is* your responsibility to bring possible abuse and other questionable situations to the attention of your pharmacist so that he or she can take the appropriate actions. Your pharmacist might know other information about the patient; after all, a pharmacist's license depends on what is dispensed, when it is dispensed, and for what reasons. Your position, however, does have its advantages, in that you may know something about the patient that the pharmacist does not know. A discussion between you and the pharmacist is, therefore, justified whenever you have questions or concerns of this nature.

SUMMARY

As you have discovered, being a knowledgeable pharmacy technician involves more than counting out pills to fill a patient's prescription. No employer should expect you to have the same background in pharmacology as your pharmacist, but they will expect you to have an understanding of basic pharmacological concepts.

If drugs are to produce their desired effects, they must be available to the cell receptors. Many variables influence how efficiently drugs are carried through the bloodstream to the target organ they are intended to affect. Of course, the route of administration plays an important part; other factors include the affinity of the drug, the transport mechanism of the target cell, and the solubility of the drug. Factors such as absorption, distribution, and ionization of the drug all contribute to how the body handles the drug once it is administered.

It is important to remember that liver function can have a significant impact on the efficacy of a drug.

Additionally, bioavailability, rate of administration, half-life, and clearance of the drug, as well as other factors, play a large role in ensuring that a sufficient amount of drug is available to produce the desired therapeutic effect. This is the main goal of pharmacotherapeutics.

Although the lines are sometimes blurred, there is a difference between drug addiction and drug dependency. Drug addiction is a disease, and it involves compulsive behavior as well as psychological and physiological dependence. Drug dependency, in contrast, usually involves only physiological dependence.

All of this knowledge is of no value unless you can utilize it. Knowing the trade and generic name for a drug is important; knowing the intended action of the drug and how the drug interacts with other drugs is far more important.

CHAPTER REVIEW QUESTIONS

1. Structures on the cells that interact with a specific drug because they have a specific structure that permits the drug to "fit" are called:
   a. neurotransmitters.
   b. receptors.
   c. stimuli.
   d. platelets.

2. How a drug works, or produces a desired or undesired effect, is referred to as:
   a. the first-pass effect.
   b. mechanism of action.
   c. potency.
   d. dose-response curve.

3. The amount of the drug that is actually available for use by the body is known as:
   a. bioavailability.
   b. affinity.
   c. processing.
   d. solubility.

4. The ability of an agonist to bind to the cell receptor is referred to as:
   a. bioavailability.
   b. affinity.
   c. processing.
   d. solubility.

5. An initial dose that may be a higher dose than the patient will take on a regular basis is called a(n):
   a. intermittent dose.
   b. STAT dose.
   c. loading dose.
   d. subtherapeutic dose.

6. The measurement of the specific amount of a drug that will achieve half of the maximal response is:
   a. ED50.
   b. drug clearance.
   c. volume of distribution.
   d. half-life.

7. The amount of time it takes a drug serum level to decrease by 50 percent is:
   a. ED50.
   b. drug clearance.
   c. volume of distribution.
   d. half-life.

8. Addiction is characterized by:
   a. compulsive behavior.
   b. physiological dependence.
   c. psychological dependence.
   d. all of the above.

9. In which of the following forms of membrane transport does the cell engulf the substance, thereby allowing the substance to enter the cell?
   a. active transport
   b. facilitated diffusion
   c. passive transport
   d. pinocytosis

10. In general, which of the following chemical forms more readily crosses the cell membrane barrier?
    a. ionized
    b. positively charged
    c. un-ionized
    d. negatively charged

CRITICAL THINKING QUESTIONS

1. Explain why it is important for you, as a pharmacy technician, to understand not only how to prepare customer prescriptions, but also the effects that the prescription drugs have on your customer's body.

2. Explain why drugs that have shorter half-lives must be dosed at more frequent intervals than drugs with longer half-lives.

3. Using what you have learned in this chapter, and drawing from your own personal experiences, how much responsibility do you believe drug-addicted persons have for causing their own drug addiction?

WEB CHALLENGE

1. Go to http://www.4um.com/tutorial/science/pharmak.htm for a tutorial on pharmacokinetics.

2. Go to http://www.mayoclinic.com to research more about drug addiction. Choose three different drugs and discuss the signs and symptoms of addiction to each.

REFERENCES AND RESOURCES

Adams, MP, Josephson, DL, & Holland, LN Jr. *Pharmacology for Nurses—A Pathophysiologic Approach*. Upper Saddle River, NJ: Pearson Education, 2005.

"Addiction Criteria" (accessed June 21, 2007): http://www.druglibrary.org/schaffer/library/addcrit.htm

Advocacy and Policy. Definitions Related to the Use of Opioids for the Treatment of Pain. A Consensus Document from the American Academy of Pain Medicine, the American Pain Society, and the American Society of Addiction Medicine (accessed June 21, 2007): http://www.ampainsoc.org

"Alcohol, Drugs and the Brain" (accessed June 22, 2007): http://www.open.org/tahana/ADA/twfadbr.htm

"Alcoholism Statistics" (accessed June 21, 2007): http://www.alcoholism-statistics.com

"Alcoholism Statistics" (accessed June 21, 2007): http://www.stopaddiction.com

Andreoli, T, Carpenter, C, Bennett, C, & Plum, F. *Essentials of Medicine* (4th ed.). Philadelphia: W.B. Saunders, 1997.

"Anxiety-Management" (accessed June 22, 2007): http://health.usnews.com/usnews/health/brain/anxiety/anx.manage.htm

Baker, R, Rakel, R, & Bope, E, eds. Psychiatric disorders: Alcoholism. In *Conn's Current Therapy 2002*. Philadelphia: W.B. Saunders, 2002.

Berkow, R. *The Merck Manual* (17th ed.). Rahway, NJ: Merck Research Laboratories, 1992.

Carmichael, BP. *Drug Abuse: Addiction vs. Dependency*. "Glossary of Terms" (accessed June 20, 2007): http://www.medsch.wisc.edu/painpolicy/glossary.htm

Harmful Interactions: Mixing Alcohol with Medicines. (Publication Number 03-5329). Bethesda, MD: National Institute on Alcohol Abuse and Alcoholism, February 2003.

Hitner, H, & Nagle, B. *Basic Pharmacology* (4th ed.). New York: Glencoe/McGraw-Hill, 1999.

Holland, N, & Adams, MP. *Core Concepts in Pharmacology*. Upper Saddle River, NJ: Pearson Education, 2003.

Koda-Kimble, MA. *Applied Therapeutics: The Clinical Use of Drugs* (5th ed.). Vancouver, WA: Applied Therapeutics, 1992.

Landry, M. *Understanding Drugs and Abuse: The Processes of Addiction, Treatment and Recovery*. Los Angeles, CA: American Psychiatric Press, 1994.

"Prescription Drugs: Abuse and Addiction" (accessed June 22, 2007): http://www.nida.nih.gov

Winter, M, & Koda-Kimble, MA, eds. Clinical pharmacokinetics. In *Applied Therapeutics: The Clinical Use of Drugs* (4th ed.). Vancouver, WA: Applied Therapeutics, 1992.

Wyngaarden, J, Lloyd Smith, L, & Bennett, C. *Cecil Textbook of Medicine* (19th ed.). Philadelphia: W.B. Saunders, 1992.

Drug Classifications

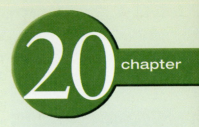

20 chapter

LEARNING OBJECTIVES

After completing this chapter, you should be able to:

- List and explain a variety of drug classifications.
- Understand the five pregnancy categories and how they affect drug classifications.
- List and describe the five schedules of controlled substances and identify drugs assigned to each schedule.

KEY TERMS

anxiety 381

depression 383

edema 384

hypertension 384

pharmacology 371

psychotic 384

seizure 381

teratogenic 393

type 1 diabetes mellitus 385

type 2 diabetes mellitus 385

pharmacology the study of drugs.

Introduction

Pharmacology is a very complex, diversified, and intriguing science. To be successful, pharmacy technicians require a basic understanding of how drugs are classified, what those classifications are, and what conditions or diseases each class of drugs treats.

Classification of Drugs

A drug may be placed into a specific category based on any one or more of the following considerations:

- chemical ingredients
- method by which the drug is used (e.g., by mouth, by injection, topical application)
- area of the body that is treated (e.g., stomach, head, heart)

These categories are also called *classifications,* and any drug fitting the designated criteria belongs to that class of drugs. Many drugs fit into more than one category because they may be indicated and used for entirely different conditions.

Although there are numerous ways to classify drugs, they are often classified into groups according to two methods. The first method is according to therapeutic classification as determined by a drug's therapeutic use. For example, *diuretic* (an agent that promotes the excretion of urine) is an example of a pharmacological classification, as it describes the drug's effect on the body. The second method is determined by mechanism of action. A therapeutic classification, such as *antinausea* drug (a drug to combat vomiting), more straightforwardly describes the clinical action of a drug.

This chapter provides an overview of the many different drug classifications. The classes discussed here are only samples of major groupings; the list is by no means all-inclusive.

Analgesics

An *analgesic* is a drug that selectively suppresses pain (see Table 20-1).

- *Narcotic analgesics* are morphine-like drugs that relieve pain and cause central nervous system (CNS) depression. Also known as *opioid analgesics,* they may cause dizziness and drowsiness. Repeated use of narcotic analgesics may lead to drug abuse and dependence.
- *Nonnarcotic analgesics* relieve pain without CNS depression. They are also known as nonopioid analgesics.

Antirheumatics

An *antirheumatic* drug is used to treat rheumatoid arthritis in patients who have not responded to more traditional methods of treatment. Salicylates and NSAIDs are examples of antirheumatic drugs.

Anti-Infectives

An *anti-infective* drug is used to treat infection by killing the infectious agent or inhibiting its growth. Anti-infective drugs can be subdivided into categories that include:

- *Amebicides*—used to treat intestinal and extraintestinal amebiasis.
- *Aminoglycosides*—bactericidal agents used to treat gram-negative infections.
- *Anthelmintics*—used to treat parasitic helminths (whipworm, pinworm, roundworm, hookworm).

Table 20-1 Analgesics

GENERIC NAME	TRADE NAME
Analgesics—Narcotic	
alfentanil HCl	Alfenta®
codeine	
codeine/acetaminophen	Tylenol® No. 2, 3, 4
fentanyl citrate	Sublimaze®
hydrocodone bitartrate/acetaminophen	Lortab®, Vicodin®
hydromorphone HCl	Dilaudid®
meperidine HCl	Demerol®
methadone	Methadose®
morphine sulfate	MS Contin®, Oramorph®, Roxanol®
oxycodone HCl	OxyContin®
oxycodone/acetaminophen	Tylox®, Percocet®
oxycodone/aspirin	Percodan®
propoxyphene	Darvon®
propoxyphene/acetaminophen	Darvocet-N®
remifentanil HCl	Ultiva®
Analgesics—Nonnarcotic	
acetaminophen	Tylenol®
clonidine	Duraclon®
acetaminophen/caffeine/butalbital	Esgic®, Esgic-Plus®
aspirin/caffeine/butalbital	Fiorinal®
diclofenac sodium/misoprostol	Arthrotec®

- *Antifungals*—used to treat local and systemic fungal infections.
- *Antimalarial* agents—used to treat malarial infections.
- *Antiprotozoals*—used to treat infections caused by protozoa.
- *Antituberculosis* agents—used to treat tuberculosis.
- *Antivirals*—used to treat viral infections by inhibiting virus replication.

See also Table 20-2. Anti-infective drugs may also be grouped by drug type:

- *Cephalosporins* are similar in structure and pharmacologic action to penicillins. They are divided into three subclassifications or "generations." As the generations go from 1 to 3, the drugs have a broader gram-negative spectrum, less efficacy against gram-positive organisms, and increased efficacy against resistant microorganisms.
- *Fluoroquinolones* are synthetic, broad-spectrum antibacterial drugs that inhibit bacterial DNA replication. Patients taking fluoroquinolones should avoid antacids containing magnesium, calcium, or aluminum, as these products will interfere with the absorption and excretion of the anti-infective drugs.

Table 20-2 Anti-Infectives

GENERIC NAME	TRADE NAME
Amebicides	
chloroquine HCl	
chloroquine phosphate	
iodoquinol	Yodoxin®
metronidazole	Flagyl®
Aminoglycosides	
gentamicin	Garamycin®
kanamycin	Kantrex®
neomycin sulfate	Neo-fradin®
paromomycin sulfate	Humatin®
streptomycin sulfate	
tobramycin	Nebcin®
Anthelmintics	
albendazole	Albenza®
diethylcarbamazine citrate	Hetrazan®
mebendazole	Vermox®
thiabendazole	Mintezol®
Antifungals	
amphotericin B desoxycholate	Amphocin®, Fungizone® IV
clotrimazole	Lotrimin® AF
fluconazole	Diflucan®
flucytosine	Ancobon®
itraconazole	Sporanox®
ketoconazole	Nizoral®
miconazole	Monistat-Derm®
nystatin	Mycostatin®
terbinafine	Lamisil®
voriconazole	V-fend®
Antimalarial Agents	
chloroquine	Aralen®
hydroxychloroquine sulfate	Plaquenil®
mefloquine HCl	Lariam®
primaquine phosphate	
quinine sulfate	
Antiprotozoals	
atovaquone	Mepron®

Table 20-2   Anti-Infectives (*continued*)

GENERIC NAME	TRADE NAME
pentamidine isethionate	Pentam® 300, NebuPent®
nitazoxanide	Alinia®
tinidazole	Tindamax®
Antituberculosis Agents	
capreomycin	Capastate Sulfate®
ethambutol	Myambutol®
isoniazid	Nydrazid®
rifabutin	Mycobutin®
rifampin	Rifadin®
rifapentine	Priftin®
Antivirals	
acyclovir	Zovirax®
amantadine	Symmetrel®
famciclovir	Famvir®
ganciclovir	Cytovene®
nevirapine	Viramune®
ribavirin	Rebetol®, Virazole®
rimantadine	Flumadine®
valacyclovir	Valtrex®
Cephalosporins	
First Generation	
cefadroxil	Duricef®, Ultracef®
cefazolin sodium	Ancef®, Kefzol®
cephalexin	Keflex®
Second Generation	
cefaclor	Ceclor®
cefamandole nafate	Mandol®
cefonicid sodium	Monocid®
cefprozil	Cefzil®
cefuroxime sodium	Ceftin®, Kefurox®, Zinacef®
Third/Fourth Generations	
cefdinir	Omnicef®
cefepime	Maxipime®
cefixime	Suprax®
cefotaxime sodium	Claforan®
ceftriaxone sodium	Rocephin®

Table 20-2 Anti-Infectives (*continued*)

GENERIC NAME	TRADE NAME
Fluoroquinolones	
ciprofloxacin	Cipro®
levofloxacin	Levaquin®
ofloxacin	Floxin®
sparfloxacin	Zagam®
Macrolides	
azithromycin	Zithromax®
clarithromycin	Biaxin®
dirithromycin	Dynabac®
erythromycin	E-mycin®, Erythrocin®
Penicillins	
amoxicillin	Trimox®, Amoxil®
amoxicillin/potassium clavulanate	Augmentin®
ampicillin	Principen®
penicillin G	Pfizerpen®
penicillin VK	Veetids®
ticarcillin	Ticar®
Tetracyclines	
demeclocycline hydrochloride	Declomycin®
doxycycline hyclate	Doryx®, Doxy®, Monodox®, Vibramycin®
minocycline hydrochloride	Dynacin®, Minocin®, Vectrin®
oxytetracycline	Terramycin®
tetracycline hydrochloride	Achromycin®, Panmycin®, Sumycin®

- *Macrolides* inhibit bacterial protein synthesis, can be either bactericidal or bacteriostatic, and are commonly used with patients who have penicillin allergies.
- *Penicillins* are bactericidal drugs that work by inhibiting bacterial cell wall synthesis. Penicillin (PCN) drugs should be taken 1 hour before or 2 hours after meals, as absorption is affected by food in the stomach.
- *Tetracyclines* are bacteriostatic, in that they inhibit bacterial growth by inhibiting protein synthesis. They are effective against both gram-positive and gram-negative microorganisms. They cause photosensitivity. Tetracyclines should be taken on an empty stomach but not with antacids.

Workplace Wisdom PCN Allergy

Because cephalosporins are similar in structure to penicillins, there is a possibility that a person with a penicillin allergy may have a cross-sensitivity to cephalosporins.

Antineoplastics

Antineoplastics (see Table 20-3) are drugs that inhibit or prevent the growth of malignant cells. They are subdivided into categories that include:

- *Alkylating agents*—cause a change in cell RNA that inhibits cell reproduction.
- *Antimetabolites*—inhibit cell growth during the S-phase of DNA synthesis.
- *Antineoplastic antibiotics*—inhibit DNA and RNA synthesis and cell division. They are not used to treat infections.
- *Hormones*—inhibit the growth of malignant cells without cytotoxic side effects; highly selective of malignant tissues related to the sex hormones (breast, prostate).

Table 20-3   Antineoplastics

GENERIC NAME	TRADE NAME
Alkylating Agents	
busulfan	Busulfex®, Myleran®
cisplatin	Platinol®, Platinol-AQ®
cyclophosphamide	Cytoxan®
Antimetabolites	
capecitabine	Xeloda®
cytarabine	Cytosar-U®
fluorouracil	Adrucil®, Carac™, Efudex®
methotrexate	Rheumatrex®, Trexall™
Antibiotics	
daunorubicin	Cerubidine®
doxorubicin	Adriamycin® RDF
epirubicin	Ellence®
Hormones	
bicalutamide	Casodex®
finasteride	Propecia®, Proscar®
megestrol acetate	Megace®
Mitotic Inhibitors	
paclitaxel	Taxol®, Onxol®, Abraxane®
vinblastine	Velban®, Velsar®
vincristine	Vincasar®, Oncovin®
vinorelbine tartrate	Navelbine®
Biological Response Modifiers	
aldesleukin	Proleukin®
BCG, Intravesical	TICE BCG®, TheraCys®
denileukin diftitox	Ontak®
levamisole	Ergamiol®

- *Mitotic inhibitors*—natural drugs for which the mechanism of action is not fully understood.
- *Biological response modifiers*—have antiviral, immunomodulating, and antineoplastic actions.

Antiseptics

Antiseptic drugs inhibit or stop bacterial growth without killing or destroying the bacteria. Examples include methylene blue, fosfomycin tromethamine (Monurol®), benzalkonium chloride, chlorhexdine gluconate (Hibiclens®, Hibistat®), hexachlorophene (pHisoHex®), and povidone iodine.

Cardiovascular Agents

Cardiovascular drugs (see Table 20-4) treat conditions of the heart and vascular systems. They are subdivided into categories that include:

- *Angiotensin-converting enzyme inhibitors*—inhibit the conversion of the enzyme angiotensin I to angiotensin II. The angiotensin II enzyme is a very strong vasoconstrictor and ACE inhibitors lower blood pressure by interfering with the conversion of the precursor enzyme.

Table 20-4 Cardiovascular Agents

GENERIC NAME	TRADE NAME
ACE Inhibitors	
benazepril	Lotensin®
benazepril + amlodipine	Lotrel®
captopril	Capoten®
captopril + hydrochlorothiazide (HCTZ)	Capozide®
enalapril	Vasotec®
enalapril + felodipine	Lexxel®
enalapril + diltiazem	Teczem®
enalapril + HCTZ	Vaseretic®
fosinopril	Monopril®
lisinopril	Prinivil®, Zestril®
lisinopril + HCTZ	Prinizide®, Zestoretic®
moexipril	Univasc®
moexipril + HCTZ	Uniretic®
perindopril	Aceon®
quinapril	Accupril®
ramipril	Altace®
trandolapril	Mavik®
trandolapril + verapamil	Tarka®
Antiarrhythmic Agents	
amiodarone	Cordarone®
bretylium tosylate	

Table 20-4 Cardiovascular Agents (*continued*)

GENERIC NAME	TRADE NAME
disopyramide	Norpace®
esmolol	Brevibloc®
flecainide	Tambocor®
mexiletine	Mexitil®
procainamide	Procanbid®
propafenone	Rhythmol®
propranolol	Inderal®
quinidine	Quinaglute®, Quinadex®
sotalol	Betapace®
Antihyperlipidemics	
atorvastatin calcium	Lipitor®
atorvastatin + amlodipine	Caduet®
cholestyramine	Questran®
colesevelam	WelChol®
colestipol	Colestid®
ezetimibe	Zetia®
ezetimibe + simvastatin	Vytorin®
fenofibrate	Tricor®
fluvastatin sodium	Lescol®, Lescol® XL
gemfibrozil	Lopid®
lovastatin	Mevacor®, Altoprev®
niacin	
pravastatin sodium	Pravachol®
rosuvastatin calcium	Crestor®
simvastatin	Zocor®
Beta-Adrenergic Blocking Agents	
clonidine	Catapres®
guanabenz acetate	Wytensin®
guanadrel	Hylorel®
guanethidine	Ismelin®
guanfacine	Tenex®
labetolol	Normodyne®
methyldopa	Aldomet®
nadolol	Corgard®
pindolol	Visken®
propranolol	Inderal®
reserpine	
timolol	Blocadren®

Table 20-4 Cardiovascular Agents (*continued*)

GENERIC NAME	TRADE NAME
Calcium Channel Blockers	
amlodipine	Norvasc®
bepridil	Vascor®
diltiazem	Cardizem®, Dilacor® XR
felodipine	Plendil®
isradipine	DynaCirc®
nicardipine	Cardene®
nifedipine	Procardia®, Adalat®
nimodipine	Nimotop®
nisoldipine	Sular®
verapamil	Calan®, Isoptin®
Vasodilators	
hydralazine	Apresoline®
isosorbide dinitrate	Isordil® Titradose, Isordil®
isosorbide mononitrate	Monoket®, Imdur®
isoxsuprine HCl	Vasodilan®, Voxsuprine®
minoxidil	
nitroglycerin	Nitrostat®, Nitro-Bid®, Nitro-Dur®
papaverine HCl	

- *Antiarrhythmic agents*—used to treat cardiac arrhythmias.
- *Antihypertensives*—a general term for drugs used in the treatment of high blood pressure. *Antihypertensive combination drugs* usually contain an antihypertensive medication in combination with a diuretic or antihyperlipidemic medication.
- *Antihyperlipidemics*—used in the treatment of elevated cholesterol levels.
- *Beta-adrenergic blocking agents (beta-blockers)*—interfere with the attachment of chemicals such as epinephrine and norepinephrine to β-adrenergic receptors. The indications for beta-blockers include hypertension and angina.
- *Calcium channel blockers*—inhibit calcium from moving across the cell membrane. The indications for CCBs include angina and hypertension.

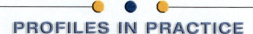

PROFILES IN PRACTICE

Todd is a pharmacy technician who works in a neighborhood pharmacy. He has a patient with a severe PCN allergy who presents a prescription for "Suprax 400 mg po daily." The prescriber was unaware of the patient's allergies, and the patient's diagnosis is uncomplicated gonorrhea.

- Do you see any potential problems with the prescription for Todd's patient? If so, what are they?
- What steps should Todd take to ensure that the patient receives the proper treatment for the condition?

- *Cardiac glycosides*—natural drugs that are indicated for the treatment of heart failure and atrial fibrillation. Digoxin (Lanoxin®) is an example.
- *Vasodilators*—dilate blood vessels and are used in the treatment of angina and hypertension.

Central Nervous System Agents

Central nervous system agent is a general term used to describe drugs that treat conditions related to the central nervous system (see Table 20-5). CNS agents are subdivided into categories that include:

- *Antianxiety* drugs—used in the treatment of **anxiety** disorders or for the short-term management of anxiety symptoms. Antianxiety drugs are further subdivided into two categories: benzodiazepines and miscellaneous. They are also indicated for acute alcohol withdrawal, **seizure** disorders, panic disorders, and as a preanesthetic for surgery.

anxiety a mental state characterized by apprehension and uneasiness stemming from the anticipation of danger.

seizure a disturbance of brain activity characterized by changes in consciousness, activity, and sensation.

Table 20-5 CNS Agents

GENERIC NAME	TRADE NAME
Antianxiety	
alprazolam	Xanax®
buspirone	Buspar®
chlordiazepoxide	Librium®
clorazepate	Tranxene®
diazepam	Valium®
lorazepam	Ativan®
oxazepam	Serax®
zaleplon	Sonata®
zolpidem	Ambien®
Anticonvulsants or Antiepileptics	
carbamazepine	Tegretol®
divalproex	Depakote®
felbamate	Felbatol®
fosphenytoin	Cerebyx®
lamotrigine	Lamictal®
phenytoin	Dilantin®
valproic acid	Depakene®
zonisamide	Zonegran®
Antidepressants	
bupropion HCl	Wellbutrin®
nefazodone HCl	Serzone®
trazodone	Desyrel®
Tricyclic Compounds	
clomipramine	Anafril®
imipramine	Tofranil®

Table 20-5   CNS Agents (*continued*)

GENERIC NAME	TRADE NAME
Serotonin and Norepinephrine Reuptake Inhibitors	
duloxetine HCl	Cymbalta®
enlafaxine HCl	Effexor®, Effexor® XR
Selective Serotonin Reuptake Inhibitors	
citalopram	Celexa®
fluoxetine	Prozac®
fluvoxamine	Luvox®
paroxetine	Paxil®
sertraline	Zoloft®
Monoamine Oxidase Inhibitors	
isocarboxazid	Marplan®
phenelzine sulfate	Nardil®
tranylcypromine sulfate	Parnate®
Antiparkinson Agents	
amantadine hydrochloride	Symmetrel®
benztropine mesylate	Cogentin®
bromocriptine mesylate	Parlodel®
carbidopa and levodopa	Sinemet®, Sinemet CR®
pergolide mesylate	Permax®
selegiline hydrochloride	Eldepryl®
trihexyphenidyl HCl	Artane®
Antipsychotics	
aripiprazole	Abilify®
chlorpromazine	Thorazine®
clozapine	Clozaril®
fluphenazine	Prolixin®, Permitil®
haloperidol	Haldol®
olanzapine	Zyprexa®
perphenazine	Trilafon®
quetiapine	Seroquel®
risperidone	Risperdal®
thioridazine	Mellaril®
thiothixene	Navane®
trifluoperazine	Stelazine®
ziprasidone	Geodon®, Zeldox®
Hypnotics	
estazolam	ProSom®
flurazepam	Dalmane®

Table 20-5 CNS Agents (*continued*)

GENERIC NAME	TRADE NAME
quazepam	Doral®
temazepam	Restoril®
triazolam	Halcion®
Sedatives	
amobarbital	Amytal®
chloral hydrate	Noctec®
eszopiclone	Lunesta®
methohexital	Brevital®
pentobarbital	Nembutal®
phenobarbital	Luminal®
secobarbital	Seconal®
thiopental	Pentothal®
zaleplon	Sonata®
zolpidem	Ambien®
Stimulants	
dextroamphetamine	Dexedrine®
dextroamphetamine sulfate, dextroamphetamine saccarate, amphetamine asparate, amphetamine sulfate	Adderall®
methylphenidate	Ritalin®, Concerta®

- *Anticonvulsants* or *antiepileptics*—suppress the neuronal activity that causes seizures.
- *Antidepressants*—used in the treatment of **depression**, obsessive-compulsive disorders, social anxiety disorders, and major depressive disorders. Antidepressants are further divided into distinctive categories, including:

  1. *Tricyclic compounds*—prevent the reuptake of serotonin or norepinephrine. Tricyclic coumpounds can be toxic, so the patient and drug regimen should be monitored.
  2. *Serotonin and norepinephrine reuptake inhibitors*—inhibit the reuptake of serotonin and norepinephrine but not dopamine.
  3. *Selective serotonin reuptake inhibitors* (SSRIs)—inhibit the reuptake of serotonin but not norepinephrine.
  4. *Monoamine oxidase inhibitors* (MAOIs)—inhibit the complex enzyme system monoamine oxidase. MAOIs have the potential to cause serious side effects.

depression a mental state characterized by lack of energy, feelings of despair, guilt, and misery, and changes in sleep pattern and eating habits.

═══ **INFORMATION** ═══

Children and adolescents with major depressive disorder, obsessive-compulsive disorder (OCD), and other psychiatric disorders who take an antidepressant are at higher risk than adults for suicidal thinking and behavior. Patients should be closely monitored for changes in behavior.

psychotic refers to a mental state characterized by a loss of orientation to reality.

- *Antiparkinson agents*—used in the treatment of Parkinson's disease.
- *Antipsychotics*—primarily used to treat **psychotic** disorders including bipolar disorder, schizophrenia, OCD, PCP-induced psychosis, psychosis/agitation in dementia, and acute porphyria. Some antipsychotics are also indicated for the treatment of nausea and vomiting, tetanus, Tourette's syndrome, acute migraines, intractable hiccups, and severe behavioral problems.
- *Hypnotics*—used to induce sleep.
- *Sedatives,* also known as *tranquilizers*—used to calm and quiet while causing a decrease in all reactions and emotions.
- *Stimulants*—increase alertness or stimulate the reticular formation of the brain.

Diuretics

edema swelling.

hypertension high blood pressure.

Diuretic drugs (see Table 20-6) are used in the treatment of **edema** and **hypertension** because they inhibit the reabsorption of sodium and chloride in the kidneys, which then causes an increase in urine output volume. Diuretics are subdivided into categories that include:

- *Thiazides*—indicated for the treatment of edema, hypertension, and renal impairment.
- *Loop diuretics*—indicated for edema, hypertension, pulmonary edema, congenital heart disease, and nephrotic syndrome.
- *Potassium-sparing diuretics*—used in conjunction with thiazide and loop diuretics to decrease potassium secretion.
- *Carbonic anhydrase inhibitors*—inhibit the enzyme carbonic anhydrase, resulting in a reduction of aqueous humor and a decrease of intraocular pressure; used in the treatment of glaucoma and for the prevention or mitigation of acute altitude sickness symptoms.

Table 20-6   Diuretics

GENERIC NAME	TRADE NAME
Thiazide and Thiazide-Like Diuretics	
chlorothiazide	Diuril®
chlorthalidone	Hygroton®
hydrochlorothiazide (HCTZ)	Hydro-Diuril®
metolazone	Zaroxolyn®
Loop Diuretics	
bumetanide	Bumex®
furosemide	Lasix®
torsemide	Demadex®
Potassium-Sparing Diuretics	
triamterene	Dyrenium®
spironolactone	Aldactone®
triamterene + HCTZ	Dyazide®
spironolactone + HCTZ	Aldactazide®
Carbonic Anhydrase Inhibitors	
acetazolamide	Diamox®
methazolamide	

Endocrine and Metabolic Agents

The general classification of *endocrine and metabolic agents* is for drugs that treat conditions and diseases of the endocrine system and metabolic processes (see Table 20-7). Subclassifications include:

- *Bisphosphonates*—inhibit bone resorption; used in the treatment of osteoporosis and Paget disease.
- *Thyroid drugs*—hormones used in the treatment of thyroid conditions such as hypothyroidism, euthyroid goiters, and thyroid cancer.
- *Antidiabetic agents*—used to lower blood glucose levels in the treatment of **type 1** and **type 2 diabetes mellitus**.

type 1 diabetes mellitus a metabolic disorder formerly called insulin-dependent diabetes mellitus (IDDM).

type 2 diabetes mellitus a metabolic disorder formerly called noninsulin-dependent diabetes mellitus (NIDDM).

Adrenocortical Steroids

Adrenocortical steroids, also referred to as *corticosteroids*, are hormones produced in the adrenal cortex. Subclassifications include:

- *Glucocorticosteroids*—steroids that also have anti-inflammatory properties. Indications include allergic reactions, GI diseases (colitis, enteritis), multiple sclerosis, ophthalmic allergies, and dermatologic diseases (dermatitis, psoriasis, urticaria). Examples include betamethasone (Celestone®), budesonide (Entcort® EC), cortisone, dexamethasone (Decadron®), hydrocortisone (Cortef®, Hydrocortone®), methylprednisolone (Medrol®, Depo-Medrol®), prednisone (Prelone®, Deltasone®), and triamcinolone (Kenalog®, Aristocort®).

Table 20-7 Endocrine and Metabolic Agents

GENERIC NAME	TRADE NAME
Bisphosphonates	
alendronate sodium	Fosamax®
ibandronate	Boniva®
pamidronate	Aredia®
risedronate	Actonel®
zolendronate	Zomig®
Thyroid Drugs	
thyroid desiccated	Armour® Thyroid
levothyroxine sodium	Synthroid®, Levoxyl®, Levothroid®
liothyronine sodium	Cytomel®, Triostat®
Antidiabetic Agents	
acarbose	Precose®
glimeprimide	Amaryl®
glipizide	Glucotrol®
glyburide	Diabeta®, Micronase®
metformin	Glucophage®
miglitol	Glyset®
nateglinide	Starlix®
pioglitazone	Actos®
repaglinide	Prandin®
rosiglitazone	Avandia®

- *Mineralocorticoids*—steroids that help to regulate the body's sodium and water balance. Fludrocortisone acetate (Florinef®) is an example.

Sex Hormones

Sex hormones are drugs that affect the growth and development of the reproductive organs and secondary sex characteristics (see Table 20-8). Subclassifications include:

- *Estrogens*—the primary female sex hormone, primarily produced in the ovaries. Synthetic estrogen is often included in hormone replacement therapy for post-menopausal women and as a component in contraceptives.

- *Selective estrogen receptor modulators (SERMs)*—drugs used in the prevention and treatment of osteoporosis. SERMs bind to estrogen receptors, activating some pathways and blocking others.

- *Contraceptive hormones*—hormones indicated for the prevention of pregnancy, emergency contraception, and (in some cases) acne vulgaris.

- *Androgens*—the primary male sex hormone; indicated in males for hypogonadism and delayed puberty and in females for metastatic cancer. Testosterone is the primary androgen produced in the testes.

- *Anabolic steroids*—synthetic drugs that imitate the male androgen testosterone; approved for use in the treatment of anemia, bone pain, protein catabolism, and weight gain.

Table 20-8   Sex Hormones

GENERIC NAME	TRADE NAME
Estrogens	
estradiol	Estrace®, Femtrace®, Estraderm®
conjugated estrogens	Premarin®
esterified estrogens	Menest®
SERMs	
raloxifene	Evista®
Contraceptive Hormones	
norethindrone	Ortho-Micronor®
norgestrel	Ovrette®
levonorgestrel (subdermal implant)	Norplant®
medroxyprogesterone (injection)	Depo-Provera®
estradiol cypionate/medroxyprogesterone acetate (injection)	Lunelle®
Androgens	
testosterone	Androderm®, Depo-Testosterone®, AndroGel®, Delatestryl®
methyltestosterone	Methitest®, Testred®, Virilon®, Oreton®
fluoxymesterone	Halotestin®
Anabolic Steroids	
nandrolone decanoate	
oxymetholone	Anadrol-50®
oxandrolone	Oxandrin®

Uterine-Active Agents

Abortifacients are used for the termination of intrauterine pregnancy. Examples include mifepristone (RU-486, Mifeprex®) and carboprost tromethamine (Hemabate®).

Oxytocics are used to induce and improve uterine contractions. Oxytocin (Pitocin®) is an example.

Uterine stimulants are indicated in the prevention and treatment of postpartum bleeding. Examples include ergonovine maleate (Ergotrate®) and methylergonovine maleate (Methergine®).

Uterine relaxants are used to stop uterine contractions. Ritodrine (Yutopar®) is an example.

Gastrointestinal Agents

Gastrointestinal agent is a therapeutic classification for drugs that are used to treat conditions and diseases affecting the gastrointestinal tract (see Table 20-9). GI agents are subdivided into categories that include:

- *Histamine H2 antagonists*—indicated for ulcers, gastroesophageal reflux disease (GERD), upper GI bleeding, and erosive esophagitis; work by blocking histamine at the H2 receptors in the stomach.

Table 20-9 GI Agents

GENERIC NAME	TRADE NAME
H2 Antagonists	
cimetidine	Tagamet®
famotidine	Pepcid®
nizatidine	Axid®
ranitidine	Zantac®
PPIs	
esomeprazole magnesium	Nexium®
lansoprazole	Prevacid®
omeprazole	Prilosec®
pantoprazole	Protonix®
rabeprazole sodium	Aciphex®
Anticholinergics/Antispasmodics	
atropine sulfate	Sal-Tropine®, AtroPen®
dicyclomine	Bentyl®
glycopyrrolate	Robinul®
Laxatives	
bisacodyl	Dulcolax®, Correctol®
cascara sagrada	
docusate calcium	Surfak® Liquigels
docusate sodium	Colace®
glycerin (suppository)	Sani-Supp®, Colace®
lactulose	Cephulac®, Enulose®
methylcellulose	Citrucel®
milk of magnesia	

Table 20-9   GI Agents (*continued*)

GENERIC NAME	TRADE NAME
mineral oil	
polyethylene glycol (PEG) solution	GlycoLax®, MiraLax®
polyethylene glycol-electrolyte solution (PEG-ES)	CoLyte®, GoLYTELY®
psyllium	Metamucil®
sennosides	ex-lax®, Senokot®
Antidiarrheals	
bismuth subsalicylate (BSS)	Pepto-Bismol®
diphenoxylate with atropine	Lomotil®
loperamide	Imodium® A-D
Antiemetics	
dimenhydrinate	Dramamine®
granisetron HCl	Kytril®
hydroxyzine pamoate	Vistaril®
meclizine	Antivert®
ondansetron HCl	Zofran®
promethazine	Phenergan®
scopolamine	Transderm Scøp®

- *Proton pump inhibitors (PPIs)*—work by inhibiting the gastric proton pump that secretes stomach acid; indicated for ulcers, erosive esophagitis, and GERD.
- *GI anticholinergics/antispasmodics*—decrease gastrointestinal motility; indicated for spastic disorders of the GI, biliary, and urogenital tracts.
- *Laxatives*—treat constipation or are used to evacuate the colon for medical examinations.
- *Antidiarrheals*—used in the treatment of nonspecific diarrhea and acute episodes of chronic functional diarrhea.
- *GI stimulants*—used to increase gastrointestinal motility; indicated in the treatment of diabetic gastroparesis and for the prevention of postsurgical and chemotherapy nausea and vomiting.
- *Antiemetics*—used in the treatment of nausea and vomiting.

Hematological Agents

Hematological agents (see Table 20-10) are drugs used in the treatment of blood-related conditions. They are subdivided into categories that include:

- *Anticoagulants*—used to prevent blood clots or thrombi.
- *Antiplatelets*—inhibit the aggregation of blood platelets in patients who have experienced a recent myocardial infarction (MI) or stroke or who have an established peripheral arterial disease.
- *Coagulants*—used to stimulate blood clotting.
- *Hematopoietic agents*—used to increase the production of blood cell components. Hematopoietic agents can be subdivided into three categories: *recombinant human erythropoietin* (increases red blood cell production), *colony stimulating factors* (increases white blood cell production), and *interleukins*

Table 20-10   Hematological Agents

GENERIC NAME	TRADE NAME
Anticoagulants	
dalteparin sodium (Na)	Fragmin®
enoxaparin Na	Lovenox®
heparin Na	
tinzaparin Na	Innohep®
warfarin Na	Coumadin®
Antiplatelets	
anagrelide HCl	Agrylin®
cilostazol	Pletal®
clopidogrel	Plavix®
dipyridamole	Persantine®
dipyridamole + aspirin	Aggrenox®
ticlopidine	Ticlid®
Hematopoietic Agents	
darbepoetin alfa	Aranesp®
epoetin alfa, recombinant	Epogen®, Procrit®
filgrastim	Neupogen®
pegfilgrastim	Neulasta®
sargramostim	Leukine®
Hemostatics	
aminocaproic acid	Amicar®
aprotinin	Trasylol®
gelatin film, absorbable	Gelfilm®
gelatin sponge, absorbable	Gelfoam®
thrombin, topical	Thrombostat®, Thrombogen®
Plasma Expanders	
albumin human	Albuminar®, Albutein®, Plasbumin®
dextran, low molecular weight	Dextran®, Gentran®
hetastarch	
Thrombolytic Agents	
alteplase recombinant	Activase®
anistreplase	Eminase®
retiplase recombinant	Retivase®
streptokinase	Strepase®
tenecteplase	Metalyse®
urokinase	Abbokinase®

(increases blood platelets). Indications include anemia, thrombocytopenia, myeloid leukemia, and bone marrow transplants.

- *Hemostatics*—used to stop bleeding; categorized as either systemic or topical.
- *Plasma expanders*—used to increase blood plasma volume in shock and burn patients.
- *Thrombolytic agents*—used to break down blood clots; indications include acute MI, acute ischemic stroke, and pulmonary embolism.

Muscle Relaxants

Muscle relaxants (see Table 20-11) are used to relax or paralyze skeletal muscles. They are subdivided into the following categories:

- *Skeletal muscle relaxants (SMRs)*—further divided into two categories, central-acting and direct-acting. The mechanism of action (MOA) for central-acting SMRs is unknown; direct-acting SMRs relax muscles by decreasing the muscle's release of calcium, which affects muscle contraction.
- *Nondepolarizing neuromuscular blockers*—injectable drugs that inhibit the neurotransmitter acetylcholine, thereby inhibiting depolarization or contraction, which stops nerve transmission; also used as an adjunct to anesthesia.
- *Depolarizing neuromuscular blockers*—injectable drugs that attach to the NII receptors, stimulating them to cause depolarization or contraction; also used as an adjunct to anesthesia.

Table 20-11 Muscle Relaxants

GENERIC NAME	TRADE NAME
SMRs—Direct-Acting	
dantrolene	Dantrium®
SMRs—Central-Acting	
baclofen	Lioresal®
carisoprodol	Soma®
chlorzoxazone	Parafon Forte DSC®
cyclobenzaprine	Flexeril®
diazepam	Valium®
metaxalone	Skelaxin®
methocarbamol	Robaxin®
orphenadrine citrate	Norflex®
tizanidine HCl	Zanaflex®
Nondepolarizing Neuromuscular Blockers	
atracurium besylate	Tracrium®
cisatracurium besylate	Nimbex®
mivacurium chloride	Mivacron®
pancuronium bromide	Pavulon®
rocuronium bromide	Zemuron®
vecuronium bromide	Norcuron®
Depolarizing Neuromuscular Blockers	
succinylcholine chloride	Quelicin®, Anectine®

Table 20-12 NSAIDs

GENERIC NAME	TRADE NAME
celecoxib	Celebrex®
diclofenac	Cataflam®, Voltaren®
etodolac	
fenoprofen	Nalfon®
flurbiprofen	Ansaid®
ibuprofen	Motrin®
indomethacin	Indocin®
ketoprofen	Orudis®, Oruvail®
ketorolac tromethamine	Toradol®
meclofenamate	Meclomen®
nabumetone	Relafen®
naproxen sodium	Naprosyn®, Anaprox®, Naprelan®
oxaprozin	Daypro®
piroxicam	Feldene®
sulindac	Clinoril®
tolmetin	Tolectin®

Nonsteroidal Anti-Inflammatory Drugs

Nonsteroidal anti-inflammatory drugs (NSAIDs) are used to treat inflammation, pain, and fever (see Table 20-12). NSAIDs reduce inflammation by blocking the prostaglandin-producing enzyme cyclooxygenase II.

Nutritional Agents

Nutritional agents are chemical compounds that the body needs to sustain proper nutrition and to prevent a variety of conditions and diseases. Nutritional agents include vitamins, minerals, and electrolytes.

Respiratory Agents

Respiratory agents treat conditions and diseases of the respiratory system (see Table 20-13). Respiratory agents are subdivided into categories that include:

- *Bronchodilators,* commonly called *antiasthmatics*—dilate the lungs; used in the treatment of asthma, bronchitis, and emphysema.
- *Antihistamines*—used in the treatment of allergies; act by blocking the chemical histamine at the H1 receptors. They are categorized as first generation (nonselectively block central and peripheral H1 receptors) and second generation (selectively block peripheral H1 receptors).
- *Nasal decongestants*—vasoconstricting drugs used in the treatment of nasal congestion; work by constricting nasal mucosa.

Other Criteria for Drug Classification

Certain drugs are classified into categories according to additional criteria, such as potential harm to a fetus or potential for abuse and dependence, for example.

Table 20-13 Respiratory Agents

GENERIC NAME	TRADE NAME
Bronchodilators	
albuterol	Ventolin®, Proventil®
albuterol + atrovent combination	Combivent®, DuoNeb®
bitolterol	Tornalate®
epinephrine	Adrenalin®
fluticasone + salmeterol combination	Advair® Diskus
formoterol	Foradil®
isoproterenol	Isuprel®
levalbuterol	Xopenex®
metaproterenol	Alupent®, Metaprel®
pirbuterol	Maxair®
salmeterol	Serevent®
salmeterol xinafoate	Serevent® Diskus
terbutaline	Bricanyl®, Brethine®
Antihistamines	
azelastine	Astelin NS®
brompheniramine	BroveX CT®
cetirizine	Zyrtec®
chlorpheniramine	Chlor-Trimeton®
clemastine	Tavist-1®
cyproheptadine	Periactin®
desloratadine	Clarinex®
diphenhydramine	Benadryl®, Banophen®, Diphedryl®
fexofenadine	Allegra®
hydroxyzine HCl	Atarax®
hydroxyzine pamoate	Vistaril®
loratadine	Alavert®, Claritin®
loratadine/pseudoephedrine	Claritin-D®
promethazine HCl	Phenergan®
Nasal Decongestants	
oxymetazoline HCl	Afrin®, Dristan®
naphazoline HCL	Privine®
phenylephrine HCl	Neo-Synephrine®
phenylephrine HCl + pheniramine maleate	Dristan® Fast Acting Formula
tetrahydrozoline HCl (Rx only)	Tyzine®
xylometazoline HCl	Otrivin®, Natru-Vent®

Table 20-14   The Five Pregnancy Categories

CATEGORY	DESCRIPTION
A (lowest risk)	No known studies proving risk or harm to fetus have been performed.
B	No known animal studies show risk. If animal studies have shown risk, no studies in women confirm risk.
C	Animal studies show risk, but controlled studies in women have not been performed.
D	These drugs may cause harm, but also may provide benefit if no other drug is available or a life-threatening situation is present.
X (highest risk)	Studies show significant risk to woman and fetus.

Pregnancy Categories

Pregnancy categories are determined on the basis of the potential harm to the unborn child. The five pregnancy categories of safety are A, B, C, D, and X, with A being the lowest risk and X being the highest (see Table 20-14).

Drug information obtained from package inserts, or reliable pharmacy references such as *Drug Facts and Comparisons,* should provide statements similar to the following indicating the potential for harm to the fetus.

- Drug is proven safe during pregnancy.
- Drug is inadequate for pregnant women because it has not been tested. (Lack of testing is often because there has been no reason to do testing.)
- Drug is proven to be **teratogenic** in animals, meaning unsafe in gestating animals. However, because there has been no reason to test the drug on humans, the drug is also considered unsafe for use by pregnant women at any point in their pregnancies.
- Drug is proven to pose a fetal risk in humans; therefore, it should not be used at any cost or for any reason.

teratogenic causing congenital malformations (birth defects).

Controlled Substance Categories

Controlled substances are classified into Schedules I, II, III, IV, or V according to their potential for abuse. The schedules or classes and descriptions are as follows:

- *Schedule I (C-I)*—drugs and chemicals that have no accepted medical use and have the highest abuse potential. Considered "street" drugs or "illicit/illegal" drugs, Schedule I drugs include:
  - heroin
  - lysergic acid diethylamide (LSD)
  - marijuana
  - peyote
  - tetrahydrocannabinol (THC)
- *Schedule II (C-II)*—drugs with accepted medical uses and that have a high abuse potential. Schedule II drugs include:
  - cocaine
  - codeine
  - fentanyl
  - hydromorphone
  - meperidine
  - methylphenidate

- morphine
- oxycodone
- secobarbital

- *Schedule III (C-III)*—drugs with an accepted medical use and a lower abuse potential as compared to C-II medications. Schedule III drugs include:
  - anabolic steroids
  - codeine with acetaminophen
  - codeine with aspirin
  - dronabinol
  - hydrocodone
  - pentobarbital
  - thiopental
- *Schedule IV (C-IV)*—drugs with an accepted medical use and a lower abuse potential than C-II and C-III medications. Schedule IV drugs include:
  - alprazolam
  - clonazepam
  - diazepam
  - flurazepam
  - lorazepam
  - meprobamate
  - phenobarbital
  - temazepam
- *Schedule V (C-V)*—drugs with an accepted medical use and the lowest abuse potential.

Schedule V drugs include liquid codeine cough preparations. Most states do not require a prescription for C-V medications.

INFORMATION

The Comprehensive Drug Abuse Prevention and Control Act of 1970 is the legislation that created the five schedules of controlled substances. The act, also known as the Controlled Substances Act (CSA), also created the Drug Enforcement Administration (DEA).

Over-the-Counter Drugs

Many medications are over-the-counter (OTC), meaning that the patient does not need a prescription for these medications. Table 20-15 lists some common OTC products.

The Food and Drug Administration (FDA) regulates both prescription and nonprescription products. Nonprescription medications must comply with FDA label requirements, which mandate the inclusion of the following information, listed in the same order, on each product label:

- active ingredient—ingredient name, including the strength per unit
- uses—the symptoms or conditions for which the drug is indicated
- warnings—including side effects, when to stop taking the medication, possible interactions, when not to use the product, and "keep out of reach of children"
- inactive ingredients—including flavors, colors, etc.
- purpose—the drug classification or category
- directions—must state age-specific doses, frequencies, and duration of therapy
- other information—including storage instructions

Table 20-15 Common OTC Products (list is not all-inclusive)

DRUG CLASSIFICATION	OTC EXAMPLES
Allergy Medications	Actifed®, Benadryl®, Claritin®, Tavist®, Triaminic®
Analgesics/Antipyretics	Advil®, Aleve®, aspirin, Motrin®, Tylenol®
Anesthetics, Local/Topical	Dermoplast®, Orajel®, Lanacaine®, Solarcaine®
Antacids	AXID® XR, Maalox®, Mylanta®, Pepcid® AC, Prilosec® OTC, Riopan®, Tagamet® HB, Tums®, Zantac® 75
Antidiarrheals	Imodium® A-D, Pepto-Bismol®, Kaopectate®
Antiemetics/Antivertigo Agents	Calm-X®, Dramamine®, Emetrol®
Antifungals	Gyne-Lotrimin®, Lamisil® AT, Lotrimin® AF, Miactin®, Monistat®, Mycelex®-7
Artificial Tears	Dry Eyes®, Murine®, Puralube® Tears, Refresh®
Contact Lens Products	Opti-Clean®, Opti-Free®, Opti-Tears®
Decongestants/Cold Remedies	Advil® Cold & Sinus, Tyenol® Cold & Flu, Thera-Flu®, Robitussin®
Diaper Rash Products	Balmex®, Desitin®, vitamin A, vitamin D
Emollients	Keri®, Lac-Hydrin®, Lubriderm®
Glucose, Blood Tests	Accu-Check® Test Strips, BD® Test Strips, OneTouch® Test Strips
Glucose, Urine Tests	Clinitest®, Chemstrip bG®, Clinistix®
Hair Loss Products	minoxidil, Rogaine®
Hemorrhoidal Agents	Preparation H®
Laxatives/Stool Softeners	Colace®, Dulcolax®, ex-lax®, Metamucil®, Fleet® laxative
Menstrual Cycle Products	Midol®, Pamprin®, Premysyn® PMS, Vitelle Lurline PMS®
Migraine Relievers	Advil® Migraine, Excedrin® Migraine, Motrin® Migraine
Muscle Aches/Pains—Liniments	Ben-Gay®, Flexall®, Tiger Balm®
Muscle Aches/Pains—Patches	Ben-Gay®
Ocular Lubricants	Dry Eyes®, HypoTears®, Lacri-Lube® NP
Pediculicides	A-200®, Pronto®, Tisit®, RID®
Poison Ivy Products, Topical	Caladryl®, Calamine®, Ivy-Dry®, Ivy Soothe®, Zanfel®
Pregnancy Tests	Clearblue Easy®, e.p.t.®, Pregnosis®, RapidVue®, QuickVue®
Smoking Cessation Products	Commit®, Nicoderm CQ®, Nicorette®, Nicotrol®
Sunscreens	Bullfrog® Sunblock, Coppertone®, Hawaiian Tropic®
Vitamins and Minerals	Most vitamins and minerals can be found in OTC formulations and strengths

SUMMARY

Drugs are classified into categories according to their chemical ingredients, the method by which the drug is used (by mouth, by injection, etc.), and the organ or system in the body that is affected by the drug (heart, eye, stomach). They are further divided into separate classes and groups. Two of the most common classifications are therapeutic use (such as analgesics, used to relieve pain), and pharmacological activity (such as diuretics, used to promote the excretion of urine). Two other important classifications of drugs are pregnancy categories, which are used to determine the potential harm to the fetus if a drug is taken by a pregnant woman; and controlled substance classes, which indicate the potential for abuse, or the addictive nature, of the drug.

Many drugs are also available OTC. It is an important pharmacy technician duty to understand drug classifications and know which drug products are available to patients without prescription. This will ensure that the patient receives the best possible care. Properly trained and educated pharmacy technicians are much more helpful to both their patients and their pharmacists.

CHAPTER REVIEW QUESTIONS

1. Drugs can be classified:
   a. according to the way they affect the body.
   b. by cost savings.
   c. by indication.
   d. a and c.

2. Which schedule of controlled substances has the most potential for abuse?
   a. C-V
   b. C-IV
   c. C-III
   d. C-II

3. Which of the following is not required on OTC product labels?
   a. active ingredient
   b. warnings
   c. directions
   d. all of the above are required

4. Which of the following is not an antidepressant drug category?
   a. SSRI
   b. MAOI
   c. tricyclic compounds
   d. CCB

5. Which of the following categories of anti-infectives can be subdivided into generations 1, 2, and 3?
   a. penicillins
   b. aminoglycosides
   c. cephalosporins
   d. macrolides

6. Which of the following types of drugs induce sleep?
   a. tranquilizer
   b. sedative
   c. stimulant
   d. hypnotic

7. Which of the following classifications of drugs is included in Schedule III controlled substances?
   a. estrogens
   b. anabolic steroids
   c. glucocorticosteroids
   d. benzodiazepines

8. Which pregnancy category has the lowest risk to the fetus?
   a. A
   b. B
   c. C
   d. D

9. Which of the following types of drugs suppresses pain?
   a. antiemetic
   b. diuretic
   c. analgesic
   d. antihypertensive

10. Which of the following types of drugs stimulates the production of blood cells?
    a. coagulants
    b. plasma expanders
    c. hematopoietics
    d. hemostatics

CRITICAL THINKING QUESTIONS

1. Why do you think anabolic steroids are a Schedule III controlled substance?

2. What impact does the FDA's new OTC label regulation have on the consumer?

WEB CHALLENGE

1. Go to http://www.fda.gov to learn more about the OTC label requirements. Write a summary of your findings.

2. Go to http://www.usdoj.gov/dea and find out more about regulations to allow electronic prescriptions for controlled substances. What are three ways these regulations would benefit both practitioners and pharmacy personnel? What are some potential risks?

REFERENCES AND RESOURCES

Adams, MP, Josephson, DL, & Holland, LN Jr. *Pharmacology for Nurses—A Pathophysiologic Approach*. Upper Saddle River, NJ: Pearson Education, 2008.

Drug Facts and Comparisons, 2006 ed. St. Louis: Wolters Kluwer Health, Inc.

Holland, N, & Adams, MP. *Core Concepts in Pharmacology*. Upper Saddle River, NJ: Pearson Education, 2007.

"The New Over-the-Counter Medicine Label: Take a Look" (accessed July 12, 2007): www.fda.gov

chapter 21

The Skin

LEARNING OBJECTIVES

After completing this chapter, you should be able to:

- List, identify, and diagram the basic anatomical structure of the skin.
- Explain the function or physiology of the skin.
- List and define common diseases affecting the skin and understand the causes, symptoms, and pharmaceutical treatments associated with each disease.

Introduction

The skin is the largest organ of the body, and has several functions. It also is subject to a wide variety (more than 1,000) of medical conditions and diseases. Skin conditions and diseases range from minor irritations to severe infections. Although creams and ointments are widely used to treat skin conditions, treatment options include oral and injectable medications as well. This chapter discusses several common skin conditions and diseases and the treatments available for these disorders.

Anatomy

Considered the largest organ of the body, the skin performs several functions:

- It acts as a mechanical barrier to infection.
- It enables and enhances the sense of touch.
- It assists in regulation of body temperature.
- It allows excretion of waste products and salt from the body.
- Through exposure to sunlight, it enables synthesis of Vitamin D for the absorption of calcium.

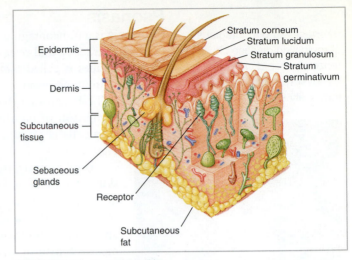

FIGURE 21-1 Structure of the skin.

The skin has three main layers: the epidermis, the dermis, and the subcutaneous layers. The skin provides protection from heat, ultraviolet radiation, and infection. Exposure of the skin to sunlight helps the body to produce Vitamin D, which is needed to make cholesterol and to absorb the calcium and phosphorus that build strong bones. As the largest sensory organ, the skin also plays a large role in the ability to feel heat, cold, pain, and pleasure (see Figure 21-1).

The *epidermis* is the outermost layer of the skin and contains *melanocytes*, where pigment is stored. It is the thinnest skin layer, and is also known as the *scarfskin* or *cuticle layer*.

The *dermis* contains fibroblasts that are responsible for secreting the proteins collagen and elastin. These proteins provide the support for and elasticity of the skin. These proteins are surrounded by a jelly-like substance called the *ground substance*, which also plays a substantial role in maintaining hydration of the skin. The dermal layer contains immune cells involved in the defense against foreign invaders that may pass through the epidermis; it also houses hair follicles, blood vessels, sweat and oil glands, and the sensory receptors for touch, pain, heat, and cold. It has an important role in maintaining body temperature at the norm of about 98.6 degrees Fahrenheit.

The dermis is attached to an underlying subcutaneous layer, also called the *hypodermis*, where the outmost part of the muscle is located. The subcutaneous layer stores **adipose** (fat) tissue, and contains the connective tissue.

adipose fat.

Diseases and Conditions of the Skin

As noted earlier, the skin is prone to more than 1,000 common problems, which may be organized into one of the nine categories discussed briefly in this section.

Rash

A **rash** is an area of red, inflamed skin, or a group of red spots, caused by irritation, allergy, infection, or defects in the skin structure, such as blocked pores or malfunctioning oil glands. Examples of rashes are contact dermatitis, and hives.

rash a skin condition characterized by redness and inflammation.

Eczema

Eczema is a skin inflammation that presents with red pimple-like bumps and is characterized by itching, blistering, or oozing areas that progress to scaly, brownish, or thickened skin. Some of the drugs that have recently been developed for eczema are also used to treat chronic plaque psoriasis. They include two FDA-approved immunomodulator creams and ointments: Elidel® (pimecrolimus) cream, used for mild to moderate atopic eczema; and Protopic™ (tacrolimus), used for severe atopic eczema. *Immunomodulators* are agents that affect the body's immune system in some way. These creams and ointments are not steroids, but are used to treat the itch and inflammation associated with atopic eczema and psoriasis.

eczema an inflammatory skin condition characterized by itching, redness, blistering, and oozing.

Psoriasis

psoriasis a noncontagious, chronic skin disease characterized by rapid skin cell turnover resulting in thick, red, scaly skin.

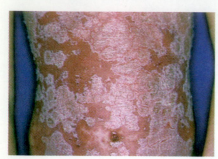

FIGURE 21-2 Psoriasis of the abdomen.

Psoriasis is a noncontagious, chronic immune disorder in which specific immune cells become overactive and release excessive amounts of proteins called *cytokines*. One of these cytokines is called tumor necrosis factor (TNF), which normally helps regulate the body's immune response to infection and inflammation. However, in patients with psoriasis, TNF causes inflammation instead of preventing it. This leads to the formation of painful, often disfiguring psoriasis plaques. The turnover of skin cells is rapid and the affected skin becomes thick, red, and scaly (see Figure 21-2).

Until recently, treatment for psoriasis only managed the patient's pain and skin inflammation. Some of the greatest discoveries—"breakthrough drugs"— in the treatment of skin disorders and diseases have been drugs for chronic plaque psoriasis and psoriatic arthritis. Some of these drugs have also been approved for use with rheumatoid arthritis. This chapter reviews some of the most recent drug discoveries that have changed the way psoriasis is treated and managed.

Treatments for Psoriasis

Enbrel® (etanercept), a subcutaneous injectable drug for psoriasis, is an anti-TNF therapy agent that works by binding to the overproduced TNF. This attachment causes the TNF to become biologically inactive, resulting in a significant reduction in inflammation. This SC injection can be self-administered.

Remicade® (infliximab) is administered by intravenous infusion under the supervision of a specialist and in combination with methotrexate (MTX), a potent antineoplastic agent used in the treatment of rheumatoid arthritis. MTX is given with infliximab to help prevent the formation of anti-infliximab antibodies.

Amevive® (alefacept), which is given IM or as an infusion by a doctor, has the severe adverse reaction of lowering T-cell count, which lessens the immune system's ability to fight cancer, infections, and other diseases. Amevive® works by binding to a specific lymphocyte antigen, CD2, and then inhibiting LFA-3/CD2 interaction, thus reducing lymphocyte (T-cell) counts and thereby treating the cause of psoriasis.

Raptiva® (efalizumab), indicated for plaque psoriasis, is an antibody that prevents activated T-cells from entering the skin. This drug is administered by subcutaneous injection once a week. Common side effects include headache, chills, fever, nausea, muscle aches, and thrombocytopenia. Efalizumab is technically described as an "immunosuppressive recombinant humanized IgG1 kappa isotype monoclonal antibody." This drug binds to a receptor that is expressed on all leukocytes. This attachment inhibits or blocks the adhesion of leukocytes to other cell types. The final result is that Raptiva® decreases the activation of T-lymphocytes and, therefore, the inflammation of psoriatic skin.

Oral Elidel® (pimecrolimus), made by Novartis, selectively inhibits inflammatory cytokine release. Limited evidence suggests the potential efficacy of 20 or 30 milligrams, taken orally twice daily, in the treatment of chronic plaque psoriasis.

Workplace Wisdom Psoriasis

Psoriasis reportedly affects up to 2 percent of the U.S. population.

infection invasion of pathogens into the body; an infection occurs when a pathogenic microbe is able to multiply in the tissues (*colonize*).

Skin Infections

Skin **infections** may be categorized into three types, grouped by causative agent: viral, bacterial, and fungal. The following provides a brief overview of each type.

Viral Infections

A viral skin infection occurs when a virus penetrates the stratum corneum and infects the inner layers of the skin. Examples include herpes simplex, warts, and shingles (herpes zoster). Temporary viral infections, such as chicken pox and measles, also affect the skin. Antibiotics and antibacterial agents cannot cure viral infections; antiviral medications and time are the only two treatments.

A new drug for treating sexually transmitted external genital and anal warts, an immunomodulator known as Aldara® (imiquimod) 5% cream, is now available. Although the warts are caused by the human papilloma virus (HPV) and are not curable, the drug can decrease their size and therefore the severity of pain. HPV is the most common sexually transmitted disease (STD).

Bacterial Infections

Bacterial skin infections are caused by many different bacteria, but the most common bacterial **pathogens** are staphylococci, streptococci, and pseudomonas. If left untreated, these infections may spread throughout the body, becoming more serious and possibly causing systemic infections. Examples include Lyme disease, impetigo, folliculitis, and cellulitis. Cellulitis, impetigo, and folliculitis are the most common bacterial skin infections.

pathogen disease-causing microorganism.

Antibiotics (abbreviated ABX) can be topically or orally administered, depending upon the microorganism and the specific ABX. Antibacterial agents are either **bactericidal** or **bacteriostatic**. Their main mechanism of action is to stop cell wall protein synthesis within the bacterium, which prevents the cell wall from growing. The inside of the cell continues to grow, and eventually bursts through the cell wall, leaking out the cytoplasm and nucleus. Thus, the microorganism explodes, collapses in on itself, and dies.

bactericidal kills microorganisms.

bacteriostatic inhibits the growth and/or reproduction of microorganisms.

Fungal Infections

Fungal skin infections, also known as *mycoses*, occur when normally harmless fungi gain entry into the skin, rather than staying on the outer layer of the skin (epidermis). These infections are usually external, affecting the skin, hair, and nails. Yeasts are a subtype of fungus, characterized by clusters of round or oval cells. Fungal infections occur in damp, dark, and warm places on the body. Examples include athlete's foot, jock itch, and ringworm. Fungal infections such as athlete's foot typically create itchy red areas that may crack or blister. These infections are common and generally mild; however, people with suppressed immune systems, or who have been taking antibiotics for a long time, are more susceptible to fungi spreading deep within the body, causing more serious systemic disease. Patients with diabetes are at highest risk.

Acne

Acne is an infection caused by a bacterium and an overproduction of **sebum** that clogs the hair follicles. The extra sebum accompanies an increase in the number and activity of hair follicles during puberty. Acne can be categorized as either noninflammatory or inflammatory.

acne a bacterial infection accompanied by an overproduction of sebum.

sebum oily substance produced by the sebaceous glands in the skin.

Noninflammatory acne consists of:

- *Whiteheads*, which occur when the trapped sebum and bacteria remain under the skin; may manifest as small white spots.
- *Blackheads*, which occur when the trapped sebum and bacteria partially break through the surface of the skin and turn black (this is due to pigmentation, not dirt).

Inflammatory acne consists of:

- *Papules*, which are formed when the wall of a follicle breaks; white blood cells rush to the site and inflammation occurs.

- *Pustules*, which occur following formation of a papule as the white blood cells move to the surface of the skin.
- *Nodules*, which occur when the follicle wall breaks and causes deep tissue inflammation. A nodule can be painful and may cause tissue damage with scarring.
- *Cysts*, which consist of a liquid- or semi-liquid-filled lesion accompanied by severe inflammation, pain, and scarring.

The exact cause of acne has not been determined, but it is *not* brought on by eating chocolate or greasy foods, as some people believe. However, several factors may increase a person's risk of developing acne:

- Heredity: If the parents had acne, the chances of their children developing acne are higher.
- Hormones: Changes during puberty and pregnancy can cause glands to plug up more frequently.
- Medications: Some drugs, such as oral or injectable steroids, can cause or worsen acne.
- Makeup: Greasy, oily, pore-clogging makeup can lead to acne.

> **INFORMATION**
>
> Acne, the most common skin disease, occurs in approximately 85 percent of all people between the ages of 12 and 24.

Cellulitis

cellulitis inflammation of the connective tissue of the skin.

Cellulitis is an acute, deep infection of the connective tissue accompanied by inflammation. The culprit is staphylococcus, streptococcus, or another bacterium. Enzymes produced by the bacteria destroy skin cells. The skin tissues of the infected area show all the cardinal signs of inflammation, becoming red, irritated, and painful. People most prone to cellulitis include those with a break in the skin from an insect bite or injury; those with a history of peripheral vascular disease (PAD), diabetes, or ischemic ulcers; those who have recently had cardiovascular, pulmonary, or dental procedures or surgeries; and those who use immunosuppressive or corticosteroid medications.

Parasitic Infestations

parasite an organism that lives on or inside another organism.

Parasitic infestations are caused by insects or worms that burrow into the skin to live and/or lay their eggs. Some infestations caused by **parasites** are scabies and lice. Parasites may enter and infect an injured or open wound, or may be transferred from one infested person or object to another person. *Scabies* is characterized by small red bumps and intense itching; it is caused by mites that burrow into the skin from bedding and mattresses.

Lice are insects that spread from person to person by close body contact and/or the sharing of clothes, hats, hairbrushes, and combs. Under the microscope, these insects look like crabs (see Figure 21-3). Three types of lice exist that infect humans: head, body, and pubic. The eggs and the adults must be killed and then removed from the hair. Although lindane-containing products can kill head and body lice, these may cause severe damage to the nervous system. The use of lindane by adults is controversial, and it is no longer used in children. A better choice for children is RID® (pyrethrins) gel or shampoo.

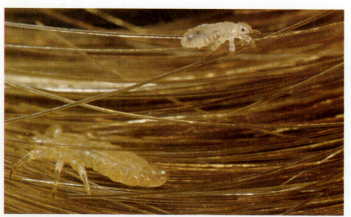

FIGURE 21-3 Parasitic infestation—head lice.

> ## Workplace Wisdom Parasitic Infestations
>
> Any patient who has a prescription to treat a parasitic infestation should be told to wash in very hot water (or dry clean) all recently worn clothing, underwear, sheets, pillowcases, and towels.

Tumors and Cancerous Growths

Tumors and cancerous growths occur when skin cells multiply or reproduce faster than normal. Those without cell mutation are considered *benign* or noncancerous, even though they may grow rapidly. In contrast, tumors or skin growths characterized by rapid reproduction and mutation of cells are considered *malignant* or cancerous.

INFORMATION

Skin cancer affects 800,000 Americans each year, and more than 90 percent of all cases are caused by continuous or early-life sun exposure. Avoiding ultraviolet rays, and early detection with regular checkups, can either prevent skin cancers or prevent benign or precancerous conditions from advancing to malignancies.

There are three main types of skin cancer: basal cell carcinoma, squamous cell cancer, and malignant melanoma.

carcinoma malignant tumor.

Basal Cell Carcinoma

Basal cell **carcinoma** is the most common and most curable skin cancer. It occurs in the epidermis, usually on the face and scalp (see Figure 21-4). The main cause of basal cell carcinoma is early, frequent, and extended sun exposure; this accounts for 25 percent of all new cancers.

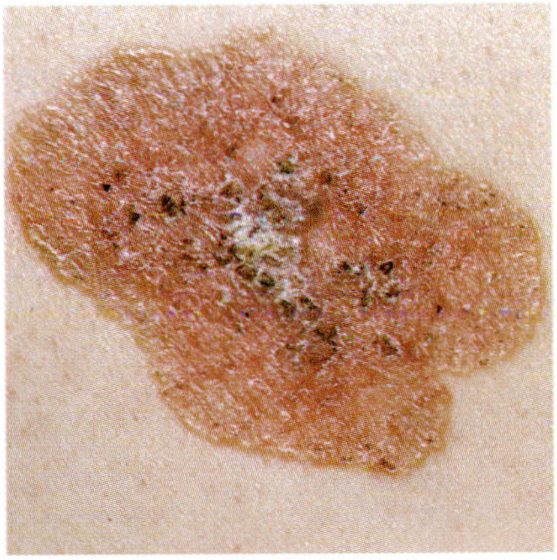

Squamous Cell Cancer

Squamous cell is the second most common skin cancer, accounting for about 20 percent of all skin cancers. It can grow and spread rapidly, often appearing on the back of the hands, on the ears, or on the edges of the lips. It usually develops in the outer layer of the epidermis. When this cancer spreads or *metastasizes*, it can invade distant organs and tissues and become fatal.

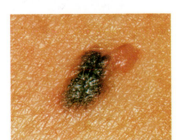

FIGURE 21-4 Basal cell carcinoma.

Malignant Melanoma

Malignant melanoma is the deadliest form of skin cancer; often, the signal is a mole that changes shape or color and may begin to bleed (see Figure 21-5). However, it can be cured if caught when the tumor is still thin and still localized in the outermost layer of the skin. At first, a melanoma is localized, and usually spreads across the skin before it moves into the deeper skin layers.

Precancerous Conditions

An *actinic keratosis (AK)*, also called a *solar keratosis*, is a scaly or crusty bump that originates on the skin surface. It may be light or dark and tan, pink, or red, and is usually rough. Although it may develop slowly, about 5 percent of AKs become squamous cell carcinomas; therefore, AK is considered a *precursor* to cancer or a precancerous growth. It may also spread to other organs and tissues on its own.

FIGURE 21-5 Malignant melanoma.

Pigmentation Disorders

The color of the skin is determined by the amount of melanin produced by the body and, to some extent, genetics. Melanocytes produce melanin. Melanocyte malfunction or absence, exposure to cold or chemicals, infections, or severe skin burns can contribute to

pigmentation color.

loss of skin **pigmentation** or hypopigmentation. An example of hypopigmentation is vitiligo. Additional or excess skin pigmentation is known as *hyperpigmentation*. Causes of hyperpigmentations include hormonal changes (especially in women using systemic birth control), aging, and metabolic disorders. Examples are freckles and age spots or "liver spots."

Miscellaneous Skin Conditions and Diseases

The skin conditions and diseases discussed next do not fall into any of the preceding nine categories.

Hyperkeratosis

Hyperkeratosis is a condition that results from having too much keratin, which is a protein of the skin, hair, and nails. It causes the skin to harden and thicken. Examples of hyperkeratosis include calluses, corns, and warts. *Warts* are small bumps on the skin surface that are caused by a human papilloma virus (HPV).

Wrinkles

Wrinkles are caused by the combination of a breakdown of the collagen and elastin within the dermis, and a reduction in size of the fat cells in the skin; these two factors result in sagging skin. Reduced production of sebum causes the moisture barrier of the skin to become thinner; consequently, more moisture is released, which results in dryer skin. When sagging, loose skin becomes dry, wrinkles are more pronounced.

Rosacea

rosacea a facial skin disorder accompanied by chronic redness and inflammation, and/or acne.

Rosacea is a chronic disorder of unknown cause, in which the skin of the face becomes red and develops pimples and lesions; these symptoms may be accompanied by enlargement of the nose. In oily, acne-prone areas, deep-seated papules and pustules cause small blood vessels to enlarge (*telangiectasia*), resulting in a flushed appearance that may last for long periods of time. There is no cure for rosacea, but with proper treatment the symptoms can be **mitigated** (controlled).

mitigate to lessen or decrease severity.

Spider Veins

Spider veins are broken blood vessels, such as capillaries, which then enlarge. As they enlarge, they become visible through the surface of the skin, varying in color from blue, purple, and orchid, to bright red. The cause may be obesity, tight stockings, exposure to sun, or natural or drug-induced hormonal changes in women.

Burns

Burns can be categorized by cause, as:

- *Thermal*—resulting from contact with fire or heat.
- *Chemical*—resulting from contact to acids, bases, or vesicants.
- *Electrical*—resulting from contact with an electrical current.
- *Friction*—resulting from harsh rubbing of the skin.
- *Sunburn*—resulting from overexposure to sunlight.

Burns are also classified by the severity, depth, or degree of injury to the skin:

- *First-degree* burns—limited damage to the epidermis; characterized by redness and pain. Considered superficial burns.
- *Second-degree* burns—damage to both the epidermis and dermis; characterized by redness, blisters, mild to moderate edema, and pain. Considered moderate burns.

- *Third-degree* burns—destruction of all the epidermis, dermis, and subcutaneous tissue; characterized by a leathery or dry white, brown, or black appearance. Blistering does not occur. These are considered critical burns, and skin grafting is usually recommended.
- *Fourth-degree* burns—destruction of the skin and underlying tissues (muscles, tendons, ligaments, and bones). Considered critical burns; skin grafts are required.

The "Rule of Nines" is used when estimating the amount of body surface area that has been burned. For an adult, the percentage of the body burned can be calculated as follows:

- Head = 9%
- Chest and abdomen = 18%
- Upper/mid/low back and buttocks = 18%
- Each arm = 9%
- Each leg = 18%
- Groin = 1%

For example, if one arm (9 percent), the groin (1 percent) and one leg (18 percent) were affected, the patient would be burned over 28 percent of the body.

The major cause of death among burn patients is not the burn itself, but the complication of infections caused by prolonged treatment and skin grafts. Burned areas are highly susceptible to infection, due to the open lesions. Silver sulfadiazine is a topical burn cream that works by acting on the cell membrane wall to inhibit microbial activity and some yeasts. In addition, when applied at the recommended 1/16-inch thickness, it allows oxygen to pass through to promote healing. The cream is applied once every 12 hours, along with a dressing change.

Workplace Wisdom Burn Statistics

Approximately 2.4 million people report burn injuries each year. Burns result in between 8,000 and 12,000 deaths annually in the United States.

Decubitus Ulcers

A *decubitus ulcer*, also known as a *pressure* or *bed sore*, is an ulceration of the skin due to pressure. These ulcers can also be caused by prolonged friction or exposure to cold. Pressure sores can range from mild (redness and/or blistering, often disappearing soon after pressure is relieved) to severe (deep tissue wounds extending to the bone or through the bone into internal organs). Sixty-seven percent of all pressure sores occur on the hip and buttock regions. The following factors increase the risk of decubitus ulcers:

- fragile skin
- being bedridden or in a wheelchair
- chronic conditions, such as diabetes or cardiovascular disease, in which circulation is impaired
- malnourishment
- older age
- urinary or bowel incontinence
- inability to move body parts without assistance

Decubitus ulcers are classified into stages by the depth or degree of injury to the tissues:

- Stage I—characterized by reddening of unbroken skin; this is an early warning that a problem exists. Usually treated by alleviating pressure, avoiding exposure to the cause, and protecting and padding the area.
- Stage II—characterized by an abrasion, blister, or superficial ulceration of the skin resulting from damage to the epidermis. Treatments include skin lotions to hydrate the tissue around the sore, as well as additional padding and relief of pressure.
- Stage III—characterized by a crater-like lesion that extends through the subcutaneous tissue. Medical care is needed to treat the sore and prevent infection.
- Stage IV—characterized by a lesion that extends through the skin into the muscle, bone, tendon, or ligaments. Can cause life-threatening infections and will not heal without proper treatment.

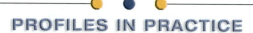

PROFILES IN PRACTICE

Travis is a pharmacy technician at Mercy General Hospital. A patient arrives in the emergency room with third-degree burns on his head, torso, left arm, groin, and both legs.

- What percentage of the patient's body has been burned?

Pharmaceutical Treatment of Various Skin Diseases

Table 21-1 lists drugs that are commonly used to treat various diseases of the skin.

Table 21-1   Drugs Used to Treat Various Skin Diseases

SPECIFIC DISEASE	TYPE OF ORGANISM OR CAUSE	DRUG CLASSIFICATION	NAME (TRADE/ GENERIC) AND DOSAGE
Acne	Bacteria: *Propionibacterium acnes*	Topical antiseptic:	benzoyl peroxide solution 2–3x/day
		Rx anti-acne therapy:	Retin-A® (retinoic acid, tretinoin) cream; apply as directed
	Overproduction of sebum; clogged pores	Topical preparation (unblocks and prevents blockage of pores)	
	Infected hair follicles	Oral/systemic acne	Accutane® (isotretinoin) PO 0.5–1 mg/kg/day × 20 weeks
		Antibiotic	TCN 250–500 mg TID × 10 days
Urticaria (hives)	Allergy or viral infection; can be idiopathic	Antihistamines	Claritin® (loratidine) 10 mg QD
		Anti-inflammatory steroids PO	Prednisone PO as directed
		Immunomodulatory agent PO	Sulfasalazine PO as directed
		Leukotriene inhibitors PO	Accolate® (zafirlukast) 20 mg BID Singulair® (montelukast) 5 mg QD

Table 21-1   Drugs Used to Treat Various Skin Diseases (*continued*)

SPECIFIC DISEASE	TYPE OF ORGANISM OR CAUSE	DRUG CLASSIFICATION	NAME (TRADE/ GENERIC) AND DOSAGE
Psoriasis	Poor immune system Infections: HIV, *H. pylori*, streptococci	Antibiotics, oral	PCN or tetracycline (TCN) PO 250–500 mg TID
		Topical steroids:	Hydrocortisone, betamethasone, fluticasone, methylprednisolone; apply as directed
		Immunosupressant: Topical	Cyclosporin Not to exceed (NTE) 5 mg/kg/day in 2 daily doses
		Immunomodulators:	Protopic® (tacrolimus) 0.03 or 0.1% ointment; apply BID Elidel® (pimecrolimus) cream; apply BID
		Oral immunomodulators:	Elidel® (pimecrolimus) PO in clinical trials
		Humanized therapeutic antibody (monoclonal antibody):	Raptiva® (efalizumab) self-administered SC injection 1/week. Conditioning dose is 0.7 mg/kg, then 1 mg/kg (maximum single dose not to exceed a total of 200 mg).
		Biological drugs (biologic response modifiers or TNF blockers): Immunosuppressive dimeric fusion protein:	Enbrel® (etanercept) SC injection, 50 mg twice weekly for 3 months, then 50 mg/week Amevive® (alefacept) 15 mg IM, once a week, for a total of 12 doses; administered by a doctor.
Arthritic psoriasis	Poor immune system	Topical immunomodulators: Biological drugs: biologic response modifiers or TNF blockers	Protopic® (tacrolimus) 0.03 or 0.1% ointment; apply BID Remicade® (infliximab), IV infusion of 3–5 mg/kg Days 1 & 2 and 6 weeks later (given with MTX).
Eczema		Topical immunomodulators:	Protopic® (tacrolimus) 0.03 or 0.1% ointment; apply BID Elidel® (pimecrolimus) cream; apply BID
Lyme disease (early stages)	Spirochete: *Borrelia burgdorferi*	Oral antibiotics:	amoxicillin 250–500 mg TID doxycycline 250–500 mg BID
Cellulitis	Staphylococcus, streptococcus	Oral antibiotics OR Intravenous (IV) antibiotics	Ancef® (cefazolin) or Dynapen® (dicloxicillin) 250–500 mg TID × 10 days IV cefazolin, oxacillin, or nafcillin; dosage varies
Impetigo (common in children 2 to 5 yrs old)	*Staphylococcus aureus*, streptococcus	Antibiotics: Erythromycin:	Zithromax® (azithromycin) 500 mg on Day 1, then 250 mg qd × 5 days

Table 21-1 Drugs Used to Treat Various Skin Diseases (*continued*)

SPECIFIC DISEASE	TYPE OF ORGANISM OR CAUSE	DRUG CLASSIFICATION	NAME (TRADE/ GENERIC) AND DOSAGE
		Cephalosporin:	Keflex® (cephalexin) 250–500 mg × 10 days
Rosacea	Acne vulgaris, along with other causes	Topical antibiotics	sodium sulfacetamide; apply as directed
		Oral antibiotics	Oral tetracycline or metronidazole (also top) 500 mg PO TID
Herpes cold sore	*Herpes simplex labialis*	Antiviral topical:	Abreva® (docosanol) cream NPT 5 apps/day
External genital and anal warts (STD)	Human papilloma virus	Topical immunomodulator:	Aldara 5% (imiquimod) cream; apply once a day, 3 days a week, leave on 6 hrs.
Ringworm fungi or tinea	*Trichophyton rubrum*	Antifungal topical:	Fulvicin® P/G (griseofulvin) Lotrimin® (clotrimazole)
Cuts	Infection prevention	Topical antibacterials:	Neosporin®, Cortisporin®, Triple Antibiotic® ointment (neomycin + polymixin b + bacitracin)
Burns	Infection prevention and oxygen promotion	Topical anti-infectives:	Silvadene® (silver sulfadiazine), Sulfamylon® (mafenide acetate); apply as directed
Athlete's foot	*Tinea pedis, Trichophyton rubrum, Epidermophyton floccosum*	Antifungal (topical cream, gel, spray, and liquid forms):	miconazole 2%, tolnaftate 1%, clotrimazole 1%, and naftifine 1% Fungizone® (amphotericin B); apply as directed
Parasites	Lice or scabies	Antiparasitic topical agents:	Kwell® (lindane) shampoo or solution [not for use with children] RID® gel (pyrethrins) Apply as directed
Hyperkeratosis	Excessive production of keratin Viruses (warts)	Keratolytics: Lactates for hardened dry skin Warts, corns, and acne	Alpha Keri Lotion®, Cetaphil®; apply as directed Salicylic or beta hydroxy acids Benzoyl peroxide creams, sol, gels Apply as directed
Pain	N/A	Topical analgesics:	Solarcaine® (benzocaine), Nupercainal®, Lidocaine®, xylocaine
Infection prevention	Various bacteria	Topical antiseptics:	Alcohol, merthiolate, Zephiran® (benzalk-onium chloride) Apply as directed
Itching	Allergic reactions, contact dermatitis, inflammation, dryness	Antihistamines, topical:	Benadryl® gel, lotion, cream (diphenhydramine)

Table 21-1   Drugs Used to Treat Various Skin Diseases (*continued*)

SPECIFIC DISEASE	TYPE OF ORGANISM OR CAUSE	DRUG CLASSIFICATION	NAME (TRADE/ GENERIC) AND DOSAGE
		Corticosteroid topical creams, ointments, solutions:	Corticaine® (hydrocortisone) Valisone®, Celestone® (betamethasone) Kenalog®, Aristocort® (triamcinonide) Lidex® (fluocinonide) Synalar® (fluocinolone) Cordan® (flurandrenolide) Apply as directed
Skin cancer	Exposure to sun, chemicals, genetic predisposition	Topical chemotherapeutic agent: Immunomodulator:	5FU (fluorouracil) cream; apply as directed Aldara® (imiquimod 5%) cream; apply once a day for 2 days a week, 3 to 4 days apart
		NSAIDs: Precancer treatment of actinic keratosis	Solaraze® (diclofenac sodium) 3% gel; apply BID

SUMMARY

The skin, considered the largest body organ, consists of three main layers: the epidermis, the dermis, and the subcutaneous layer. The skin performs several important functions, serving as a barrier to foreign organisms and debris, managing and regulating the body temperature, excreting salts and excess water, and acting as a shock absorber to protect the underlying organs.

Diseases of the skin can range from simple rashes to deadly cancers (malignant melanoma). The most common skin disease, acne, affects approximately 17 million Americans. Fortunately, a large array of pharmaceuticals is available to treat skin conditions and diseases.

CHAPTER REVIEW QUESTIONS

1. Which layer of skin contains blood vessels and hair follicles?
   a. dermis
   b. epidermis
   c. subcutaneous layer
   d. both b and c

2. Which of the following drugs indicated for psoriasis is administered intramuscularly?
   a. Amevive®
   b. Enbrel®
   c. Remicade®
   d. none of the above

3. Cellulitis is characterized by inflammation of the:
   a. dermis.
   b. epidermis.
   c. subcutaneous layer.
   d. deep connective tissue.

4. Which of the following is considered the deadliest form of skin cancer?
   a. basal cell carcinoma
   b. malignant melanoma
   c. squamous cell cancer
   d. benign skin tumors

5. The cause of the skin condition _____ is unknown.
   a. cellulitis
   b. hyperkeratosis
   c. rosacea
   d. spider veins

6. Elidel® cream is used to treat which of the following skin conditions?
   a. acne
   b. rosacea
   c. eczema
   d. urticaria

7. Herpes simplex, herpes zoster, and warts are classified as what type of skin disease?
   a. bacterial skin infection
   b. fungal skin infection
   c. parasitic skin infestation
   d. viral skin infection

8. Patients with diabetes are considered at high risk for fungal skin infections.
   a. true
   b. false

9. Skin cancer affects approximately _____ in the United States each year.
   a. 2 percent of the population
   b. 800,000 people
   c. 17 million people
   d. 50 percent of the population

10. Which of the following drugs is used to treat lice infestations in children?
    a. griseofulvin
    b. lindane
    c. miconazole
    d. pyrethrins

CRITICAL THINKING QUESTIONS

1. What type of precautions should a caregiver use when administering treatment to a patient with severe burns, or when applying medication to burns?

2. Discuss what can be done to prevent the spread of parasite infestations?

3. Why do you believe acne affects so many people? What do you think can be done (outside of medication) to help reduce the number and severity of acne outbreaks?

WEB CHALLENGE

1. Visit The American Cancer Society's website at http://www.cancer.org to learn more about skin cancer. Write a summary of ways to prevent basal and squamous cell cancer.

2. To learn more about adult and pediatric dermatological conditions, go to http://www.healthsystem.virginia.edu. At the home page, click on the "Patients & Visitors" tab and then choose *patient information*. Then, from the drop-down menu (under adult or children health topics), choose dermatology. Write a short summary of three conditions you find discussed at this Web site; include treatment options.

3. Visit http://www.acne.org to learn more about the causes of acne.

REFERENCES AND RESOURCES

"About Aldara® (imiquimod)—Package Insert for Both External Genital Warts and Actinic Keratoses" (accessed July 7, 2007): http://www.3m.com/us/healthcare/pharma/aldara/AKPI.pdf

"About Amevive® (alefacept) Doctor's Guide: Amevive (Alefacept), Treatment for Psoriasis, Approved in Israel, Receives 'Positive Opinion' from Swiss Regulatory Authority, May 3, 2004" (accessed July 7, 2007):
http://www.pslgroup.com/dg/243fd2.htm;
http://www.rxlist.com/cgi/generic3/amevive.htm;
http://www.centerwatch.com/patient/drugs/dru820.html

"About Commonly Sexually Transmitted Diseases: HPV" (accessed July 7, 2007): http://www.princeton.edu/puhs/SECH/hpv.html

"About Elidel® 1% (pimecrolimus) cream for eczema by National Eczema Society" (accessed July 7, 2007):
http://www.eczema.org/PIMECROLIMUSCREAM.pdf

"About Enbrel® (etanercept) FDA approval of Enbrel (etanercept) for psoriasis on April 30, 2004" (accessed July 3, 2007):
http://www.amgen.com/news/viewPR.jsp?id=521767;

http://www.enbrel.com/news/pdf/Enbrel_Psoriasis_Approval.pdf;
http://my.webmd.com/content/article/86/99063.htm

"About Raptiva® (efalizumab)" (accessed July 1, 2007):
http://www.thedrugdatabase.com/directory/R/Raptiva;
http://www.raptiva.com/about/faqs.jsp#Q7

"About Raptiva: Genetech Patient and Professional Information Website" (accessed June 29, 2007): http://www.drugs.com/raptiva.html

"About Remicade® (infliximab)" (accessed June 29, 2007): http://www.dermnetnz.org/dna.psoriasis/infliximab.html

"About Skin Anatomy and Physiology" (accessed June 29, 2007): http://www.essentialdayspa.com/Skin_Anathomy_and_Physiology.htm

"About Skin Cancer: The Skin Cancer Foundation" (accessed June 20, 2007): http://www.skincancer.org

"About Tacrolimus for Eczema and Psoriasis: AAD: Tacrolimus Ointment Safe and Effective in All Ages for Mild to Moderate Eczema, by Bruce Sylvester" (accessed June 29, 2007):
http://www.docguide.com/news/content.nsf/news/

8525697700573E1885256E37006578F2?OpenDocument&id=48d de4a73e09a969852568880078c249&c=Dermatitis&count=10

"Acne" (accessed September 17, 2007): http://www.medicinenet.com

Adams, MP, Josephson, DL, & Holland, LN Jr. *Pharmacology for Nurses—A Pathophysiologic Approach*. Upper Saddle River, NJ: Pearson Education, 2005.

American Association of Family Physicians. "Common Bacterial Skin Infections" (accessed June 29, 2007): http://www.aafp.org/afp/20020701/119.html

"Decubitus Ulcer Information and Wound Stages." LDHP Medication Review Services Corporation, December 1999 (accessed September 17, 2007): http://www.expertlaw.com

"Degree of Burns" (accessed September 15, 2007): http://www.burnsurvivorsttw.org

"Food, Drug and Cosmetic Act" (accessed July 7, 2007): http://www.fda.gov/opacom/laws/fdcact/fdcact1.htm

"Healthepic Anatomy of Skin" (accessed June 29, 2007): http://www.healthepic.com/hers/static/hers_beauty_skindeep_anatomy.htm

Holland, N, & Adams, MP. *Core Concepts in Pharmacology*. Upper Saddle River, NJ: Pearson Education, 2003.

"How to Treat Burns of All Degrees" (accessed September 15, 2007): http://www.med-help.net

Kamel, MN. "Anatomy of the Skin" (accessed June 27, 2007): http://www.telemedicine.org/anatomy.htm#functions

Moyer, P. "About ORAL Elidel® AAD: Oral Pimecrolimus Effective in Treating Psoriasis" (accessed June 29, 2007): http://www.pslgroup.com/dg/22ebd2.htm

"Pressure Ulcer" (accessed September 17, 2007): http://www.nlm.nih.gov

Revis, DR. "Decubitus Ulcers." October 25, 2005 (accessed September 17, 2007): http://www.emedicine.com

"What is Acne?" (accessed September 17, 2007): http://www.skincarephysicians.com

"What is Acne? Fast Facts: An Easy-to-Read Series of Publications for the Public" (accessed September 17, 2007): http://www.niams.nih.gov

LEARNING OBJECTIVES

After completing this chapter, you should be able to:

- List, identify, and diagram the basic anatomical structure and parts of the eye and ear.

- Describe the function or physiology of the ears and eyes.

- List and define common diseases affecting the eyes and understand the causes, symptoms, and pharmaceutical treatments associated with each disease.

- List and define common diseases affecting the ears and understand the causes, symptoms, and pharmaceutical treatments associated with each disease.

Introduction

Chapter 21 discussed the largest sensory organ, the skin. This chapter explores the sense of sight, the sense of hearing, and the respective sensory organs, the eye and the ear. Vision is the most basic and primary of our senses, and we tend to value it more than any other sense. Loss of sight usually means that a person will rely more acutely on the sense of hearing. Many parts of the eye contribute to the perception of a good image, but it is the retina, a piece of brain tissue, that is most vital for vision; it takes direct stimulation from the world outside the body, in the form of light, and begins the process of translating that stimulation into images.

The ear is responsible for hearing. Sound waves travel from the outer ear down the external auditory canal, striking the eardrum and making it vibrate. These vibrations cause three tiny bones in the middle ear to amplify the sound to the cochlea of the inner ear. From here, nerves ultimately transmit the sound to the brain where it's interpreted. Disorders of the ear include infection of the Eustachian tube, or *serous otitis media*, complications of earwax buildup, and types of hearing loss.

Anatomy and Physiology of the Eye

The main structures of the eye include the cornea, sclera, conjunctiva, iris, pupil, lens, retina, optic nerve, macula, vitreous humor, choroid, and the extraocular muscles (see Figure 22-1).

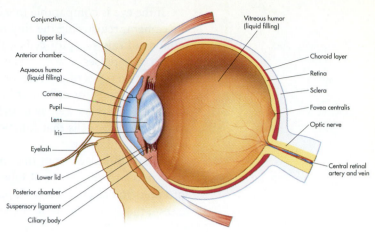

FIGURE 22-1 Anatomy of the eye.

- The *cornea* is the clear or transparent outer "window" of the eye, made up primarily of connective tissue. It focuses light as the light enters the eye.

- The opaque, white portion around the circumference of the cornea is the *sclera*.

- The thin, transparent layer that extends from the edge of the cornea and covers the sclera and lines the inside of the eyelids is the *conjunctiva*.

- The colored disc visible through the cornea is the *iris*. The opening in the iris is the *pupil*.

- The *lens* (or *crystalline lens*) is located directly behind the iris. The lens focuses light onto the retina.

- Often referred to as the "film" of the camera, the *retina* lines the back of the eye. The retina is composed of sensory tissue that converts light rays into impulses that move along the optic nerve.

- The *optic nerve* is the visual pathway by which electrical impulses move from the retina to the brain and back.

- The *macula* is a small yellowish area in the retina that provides the most central and acute vision.

- The *vitreous* **humor**, composed mostly of water, occupies about 80 percent of the interior of the eye between the lens and the retina.

humor a body fluid.

- The *choroid* is the layer between the sclera and the retina. The choroid is composed of layers of nourishing blood vessels.

Three pairs of extraocular muscles regulate the motion of each eye: the medial/lateral rectus muscles, the superior/inferior rectus muscles, and the superior/inferior oblique muscles. Cranial nerve III stimulates four of the six extraocular muscles: medial rectus, superior rectus, inferior rectus, and inferior oblique. The eye orbit is surrounded in layers of soft, fatty tissue, which protect and cushion the eye and enable it to turn easily.

How the Eye Works

Understanding of specific eye diseases begins with knowledge of how the eye works. As you know, the function of the eyes is to allow the person to see. Vision occurs as light waves reflected from an object, such as a building, enter the eye through the cornea and then through the pupil. The light waves *converge*, or come together, first at the cornea, and then are further focused by the crystalline lens, to a nodal point called "N" that is located on the immediate backside surface of the lens. This is the point where the image becomes *inverted* (turned upside-down). In a young pair of eyes, the lens of the eye can modify its shape to change focus from far distance to near distance.

The light progresses through the vitreous humor and then back to a clear focus on the retina and macula (see Figure 22-2).

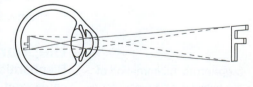

FIGURE 22-2 The eye as a camera.

If the eye is comparable to a camera, the retina would be considered the film inside the camera, registering the tiny photons of light that interact with it. Inside the retina, millions of tiny receptor cells, called *photoreceptors*, absorb the light energy and trigger nerve impulses.

The two types of photoreceptors are called rods and cones. *Rods* are the elongated, rod-shaped receptor cells that function best in low light. They are used for peripheral and night vision as well as in the perception of shape, size, and brightness. *Cones* are conical receptor cells that function best in bright light; they enhance the perception of fine detail and color.

Nerve impulses from the cones and rods are sent as electrical signals along the optic nerve to the occipital lobe at the posterior of the brain. This part of the brain interprets the electrical signals as visual images. Therefore, it is actually the brain that "sees"; the eyes only aid in the visual process (primarily as light collectors).

Diseases of the Eyes

ophthalmic pertaining to the eye.

The eyes are prone to many diseases and disorders, including infection, vision problems, and allergic reactions. With most common **ophthalmic** products, side effects are minimal, but may include localized ocular toxicity and hypersensitivity, including eyelid itching and swelling, and conjunctival redness. Ophthalmic products must be sterile, pH-balanced, clear, and particle-free; they are typically used for dry eyes, infection, inflammation, and allergies. This chapter discusses infections and vision disorders. The treatment of allergic reactions involving the eyes, with anti-allergenic agents, antihistamines, artificial tears, and anti-inflammatory products, is addressed in Chapter 25, in a section on allergies.

Eye Infections and Pharmaceutical Treatment

This section describes some common infections of the eye and the pharmaceutical treatment of those infections.

Stye

stye an infection of one (or more) of the sebaceous glands of the eye.

hordeolum an infection of one (or more) of the sebaceous glands of the eye.

A **stye** or **hordeolum** is a localized infection of the sebaceous gland in a hair follicle at the base of an eyelash. Although visual acuity is unchanged, a stye is accompanied by redness, swelling, and eyelid pain. If the infection is deep within the lid, it is called a *meibomianitis* or *internal hordeolum*, and is sometimes accompanied by conjunctivitis and purulent drainage. Anti-infective eye drops are instilled into the lower conjunctival sac, and warm tap water or cold compresses can be applied for 10 minutes per hour, or 20 minutes four times a day, to control inflammation.

Staphylococcus aureus and *Staphylococcus epidermidis* are the most likely culprits, so treatment is with antibiotics. Topical antibiotics are usually ineffective. Styes typically disappear on their own, and therefore oral antibiotic therapy is usually not warranted. In rare cases, though, oral antibiotic therapy could include a 10-day course of one of the following:

- dicloxacillin 250 mg PO q6h
- erythromycin 250 mg PO qid
- tetracycline 250 mg PO qid
- amoxicillin 500 mg PO tid

Blepharitis

blepharitis inflammation of the eyelid margins accompanied by redness.

Blepharitis is an inflammation of the eyelid margins, accompanied by redness, thickening, and possibly the formation of scales and crusts or shallow marginal ulcers. Ulcerative blepharitis is considered acute, whereas seborrheic blepharitis and meibomian gland dysfunction (meibomitis) are chronic types of blepharitis. The latter is often associated with acne rosacea. To treat ulcerative blepharitis, use one of the following antibiotic ointments for seven to ten days:

- bacitracin/polymyxin B
- gentamicin 0.3% qid

To treat seborrheic blepharitis, improve hygiene; use diluted baby shampoo to clean the eyelids and remove greasy buildup.

To treat for meibomian gland dysfunction, use oral antibiotic: doxycycline 100 mg PO bid, over 3 to 4 months tapered down over the course of therapy.

Conjunctivitis

Conjunctivitis is the acute or chronic inflammation of the conjunctiva caused by a virus, bacteria, allergy, or irritant wind, smoke, or snow. Conjunctivitis has four major causes: allergies, bacteria, viruses, and chlamydia. Conjunctivitis can accompany the common cold and *exanthems* (viral rashes), such as rubella, measles, chickenpox (varicella), and mumps.

conjunctivitis acute or chronic inflammation of the eye conjunctiva.

Allergic Conjunctivitis

Allergic conjunctivitis or "redeye," is caused by hay fever, dust, mite dander, or animal dander. Allergic conjunctivitis usually affects both eyes; symptoms include itching, swelling, and tearing. Allergic conjunctivitis is usually seasonal and is not contagious.

Bacterial Conjunctivitis

Bacterial conjunctivitis often starts in one eye but soon spreads to the other. It usually includes a thick, sticky **mucopurulent** discharge that causes the eyelids and eyelashes to be matted or pasted shut upon awakening. There may be mild sensitivity to light (*photophobia*) with some discomfort, but usually no pain. Visual function is normal in most cases. The eye creates its own bacteriostatic lysozymes and immunoglobulins in the tear film, contributing to its strong immune defense. The eye will fight to return to homeostasis and the infecting bacteria will eventually be destroyed.

mucopurulent containing or composed of mucus and pus.

However, an extra-heavy load of external organisms can overpower the immune system, causing a conjunctival infection and setting the eye up for potential corneal infection. Therefore, antibiotics should be given to avoid such a possibility. A broad-spectrum ophthalmic antibiotic, treating both gram-positive and gram-negative organisms, and an anti-inflammatory will treat both the infection and the inflammation (see Table 22-1). A wet, sticky, matted-shut eyelid is usually indicative of bacterial conjunctivitis that is highly contagious (see Figure 22-3).

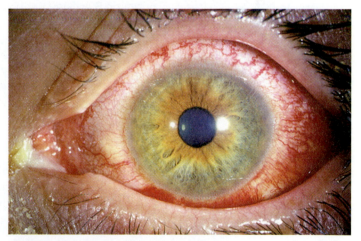

FIGURE 22-3 Bacterial conjunctivitis. (Phototake NYC.)

Workplace Wisdom Contagious Conjunctivitis

Patients with contagious conjunctivitis should take the precautions necessary to avoid passing the infection to others or reinfecting themselves. Precautions include frequent handwashing and avoidance of swimming, shaking hands, or touching the face, as well as disinfecting counters and doorknobs, and not reusing towels, handkerchiefs, or tissues.

Table 22-1 Various Topical Ophthalmics Used for Ocular Infections

TRADE NAME	GENERIC NAME	INDICATION	SIG
Antibacterials (ABs)			
Aminoglycosides			
Tobrex®	tobramycin, 0.3% solution or ointment	bacterial conjunctivitis, corneal infections	1 to 2 gtts q4 hr Severe infections: 2 gtts q1 hr until improvement, then the above regimen. Apply $\frac{1}{2}$-inch ribbon ung q3–4 hr
Genoptic®	gentamicin	bacterial conjunctivitis, corneal infections	1 to 2 gtts q4 hr
Garamycin Ophthalmic®	gentamicin, ophthalmic solution, 0.3%	bacterial conjunctivitis, corneal ulcers, blepharitis	Severe infections: 2 gtts q1 hr
Erythromycins (ABs)			
Ilotycin®	erythromycin, ophthalmic ointment, 0.5%	neonatal inclusion or chlamydial, *Neisseria gonorrhea*, or swimming pool conjunctivitis	Apply approx. 1 cm ribbon ung not to exceed (NTE) 6 times/day
Sulfur-Based Antibacterials			
Bleph-10®	sulfacetamide sodium, ophthalmic solution, 10%	bacterial infections that may or may not accompany viral infection (secondary infections)	1 to 2 gtts q2–3 hr, tapered down for 7–10 days
Combination Antibiotics			
Maxitrol®	polymixin B sulfate, neomycin, and bacitracin zinc (ointment)	blepharitis, nongonococcal bacterial and adult gonococcal conjunctivitis	Apply 1 cm ribbon ung, q2 hr qid. In addition, single dose of ceftriaxone 1 g IM or ciprofloxacin 500 mg bid PO for 5 days
Polytrim®	polymixin B sulfate, trimethoprim sulfate, and gentamicin 0.3%	bacterial infections, blepharitis, nongonococcal bacterial and adult gonococcal conjunctivitis	Apply 1 cm ribbon ung, q2 hr qid
Fluoroquinalones (ABs)			
Ciloxan®	ciprofloxacin	bacterial infections caused by stubborn resistant pseudomonas	1–2 gtt qid to q1 hr for the first few days
Ocuflox®	ofloxacin, 0.3% solution	same as above	1–2 gtts q2–4 hr for 2 days, then 1–2 q4 hr for 7 days
Chibroxin®	norfloxacin, 0.3%	same as above	1–2 gtts q4 hr NTE 7 days
Combination Drugs			
Tobradex®	tobramycin and dexamethasone; antibacterial and steroid combinations for infection and inflammation	bacterial conjunctivitis, corneal ulcers	Apply approx. $\frac{1}{2}$-inch ribbon ung, NTE 4 times/day. 1 to 2 gtts q4–6 hr

Table 22-1 Various Topical Ophthalmics Used for Ocular Infections (*continued*)

TRADE NAME	GENERIC NAME	INDICATION	SIG
Antivirals			
Viroptic®	trifluridine solution 1% (a pyrimidine (thymidine) analog activated by cellular thymidine kinase)	epithelial keratitis caused by herpes simplex virus and keratoconjunctivitis; (works by inhibition of DNA polymerase; DOC in United States for topical ophthalmic antiviral therapy as it is least vulnerable to resistant strains)	To cornea: 1 gtt q2 hr NTE 9 gtts/day, then 1 gtt q4 hr and tapered thereafter
Vira-A®	vidarabine, ointment 3%	acute keratoconjunctivitis, epithelial keratitis caused by herpes simplex virus 1 & 2 (interferes with early steps of viral DNA synthesis; rapidly metabolizes to Ara-Hx)	$\frac{1}{2}$-inch ribbon q3 hr, NTE 5 doses/day
Herplex® (halogenated pyrimidine derivatives)	idoxuridine, solution 0.1% and ointment	acute keratoconjunctivitis, epithelial keratitis caused by herpes simplex virus 1 & 2 (slows growth of viruses by blocking reproduction; produces incorrect DNA copies, thus preventing the virus from replicating and infecting or destroying tissue)	Ointment: $\frac{1}{3}$-inch ribbon q4 hr. Solution: 1 gtt q1 hr during a.m., q2 hr during p.m.
Antihistamines			
Emadine®	emedastine difumarate, ophthalmic solution 0.05%	allergic conjunctivitis (antihistamine prevents H-1 from binding on the eye cell, thus preventing itching, watering, and redness)	1 gtt in the affected eye, NTE 4 times daily
Livostin™ 0.05%®	levocabastine suspension, 0.05%	allergic conjunctivitis (antihistamine for seasonal allergic conjunctivitis. MOA same as above)	1 gtt qid
Patanol®	olopatadine, 0.1%	allergic conjunctivitis (antihistamine. MOA same as above)	1 drop, bid or q6–8 hr
Mast Cell Stabilizers			
Alomide®	lodoxamide, solution 0.1%	allergic conjunctivitis (mast cell inhibitors prevent allergic reactions) and for vernal keratoconjunctivitis, vernal conjunctivitis	1–2 gtts qid, NTE 3 months
Crolom®	cromolyn sodium, 4%	allergic conjunctivitis	1–2 gtt qid
Alamast®	pemirolast potassium, 0.01%	allergic conjunctivitis	1–2 gtt qid

Table 22-1   Various Topical Ophthalmics Used for Ocular Infections (*continued*)

TRADE NAME	GENERIC NAME	INDICATION	SIG
Anti-inflammatory Agents			
Acular®	ketorolac	any conjunctivitis (for NSAID anti-inflammatories MOA, see Chapter 9 re inflammation process and site of action of ASA, NSAIDs, and COX-2 inhibitors)	1 drop qid
Eflone®, Forte Liquifilm®, FML Liquifilm®, FML S.O.P.® 0.1% ointment	fluorometholone, 0.1% suspension or ointment	any conjunctivitis (MOA of topical corticosteroids for inflammation in stubborn cases of conjunctivitis, keratitis, iritis MOA: inducing phospholipase A2 inhibitory proteins responsible for controlling the biosynthesis of prostaglandins and leukotrienes, thereby reducing or inhibiting the release of arachidonic acid and interfering with the inflammation cycle)	1–2 gtt bid, tid, and qid
Pred Forte®	prednisolone acetate, 0.12 to 1.0%	any conjunctivitis (MOA of topical corticosteroids for inflammation in stubborn cases, same as above)	1 drop every 1–6 hr. Caution: Use may cause glaucoma
Decongestants/Vasoconstrictors			
Naphcon®, Allerest®, Clear Eyes®	naphazoline HCl, 0.1% solution	allergic conjunctivitis (decongestant vasoconstrictor returns blood to its origin, reducing redness)	1 drop, bid to qid, NTE 5 days
OcuClear®, Visine LR®	oxymetazolone, 0.025% solution	same as above	1–2 gtts qid
Visine®, Murine Plus®	tetrahydrozoline 0.05% solution	same as above	1–2 gtts bid–tid
Combination Drugs			
Naphcon-A®	naphazoline HCl/ pheniramine maleate, 0.1% solution (decongestant with an antihistamine)	allergic conjunctivitis (MOA—vasoconstriction, while antihistamine prevents H1 binding on eye cells)	1 drop, bid–qid, NTE 5 days
Zaditor®	ketotifen fumarate, 0.025% (antihistamine-mast cell stabilizer with anti-inflammatory properties)	allergic conjunctivitis (MOA— antihistamine binds to H-1 receptors of the eyes, preventing allergic response; mast cell stabilizer prevents H-1 release, decreasing chemotaxis and activation of eosinophils; inhibits pro-inflammatory mediators)	1 drop q8–12 hr (patients over 3 years of age)

Viral Conjunctivitis

Viral conjunctivitis or "pinkeye" has a short duration and is usually self-limiting, about one week in mild cases and up to three weeks in severe cases. It usually follows an upper respiratory infection or results from contact with someone who is infected. No treatment or cure is currently available. Symptoms, however, can often be relieved with lubricants and cool compresses. If it is suspected that a bacterial infection is also present, treat with ophthalmic antibiotics, such as sulfacetamide sodium 10% drops or trimethoprim/polymyxin B for seven to ten days. A matted-down, shut eyelid with a crust is indicative of viral conjunctivitis, which is contagious.

Conjunctivitis Caused by Chlamydia

Conjunctivitis may be caused by the sexually transmitted disease chlamydia. Often referred to as *neonatal inclusion conjunctivitis* or *swimming pool conjunctivitis*, newborns can acquire the infection from their mothers as they pass through the birth canal. Neonates are treated with erythromycin 12.5 mg/kg PO or IV qid for 14 days, because pneumonia and other complications may result from untreated conjunctivitis.

Infected mothers and their sexual partners are also treated to cure the conjunctivitis and concomitant genital infection with one of the following:

- azithromycin 1 g PO once
- doxycycline 100 mg PO bid for 1 week
- erythromycin 500 mg PO qid for 1 week

Eye Disorders That Affect Vision

Eye infections are usually self-limiting; only severe infections require treatment with antibiotics. Infections rarely contribute to vision problems. This section addresses eye diseases that affect the function of the eye and contribute to irreversible vision problems; we also discuss treatments available for these diseases and conditions.

Glaucoma

Glaucoma is one of the leading causes of permanent blindness, affecting more than 2 million Americans. Glaucoma is a slow, progressive disease that increases the **intraocular** pressure of the aqueous humor and decreases the outflow of aqueous humor. Visual impairment is irreversible and permanent. Blindness from glaucoma is inevitable, as there is no cure for glaucoma. However, its progress can be slowed with proper care.

glaucoma a group of eye diseases characterized by an increase in intraocular pressure.

intraocular within the eye.

Groups at high risk include:

- African Americans
- Asians
- patients who have family members with glaucoma
- patients who have had eye injury
- steroid users
- persons over the age of 60

Other risk factors include:

- nearsightedness
- diabetes
- hypertension

Glaucoma is usually **asymptomatic**. In most cases, detection and prevention of the disease is through glaucoma screening during routine eye examinations.

asymptomatic showing no evidence of disease or disordered condition.

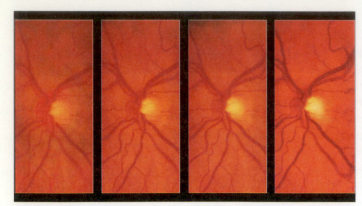

FIGURE 22-4 Open-angle glaucoma: Four retinal images of a glaucomatous optic disk taken over a six-year period (left to right). (Phototake NYC.)

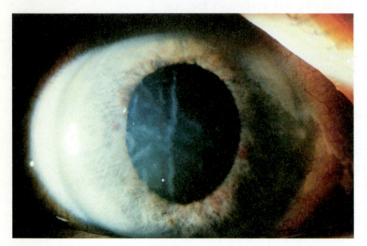

FIGURE 22-5 Closeup of an eye with narrow-angle glaucoma, shown as a cloudy, steamy cornea. (Phototake NYC.)

There are two main types of glaucoma: open angle and closed angle. Patients with glaucoma should consult with their physician before taking any OTC medication. Antihistamines, decongestants, and vasoconstrictors may worsen their condition, as these drugs can increase intraocular pressure (IOP).

Open-Angle Glaucoma

Open-angle glaucoma, or *wide-angle glaucoma*, constitutes about 90 percent of all cases of glaucoma (see Figure 22-4). It is defined as an increase in intraocular pressure due to abnormality in the trabecular meshwork that controls flow of aqueous humor between the anterior chamber and the canal of Schlemm. In this disorder, the canal is impaired and does not allow the fluid to return to the blood system. Because the fluid does not drain fast enough, IOP builds up and creates pressure against the optic nerve. If not treated, the condition can lead to a gradual loss of vision. Three basic treatments are available: medication, laser surgery, and filtration surgery. The goal of treatment is to lower the pressure in the eye.

Closed-Angle Glaucoma

In *closed-angle* or *narrow-angle glaucoma*, the anterior chamber of the eye (the space between the cornea and iris) fills with aqueous humor and the iris becomes misshapen (see Figure 22-5). The edge of the iris blocks drainage of the humor, causing an increase in pressure. Closed-angle is the least common and most devastating form of glaucoma.

Although patients with open-angle glaucoma do not experience symptoms, those with closed-angle glaucoma may. Symptoms can come on rapidly, and should be considered an emergency, as blindness can occur within three to five days if left untreated. Symptoms include:

- sudden intermittent changes in IOP due to extensive and prolonged pupil dilation
- ocular pain or inflammation
- blurred vision
- headache
- pressure over the eye
- a cloudy cornea
- extreme sensitivity to light, or seeing halos around lights
- nausea and/or vomiting
- moderate pupil dilation that is not reactive to light

The cause is usually an inherited anatomic deformity of the anterior chamber, which predisposes it to be or to become narrow so that aqueous humor cannot freely flow or drain. In addition to heredity, any one of the following may precipitate closure of the anterior chamber:

- defect in the eye chamber
- anything that causes the pupil to dilate (dim lighting, dilation, drops for eye examinations)

- certain oral or injected medications
- blow to the eye
- diabetes-related growth of abnormal blood vessels over the angle
- most at risk are Asian, farsighted, or over the age of 60. People in these groups should have their pressure checked every year or two.

Secondary Glaucoma

Secondary glaucoma occurs as the result of an eye injury, inflammation, tumor, advanced cases of cataracts, or diabetes, or it can be induced by use of drugs such as steroids. This form of glaucoma may be mild or severe, and may be either open-angle or closed-angle glaucoma. Treatment is the same as for primary glaucoma.

Many cortisone-like drugs are widely used to treat a variety of conditions, such as asthma, poison ivy, arthritis, and other inflammatory conditions. Such drugs as ingredients in eyedrops or eye ointments may cause secondary glaucoma; people with existing primary glaucoma must be sure not to use them. Corticosteroids that are injectable, oral, or topically applied to the skin are not a danger to most patients. However, after glaucoma patients undergo a guarded filtration procedure, in which a new drain is made, postsurgical use of such corticosteroids will be required for approximately one month to reduce inflammation and prevent scarring that could close the new drain.

Oral medications taken for high blood pressure can cause problems for people with glaucoma. Therefore, it is advisable for glaucoma patients to try to control their blood pressure by nonmedicinal means, such as weight reduction and exercise. When lifestyle changes are not effective, antihypertensive medications will be indicated, but the glaucoma must be carefully monitored and can worsen.

Fluid is constantly flowing into and out of the eye. If that flow is blocked, the pressure inside the eye rises. Oral cold remedies may contain drugs that enlarge or dilate the pupil by causing the iris to constrict. These prescription drugs are atropine or atropine-like products. (The same compound can be found in Lomotil® for diarrhea.) The dilated pupil places pressure on the drain, preventing the release of aqueous humor, because outflow channels are blocked by the iris when the pupil is enlarged. Psychotropic agents and "tranquilizers" also dilate the pupil. Therefore, people with narrow anterior chamber angles are at risk for developing elevated IOP when their pupils are dilated (as in the dark, or from use of eyedrops or oral medications that dilate the pupil). The FDA requires labels on these agents to warn consumers that the medications may cause glaucoma and should not be used by persons with existing glaucoma. Those who have had **iridotomy** are not at risk of new closure by such drugs.

Drugs for glaucoma either decrease the formation of aqueous humor, increase the outflow of aqueous humor, or both (see Table 22-2). The newest type of antiglaucoma agent, a prostanoid selective FP receptor agonist, works by increasing the outflow of aqueous humor by two routes: the canal of Schlemm and trabecular meshwork, and the uveoscleral route.

Cataracts

A **cataract** is a condition in which the lens becomes opaque and interferes with the transmission of light to the retina; the vision becomes less sharp, less colorful, and less intense. It is a myth that a "film" grows on the eyes; rather, a cataract develops within the eye. The lens becomes opaque when old cells of the lens die and become trapped within the capsule that contains the lens. The cells then accumulate over time, causing the lens to cloud and images to look blurred or doubled. Cataracts are usually a natural result of aging; however, eye injuries, diseases (diabetes and alcoholism), and certain medications can cause cataracts. They can be treated only with surgery

iridotomy an incision made in the iris of the eye to enlarge the pupil.

cataract an ocular opacity or obscurity in the lens of the eye.

Table 22-2   Drugs for Glaucoma with Various Mechanisms of Action

TRADE NAME	GENERIC NAME	MOA	INDICATIONS	SIDE EFFECTS	SIG
Beta-Blocking Agents		MOA unknown, but may reduce aqueous humor formation and increase drainage	chronic open-angle glaucoma, ocular hypertension	stinging, oral dryness, ocular pruritus, drowsiness, blurring of the eyes	1. Stinging or irritation of eye when medicine is applied 2. Redness of eye or inside of eyelid 3. Decreased night vision 4. Blurred vision
Timolol®, Betimol®, OcuDose®, Timoptic-XE®	timolol maleate, ophthalmic solutions 0.25% and 0.5%		nonselective (Beta 1 and 2)		1 gtt 0.25% bid, NTE 1 gtt 0.5% bid
Betoptic®	betaxolol HCl, solution 0.5% and 0.25% suspension		Beta 1 selective		1–2 gtts bid
Betoptic-S®	betaxolol HCl, 0.25% suspension		Beta 1 selective		1–2 gtts bid
Betagan®	levobunolol HCl, solution 0.25% or 0.5%		nonselective (Beta 1 and 2)		1–2 gtts 0.5% solution qd, NTE 2 gtts 0.5% sol. bid 1–2 gtts 0.25% solution bid
Ocupress®	carteolol HCl, solution 1%		nonselective (Beta 1 and 2)		1 gtt q12 hr (or bid)
OptiPranolol®	metipranolol HCl, solution 0.3%		nonselective (Beta 1 and 2)		1 gtt q12 hr or bid
Adrenergic Agonists		Reduce aqueous humor production and increase aqueous humor outflow	selective alpha-2 adrenergic agonist	stinging, oral dryness, ocular pruritus, drowsiness, conjunctival follicles, blurring of the eyes	
Alphagan®	brimonidine, 0.2%			pressure-lowering effects of brimonidine may decrease over time; patient must be monitored	1 gtt bid or tid
Lopidine®	apraclonidine, 0.5% and 1%				1–2 gtts q8 hr
Miotics		Pull on the ciliary muscle, causing the spaces within the meshwork to open more and thus increasing the flow of fluid	various purposes	small pupil, headache, blurred vision, change in refraction, decreased visual field, retinal detachment	

Table 22-2   Drugs for Glaucoma with Various Mechanisms of Action (*continued*)

TRADE NAME	GENERIC NAME	MOA	INDICATIONS	SIDE EFFECTS	SIG
		out of the eye. Decrease the size of the pupil, relaxing the iris, thus increasing fluid outflow through the trabecular meshwork only. Constrict the pupil.			
Miostat®, Carbastat®	carbachol, solution 0.01%	Cholinergic (parasympathomimetic) agent; constricts the iris and ciliary body, results in reduction of IOP. Exact MOA is not precisely known.	to obtain miosis during surgery		no more than 0.5 mL instilled into the anterior chamber for miosis
Cholinergic Agents					
Isoptocarpine®, Pilocar®	pilocarpine, 0.25%, 0.5%, 1%, 2%, 3%, 4%, 5%, 6%, 8%; ophthalmic gel, 4%	Direct-acting cholinergic agent.	chronic simple open glaucoma, chronic angle-closure glaucoma	painful contraction of ciliary muscle, painful eye or brow, blurred vision, spasms, twitching, darkened vision, headaches	open-angle glaucoma. 1 gtt 0.5%–4% sol. qid Acute closed-angle glaucoma: 1 gtt 1%–2% sol. q5–10 min for 3 doses, then 1 gtt q1–3 hr until IOP is decreased; $\frac{1}{2}$-inch ribbon qhs only
Phospholine Iodide®	echothiophate iodide, ophthalmic solution 0.03%, 0.06%, 0.125%, and 0.25%	Long-acting cholinesterase inhibitor of endogenous ACH in iris, ciliary muscle; decreases aqueous humor outflow.	chronic angle-closure glaucoma		lowest dose possible with least potent medication: qd or bid, NTE bid (as it is long-acting)
Carbonic Anhydrase Inhibitors		Carbonic anhydrase inhibitors (CAIs) reduce aqueous humor production, thus lowering pressure in the eye.	open-angle glaucoma, ocular hypertension	1. Blurred vision 2. Bitter, sour, or unusual taste 3. Dermatitis 4. Chest pain 5. Conjunctivitis 6. Diarrhea 7. Dizziness 8. Double vision 9. Dry eye 10. Dry mouth	
Azopt®	brinzolamide, 1% solution			chest pain, jaundice	1 gtt q8 hr

Table 22-2 Drugs for Glaucoma with Various Mechanisms of Action (*continued*)

TRADE NAME	GENERIC NAME	MOA	INDICATIONS	SIDE EFFECTS	SIG
Trusopt®	dorzolamide HCl, 2% solution			allergic reactions in patients who are also allergic to sulfonamides	1 gtt q8 hr
Diamox®	acetazolamide, 125 mg, 250 mg, 500 mg (sustained-release)		do not give to those allergic to sulfa drugs	loss of appetite, metallic taste, diarrhea, weakness, tingling sensation in hands or feet or mouth area, hearing impairment or ringing in the ears, convulsions, shortness of breath or difficulty breathing	125 mg or 250 mg 1–4 times per day ud Diamox Sequels 500 mg: 1 cap bid
Combination Products		Dual action of beta blocker and carbonic anhydrase inhibitor.		eye pain, tearing, itching, blurred or cloudy vision, ocular burning	
Cosopt®	dorzolamide HCl and timolol maleate	Dorzolamide, a CAI, and timolol, a beta blocker, both decrease aqueous humor production; timolol also increases drainage.		same as preceding, plus keratitis, blepharitis, conjunctival edema, discharge from follicles, corneal erosion, corneal cataracts, dizziness, bronchitis, dyspepsia, abdominal pain, back pain; bitter, sour, or unusual taste	1 gtt bid
Osmotic Diuretics			head or eye injury, before or after surgery; acute closed-angle glaucoma		
Ophthalagen®	glycerin anhydrous	Clears the edema and enables outflow.	eye surgery in cases of head or eye injury	diarrhea, back pain, confusion, hyperosmolar coma	PO 1 to 1.8 g/kg, 1–1.5 hr before surgery, q5 min
Osmitrol®	mannitol	Increases glomerular filtration with minimal reabsorption of water in the tubules, enhances secretion of Na^+ and Cl^- ions.	to lower IOP when other means and agents have failed	rebound urinary retention, headache, back/chest pain, chills/rigors, nausea and vomiting, confusion, pulmonary edema, hypokalemia, hyponatremia	IV infusion: 1.5–2 mg/kg (15–20% sol), 30–50 min/hr, over 30 to 60 min; NTE 50 to 200 g in a 24-hour period

Table 22-2   Drugs for Glaucoma with Various Mechanisms of Action (*continued*)

TRADE NAME	GENERIC NAME	MOA	INDICATIONS	SIDE EFFECTS	SIG
Prostamides and Prostaglandins		Exact MOA unknown, but believed to increase uveoscleral outflow of aqueous humor.	open-angle glaucoma	change of iris color, red eye, eye irritation or inflammation, flu-like syndrome, arthritis	
Lumigan®	bimatoprost, ophthalmic solution, 0.03%	Dual action improves natural flow of fluid through both the trabecular meshwork and the uveoscleral route (tissue and eyelid).	open-angle glaucoma	in addition to preceding, may increase growth of eyelashes and increase pigmentation of the iris and periorbital area	1 gtt qd dosing only
Rescula®	unoprostone isopropyl solution 0.15%	Inactive biosynthetic cyclic derivative of arachidonic acid; MOA is unknown, but does increase outflow of aqueous humor.	open-angle glaucoma	may gradually change eye color, increasing the amount of brown pigment in the iris	1 gtt bid
Travatan®	trovoprost, solution 0.004%	Prostaglandin F2 alpha analogue (synthetic): Selective FP prostanoid receptor agonist, causing release of MMP (metalloproteiniases) that degrade the cellular matrix and thus increasing outflow; exact MOA unknown, believed to decrease IOP by increasing uveoscleral outflow of aqueous humor.		may gradually change eye color, increasing the amount of brown pigment in the iris; may increase growth of eyelashes	1 gtt q p.m. ONLY, NTE 1 gtt qd
Xalatan®	latanaprost, 0.005% solution	Prostanoid selective FP receptor agonist; MOA same as Travatan®.		may gradually change eye color, increasing the amount of pigment in the iris; may increase growth of eyelashes	1 gtt q p.m. only, NTE 1 gtt qd

in which the clouded lens is replaced with a clear, plastic lens. The four causes of cataracts are:

1. Congenital—hereditary, or measles infection during the first trimester.
2. Trauma—injury to the lens.
3. Age—85 percent of people over 80 years of age have some clouding of the lens.
4. Metabolic and toxic agents—induced by diabetes, smoking, or taking certain drugs (digoxin, alcohol).

Vascular Retinopathies

retinopathy a noninflammatory disease in which the retina of the eye is damaged.

Vascular **retinopathy** is a noninflammatory disease in which the retina has become damaged. It is important to understand that there are many causes, including diabetes and hypertension. There is no pharmaceutical treatment for the many different types of retinopathies; however, some retinopathies may respond to laser treatment.

A technician should pay attention and listen to a patient who mentions visual disturbances while taking specific medications. Report all discussions to the pharmacist, who has better knowledge and understanding of the side effects and interactions of the drugs and may contact the patient's physician about further observation and testing.

Types of Retinopathies

1. *Simple or nonproliferative* retinopathies are characterized by defective bulging of vessel walls, which causes bleeding into the eye. The bulging is caused by small clumps of dead retinal cells, called *cotton wool exudates*, and by closed vessels. This form of retinopathy is considered mild.
2. *Proliferative* retinopathies are severe forms characterized by newly grown blood vessels and scar tissue formed within the eye, by closed-off blood vessels that are badly damaged, and by the retina breaking away or detaching from the surrounding mesh of blood vessels that nourish it.

In general, many retinopathies occur due the following sequence of events. Blood flow to the retina is disrupted, either by blockage or breakdown of the various vessels. Bleeding or hemorrhage occurs, and fluid, cells, and proteins known as *exudates* leak into the area. A lack of oxygen to surrounding tissues (*hypoxia*) or decreased blood flow results; ischemia may lead to necrosis of the retina or other ocular tissue. This stimulates production of certain chemicals by the body, which in turn cause new blood vessels to grow. This new growth is called *neovascularization*. However, these new vessels generally leak blood, causing further problems. The retina may swell, and adversely affect vision, or the retina may detach completely. The following are common causes of retinopathies:

- Certain medications, such as chloroquine, thioridazine, and large doses of tamoxifen, can cause the arteries and veins to become blocked, resulting in a retinal artery or vein occlusion.
- Microaneurysms or bleeding into the vitreous humor.
- Direct sunlight exposure, such as looking directly at the sun during an eclipse, can cause *solar retinopathy*.
- Neovascularizations or the formation of new blood vessels; these tend to be fragile, leak protein, and bleed.
- Diabetes. Diabetic retinopathies are confined to the retina and involve thickening of capillary walls and microaneurysm formation, followed by rupture and bleeding into the retina. In proliferative diabetic retinopathies, the retina bleeds into the vitreous humor.
- Central vein occlusion. This is often secondary to hypertension (HTN), diabetes mellitus, or sickle cell anemia; it causes a rapid deterioration of visual acuity.
- Atherosclerosis. *Atherosclerotic retinopathy* is the hardening or thickening of the retinal arteries.

- Retinal artery occlusion, which is the complete blockage of an artery to the retina; it results in sudden, unilateral blindness (one-eye or one-sided anopsia).
- Hypertension. *Hypertensive retinopathy* is damage to the retinal arteries caused by high blood pressure.
- Syphilis. *Syphilitic retinopathy* occurs when the retina becomes infected by the spirochete that causes syphilis.

Cycloplegic Drugs, Mydriatic Drugs, and Lubricants

Certain drugs help ophthalmologists examine their patients' eyes. Drugs that relax the ciliary muscle are **cycloplegic** drugs. Drugs that dilate the pupils are **mydriatic** drugs. People with dilated pupils may experience blurred vision for approximately two to four hours. When pupils are dilated, brilliant lights may be bothersome. Dark glasses should be worn until the dilation subsides.

cycloplegic causing relaxation and paralysis of the intraocular muscles.

mydriatic causing dilation of the pupil of the eye.

Lubricants restore moisture to a dry eye. Dry eyes may result from exposure to the elements, such as sun or wind; to chemicals, such as chlorine; to allergens; or to some medications.

Originally responding to possible injury or infection, the immune system sends white blood cells and other mediators in the blood to the eye. With more blood, the whites of the eye get redder as blood vessels dilate (open up) to accommodate the influx of blood. Vasoconstrictors or decongestants return blood when the mediators are no longer needed. Vasoconstriction therapy should be short-term, as a rebound effect will occur with long-term use.

The rebound effect happens after the swelling subsides and the redness goes away. At that point, the blood vessels become dilated again to counter the vasoconstrictive effect of the medication. This paradoxical overcompensation, or "self-correcting" action, causes the blood vessels to dilate even more, resulting in a tolerance after two to five days. Because the blood vessels have dilated so much, they tend not to constrict well anymore, and the patient needs more drug to counter this residual dilation. The rebound effect will continue with prolonged use of vasoconstricting medications; therefore, long-term use of vasoconstrictors should be avoided. In fact, some research suggests a connection between long-term use of vasoconstrictors and glaucoma.

PROCEDURE 22-1

General Guidelines for Using an Ophthalmic Product

Patients should be advised to follow these basic precautions and standards when placing eyedrops or ointment into the eye.

1. Wash hands thoroughly with soap and water.
2. Remove contact lenses before putting in ophthalmic medication. Wait 15 minutes after administering the medication before putting lenses back in.
3. Never touch the tip of the tube to the eye or to anything else.
4. Wipe any excess medication from the eyelids and lashes by using a tissue. Recap the medication container and store it in a proper location at the correct temperature.
5. Wash hands immediately to remove any medication.
6. If more than one type of eye medication is used, wait 5–10 minutes before administering the second medication.
7. Sometimes eye medications can cause a few moments of blurry vision; wait until the vision completely clears before resuming activities such as driving.

PROCEDURE 22-2

Applying an Ophthalmic Ointment

In addition to the basic guidelines for applying an ophthalmic medication described in Procedure 22-1, patients should follow these instructions when using an ophthalmic ointment. Note that the stream of oil-based ointment is measured by the length of the "ribbon" that comes out of the tube. The measurement can be stated in either centimeters or inches.

1. Hold the tube between your thumb and forefinger. Place it near the eye, but not touching any part of the eye or the eyelid. Tilt your head forward slightly.

2. With the index finger of your other hand, pull the lower eyelid down to form a "V" pocket. Squeeze the tube and place a ribbon of ointment or gel into the "V" pocket made by the opened lower eyelid. Do not let the tip of the tube touch the eye.

3. Blink the eye gently; do not squeeze lids together. Close the eye for 1–2 minutes.

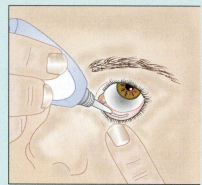

FIGURE 22-6 Applying an ophthalmic ointment.

PROCEDURE 22-3

How to Instill an Ophthalmic Solution

Ophthalmic liquid medications must be instilled; otherwise, the medication will immediately drain from the tear duct area. In addition to the basic instructions described in Procedures 22-1 and 22-2, patients should follow these specific instructions for instilling a liquid into the eye.

1. Uncap the container, tilt the head back slightly, and look at the ceiling.

2. Use the index finger to gently pull down on the lower eyelid to form a pocket.

3. Position the dropper above the eye. Look up and away from the dropper.

4. Squeeze out the prescribed number of drops and gently close the eye.

5. Apply gentle pressure to the inside –corner of the closed eye (near the nose) for about one minute to prevent the liquid from draining down from the tear duct.

7. If using drops in both eyes, repeat the process in the other eye.

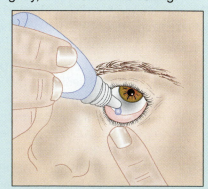

FIGURE 22-7 Instilling ophthalmic drops.

⚫ ⚫ ⚫

PROFILES IN PRACTICE

Duane is a pharmacy technician in a retail pharmacy. A customer requests a refill of a Tobradex® ophthalmic suspension, which was prescribed for bacterial conjunctivitis. The patient informs Duane that although the medication was used as prescribed, the infection returned.

• What are some possible reasons for the return of the customer's infection?

The Ear

Hearing starts at the outer ear, as sound waves or vibrations travel down the external auditory canal and strike the eardrum. When the eardrum vibrates, the vibrations are passed to three tiny bones in the middle ear. These bones amplify the sound and send the sound waves to the inner ear and into the fluid-filled hearing organ, the *cochlea*. The cochlea is lined with cells that have thousands of tiny hairs (*cilia*) on their surfaces. The sound vibrations make the tiny hairs move. By their movement, the hairs translate the sound vibrations into nerve signals, so your brain can interpret the sound. The signals travel to the brain along special nerves. After the sound waves reach the inner ear, they are converted into electrical impulses, which the auditory nerve sends to the brain. The brain recognizes these electrical impulses as sound.

Anatomy and Physiology of the Ear

The ear has three major areas: the outer, middle, and inner ear (see Figure 22-8). The outer ear structures, commonly called the *flaps* and *ear lobes*, are the cartilaginous portion known technically as the *pinna* or *auricle*. The pinna acts as a preamplifier that enhances the sensitivity of hearing.

The *tympanic membrane* or *eardrum* receives the vibrations that travel up through the auditory canal. These vibrations are transferred to three of the smallest bones in the body, the *ossicles*, then to the oval opening into the inner ear. The *malleus* or hammer, the *incus* or anvil, and the *stapes* or stirrup form the connection between the vibration of the eardrum and the forces exerted on the oval opening of the inner ear. The eardrum provides amplification of about 15 times more than the aural opening. The auditory canal acts as a closed-tube resonator, which boosts and improves sounds in the 2–5 kilohertz range. At the eardrum, sound energy (air pressure changes) are converted into the mechanical energy of eardrum movement.

Eustachian Tube

The *eustachian tube* connects the middle ear with the nasopharynx of the throat. When a person swallows or coughs, this tube acts to equalize the pressure between the middle ear and the outer ear. Proper transfer of sound waves occurs when the pressure is the same. The eustachian tube is shorter in children, and often oriented more horizontally. It is therefore less likely to open and more likely to become blocked by enlarged adenoids. Fluid may collect within the middle-ear area of young children, causing temporary hearing loss and/or a feeling of fullness and pain. This condition is called *serous otitis media (SOM)*. SOM may occur shortly after or during an upper respiratory infection

FIGURE 22-8 Anatomy of the ear.

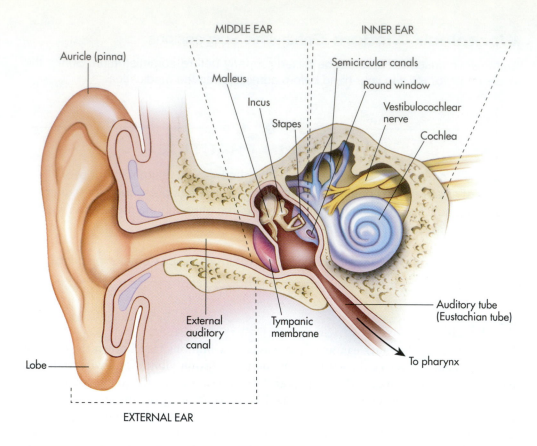

when the child has nasal congestion. Allergy-induced congestion or SOM may require antihistamines to dry out the congestion and to stop the allergic response that is causing it. SOM is most common among children younger than five years old.

Sometimes a person with SOM needs a *myringotomy*—the surgical relief of fluid pressure—or the surgical insertion of ventilation tubes into the middle ear. A patient with these tubes should avoid swimming, as water may contaminate the surgical site and cause a potentially serious infection.

The middle ear serves as an equalizer, matching the impedance of air in the ear canal to the impedance of the *perilymph* of the inner ear. Perilymph has the same makeup as cerebrospinal fluid (CSF), with a low potassium (K^+) concentration and a high sodium (Na^+) concentration. The scala tympani also contain perilymph.

Cochlea

The snail-shaped *cochlea* is the sensory organ of hearing, as it contains the auditory nerves. The wavelike patterns initiated by vibration of the stapes footplate causes a shearing of the cilia of the outer and inner hair cells. This process causes hair-cell depolarization, which occurs in the organ of Corti within the scala media of the cochlea. This changes the vibrational energy into neural energy that is transmitted along the eighth cranial nerve to the brain, which interprets these impulses as sound.

Vestibular Labyrinth

The *vestibular labyrinth* is composed of the *saccule* and *utricle*, which are the sense organs for balance. The vestibular labyrinth contains the receptors for balance and notifies the brain about an individual's linear and rotational orientation and movement in space.

Disorders and Diseases of the Ear

This section discusses some common disorders and diseases of the ear.

Complications of Earwax Buildup

The skin of the outer part of the ear canal contains the ceruminous and sebaceous gland that produces earwax (*cerumen*). The purposes of earwax are to:

- trap dust, dirt, insects, sand, and other particles, preventing them from getting into the eardrum.
- keep the eardrum moist.
- act as a water repellent.
- inhibit the growth of bacteria in the eardrum.

In most cases, earwax accumulates in small quantities for a short period of time, carrying particles along with it as it dries and comes out of the ear. Earwax can migrate to the pinna, where it is easily wiped off. Earwax does not form in the deep part of the ear canal near the tympanic membrane. Normal amounts of earwax are healthy.

Dry, itchy ears may be a result of wax deficiency. The homeostasis of self-cleaning—that is, the process of producing earwax, which then dries, flakes, and falls out of the ear canal, is slow and constant. Sometimes homeostasis is interrupted when the wax builds up against the eardrum. Using cotton swabs or other objects to "clean out" the ear serves only to push the earwax further inside. Continuous scratching of the ear canal, which has very thin skin and is easily injured, can lead to pain and infection. Hearing aids can prevent the migration of earwax out of the canal.

Annual ear exams can prevent some temporary hearing loss. The audiologist may wash the ear out, vacuum it, or physically remove the wax with special instruments. OTC eardrops may be used to soften the earwax before the wash or suctioning.

Workplace Wisdom Perforated Eardrums

If the eardrum has been punctured or perforated, infection may result from the use of water or presoftening eardrops. Examples of earwax softeners are Debrox® and Murine Ear Drops® (carbamide peroxide).

Types of Hearing Loss

Hearing loss may be caused by a number of factors. The most typical hearing losses, and the ones discussed in this section, are conductive, sensory, drug-induced, neural, and presbycusis.

Conductive Hearing Loss

Conductive hearing loss occurs when a problem exists with a part of the outer or middle ear. Usually this is a mild and temporary hearing loss, because, in most cases, medical treatment can help. Causes may include a blow to the head or ear, birth defects, malformation of parts of the outer or middle ear, a tiny hole or perforation in the eardrum, wax buildup in the ear canal, and middle-ear infections.

Sensory Hearing Loss

Sensory hearing loss occurs when the cochlea is not working correctly because cilia have been damaged or destroyed. This problem can affect one ear or both ears. Depending on the extent of loss, sound may be muffled (mild loss), some sounds might become slightly inaudible (moderate loss), or no sounds at all may be heard (severe/profound loss). Speech may also be affected. Sensory hearing impairment is almost always permanent. It may be due to heredity factors, or may occur during fetal developmental stages if the pregnant mother gets certain kinds of diseases, such as rubella (German measles). Other possible causes are certain medications, severe injury to the head, frequent listening to extremely loud music, and exposure to other loud noises (factory machinery, race cars, airplane engines).

" **Workplace Wisdom** Hearing Impairments

According to the National Institute on Deafness and Other Communication Disorders, approximately 28 million Americans have some type of hearing impairment, and 2 to 3 out of every 1,000 infants born in the United States are deaf or hearing-impaired. "

Drug-Induced Hearing Loss

Drug-induced hearing loss can occur with use of some ototoxic drugs that impair hearing and balance. Hearing loss can be reversible (temporary) or irreversible (permanent). Drugs that may cause hearing loss (see Table 22-3) are found in several classifications, such as:

- IV aminoglycosides
- Loop diuretics
- Antineoplastic agents (anticancer drugs)
- Quinine-containing drugs

tinnitus ringing or buzzing in the ear that is not caused by an external source; may be caused by infection or a reaction to a drug.

In addition, large doses of aspirin can cause ringing in the ears, or **tinnitus**.

Neural Hearing Loss

Neural hearing loss occurs when there is a problem with the connection from the cochlea to the brain. For example, when the nerve that carries the messages from the cochlea to the brain is damaged, neural hearing loss may result. This type of hearing loss is permanent.

Presbycusis

Presbycusis is the permanent loss of hearing due to damaged hearing nerves. When hearing deteriorates with age, sensitivity to high-pitched sounds fades first. This is

Table 22-3 Drugs That May Cause Sensory Hearing Loss

TRADE NAME	GENERIC NAME
Antibiotics	
Amikin®	amikacin IV
Garamycin®	gentamicin IV
Nebcin®	tobramycin IV
Loop Diuretics	
Bumex®	bumetanide
Demadex®	torsemide
Edecrin®	ethacrynic acid
Lasix®	furosemide
Antineoplastic Agents	
Paraplatin®	carboplatin
Platinol®	cisplatin
Quinine Products (selected)	
Aralen®	chloroquine
Quinaglute Dura-tabs®, Quinidex Extentab®	quinidine
Quinine	quinine sulfate
Tonic water	

why people often say that they can hear sounds but cannot understand what is being said. Presbycusis develops slowly and gradually. *Recruitment*, a progression of presbycusis, is a loss of sensitivity to soft sounds and a decreased ability to tolerate loud sounds.

Otitis Media

One of the most common causes of conductive hearing loss is **otitis media**, an inflammation and infection of the middle ear that usually presents in one out of three children. Acute otitis media is an infection that produces pus, fluid, and inflammation within the middle ear; it is usually quite painful. Older children may complain of ear pain, a feeling of fullness in the ear, or hearing loss. Younger children may present with irritability, fussiness, or difficulty in sleeping, feeding, or hearing. Fever is usually present.

These symptoms are frequently associated with signs of upper respiratory infection, such as a runny or stuffy nose or a cough. Otitis media, the most common childhood illness, usually appears four to seven days after the respiratory infection. Severe ear infections may cause the eardrum to rupture. Immediate medical treatment is then necessary. More than 80 percent of all children will have at least one middle-ear infection before they are 3 years old. Usually, otitis is easily treatable; however, a temporary hearing loss may result. This conductive hearing loss may cause delays in speech and language development and lead to learning difficulties. If left untreated, permanent hearing loss, rupture of the tympanic membrane, and/or meningitis may develop (see Table 22-4).

otitis media infection and inflammation of the middle ear.

Table 22-4   Antibiotic Treatment of Otitis Media in Children

Prophylaxis	
Amoxil®, Trimox®, Wymox®	amoxicillin
	sulfisoxazole (DOC)
First-Line Therapy	
Bactrim®	trimethoprim-sulfamethoxazole (TMP-SMX)
Septra® (used for patients with penicillin allergy)	amoxicillin
Amoxil®, Trimox®, Wymox®	amoxicillin
Second-Line Therapy	
Augmentin®	amoxicillin and clavulanate potassium
Biaxin®	clarithromycin
Cedax®	ceftibuten
Ceftin®	cefuroxime axetil
Cefzil®	cefprozil
Lorabid®	loracarbef
Vantin®	cefpodoxime proxetil
Zithromax®	azithromycin
Third-Line Therapy	
Cleocin® (used for resistant pneumococci)	clindamycin
Rocephin®	ceftriaxone sodium

SUMMARY

The most basic of all of our senses is sight. The anatomy and physiology of the eye are discussed extensively in this chapter.

The eyes are prone to many diseases, but eye infections are usually self-limiting and treatable; only on rare occasions do they lead to vision problems. More serious diseases, such as glaucoma, can cause irreversible vision problems.

A wide variety of treatment modalities is available to treat eye disorders. However, it is important that ophthalmic products be used safely and properly. One of your most important responsibilities as a pharmacy technician is to thoroughly understand the basics of safe use of ophthalmic remedies, so you can properly

handle these medications and help educate patients about their use.

The ear consists of three major areas: the outer, middle, and the inner ear. The functions of the ear include hearing and the maintenance of equilibrium or balance. Like the eye, the ear is susceptible to a variety of disorders; most can normally be prevented, controlled, or reversed with treatment. Although easily treatable, common problems such as otitis media (a middle-ear infection) can lead to permanent hearing loss if left untreated. It is estimated that more than 80 percent of children will be affected with this disorder before they reach the age of 3 years.

CHAPTER REVIEW QUESTIONS

1. _____ is an inflammation of the eyelid margins accompanied by redness.
   a. Conjunctivitis
   b. Blepharitis
   c. Retinopathy
   d. Glaucoma

2. Which part of the eye is composed of light-sensitive nerve endings that take visual impulses to the optic nerve?
   a. macula
   b. vitreous humor
   c. choroid
   d. retina

3. Inflammation of the thin lining that covers the white of the eyeball and inner surface of the eyelid is known as:
   a. conjunctivitis.
   b. blepharitis.
   c. retinopathy.
   d. glaucoma.

4. Treatment options for open-angle glaucoma include:
   a. laser surgery.
   b. medication.
   c. filtration surgery.
   d. all of the above.

5. The most common childhood illness is:
   a. conjunctivitis.
   b. glaucoma.
   c. otitis media.
   d. pink eye.

6. The first line of therapy for otitis media includes which of the following drugs?
   a. clindamycin
   b. azithromycin
   c. clarithromycin
   d. amoxicillin

7. Ototoxicity caused by medications can lead to:
   a. hearing impairment.
   b. balance impairment.
   c. infection.
   d. a and b.

8. Otitis media is:
   a. a blockage in the tear ducts.
   b. the first sign of the onset of glaucoma.
   c. not curable.
   d. an inflammation and infection of the middle ear.

9. Which of the following statements is/are true?
   a. Ophthalmic medication must be sterile.
   b. The ophthalmic medication container must remain sterile.
   c. Contact lenses must be removed before administering an ophthalmic medication.
   d. All of the above are true.

10. Which of the following drugs is not indicated for glaucoma?
    a. betaxolol
    b. latanoprost
    c. carbamide peroxide
    d. brinzolamide

CRITICAL THINKING QUESTIONS

1. State which sense, eyesight or hearing, is more important to you, and explain why you would rather lose the other sense.

2. Explain why the eye is considered the body's camera.

3. Why do doctors often tell their patients not to "stick anything smaller than an elbow" in the ear?

WEB CHALLENGE

1. Visit http://www.glaucoma.org/ and find out what researchers are doing to find a cure for glaucoma. Write a one-page summary of your findings.

2. Go to http://visionsimulator.com to see how various eye diseases actually affect a person's vision.

   Select one disease and write a one-page description of its effects on vision along with treatment options.

3. Go to http://www.nidcd.nih.gov/ to learn more about diseases and conditions affecting the ear.

REFERENCES AND RESOURCES

Adams, MP, Josephson, DL, & Holland, LN Jr. *Pharmacology for Nurses—A Pathophysiologic Approach*. Upper Saddle River, NJ: Pearson Education, 2005.

"Anatomy, Physiology and Pathology of the Human Eye" (accessed June 23, 2007): http://www.tedmontgomery.com/the_eye/

Beltone interactive Internet site for the anatomy of the ear (accessed June 24, 2007): http://www.beltone.com/ear_anatomy/ear_anatomy.asp#

"Eye Anatomy" (accessed June 24, 2007): http://www.stlukeseye.com

Holland, N, & Adams, MP. *Core Concepts in Pharmacology*. Upper Saddle River, NJ: Pearson Education, 2003.

Lumigan® package insert (accessed June 25, 2007): http://www.lumigan.com/pdfs/PI.pdf

The Merck Manual of Diagnosis and Therapy (accessed June 25, 2007): http://www.merck.com/mrkshared/mmanual/section8/chapter94/94c.jsp

"Review of Anatomy: The Ear and Temporal Bone" (accessed June 25, 2007): http://www.bcm.tmc.edu/oto/studs/anat/tbone.html#EAR

"Statistics about Hearing Disorders, Ear Infections, and Deafness" (accessed June 25, 2007): http://www.nidcd.nih.gov/

"Timolol®" (accessed June 25, 2007): http://www.rxlist.com/cgi/generic/timolol_cp.htm

"What is Glaucoma?" (accessed June 25, 2007): http://www.glaucoma.org

The Gastrointestinal System

LEARNING OBJECTIVES

After completing this chapter, you should be able to:

- Identify the basic anatomical and structural parts of the digestive system.
- Describe the physiology of the digestive system.
- List and describe the three main categories of nutrients.
- Identify the functions and AMDR of the macronutrients.
- State the difference between essential and nonessential amino acids.
- Identify the functions, symptoms of deficiencies, and Reference Daily Intakes (RDIs) of the micronutrients.
- Understand the importance of water to the body.

Introduction

The digestive system is responsible for adequate nourishment and hydration of the body. Without proper nourishment and hydration, body cells would die and, eventually, the body itself would die. The main purpose of the digestive system is to fuel the body so that it can continue to survive and function properly.

Lack of proper nutrition and digestion can lead to numerous disease states. The body needs the right amounts of macronutrients, micronutrients, and water to function properly. Nutrition guidelines and recommendations have been established to help educate the public and make sure people receive the correct amount of nutrients.

Anatomy and Physiology of the Digestive System

The digestive system, which extends from the mouth to the anus, is a long tube that twists and turns, with a series of hollow organs along its length (see Figure 23-1). This tube is lined with protective mucosa that prevents acid from causing sores or ulcers. In the mouth, stomach, and small intestine, the mucosa also contains tiny glands that produce the liquid digestive juices that help digest food. These liquids contain enzymes and acids.

The liver and pancreas produce digestive juices that are sent to the intestine through small ducts. The liver produces *bile*, which is stored in the gallbladder, and the pancreas produces enzymes. In addition, accessory organs, nerves, and blood play a major role in the digestive system.

Rings of smooth muscle along the digestive tract produce a wave of synchronized contractions, called *peristalsis*, that help propel the food down the tube. The six main parts or organs of the digestive system are the:

- mouth
- esophagus
- pharynx
- stomach
- small intestine
- large intestine

The six accessory organs of the digestive system are the:

- teeth
- tongue
- salivary glands
- liver
- gallbladder
- pancreas

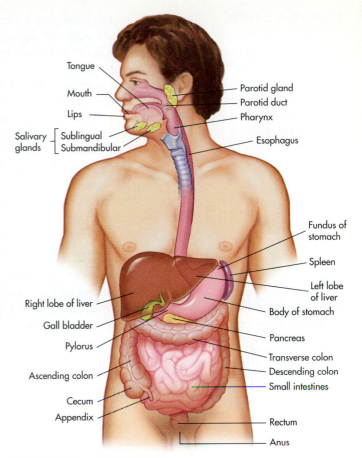

FIGURE 23-1 The digestive system.

Digestion

The body uses digestion to accomplish the following functions:

- Break up food particles into smaller pieces.
- Break down food substances into nutrients that the body can use in body processes, as energy or building materials.
- Transfer what it cannot use out of the body, as waste; this elimination process is known as *excretion*.
- Reabsorb water into the body's tissues to prevent dehydration.

Digestion involves many different body organs and structures. This section takes you through the digestive process one step at a time.

The Mouth

Digestion begins in the opening of the alimentary tract, or *mouth*, where the teeth, tongue, and saliva aid in physical digestion (see Figure 23-2). **Mastication** occurs as the teeth

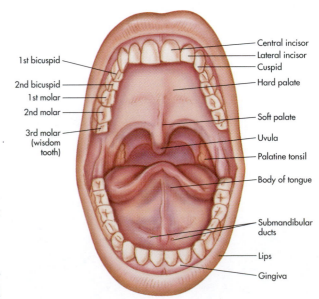

FIGURE 23-2 The mouth.

mastication chewing.

monosaccharide simplest form of carbohydrate (e.g., glucose, fructose).

break up the food pieces into smaller particles. Saliva moistens the food to ease swallowing, and adds predigestive enzymes to the mix. The tongue moves the ball of chewed food, or *bolus*, to the uvula, and both assist in swallowing. Food then passes through the throat (*pharynx*) into the esophagus as the windpipe or *trachea* is closed off by the epiglottis. Before the food is swallowed, the carbohydrate content of the food is chemically broken down by an enzyme into simple sugars or **monosaccharides**. This enzyme is an amylase known as *ptyalin*.

Monosaccharides are the building blocks of carbohydrates. Because food is usually swallowed before being completely chewed or moistened with enzymes, physical and chemical digestion have not been completed. The bolus passes through the approximately 10-inch-long esophagus, which runs behind the heart before meeting the stomach. Before entering the stomach, the bolus must pass through the cardiac sphincter, also referred to as the *lower esophageal sphincter (LES)*.

The Stomach

The three parts of the stomach are the fundus, body, and pylorus (see Figure 23-3). The smooth muscles of the stomach continue peristalsis, which moves the foodstuff, now called **chyme**, along the digestive tract to break up the food into even smaller pieces. Chyme has the consistency of a thick, soupy liquid. Chemical digestion in the stomach occurs when the walls of the stomach sense the weight or presence of the food and get stretched out. In response, the parietal cells make and secrete hydrochloric acid, which converts **pepsinogen** into the enzyme **pepsin**. The proteolytic enzyme pepsin chemically breaks down protein into amino acids. Amino acids are the building blocks of all proteins. About four hours later, peristalsis continues to move the chyme, consisting of carbohydrates, monosaccharides, proteins, and amino acids, through the pyloric sphincter.

chyme the liquid that food turns into before it passes into the small intestine.

pepsinogen precursor to pepsin.

pepsin digestive enzyme needed to break down food proteins.

The Small Intestine

The three parts of the small intestine are the duodenum, jejunum, and ileum (see Figure 23-4). The *duodenum* is the first part of the small intestine, where about 80 percent of all food is chemically digested. As a result, about 80 percent of all ulcers are found in the duodenum. As the highly acidic chyme enters the duodenum, it must be

FIGURE 23-3 The stomach.

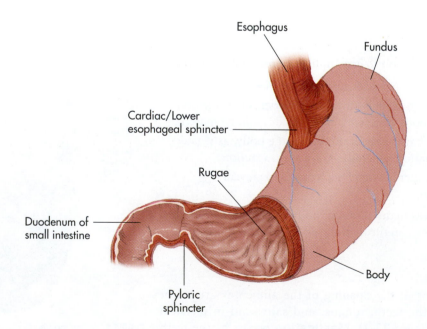

Esophagus

Fundus

Cardiac/Lower
esophageal sphincter

Rugae

Duodenum of
small intestine

Body

Pyloric
sphincter

neutralized by an alkaline substance, bicarbonate. Otherwise, a duodenal ulcer will result. The strong acidity of the chyme signals the pancreas to secrete bicarbonate along with its starch-, protein-, and fat-digesting enzymes. Secreted bicarbonate neutralizes the stomach acids and raises the pH in the small intestine to slightly acidic (about 5.5); this is the chemical environment in which the pancreatic enzymes work best.

The small intestine calls upon the liver to make and secrete bile to help in digesting **lipids**. Stored bile from the gallbladder is sent to the small intestine to break up large molecules of fats into smaller ones, a process called *emulsification*. Emulsification occurs so that fat and fat-soluble vitamins can be absorbed in the intestine after enzymes break down the smaller globules into absorbable nutrients.

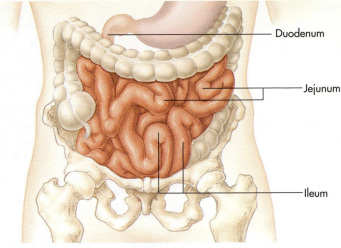

FIGURE 23-4 The small intestine.

While food is in the small intestine, the pancreas sends out all three of its enzymes in a juice or secretion. Trypsin, a **protease**, further breaks down any remaining proteins or amino acids into the simplest of amino acids. Amylopsin, an amylase, breaks down any remaining carbohydrates and simple sugars into the simplest of sugars (monosaccharides). Finally, a lipase called steapsin, not produced elsewhere in the digestive tract, breaks down the smaller molecules of fat into fatty acids and glycerol (the building blocks of fats). At this point all food sources—carbohydrates, proteins, and fats (lipids)—have been broken down into their simplest constituent nutrient substances and are ready to enter the bloodstream, so the body can use them as energy to power other body processes. The four nutrients—monosaccharides, amino acids, fatty acids, and glycerol—are then absorbed into the capillaries of the blood system and small lymph vessels by finger-like projections in the small intestine, called *villi* and *microvilli*. Whatever is not absorbed there is then passed out of the small intestine into the large intestine and out of the body as waste.

The small intestine is where the majority of absorption occurs. The nutrients are absorbed into tiny lymph vessels called *lacteals* and are passed through a large portal vein to the liver. The liver breaks down any toxins that may be present and prepares the nutrients for release into the bloodstream. The bloodstream carries the nutrients to every cell in the body, where they are used for energy and for tissue building and repair.

Table 23-1 shows the chemical breakdown of specific foods in a typical sandwich and the function of the nutrient building blocks produced during digestion.

lipid fat.

protease enzyme that begins protein breakdown.

Table 23-1   Comparison of Nutrient Functions within the Body

FOOD SOURCE	CHEMICAL BASE OF FOOD SOURCE	BUILDING BLOCK (NUTRIENT PRESENT AT THE END OF DIGESTION OR HYDROLYSIS)	FUNCTION OF THE BUILDING BLOCK OR NUTRIENT
bread or bun	complex carbohydrates	simple sugars or monosaccharides	quick energy
hamburger patty	protein	amino acids	growth and repair of all cells, tissues, organs, structure (especially muscle)
mayonnaise	lipids (fats)	fatty acids and glycerol	stored energy, lubrication, protection/ padding, insulation

FIGURE 23-5 The large intestine.

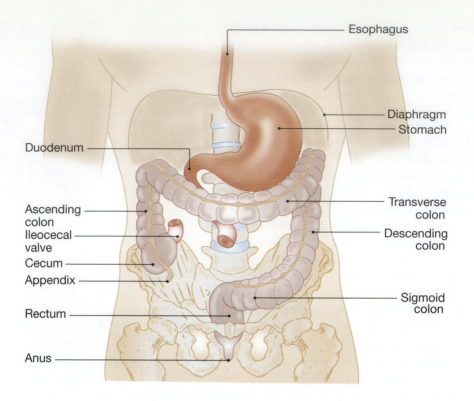

The Large Intestine

The large intestine, or *colon*, is divided into the following seven sections (in order) (see Figure 23-5):

1. cecum
2. ascending colon
3. transverse colon
4. descending colon
5. sigmoid colon
6. rectum
7. anus

Waste (material or residue that is not absorbed) is moved through the ileocecal valve that connects the lower ileum of the small intestine to the cecum. The large intestine utilizes smooth muscle to mix the waste and allows the water to be reabsorbed. The motility of the colon is considered to be unsynchronized or nonperistaltic. A second and very important type of motility that occurs in the large intestine is the high-amplitude propagating contraction (*HAPC*). These extremely strong contractions occur about six to eight times per day in healthy people, are longitudinal, and sweep from the cecum to stop just above the rectum. They move the waste down the large intestine and trigger bowel movements. Food waste, along with bacteria, remains in the large intestine for about 30 hours.

Disorders of the Digestive System

The following section discusses some common disorders of the digestive system.

Gastroesophageal Reflux Disease

Commonly called *heartburn* or *acid reflux*, *gastroesophageal reflux disease (GERD)* occurs because the lower esophageal sphincter relaxes when it should contract. Therefore, stomach acid can regurgitate or back up from the stomach into the esophagus.

The primary goal in GERD treatment is to reduce the overproduction of acid and contract the lower esophageal sphincter. Reglan® (metoclopramide) 10 to 15 mg PO qid 30 min ac and qhs is indicated for serious GERD that cannot be alleviated by OTC drugs. Metoclopramide can act as a GI stimulant or as an antiemetic/antinauseant.

- **GI Stimulant—Dopamine Receptor Antagonist.** MOA 1—Stimulates peristalsis of the upper GI tract without causing more acid production; causes relaxation of the pyloric sphincter and increased resting tone of the LES (that is, it helps the muscle of the LES stay tighter even in its relaxed state). Relaxing the pyloric sphincter and contracting the LES allow a quicker elimination process, or emptying time, so that food goes through the stomach faster.

- **Antiemetic or Antinauseant.** MOA 2—The antiemetic action of metoclopramide is unknown, but is believed to be a result of its antagonism of central and peripheral dopamine receptors. Dopamine causes nausea and vomiting by stimulation of the medullary chemoreceptor trigger zone (CTZ). Metoclopramide promotes proper sphincter function by blocking stimulation of the CTZ by agents like L-dopa or apomorphine, which are known to increase dopamine levels and to have dopamine-like effects.

Side effects include drowsiness and urinary incontinence. Drug interactions may occur with anticholinergic drugs, such as atropine and scopolamine, and narcotic analgesics, such as Tylenol #3® and Vicodin®. Additive sedative effects can occur when metoclopramide is given with alcohol, sedatives, hypnotics, narcotics, or tranquilizers such as Valium®, Dalmane®, Percocet®, or Tofranil®.

" Workplace Wisdom Digestive Disorders

An estimated 70 million Americans are said to have one or more digestive disorders, which account for 13 percent of all hospitalizations. "

Nausea and/or Vomiting

Nausea precedes vomiting and is a feeling of awareness that something is stimulating the vomit center and that vomiting is going to occur. Vomiting, or *emesis*, is produced by involuntary contraction of the abdominal muscles when the fundus and LES are relaxed, causing a strong ejection of gastric contents. If left untreated, chronic vomiting can cause malnutrition, dehydration, potassium chloride (KCl) electrolyte deficiency, heart problems, and arrhythmias. Nausea and vomiting occur when the vomiting center in the brain is activated by any of the following causes:

- Migraines.
- Gallstones.
- Intestinal obstructions.
- Irritation of the stomach.
- Overeating.
- Food poisoning.
- Overconsumption of alcohol.
- Food allergies.
- Reactions to medications such as NSAIDs and chemotherapy drugs.
- Illness.
- Various conditions of the body or disease states.
- Pyloric stenosis—a blockage at the stomach outlet that produces projectile vomiting in infants and must be treated immediately.

Table 23-2 Postoperative Vomiting Drugs

TRADE NAME	GENERIC NAME	AVAILABLE STRENGTH AND DOSAGE FORMS	DOSAGE
Compazine®	prochlorperazine	Tab: 5 mg, 10 mg, 25 mg	5–10 mg po tid–quid
		Supp: 2.5 mg, 5 mg, 25 mg	50 mg pr bid
		Inj: 5 mg/mL	Not to exceed (NTE) 40 mg/day IV
Phenergan®	promethazine	Tab: 12.5 mg, 25 mg, 50 mg	12.5 mg–25 mg q4–6 hr
		Supp: 12.5 mg, 25 mg, 50 mg	
		Inj: 25 mg/mL, 50 mg/mL	
Tigan®	trimethobenzamide	Cap: 300 mg	300 mg po tid–quid
		Supp: 100 mg, 200 mg	100–200 mg pr tid–qid
		Inj: 100 mg/mL	200 mg IM tid–qid

- Anesthesia—postoperative vomiting is generally caused by the decreased amount of narcotic or opium derivative in the body after surgery (see Table 23-2).
- Pregnancy—no drugs have been approved for "morning sickness," but Vitamin B6 may help to reduce the emotional stress that may accompany it. No nutritional deficiencies are associated with nausea and vomiting during pregnancy.
- Bacterial or viral gastroenteritis—acute-onset gastroenteritis is most commonly caused by some type of bacteria or virus. This could result from eating contaminated food or catching influenza. Gastroenteritis usually causes a one-time attack of sudden projectile vomiting that does not require medication. The patient generally feels much better after the attack.
- Psychogenic vomiting—some nausea/vomiting is due to depression, anxiety, and emotional stress.
- Motion sickness (*vertigo*)—occurs when the body is subjected to accelerations of movement in different directions or under conditions where visual contact with an actual outside horizon is lost. The balance center of the inner ear then sends information to the brain that conflicts with the visual clues of being still; the resulting confusion causes nausea.

Treatment to relieve nausea and vomiting is typically through medication. Which medication is prescribed depends on the particular patient's problem (see Table 23-3).

Antihistamines work by competitive inhibition or by blocking H1 receptor sites, slowing the response to the stimuli causing the nausea and vomiting (see Table 23-3).

Table 23-3 Antihistamines Used as Antiemetics

TRADE NAME	GENERIC NAME	DOSAGE
Antivert®	meclizine	25 mg–50 mg 1 hour prior to travel
		25 mg–100 mg daily in divided doses (for vertigo)
Dramamine®	dimenhydrinate	50 mg tabs: 1–2 tablets q4–6 hr, NTE 300 mg/6 tablets in 24 hours
Transderm-scop®	scopolamine	one patch q3 days

Antihistmines are thought to block excitatory labyrinthine impulses at cholinergic synapses in the region of the vestibular nuclei. Side effects include drowsiness and dry mouth. Listed warnings advise patients with glaucoma or urinary disturbances not to take antihistamines.

Nausea and/or vomiting may occur as a side effect of chemotherapy, either during or after administration of chemotherapeutic drugs. Serotonin receptors of the 5-HT$_3$ type are located peripherally on vagal nerve terminals and centrally in the chemoreceptor trigger zone of the area postrema of the brain. During chemotherapy that induces vomiting, mucosal enterochromaffin cells release serotonin that stimulates 5-HT$_3$ receptors. This evokes vagal afferent discharge, or firing, which induces vomiting.

Drugs used for post-emetogenic nausea are called 5-HT$_3$ antagonists. These drugs block serotonin from binding with and stimulating the 5-HT$_3$ receptors, and thus prevent nausea and vomiting (N/V). There are no listed drug interactions for 5-HT$_3$ antagonists. Side effects are minimal, but may include headache, diarrhea, or constipation (see Table 23-4).

❝ Workplace Wisdom Herbal Remedy

Ginger root is an herb that is known to aid in combating nausea and vomiting. A minor side effect of ginger root is a burning stomach. ❞

Ulcers

Ulcers are sores on the inside "flesh" wall of the stomach or intestines caused by overproduction and secretion of the parietal cells. A *peptic ulcer* is a sore that forms in the lining of the stomach or the duodenum. Ulcer symptoms can include burning pain in

Table 23-4　Drugs Used for Post-Emetogenic Nausea

TRADE NAME	GENERIC NAME	DOSAGE	
5-HT$_3$ Antagonists			
Aloxi®	palonosetron HCl	Inj: 0.25 mg/5 mL	0.25 mg as a single dose 30 min before administration of chemotherapy
Anzemet®	dolasetron mesylate	Tab: 50 mg, 100 mg Inj: 20 mg/mL	100 mg po within 1 hr before chemotherapy 1.8 mg/kg as a single dose 30 min before chemotherapy
Kytril®	granisetron HCl	Tab: 1 mg Liq: 1 mg/5 mL In: 1 mg/mL	2 mg po daily or 1 mg po bid 10 mcg/kg IV within 30 min before chemotherapy
Zofran®	ondansetron HCl	Tab: 4 mg, 8 mg, 24 mg Inj: 2 mg/mL Premix IV: 32 mg/50 mL	8 mg po bid 0.15 mg/kg IV × 3 doses *or* 32 mg IV × 1 dose

the upper abdomen, nausea, vomiting, loss of appetite, weight loss, fatigue, deep recurring ache relieved with food or antacids, gastric pain aggravated by general irritants, and nocturnal (nighttime) pain.

" Workplace Wisdom Peptic Ulcers

More than 400,000 new cases of peptic ulcers are diagnosed each year, and ulcers are the reason for nearly 40,000 surgeries annually.
"

Peptic ulcer disease can affect all age groups, but is less common in children. In the past, it was believed that men were at twice the risk for ulcers as women, due to unhealthy diets and high stress levels. However, it is now known that most ulcers are caused by bacterial infections or medications. Therefore, women and men are at equal risk of developing ulcers. The risk of duodenal ulcers tends to begin around age 25 and continues until age 75. Gastric ulcers peak in people between the ages of 55 and 65. There is an 80 percent incidence of duodenal ulcers (see Figure 23-6).

Nonsteroidal Anti-Inflammatory Drugs

Some peptic ulcers can be caused by the extended use of nonsteroidal anti-inflammatory drugs (NSAIDs), such as ibuprofen and naproxen sodium. Many NSAID medications can be found in most stores and are available OTC. Other NSAIDs, such as Celebrex®, require a prescription.

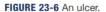

FIGURE 23-6 An ulcer.

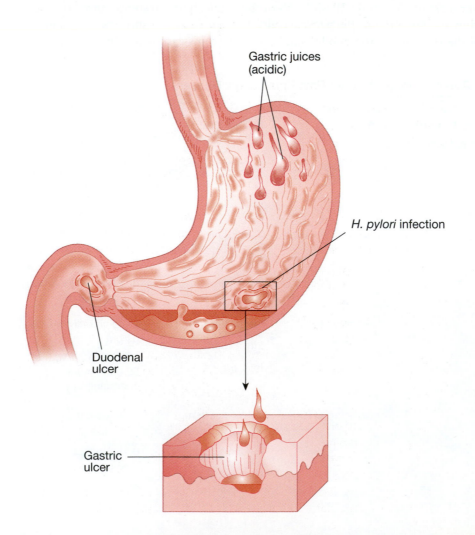

Gastric juices (acidic)

H. pylori infection

Duodenal ulcer

Gastric ulcer

NSAIDs are prescribed to reduce inflammation and fever, but are also effective for analgesia (pain reduction). However, use of NSAIDs does increase the risk of stomach ulcers. NSAIDs work by blocking the effect of the enzyme cyclooxygenase (COX). Prostaglandins are produced within the body's cells by one of two COX enzymes, COX-1 and COX-2. Prostaglandins promote inflammation, pain, and fever. However, they also protect the lining of the stomach from the damaging effects of acid, by stimulating the *gastric mucosa* to secrete a protective fluid. Only COX-1 produces prostaglandins that support platelets and protect the stomach. NSAIDs block all COX enzymes, and thus reduce prostaglandin production throughout the body. This can reduce the stomach's natural defenses and promote ulcer development.

Workplace Wisdom NSAIDs

Nearly 4 percent of regular NSAID users develop serious gastrointestinal conditions. Patients are advised to always take NSAID medications with food to help prevent stomach problems. NSAID-induced ulcers usually heal once the person stops taking the medication.

Other Causes of Ulcers

Other factors that can induce the overproduction of acid and cause ulcers include the following:

Infection.   A major cause of peptic ulcers is infection with the bacterium *Helicobacter pylori (H. pylori),* a spiral-shaped bacterium found in the gastric mucous layer or adhering to the epithelial lining of the stomach. It can multiply readily in the right conditions. A by-product of its cell division is an acid that leads to overacidification of the stomach and intestines. *H. pylori* is responsible for about 90 percent of duodenal ulcers and 80 percent of gastric ulcers. Many people have *H. pylori* infections, but not everyone with an infection develops a peptic ulcer.

Smoking.   Ulcers are more likely to occur, less likely to heal, and more likely to cause death in smokers than in nonsmokers. Some studies show that smoking reduces the bicarbonate produced by the pancreas, interfering with the neutralization of acid in the duodenum. Other research shows that smoking lessens the power of the immune system to fight the *H. pylori* bacteria. The best advice is to discontinue smoking.

Alcohol.   Research reports are mixed, but some results show that alcohol may aggravate *H. pylori* infections and cause more bleeding. The advice is to decrease alcohol consumption or discontinue consumption completely in severe cases.

Excessive peristalsis.   Motility stimulates the parietal cells to secrete more acid, and some researchers believe that the peristalsis that accompanies stress can lead to this. Diarrhea may be caused by an increase in motility and peristalsis, or "spasms of the colon," so antidiarrheals may help in alleviating the overproduction of acid by reducing motility. Antispasmodics, also known as *muscarinic receptor antagonists*, that have a direct effect on smooth muscle are usually prescribed. An example is Donnatal®, which contains belladonna alkaloids.

Anticholinergics.   These medications inhibit the actions of acetylcholine at the postganglionic parasympathetic neuroeffector sites. Large doses block nicotinic sites, inhibit gastric acid secretion, and decrease GI and urinary tract motility. Moderate doses dilate the pupils and increase heart rate; small doses inhibit salivary and bronchial secretions. Drugs prescribed for this include prostaglandin replacement. An example is Cytotec® (misoprostol). Available in 100 and 200 mg tablets, a common dosage is 100 to 200 mcg qid with food. Dose can be reduced to 100 mcg if the larger dose cannot be tolerated. Because misoprostol is a prostaglandin-like substance or agonist, it stimulates production of prostaglandins by the mucosal lining. By increasing the viscosity of the gastric mucosa, it offers greater protection from the acid when the patient takes an NSAID that blocks prostaglandins. Adverse reactions include diarrhea, cramping, miscarriage, premature labor, and birth defects.

hypersensitivity allergy.

Food hypersensitivities. **Hypersensitivities** to foods, such as peanut butter, shrimp, and milk, can cause the mast cells to release histamine2 (H2). H2 binds to the H2 receptor site of the parietal cells that line the stomach wall, thus triggering the production and release of acid. As the lock-and-key theory suggests, H2 antagonists enter the H2 receptors in the parietal cells, thus preventing H2 from binding there. This blocks both acid production and secretion. This is called *competitive inhibition* (see Table 23-5).

Ulcer Therapy

Therapy for *H. pylori* infection consists of 10 to 14 days of one or two antibiotics, such as amoxicillin, tetracycline (not to be used for children under 12 years old), metronidazole, clarithromycin, plus ranitidine bismuth citrate or bismuth subsalicylate, or a proton pump inhibitor (PPI). Acid suppression by the H2 blocker or proton pump inhibitor, in conjunction with the antibiotics, helps alleviate ulcer-related symptoms, heal gastric mucosal inflammation, and may enhance efficacy of the antibiotics against *H. pylori* (see Table 23-5 and Table 23-6).

Adverse reactions to H2 antagonist drugs include fatigue, hypertension, muscle pain, bronchiospasm, grand mal seizures, impotence, and *gynecomastia* (development of breasts in males).

Proton pump inhibitors block the enzyme that turns on the H+–ATPase enzyme system. When this enzyme is blocked, the parietal cells will not secrete hydrogen, which is the last step in making HCl. Side effects include headache, nausea, and vomiting. Drugs with adverse interactions include digoxin (PPIs can cause an increase in plasma levels of digoxin) and ketoconazole (PPIs can cause a decrease in plasma levels of ketoconazole) (see Table 23-7).

Table 23-5   H2 Antagonist Drugs Used for Ulcer Treatment

TRADE NAME	GENERIC NAME	AVAILABLE STRENGTH AND DOSAGE FORM	DOSAGE
Axid®	nizatidine	Tab: 150 mg, 300 mg	150 mg po bid or 300 mg po qhs
Pepcid®	famotidine	Tab: 20 mg, 40 mg	20 mg–40 mg po daily
		Susp: 40 mg/5 mL oral	
Tagamet®	cimetidine	Tab: 200 mg, 300 mg, 400 mg, 800 mg	300 mg po qid or 400 mg po bid or 800 mg po qhs
		Inj: 300 mg/2 mL	300 mg IV q6–8 hr
Zantac®	ranitidine	Tab: 150 mg, 300 mg; 25 mg, 150 mg effervescent tablets	150 mg po bid or 300 mg po qhs
		Syrup: 75 mg/5 mL	
		Inj: 25 mg/1 mL premixed IVPB: 50 mg	50 mg IM or IV q6–8 hr

Table 23-6 Multiple Drug Therapy Used for *H. pylori* Infection

DRUG REGIMENS	
Non-PPI Drug Regimen	
bismuth subsalicylate (Pepto-Bismol®) 525 mg qid	+ metronidazole (Flagyl®) 250 mg qid + tetracycline 500 mg qid* × 2 wks + H2 receptor antagonist therapy as directed × 4 wks
Double-Drug Theory	
lansoprazole 30 mg tid	+ amoxicillin 1 g tid × 2 wks
Triple-Drug Theory	
1. omeprazole 20 mg bid + clarithromycin 500 mg bid + amoxicillin 1 g bid × 10 days	
2. lansoprazole 30 mg bid + clarithromycin 500 mg bid + amoxicillin 1 g bid × 10 days	

Table 23-7 PPI Drugs Used for Ulcer Treatment

TRADE NAME	GENERIC NAME	AVAILABILITY	DOSAGE
Aciphex®	rabeprazole sodium	20 mg delayed-release tablets	20 to 40 mg daily
Nexium®	esomeprazole magnesium	20 mg, 40 mg delayed-release capsules	20 or 40 mg daily
Prevacid®	lansoprazole	15 mg, and 30 mg enteric-coated delayed-release capsules	15 or 30 mg daily
Prilosec®	omeprazole	10 mg, 20 mg, and 40 mg delayed-release capsules	20 or 40 mg daily
Protonix®	pantoprazole	20 mg, 40 mg delayed-release tablets	40 mg daily

Constipation

Constipation is a GI condition characterized by hard, dry, small-sized stools that are difficult to pass. People with constipation usually have fewer than three bowel movements per week, along with other symptoms that may include straining, bloating, abdominal pain and distention, or the sensation of incomplete emptying. Constipation is a symptom, not a disease, and in most cases results from a diet that is high in fat and low in fiber. Other causes of constipation are:

- lack of physical activity
- medications such as loperamide, codeine, morphine, and iron supplements
- abuse of laxatives
- suppression of defecation
- milk
- diseases such as multiple sclerosis, stroke, and diabetes
- changes in lifestyle, such as aging, pregnancy, and travel

Laxatives are drugs used to treat constipation or evacuate the colon for medical examinations (see Table 23-8). They include the following types:

- *Bulk-forming*, which work in the intestine by absorbing water to make the stool softer. Considered the most common and safest type of laxative.
- *Emollients*, which work by stopping the colon from absorbing fecal water, and thereby softening the stool.
- *Evacuants*, used for bowel cleansing before medical exams.
- *Fecal softeners/surfactants*, which work in the intestines and help mix fat and water to soften stool.
- *Hyperosmotics*, which cause colon fluid retention and thereby increase peristalsis.
- *Saline*, which draws water into the colon, making it easier to pass stools.
- *Stimulants/irritants*, which work by causing rhythmic intestinal contractions.

Table 23-8 Types of Laxatives

TYPE	ONSET OF ACTION	TRADE NAME	GENERIC NAME
Bulk-forming	12–72 hours		psyllium
		Metamucil®	polycarbophil
		FiberCon®	methylcellulose
Emollient	6–8 hours	Citrucel®	mineral oil
Evacuant	1 hour		Polyethylene glycol-electrolyte solution (PEG-ES)
		CoLyte®	Polyethylene glycol (PEG) solution
		GoLYTELY®	
Fecal softener/ surfactant	raise 12–72 hours	GlycoLax®	docusate sodium
		MiraLax®	
		Colace®	docusate calcium
Hyperosmotic	15 min–1 hour	Surfak® Liquigels	glycerin supp
	24–48 hours	Sani-Supp®	lactulose
		Colace®	
Saline	30 min—3 hours	Cephulac®	magnesium sulfate
		Enulose®	(Epsom Salt)
			milk of magnesia
			monobasic sodium phosphate/dibasic sodium phosphate
Stimulant/irritant	6–8 hours	Fleets Phospho-Soda®	cascara sagrada
	6–10 hours		sennosides
	supp: 15 min–1 hour	ex-lax®	bisacodyl
	tab: 6–10 hours	Senokot®	
		Dulcolax®	
		Correctol®	

Nutrition

Modern daily food intake recommendations are based on *Nutrition and Your Health: Dietary Guidelines for Americans*. This publication was first developed in 1980 by the U.S. Department of Agriculture (USDA) and the Department of Health and Human Services (DHHS) for use in consumer nutrition education efforts with healthy Americans aged 2 years and older. The guidelines are revised every five years to include analysis of the most recent research of the Dietary Guidelines Advisory Committee (DGAC).

The Recommended Dietary Allowances (RDAs) were established to define the nutritional needs of healthy persons living in the United States. The Food and Nutrition Board of the National Academy of Sciences set the values for the RDAs on the basis of human and animal research.

The RDAs have been revised and are now being replaced by the **Dietary Reference Intake (DRI)**. The DRIs include both recommended intakes and tolerable upper intake levels. The National Information Resource Center states that the DRIs are based on the evaluation of the four following categories:

1. Estimated Average Requirement—the nutrient value that is estimated to meet the needs of 50 percent of the population.

2. Recommended Dietary Allowance—the nutrient value that prevents deficiencies in 98 percent of the population.

3. Adequate Intake—the value set for nutrients that do not have an RDA.

4. Tolerable Upper Intake Level (UL)—the highest value of a nutrient that is not likely to pose adverse effects in 98 percent of the population.

The nutrients needed by the body fall into one of three categories: macronutrients, micronutrients, and water.

> **Dietary Reference Intakes (DRI)** nutritional guidelines that include both recommended intakes and tolerable upper intake levels.

Macronutrients

Macronutrients are nutrients that the body requires in relatively large quantities; the three types are carbohydrates, proteins, and fats. **Kilocalories (kcal)** are the units of measure of the energy needed to digest and utilize food and the energy expended with exercise. Fats are the most concentrated source of food energy. One gram of fat supplies about 9 kcal, as compared to the 4 kcal supplied by carbohydrates and protein. The micronutrients—vitamins, minerals, and water—provide no calories or energy.

> **kilocalories (kcal)** unit of measurement for food energy.

Carbohydrates

Sources of carbohydrates include fruits, vegetables, whole grains, and legumes, all of which contain fiber, starch, and some vitamins and minerals. Carbohydrates can be classified as either simple or complex. Simple carbohydrates are sugars and contain no energy-yielding calories. They are considered "empty calories," like candy, for example. Complex carbohydrates are starches, take longer to be broken down in the digestive tract, and have more nutritional value than simple sugars. Whole-grain bread is an example of a complex carbohydrate.

Carbohydrates provide immediate energy and are the most readily available sources of food energy. During digestion and metabolism, carbohydrates are broken down to the simple sugar glucose to be used as the body's principal energy source. Glucose is stored in the liver and muscle tissue as glycogen. A carbohydrate-rich diet is necessary to maintain muscle glycogen, the preferred fuel for most types of exercise. The **Acceptable Macronutrient Distribution Range (AMDR)** for carbohydrates is 45 to 65 percent of daily caloric intake. The AMDR is the range associated with the reduced risk of disease while providing needed nutrients. Of course, most health benefits will be derived from ingestion of more complex carbohydrates and fewer simple carbohydrates.

> **Acceptable Macronutrient Distribution Range (AMDR)** the range of intake levels that provide adequate amount of a nutrient and are associated with a reduced risk of disease.

Fats

Lipids play an important role in the body. The main functions of body fat are to:

- help to provide lubrication
- store energy reserves
- act as insulation to provide and retain warmth
- provide a cushion and protect vital organs by acting as a shock absorber
- help metabolize carbohydrates and proteins more efficiently
- help absorb and transport fat-soluble vitamins such as Vitamins A, D, E, and K

Dietary fats (lipids) are the body's only source of the fatty acid linoleic acid, which is essential for growth and skin maintenance. Fats are divided into two categories: saturated and unsaturated (including monounsaturated and polyunsaturated fatty acids). These fatty acids differ from each other chemically based on the nature of the bond between the carbon and hydrogen atoms.

As a general rule, saturated fat is solid at room temperature; most saturated fat is derived from animal sources. Unsaturated fat, which is liquid at room temperature, is derived primarily from plants. Monounsaturated and polyunsaturated fats should be emphasized in the diet, as they tend to lower the blood cholesterol level. Saturated fats tend to raise the level of blood cholesterol. High blood cholesterol levels are associated with an increased risk of coronary heart disease.

Of the two types of fat, saturated is considered "bad" fat because the entire lipid chain has hydrogen atoms covering it, which leads to increased **low-density lipoprotein (LDL)** and total cholesterol levels. Saturated fats contain more cholesterol because they are derived from animal sources such as meat and dairy products. Butter, skin of the animal, and mayonnaise are also saturated fats. Some saturated oils, such as palm and coconut oil, may actually cause the body to overmanufacture cholesterol.

Unsaturated fat is considered good or better dietary fat because it is less hydrogenated. Examples of monounsaturated fat are olive oil and canola oil. Polyunsaturated fats are found in most other vegetable oils and nuts, but deep cold-water fish, such as salmon, mackerel, tuna, and bluefish, are also all sources of "good" dietary fat.

low-density lipoprotein (LDL) bad cholesterol.

" Workplace Wisdom Dietary Risks

Current studies show diets containing a higher amount of a certain type of polyunsaturated fatty acid are associated with a decreased risk for heart disease in certain people. "

Hydrogenated fats are created when an oil or fat that is largely unsaturated, such as corn oil, has hydrogen added to it. Chemically saturating an unsaturated fat, by adding hydrogen atoms, produces trans-fatty acids, which act like saturated fats in the body and have the same capacity to do harm as saturated fats. Research shows that trans-fatty acids increase LDL cholesterol levels, decrease the levels of **high-density lipoprotein (HDL)** cholesterol, and thus increase the risk of coronary heart disease. Hydrogenated fat, like margarine, is solid or semi-solid at room temperature; it is used in many processed foods because it is more stable and goes rancid more slowly than unprocessed, unhydrogenated fats and oils.

In addition, trans-fatty acids, which are chemically altered (processed) fats, are also found in many packaged foods, and may be listed on the labels as partially hydrogenated or hydrogenated oil. The more solid and hydrogenated the fat is, the more trans-fatty acids there are in the product. Commercial peanut butter is an example.

high-density lipoprotein (HDL) good cholesterol.

Palm and coconut oils are also high in saturated fats, even though they stay liquid at room temperature. They will raise blood levels of bad cholesterol (LDL and *VLDL*, which is very low-density lipoprotein) and lower good cholesterol (HDL).

Essential fatty acids, omega-3 and omega-6, are fats that are needed by the body but are not produced internally; they must be taken in from foods. Omega-3 fatty acids, found primarily in fish, helps prevent heart disease, arthritis, and cancer growth and development.

The AMDR for fats is 20 to 35 percent of caloric intake—but not more than 10 percent of calorie intake should be saturated fat. Saturated fats, hydrogenated or partially hydrogenated fats or oils, trans fats (chemically altered), and palm and coconut oils that raise blood bad cholesterol (LDL and VLDL) should be avoided and replaced with healthier fats such as olive and canola oil.

Protein

Proteins make up almost all cells, tissues, and organs of the body and are considered the body's main building blocks. Hormones, enzymes, and blood-plasma transport systems are also composed of proteins. Protein is necessary to make and repair body cells, tissue, and muscle.

Proteins are composed of complex strings of amino acids.

Proteins can be divided into two groups: complete and incomplete. *Complete* or *essential proteins* have the essential amino acids necessary to build other proteins. Complete proteins can be found in animal muscle (e.g., beef, chicken, pork, fish). Incomplete proteins are missing one or more of the amino acids needed to build other proteins. *Incomplete protein* can be found in plant-based foods such as beans and peanuts.

The body requires 20 different amino acids, both essential and nonessential, to maintain proper nutrition. Essential amino acids are not produced within the body. Therefore, essential amino acids have to be derived from food intake. The remaining 11 nonessential amino acids can be produced by the body (see Table 23-9).

Protein is not normally a significant energy source, during either rest or exercise. However, the body will use protein for energy when calorie or carbohydrate intake is inadequate (during fasting or a low-carbohydrate diet). The AMDR for protein is 10 to 35 percent of total caloric intake.

When a person eats excessive amounts of protein, the body must excrete the extra nitrogen. Therefore, the body produces extra urine, requiring extra fluid. This places

Table 23-9   Essential and Nonessential Amino Acids

ESSENTIAL	NONESSENTIAL
histidine	alanine
isoleucine	arginine
leucine	asparagine
lysine	aspartic acid
methionine	cysteine
phenylalanine	glutamic acid
threonine	glutamine
tryptophan	glycine
valine	proline
	serine
	tyrosine

many athletes, and others who are less than amply hydrated, at risk of dehydration. In extreme cases, excess protein or amino acid intake can lead to kidney damage. In addition, excessive protein intake can cause urinary calcium loss. However, severe restriction of protein intake often results in decreased iron intake.

Micronutrients

Micronutrients are nutrients that the body requires in only small quantities. Micronutrients include both vitamins and minerals.

Vitamins

Following the DRI suggestions for vitamins may help to prevent diseases and maintain good health. Good food sources are preferred to vitamin supplements because food also is a good source of fiber and other nutrients. Vitamins are classified as either fat-soluble or water-soluble. The Reference Daily Intakes (RDIs) mentioned in the following sections are for the average adult male and female 19 to 70 years old.

Fat-Soluble Vitamins

The fat-soluble vitamins, A, D, E, and K, are found in the fat and oily parts of foods. They tend to be stored in the liver and adipose tissue and remain there, rather than being excreted like most water-soluble vitamins. The storage of fat-soluble vitamins in the body makes it possible to survive long periods of time without having to include them in the diet. However, because they are stored so efficiently in the body, fat-soluble vitamins carry a high risk of toxicity.

Vitamin A.   Vitamin A (retinol) is found in orange, yellow-orange, and green leafy vegetable foods, such as carrots, pumpkin, apricot, squash, peaches, and spinach. Vitamin A is also found in beef liver and fish liver oil.

Most of the body's vitamin A is stored in the liver as retinyl palmitate and released into the bloodstream as retinal. It binds to retinol-binding protein and prealbumin (transthyretin). It helps with eyesight and epithelial cells and tissues (skin cells).

Deficiencies in vitamin A may cause night blindness; xerosis (dryness) of the conjunctiva and cornea; xerophthalmia and keratomalacia; keratinization of lung, GI tract, and urinary tract tissues; and increased susceptibility to infection. Follicular hyperkeratosis of the skin (raised pink bumps where hair exits) is common in vitamin A deficiency.

Acute toxicity occurs in children taking vitamin A doses greater than 100,000 micrograms (300,000 International Units), resulting in increased intracranial pressure and vomiting. Death may ensue unless ingestion is discontinued. Women who take 13-*cis*-retinoic acid (isotretinoin) for skin conditions during pregnancy may cause birth defects in infants. Adults may also exhibit *carotenosis*, in which the skin (not including the sclera) becomes deep yellow or orange-yellow, especially on the palms and soles. Early warning signs may include sparse or coarse hair, thinning eyebrows, dry rough skin, and cracked lips. The DRI is 900 micrograms (**μg**)/day for males and 700 μg/day for females.

μg microgram.

Vitamin D.   Sunlight enables the skin to make vitamin D with cholesterol. Milk is often **fortified** with vitamin D, as are canned salmon and tuna. The main function of vitamin D is to improve the absorption of calcium from the intestine, to make stronger bones and teeth. Deficiency causes metabolic bone softening called *rickets* in children and *osteomalacia* in adults. The DRI is 5 μg/day (ages 19–50) and 10 μg/day (ages 51–70) for both males and females.

fortified with an added nutrient for enrichment.

Vitamin E.   Vitamin E is found in wheat germ oil, sunflower seeds, eggs, butter, nuts, and leafy green vegetables. Vitamin E is a strong antioxidant for lipids.

Deficiency is generally caused by **malabsorption**, not by lack of ingestion. Vitamin E deficiency may cause disorders of the reproductive system; abnormalities of muscle, liver, and bone marrow; hemolysis of red blood cells; defective embryo genesis; brain dysfunction; and disorder of capillary permeability. The DRI is 15 mg/day for both males and females.

Vitamin K. Vitamin K (phytonadione) is found primarily in dark-green leafy vegetables. Vitamin K is necessary for blood coagulation; it controls the formation of coagulation factors II (prothrombin), VII (proconvertin), IX (Christmas factor, plasma thromboplastin component), and X (Stuart factor) in the liver. Vitamin K is also needed for calcium uptake in the bones. It is used as an antidote for coumadin overdoses.

Deficiency is rare in adults because the microbiologic flora of the normal gut synthesize menaquinones (from Vitamin K). However, the following can contribute to an increased need for Vitamin K: trauma, extensive surgery, long-term parenteral nutrition with or without treatment with broad-spectrum antibiotics, and overdoses of coumadin. Drugs that contribute to vitamin K-related hemorrhagic disease are anticonvulsants, anticoagulants, certain antibiotics (particularly cephalosporins), salicylates, and megadoses of vitamin A or E. The DRI is 120 µg/day for males and 90 µg/day for females.

> **malabsorption** an abnormality in digestion that causes nutrients to be absorbed poorly or not at all.

INFORMATION

In infants, the liver, where vitamin K is stored, is not fully developed. Thus, vitamin K deficiency in breastfed infants remains a major worldwide cause of infant morbidity and mortality. One to seven days postpartum, the vitamin-deficient infant may have skin, GI, or chest hemorrhage.

Water-Soluble Vitamins

Water-soluble vitamins, for the most part, are carried in the bloodstream and excreted in the urine. Although they are required only in small doses, intake is needed on a daily basis. Vitamins B1, B2, B6, B12, and C are water-soluble vitamins. Water-soluble vitamins are unlikely to be toxic, but excess intake of Vitamins C and B6 may have serious side effects. These vitamins are easily destroyed during storage or preparation.

Vitamin B1. Vitamin B1 (thiamine) can be found in fortified bread and cereals, sunflower seeds, peanuts, wheat bran, beef liver, pork, seafood, egg yolk, and beans. Vitamin B1 is necessary for carbohydrate metabolism.

Deficiency causes the disease *beriberi,* which affects the peripheral neurologic, cerebral, cardiovascular, and GI systems. Those most at risk are breastfeeding infants whose mothers are thiamine-deficient, adults with high consumption of polished rice, alcoholics, patients on renal dialysis, patients on total parenteral nutrition (TPN) (high concentrations of dextrose infusions or frequent or long-term infusions can lead to increased need for B1, especially if vitamin B1 is not administered), and patients with **hypermetabolic** states in which more carbohydrate is needed or metabolized (for example, fever, infection, pregnancy, and strenuous exercise). The DRI is 1.2 mg/day for males and 1.1 mg/day for females.

> **hypermetabolic** metabolizing at an increased rate.

Vitamin B2. Vitamin B2 (riboflavin) is found in liver, kidney, heart, nuts, cheese, eggs, milk, green leafy vegetables, whole grains, and fortified cereals. Vitamin B2 is needed for the health of the mucous membranes in the digestive tract and aids in absorption of iron and vitamin B6.

Deficiency of vitamin B2 leads to oral, eye, skin, and genital lesions; dizziness; hair loss; insomnia; light sensitivity; poor digestion; retarded growth; slow mental responses; and burning feet. The DRI is 1.3 mg/day for males and 1.1 mg/day for females.

Vitamin B3. Vitamin B3 (niacin) is found in lean meats, poultry, fish, liver, and peanuts. Vitamin B3 is very important in oxidation-reduction reactions and is vital in protein metabolism.

Deficiency of niacin and tryptophan, an amino acid that allows the body to synthesize niacin, leads to the disease *pellagra*. Pellagra affects the skin, mucous membranes, GI and brain/CNS systems, with photosensitive rash, scarlet stomatitis, glossitis, diarrhea, and mental aberrations. Common in India and Central and South America, deficiency is found in diets high in corn. The DRI is 16 mg/day for males and 14 mg/day for females.

Vitamin B5. Vitamin B5 (pantothenic acid) can be found in beef, brewer's yeast, eggs, fresh vegetables, kidney, legumes, liver, mushrooms, nuts, pork, fish, whole rye flour, and whole wheat. Vitamin B5 is important for the secretion of hormones such as cortisone, and for maintenance of healthy skin, muscles, and nerves. Pantothenic acid is used in the release of energy; in the metabolism of fat, protein, and carbohydrates, and in the manufacture of lipids, neurotransmitters, steroid hormones, and hemoglobin.

Although vitamin B5 deficiency is extremely rare, symptoms include insomnia, depression, nausea, headache, and muscle spasm. The DRI is 5 mg/day for both males and females.

" Workplace Wisdom Vitamin Abbreviations

It is important for pharmacy technicians to know both the vitamin letter and its corresponding generic name. This is because vitamin names written without the generic name raise the risk of transcription and/or filling errors. "

Vitamin B6. Vitamin B6 (pyridoxine) is found in fortified cereals, beans, meat, poultry, fish, and some fruits and vegetables. Vitamin B6 is needed for red blood cell formation, antibody production, and cell respiration and growth, as well as for the conversion of tryptophan to niacin. When caloric intake is low, the body needs B6 to help convert stored carbohydrate or other nutrients to glucose to maintain normal blood sugar levels. Vitamin B6 helps maintain the normal range of blood glucose and the health of lymphoid organs (thymus, spleen, and lymph nodes) that make white blood cells. It is needed for the synthesis of the neurotransmitters required for normal nerve cell communication, such as serotonin and dopamine.

" Workplace Wisdom Pyridoxine Supplements

Although a shortage of vitamin B6 will limit the functions discussed here, supplements do not enhance them in well-nourished individuals without vitamin B6 deficiencies. "

Vitamin B6 deficiency can result in a form of anemia that is similar to iron-deficiency anemia. B6 deficiency can decrease antibody production and suppress the immune response. Signs and symptoms include dermatitis, glossitis (a sore tongue), depression, confusion, and convulsions.

Toxicity of vitamin B6 may cause sensory ataxia, profound impairment of position and vibration sense in the lower limbs, and nerve damage to the arms and legs. This neuropathy is usually related to high intake of vitamin B6 from supplements, and can be reversed by stopping supplementation. Senses of touch, temperature, and pain are only somewhat affected. The RDI is 1.3 mg/day for males and females aged 19 to 50 and 1.7 mg/day males and 1.5 mg/day for females over the age of 51.

Vitamin B9. Vitamin B9 (folic acid) is found in barley, beef, bran, brewer's yeast, brown rice, cheese, chicken, dates, green leafy vegetables, lamb, legumes, lentils, liver, milk, mushrooms, oranges, split peas, pork, root vegetables, salmon, tuna, wheat germ, whole grains, and whole wheat. Vitamin B9 is important for energy production and the formation of red blood cells. It strengthens immunity, promotes healthy cell division and replication, assists in protein metabolism, and prevents depression and anxiety.

Folic acid deficiency can be serious and may result in sore, red tongue, anemia, apathy, digestive disturbances, fatigue, graying hair, growth impairment, insomnia, labored breathing, memory problems, paranoia, and weakness. Spina bifida can occur in the infant if a pregnant woman does not get enough folic acid, especially in the first trimester. The RDI is 400 µg/day for both males and females.

● ● ● PROFILES IN PRACTICE

A doctor orders TPN for an inpatient; the solution is to contain 20 g of lipids 20% (fat), 50 g of amino acids 10% (protein), and 350 g of dextrose 70% (carbohydrate) per TPN bag.

_____

• What is the total number of kcals provided to the patient by one TPN bag?

Vitamin B12. Vitamin B12 (cyanocobalamin) is found in mollusks, clams, beef liver, rainbow trout, and fortified cereals. Vitamin B12 is needed for healthy nerve cells, to make DNA, and for the formation of red blood cells. Vitamin B12 is bound to the protein in food, and hydrochloric acid in the stomach releases B12 from the protein during digestion. Once released, B12 combines with a substance called intrinsic factor (IF) before it is absorbed into the bloodstream.

Deficiency is a very serious problem, ultimately leading to irreversible nerve damage signified by numbness and tingling in the hands and feet. Signs and symptoms include fatigue, weakness, nausea, constipation, flatulence, loss of appetite, weight loss, difficulty in maintaining balance, depression, confusion, poor memory, and soreness of the mouth or tongue. The RDI is 2.4 µg/day for both males and females.

● INFORMATION ●

Vitamin B12 binds with intrinsic factor before it is absorbed and used by the body. An absence of IF prevents normal absorption of B12 and results in *pernicious anemia*. Patients with pernicious anemia need IM injections of B12, as it is a chronic condition requiring monitoring by a physician and lifelong supplementation of vitamin B12.

Vitamin C. Vitamin C (ascorbic acid) is found in citrus fruits, including oranges, lemons, limes, and grapefruits. Vitamin C is an **antioxidant**, and is essential for collagen formation and for maintaining the integrity of connective tissue, bone, and teeth. Important for wound healing and recovery from burns, vitamin C helps the absorption of iron. Vitamin C functions as a reduction/oxidation system in the cells of the body. It also activates enzymes that hydroxylate procollagen proline and lysine to procollagen hydroxyproline and hydroxylysine.

antioxidant molecule that slows or prevents the oxidation of other molecules.

Severe deficiency results in *scurvy*, a condition characterized by general weakness, bleeding gums, anemia, and skin bleeding. The DRI for vitamin C is 90 mg/day for males and 75 mg/day for females.

Minerals

Minerals are inorganic compounds that are much smaller than vitamins and occur in much simpler forms. Like vitamins, minerals have no calories and do not provide energy to the body. Dozens of minerals are found in nature, and 21 of them are essential for human nutrition. Minerals also act as helpers in delivering nutrients and aiding in certain functions in the body. They differ from vitamins in that they are indestructible; they act as catalysts in body processes, but are not consumed or broken down in these processes. Minerals are not made by the body; therefore, **exogenous** sources must be used.

exogenous from outside the organism.

Some minerals, such as calcium and phosphorus, are used to build bones and teeth. Others are important components of hormones, such as iodine in thyroxine. Sodium and potassium are minerals called *electrolytes* that help regulate muscle contraction, conduction of nerve impulses, and normal heart rhythm.

Minerals are classified into two groups, based on the body's need. The *major minerals*, or *macrominerals*, are needed by the body in larger quantities; in general, more than 100 mg per day. Calcium, chlorine, magnesium, phosphorus, potassium, sodium, and sulfur fall into this category. *Minor minerals*, or *trace elements*, are needed in amounts of less than 100 mg per day. Iron, zinc, selenium, copper, and iodine are minor minerals.

Minerals are very important in regulation of numerous body functions. Some common minerals, their main functions, and DRIs are listed in Table 23-10.

Table 23-10   Mineral Functions and DRIs

MINERAL	MAIN FUNCTION	DRI (MALES)	DRI (FEMALES)
Calcium	bone, muscle, nerve, and blood development	1,000 mg/day (ages 19–50) 1,200 mg/day (ages 51 & up)	1,000 mg/day (ages 19–50) 1,200 mg/day (ages 51 & up)
Iron	maintains oxygen levels in blood	8 mg/day	18 mg/day (ages 19–50) 8 mg/day (ages 51 & up)
Magnesium	aids in energy metabolism, protein synthesis, maintenance of muscle and nerve function. Needed for more than 300 biochemical reactions in the body.	400 mg/day (ages 19–30) 420 mg/day (ages 31 & up)	310 mg/day (ages 19–30) 320 mg/day (ages 31 & up)
Potassium	maintains proper muscle memory function	4.7 g/day	4.7 g/day
Selenium	supports immune system and thyroid, and helps make antioxidants	55 μ/day	55 μ/day
Sodium	regulates body fluids	1.5 g/day (ages 19–30) 1.3 g/day (ages 31–70)	1.5 g/day (ages 19–30) 1.3 g/day (ages 31–70)
Zinc	aids in the healing process	11 mg/day	8 mg/day

Water

Water makes up 60 percent of an adult's body weight. The average adult male should drink 3 liters of fluids per day while women need 2.2 liters per day. Most water should come from liquids and foods. Water is an indispensable component of the body: it actually forms a major portion of every tissue and provides the medium in which most of the body's activities are conducted. It also facilitates many of the metabolic reactions that occur in the body and helps transport vital materials to the cells. One highly important function of water is to serve as the vehicle in which glycogen is transported into muscle cells. *Glycogen* is often referred to as muscle fuel, because it powers muscle contractions.

INFORMATION

Use the following formula to determine your water requirements.

Body weight $\times$ 0.6 $\div$ 12

Example

200 lb. $\times$ 0.6 $\div$ 12 = 10 (8-oz. glasses of water a day)

Regular intake helps maintain normal functions of the body. Thirst is a signal to drink water. Lack of water can lead to dehydration.

USDA MyPyramid Food Guidance System

The traditional food guide pyramid was developed by the USDA with support from the Department of Health and Human Services. With the understanding that "one size does not fit all," the food pyramid was recently revised to reflect more individual dietary needs. Now called MyPyramid, the USDA guidance system is designed to help people to:

- make healthy food choices
- find balance between food and exercise
- stay within the recommended caloric intake
- get the most nutrition from their caloric intake

Food Allergies

People develop allergies to all different kinds of foods. Approximately 2 percent of American adults and 5 percent of infants and children have a food allergy, and 90 percent of all food-related allergic reactions are caused by one of the following eight foods: milk, eggs, fish, shellfish, tree nuts, peanuts, wheat, and soybeans. Food allergies involve the immune system and can be quite troublesome for those who experience common symptoms, such as swelling, hives, rashes, nasal congestion, asthma, nausea, diarrhea, and gas. Symptoms can be immediate or delayed up to 48 hours after ingestion of the offending food. Allergic reactions can be severe and life-threatening, causing anaphylactic shock and even death.

Food *intolerances* cause the same symptoms as food allergies, but without involving the immune system. For example, a lactose intolerance can cause symptoms similar to mild allergy, such as gas and diarrhea. However, lactose intolerance may also cause thinning of the GI mucous lining, cramping, and bleeding during defecation; an allergy to milk would not produce these effects. All unexpected food reactions should be evaluated by an expert.

SUMMARY

The gastrointestinal system is the system whereby food travels through the body and digestion is accomplished. Food is broken down, absorbed, or chemically modified into substances that are required by the cells to survive and function properly. Waste products that the body cannot use are eliminated. The gastrointestinal system extends from the mouth to the anus. Its six main parts are the mouth, esophagus, pharynx, stomach, and small and large intestines. Various supportive structures, accessory glands, and accessory organs are also parts of the complete digestive system. The main purpose of the digestive system is to fuel the body.

An estimated 70 million Americans suffer from one or more digestive disorders; these disorders account for 13 percent of all hospitalizations. More than 400,000 new cases of peptic ulcer are diagnosed each year, resulting in nearly 40,000 surgeries annually. As a pharmacy technician, you should be aware of the important digestive disorders discussed throughout this chapter.

Many over-the-counter remedies are available to treat the "milder" forms of digestive disease. More serious gastrointestinal diseases often require more aggressive therapies, including surgery.

As with any disease, the primary goal is prevention. Pharmacy technicians need to be prepared to assist the pharmacist in providing information to clients about proper nutrition, and should have an understanding of USDA recommendations and the current Dietary Reference Intakes.

CHAPTER REVIEW QUESTIONS

1. Most ulcers are found in the:
   a. stomach.
   b. duodenum.
   c. jejunum.
   d. ileum.

2. The waves of synchronized contractions that move food along the GI tract are known as:
   a. villi.
   b. emulsification.
   c. motility.
   d. peristalsis.

3. Which of the following is not part of the large intestine?
   a. cecum
   b. transverse colon
   c. duodenum
   d. sigmoid colon

4. Reglan® is used:
   a. as a GI stimulant.
   b. as an antiemetic.
   c. in the treatment of GERD.
   d. for all of the above.

5. The three parts of the small intestine are:
   a. esophagus, stomach, duodenum.
   b. jejunum, duodenum, ileum.
   c. duodenum, diaphragm, ileum.
   d. stomach, esophagus, jejunum.

6. Which of the following promotes inflammation, pain, and fever?
   a. cyclooxygenase
   b. NSAIDs
   c. 5-HT$_3$ antagonists
   d. prostaglandins

7. Which of the following can induce the overproduction of stomach acid?
   a. alcohol
   b. NSAIDs
   c. smoking
   d. all of the above

8. Current dietary daily recommendations are based on:
   a. RDA.
   b. HDL.
   c. DRI.
   d. USDA.

9. Carbohydrates should make up what percentage of a person's dietary intake?
   a. 10–35%
   b. 20–35%
   c. 45–65%
   d. 50–75%

10. Saturated fat intake should not exceed _____ of a person's total fat intake.
    a. 2%
    b. 5%
    c. 10%
    d. none of the above

11. Bile is stored in the:
    a. pancreas.
    b. liver.
    c. gallbladder.
    d. small intestine.

12. The fat-soluble vitamins are:
    a. vitamin A, vitamin B, vitamin C, vitamin D.
    b. vitamin A, vitamin C, vitamin D, vitamin K.
    c. vitamin A, vitamin D, vitamin E, vitamin K.
    d. vitamin B, vitamin C, vitamin D, vitamin K.

13. Vitamin B3 is also known as:
   a. pyridoxine.
   b. thiamine.
   c. folic acid.
   d. niacin.

14. Vitamin B6 is also known as:
   a. pyridoxine.
   b. thiamine.
   c. folic acid.
   d. niacin.

15. Macrominerals are generally required by the body in:
   a. trace amounts.
   b. amounts less than 100 mg/day.
   c. amounts greater than 100 mg/day.
   d. amounts greater than 500 mg/day.

CRITICAL THINKING QUESTIONS

1. Why are many vitamin deficiencies more prevalent in underdeveloped countries than in the United States?

2. No-/low-carbohydrate and high-protein diets are very popular. Do you think these types of diets are nutritionally sound?

3. What can people do to help reduce their risk of developing ulcers?

WEB CHALLENGE

1. Go to http://www.mypyramid.gov to assess your dietary intake and physical activity levels.

2. Visit http://www.nlm.nih.gov/medlineplus/gerd.html to learn more about GERD.

REFERENCES AND RESOURCES

Adams, MP, Josephson, DL, & Holland, LN Jr. *Pharmacology for Nurses—A Pathophysiologic Approach*. Upper Saddle River, NJ: Pearson Education, 2005.

Arthritis Today 2004 Drug Guide DMARDs (accessed July 15, 2007): http://www.arthritis.org/conditions/DrugGuide/about_dmards.asp

"Carbohydrates, Proteins, and Fats" (accessed June 27, 2007): http://www.merck.com/mmhe/sec12/ch152/ch152b.html

Drug Facts and Comparisons, 2006 ed. St. Louis: Wolters Kluwer Health.

"Food Allergens" (accessed September 11, 2007): www.fda.gov

Holland, N, & Adams, MP. *Core Concepts in Pharmacology*. Upper Saddle River, NJ: Pearson Education, 2007.

Mayo Clinic. "Water: How much should you drink every day?" (accessed 4/12/2008). http://www.mayoclinic.com/health/water/NU00283

The Merck Manual of Diagnosis and Therapy: http://www.merck.com/mrkshared/mmanual/section5/chapter57/57a.jsp

MOA of APAP News on APAP (accessed July 15, 2007): http://www.pharmweb.net/pwmirror/pwy/paracetamol/pharmwebpicmechs.html

National Digestive Diseases Information Clearinghouse (NDDIC) (accessed September 14, 2007): http://digestive.niddk.nih.gov

National Institutes of Health Office of Dietary Supplements (accessed June 26, 2007): http://ods.od.nih.gov/index.aspx

National Library of Medicine. "A Review of SERMs and National Surgical Adjuvant Breast and Bowel Project Clinical Trials" (accessed July 15, 2007): http://www.ncbi.nlm.nih.gov/entrez/query.fcgi?cmd=Retrieve&db=PubMed&listuids=14613021&dopt=Abstract

United States Department of Agriculture (accessed June 30, 2007): http://www.mypyramid.com

The Musculoskeletal System

LEARNING OBJECTIVES

After completing this chapter, you should be able to:

- List, identify, and diagram the basic anatomical structure and parts of the muscles and bones.

- Describe the functions and physiology of the muscles and bones.

- List and define common diseases affecting the muscles and bones and understand the causes, symptoms, and pharmaceutical treatments associated with each disease.

- Describe the mechanisms and the complications of the following musculoskeletal diseases and comprehend how each class of drugs works: osteomyelitis, osteoporosis, osteoarthritis, gout, inflammation, multiple sclerosis, and cerebral palsy.

- List the indications for use and mechanisms of action of ASA, NSAIDs, COX-2 inhibitors, antigout agents, calcitonin, bisphosphonates, SERMs, and skeletal muscle relaxants.

Introduction

The musculoskeletal system is extremely important, as it provides the framework of the human body for both support and movement. All body movement is coordinated between the nervous system and the bones, joints, muscles, ligaments, cartilage, and tendons. Whether you are eating, riding a bike, eliminating waste, or simply breathing, the musculoskeletal system underlies that action.

Anatomy of the Muscles

Skeletal **muscles** are attached to bones and enable body movement (*kinetics*). Skeletal muscles are voluntary, striated in shape, and contain multiple peripheral nuclei.

The heart is made up of cardiac muscle known as the *myocardium*. This muscle contracts rhythmically, and its action is coordinated by the transmission of electrical impulses from nerve to muscle fibers. The cadence and rhythm of the heart, as well as the force of contraction, are dependent on this muscle.

Smooth muscle, or *visceral muscle,* is attached to, or lines, organs such as the stomach, intestines, lungs, and blood vessels. Figure 24-1 shows the three types of muscle.

Muscle Action

A muscle's thick and thin filaments do the actual work of the muscle. The thick filaments are made of a protein called *myosin*, formed as a shaft of myosin molecules arranged in the shape of a cylinder. There are about 300 molecules of myosin per thick filament. The enzyme ATPase hydrolyzes adenosine triphosphate (ATP), which is required for myosin and actin cross-bridge formation. The thin filaments are composed of three different proteins—actin, tropomyosin, and troponin—and look like two strands of pearls twisted around each other. Together these are termed the *regulatory protein complex.*

The thick myosin filaments grab onto the thin actin filaments by forming cross-bridges during contraction of the muscle. The thick filaments grab and pull the thin filaments past them, which shortens the **sarcomere**. The signal for contraction in a muscle fiber is synchronized over the entire fiber so that all of the myofibrils that make up the sarcomere shorten at the same time. Two proteins in the grooves of each thin filament enable the thin filaments to slide along the thick ones. These proteins are *tropomyosin*, a long rod-like protein, and *troponin*, a shorter bead-like protein complex. Troponin and tropomyosin are the molecular chemicals or "switches" that control the interaction of actin and myosin during muscle contraction.

Chemical and physical interactions between actin and myosin cause the sarcomere length to shorten, and therefore the **myocyte** (muscle cell), to contract, during the process of excitation-coupling contraction.

The Functions of Muscles

The main functions of the muscles include:

- Providing movement of and within the body through contraction. This includes large movement, such as running or walking, and finer movement such as smiling or wincing.
- Stabilizing the joints.
- Maintaining body posture.
- Producing heat within the body to maintain body temperature. About 85 percent of the heat produced inside the body occurs as a result of muscle contraction.

The Bones

A newborn has about 300 "soft" **bones**, which eventually grow together, or *fuse*, to form the 206 adult bones. Some baby bones are made of **cartilage**, which is a soft and flexible cushion. During childhood, the cartilage grows and slowly hardens into bone, as calcium is deposited. At about the age of 25, the cartilage will have finished hardening into bone. After the cartilage has hardened, there can be no more bone growth. Bones are classified into one of the following five categories.

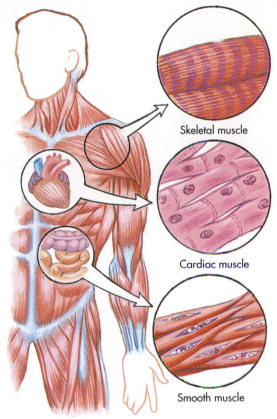

FIGURE 24-1 Types of muscle.

Skeletal muscle

Cardiac muscle

Smooth muscle

muscle specialized tissue that contracts when stimulated.

sarcomere one of the segments into which a fibril of striated muscle is divided.

myocyte a muscle cell.

bones specialized form of dense connective tissue consisting of calcified intercellular substance that provides the shape and support for the body. Bones are made of calcium and phosphate. Injuries can result in fractures.

cartilage soft tissues that line every joint and give shape to the ears and nose. Injuries can result in tears or degeneration of the cartilage and arthritis.

FIGURE 24-2 The long bone.

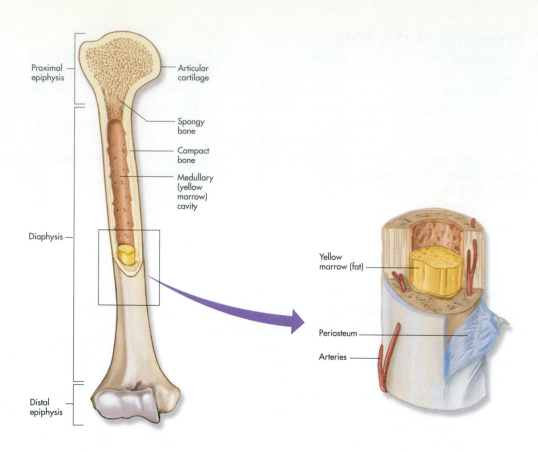

1. *Flat* bones are generally more flat than round. Examples are the cranial bones and the rib bones.

2. *Irregular* bones have no defined shape. Examples are the scapula and the vertebrae.

3. *Sesamoid* bones often have cartilage and fibrous tissue mixed in. These bones are found in the joints and help to lower friction and enhance joint movement. One examples is the patella (kneecap).

4. *Short* bones are more cube-shaped. Examples are the carpals of the hand.

5. *Long* bones are the most common (see Figure 24-2). One example is the femur of the leg. The inside of a long bone is divided into two areas: the *epiphysis* (the rounded end of the bone) and the *diaphysis* (the main shaft or central part of the bone).

The epiphysis is covered with smooth, slippery articular cartilage, which helps bones move against each other at the joints. The inside of the epiphysis is made up of spongy or *cancellous* bone, which is made from criss-crossed strands of bone; the spaces between these strands are filled with bone marrow.

The diaphysis has a hollow core, the *medullary cavity*, that is filled with red marrow in children and yellow marrow in adults. The walls of the diaphysis are made of a second type of bone called *compact bone*, which is much harder and more solid than spongy bone. The outermost layer of the long bone is the *periosteum*, which covers the diaphysis and part of the epiphysis, but does not cover the articular cartilage. This layer contains cells called *osteoblasts*, which make new bone to replace older bone cells (*osteoclasts*), and also provide nourishment for the bone.

Bone Marrow

Bone marrow is the gelatinous substance inside bones (see Figure 24-3) and occurs in two types: red and yellow. Red marrow is a red, jelly-like substance that contains blood cells and is usually found only in the sternum, vertebrae, ribs, hips, clavicles, and cranial bones. Red

bone marrow the spongy type of tissue found inside most bones; responsible for the manufacture of red blood cells, some white blood cells, and platelets. Also acts as storage area for fat.

bone marrow produces red blood cells, white blood cells, and blood platelets. In infants, red marrow is found in the bone cavities. As one ages, red marrow converts to yellow, has less fat, and is high in *erythrocytes* (red blood cells or RBCs).

Yellow marrow is a fatty yellow substance that replaces red marrow in the long bones of adults; it does not produce blood cells. Yellow bone marrow has fewer pluripotential hematopoietics (stem cells), and what stem cells it does contain are inactive.

The Functions of Bones

The main functions of the bones include:

- Providing the framework or foundation of the body.
- Supporting the body against the pull of gravity to keep it in an upright position (see Figure 24-4).
- Protecting the internal organs—heart, lungs, brain, liver—by enveloping them in a "cage."
- Allowing the exchange of nutrients and waste products, via the tunnels within the bone's living tissue.
- Acting as the components of a mechanical lever system that works with the muscular system to allow movement.

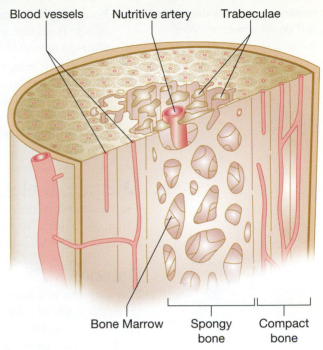

FIGURE 24-3 Bone marrow.

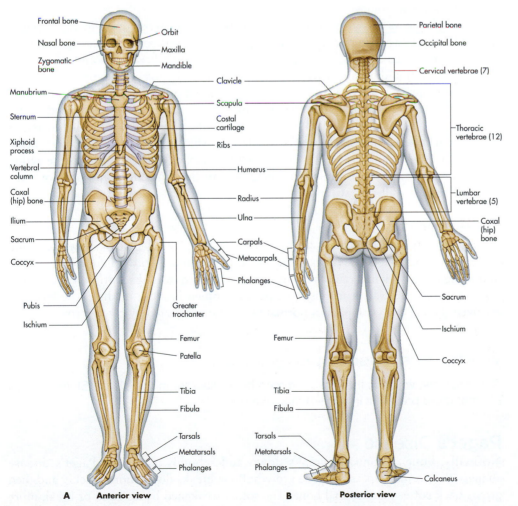

FIGURE 24-4 The skeleton.

hematopoiesis the formation and development of blood cells.

- Producing **hematopoiesis** in the red marrow. Bone marrow produces red blood cells to transport oxygen, white blood cells to fight disease-causing organisms, and platelets to stop bleeding; it also makes new cells to replace old, worn-out cells.
- Storing nutrients, such as calcium and phosphorus, in bone marrow. When calcium levels in the blood decrease below normal, the bones release calcium so that there will be an adequate supply for metabolic needs. When blood calcium levels increase, the excess calcium is stored in the bone matrix. The dynamic process of releasing and storing calcium goes on almost continuously, to maintain homeostasis.

Musculoskeletal Disorders

Diseases and disorders of the muscles and bones range from minor discomfort to debilitating conditions. This section discusses several of the most common diseases and disorders of the musculoskeletal system.

Osteomyelitis

Osteomyelitis is a bacterial infection inside the bone that destroys bone tissue. Often the original site of infection is in another part of the body, but the infection spreads to the bone via the blood.

Pharmacokinetics plays an important role in selecting anti-infective agents to combat osteomyelitis. The physician generally chooses the drug that exhibits the highest bactericidal or fungicidal activity with the least toxicity at the lowest cost. A penicillinase-resistant semisynthetic penicillin (PCN), such as nafcillin or oxacillin, and an aminoglycoside should ameliorate osteomyelitic infections, at least until culture results and sensitivities are determined.

Staphylococcus aureus is the usual culprit behind spinal osteomyelitis; it responds well to IV clindamycin in penicillin-allergic patients. Antimicrobial IV therapy may last six weeks or longer. Surgical debridement of infected, devitalized bone and tissue must be performed in addition to the IV therapy. Occasionally, hyperbaric oxygen therapy (HBO) is required. HBO therapy is a medical treatment in which patients breathe pure oxygen inside a pressurized chamber. The hyperbaric chamber is pressurized to 2.5 times normal atmospheric pressure, and delivers 100 percent oxygen. This increases the amount of oxygen being carried by the blood, which results in more oxygen being delivered to the organs and tissues in the body. This extra oxygen improves the action of certain antibiotics, activates white blood cells to fight infection, and promotes the healing process in chronic wounds.

Osteoporosis

Osteoporosis is bone brittleness due to lack of calcium. Estrogen helps to keep calcium in the bone and blood; parathyroid hormone (PTH) and calcitonin contribute to the homeostasis of calcium; and vitamin D is required for absorption of calcium. Osteoporosis is prevalent in postmenopausal women because of their low levels of estrogen. Figure 24-5 compares a normal bone to one affected by osteoporosis.

> ### Workplace Wisdom Osteoporosis
>
> Osteoporosis, which is the most common bone disorder in the United States, is 400 percent more prevalent in women than in men.

Paget's Disease

Normally, bone continually breaks down and rebuilds itself, but Paget's disease changes the normal process of bone growth: Bone breaks down more quickly and then grows back softer than normal bone. The softer, weakened bones bend or break more

FIGURE 24-5 Bone density.

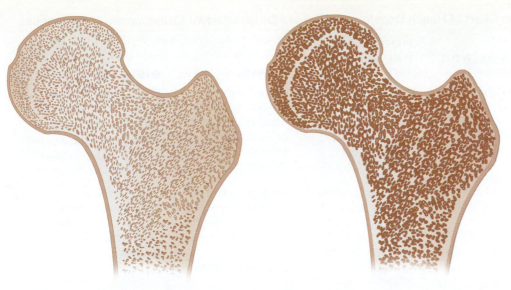

Normal Bone Tissue   Bone Tissue with Osteoporosis

easily, and may grow larger than before. Although this disease can affect any bone, it is more common in the skull, vertebra, hip, pelvis, and leg bones.

Treatment of Weak, Fragile, or Soft Bones

As discussed previously, osteoporosis is a major cause of bone fractures, affecting 20 million Americans. Women over the age of 45 commonly suffer fractures of the hip, wrist, or spine due to loss of bone mass from osteoporosis. Think of bone remodeling as a ditch digger digging a ditch and another person right beside him filling up the ditch. As old bone is worn away or removed, new bone is made. As calcium removal leaves a hole in the bone, new calcium is laid to fill in the holes, making new bone. PTH and calcitonin hormones from the parathyroid gland and thyroid gland, respectively, contribute to this homeostasis.

In addition to vitamin D and mineral calcium replacement therapy, weak, fragile, and soft bones may respond to hormonal therapy (estrogen, calcitonin) and bisphosphonates. Estrogen hormonal therapy (estrogen replacement therapy or ERT, hormone replacement therapy or HRT) is used for osteoporosis, while bisphosphonates and calcitonin are used for both Paget's disease and osteoporosis (also see Tables 24-1 and 24-2).

Table 24-1   Bone Resorption Inhibitors

BONE RESORPTION INHIBITOR	TRADE AND GENERIC NAMES	NOTES
bisphosphonates, nitrogen side-chain	Actonel® (risedronate) Aredia® (pamidronate) Boniva® (ibandronate) Fosamax® (alendronate) Zometa® (zoledronic acid)	The newer, more potent bisphosphonates are also called third-generation bisphosphonates Hypercalcemia with metastases, menopausal osteoporosis
bisphosphonates, nonnitrogen side-chain calcitonin— polypeptide hormone	Didronel® (etidronate) Skelid® (tiludronate) Miacalcin Nasal Spray®	first- and second-generation Paget's disease Reduces the risk of vertebral fracture, but not hip or wrist, in postmenopausal women with osteoporosis

Table 24-2 Comparison Chart of Health Benefits and Risks of Drugs Used for Osteoporosis in Menopause

	PARATHYROID HORMONE	HORMONE REPLACEMENT THERAPY	SERMs	BISPHOSPHONATES
Selected Examples	Forteo® (teriparatide, rDNA origin)	Premarin®, Climara®	Evista® (raloxifene), the only SERM approved for osteoporosis. Others in the investigational pipeline as of 2007.	**Oral agents:** Fosamax® (alendronate), Actonel® (risedronate). **Injected agents:** Aredia® (pamidronate), Zometa® (zoledronic acid).
Osteoporosis and Fracture	Increases bone mineral density; reduces risk of fracture	Increases bone density; reduces risk of fracture, although not significantly in women over age 60. Not currently recommended for prevention of osteoporosis in most women.	Increases bone density; reduces risk of spinal fractures. Does not appear to prevent hip fractures as bisphosphonates do.	Drug of choice (DOC) for most women. Proven to increase bone mass and prevent fractures, including hip, spine, and wrist.
Heart Disease	Unknown	No overall benefit; increased risk of myocardial infarction (MI) and stroke within the first two years in women with existing heart disease.	Possible protection, according to a 2002 study, in women with existing heart disease.	No known effects.
Cancer	Animal studies report higher risk of bone tumors; human cancer risk unknown	Increased risk of breast cancer. Estrogen without progesterone increases risk of uterine cancer. Possible protection against colon cancer.	Tamoxifen and raloxifene reduce breast cancer risk. Tamoxifen increases risk of uterine cancer.	May have antitumor properties. May slow metastasis to the bone in cancer patients.
Other Positive Effects	Unknown	Possible protection against urinary tract infections with vaginal application *only*, incontinence, glaucoma, macular degeneration	No vaginal bleeding. Fewer side effects than HRT or bisphosphonates.	Unknown.
Other Negative Effects	Injectable only (pain)	Increases risk of blood clots, vaginal bleeding, breast pain, asthma, endometriosis, fibroids, TMJ, varicose veins, gallstones. Mixed studies on Alzheimer's, osteoarthritis, migraines, and cataracts.	Increases risk of blood clots. Side effects include menopausal symptoms of hot flashes, leg cramps. Swelling in the legs.	Increases risk of GERD. Possible long-term risk of ulcers, especially in combination with NSAIDs or ASA. Administration of some requires empty stomach and 30 minutes of sitting up.

Cholesterol in the skin, along with sunlight, generates the inactive form of vitamin D that becomes cholecalciferol. This is released into the blood system, where it becomes calcifediol. Finally it is sent to the kidneys, where it is changed by enzymes to an active form of vitamin D called *calcitriol*.

The parathyroid gland and the thyroid gland work together to ensure that the bone-building and bone-demineralization (dissolution) processes maintain homeostasis. *Osteoclasts*, bone cells that arise from marrow stroma cells and found on the surfaces where bone is being formed, are generally regarded as bone-forming cells. Osteoclasts, enriched with identifier acid phosphatase, are large, multinucleated cells that play an active role in bone resorption or breakdown. Parathyroid hormone from the parathyroid gland and calcitonin from the thyroid gland work in tandem to accomplish this. When PTH is released, it stimulates bone demineralization, or the breakdown of bone. This is the process called *bone resorption* (not to be confused with absorption or reabsorption) in which the smaller minerals enter the bloodstream. One of the minerals that enters the blood system is calcium. Calcium is necessary for proper nerve and muscle function. PTH allows the kidneys to change the calcifediol to calcitriol.

Too much calcitriol released from the kidneys back into the bloodstream would cause hypercalcemia. When this happens, the thyroid gland (if functioning normally) will secrete calcitonin to counter the increase of calcium ions (Ca^{++}) in the blood. While calcium is coming out of the bone into the blood, the bone is left with "holes" in it that may contribute to osteoporosis if the calcium is not replaced—that is, if the bone is not rebuilt.

Bisphosphonates

Bisphosphonates are a very common treatment for osteoporosis, as they mimic the natural organic bisphosphonate salts found in the body, inhibiting bone resorption and osteoclast activity and restoring bone mass and density. There are two types of bisphosphonates: nonnitrogen side-chain and nitrogen side-chain bisphosphonates. The nitrogen side-chain type is preferred because they are more potent. Bisphosphonates irreversibly bind and inactivate osteoclasts and induce apoptosis of the osteoclast. In addition, they decrease osteoclast action. Bisphosphonates work by inhibition of the mevolonate pathway, the pathway responsible for cholesterol synthesis. The inactivated osteoclast is then incorporated into the bone matrix.

Calcitonin

Calcitonin inhibits bone resorption, and decreases the number of bone fractures from low bone density, by increasing bone growth and the number and action of osteoblasts. It blocks the bone-mineral-absorbing activity of the osteoclasts (bone cells), increases calcium excretion by the kidneys, and slows bone resorption—the speed at which bone is broken down before it is replaced.

Calcitonin is a polypeptide hormone that is a potent inhibitor of osteoclastic bone resorption, but its effects are only temporary. It acts directly on osteoclasts (via receptors on the cell surface for calcitonin). The calcitonin receptor is specific for osteoclasts and causes rapid shrinkage of the osteoclasts with initial exposure. Osteoclasts avoid the inhibitory effects of calcitonin following continued exposure.

Calcitonin is available in a nasal spray or injection. Often, calcitonin from eel or salmon is used, as it is many times stronger and longer-lasting than the human form. Calcitonin produces small, incremental increases in the bone mass of the spine, with a modest reduction of bone turnover in women with osteoporosis. Although calcitonin reduces the risk of vertebral fracture in postmenopausal women with osteoporosis, it does not show much sign of helping nonverterbral fractures, such as in the hip or wrist. Calcitonin may also have an analgesic benefit. Miacalcin Nasal Spray® has a new delivery system via the nose, as opposed to injection. Inhalation of 200 units/day may cause the minor side effect of nasal irritation.

Selective Estrogen Receptor Modulators

Another option for postmenopausal women is the class of drugs called selective estrogen receptor modulators (SERMs). SERMs have a protective effect on the bones and heart; however, they do not control the hot flashes associated with menopause. Early studies report a significant reduction in the number of cases of breast cancer detected in women using SERMs. Because SERMS do not stimulate the uterus, there is no increased risk of endometrial cancer and no vaginal bleeding. The most common side effects are leg cramps and hot flashes that are worse than without the drug. Contraindications include a history of breast cancer, liver problems, or blood clots; or if the patient is on HRT.

Nonpharmacologic Treatments of Osteoporosis

Nonpharmacologic treatments for osteoporosis include weight-bearing exercise, such as daily walking. Lifestyle changes include smoking cessation and reduced intake of caffeinated and alcoholic beverages. Calcium intake from diet and supplements should total about 1,500 mg per day for a postmenopausal woman, or 1,000 mg per day if she is receiving hormone replacement therapy.

Bursitis

Bursitis is an inflammation of the *bursae*, which are the small, fluid-filled pouches between bones and **ligaments**, or between bones and muscles, that serve as cushions.

Tendonitis

Tendonitis is an inflammation of the **tendons**, which are cords of connective tissue that attach muscle to bone.

Myalgia

Myalgia is muscle pain. It can be caused by many things, and range from very minor to severe and acute to chronic.

Bone Marrow Disorders

Any disease or condition that affects blood cell production is considered a bone marrow disorder. This section briefly describes a few of the most common ones.

Anemia

Anemia is failure of the bone marrow to produce the components of the red blood cells. The most common cause is a lack of iron, which causes a lack of oxygen inside the erythrocyte and leads to fatigue. However, blood loss or hemolysis (red blood cell destruction) can also cause a variety of anemias, such as microcytic and normocytic.

Leukemia

Leukemia begins when one or more white blood cells experience deoxyribonucleic acid (DNA) loss or damage. The damaged DNA is then copied and passed on to subsequent generations of cells. These abnormal cells do not die off like normal cells, but instead multiply and accumulate within the body. No one really knows why such changes occur, but some factors that increase the risk of this disorder include genetics, age, environment, and lifestyle. All cancers, including leukemia, begin as a mutation in the genetic material—the DNA within certain cells.

Arthritis

Arthritis is the inflammation of a **joint**. There are several different types of arthritis, which vary in onset, action, and treatment possibilities.

Rheumatoid Arthritis

Rheumatoid arthritis (RA) is a progressive form of arthritis that has devastating effects on the joints, body organs, and general health. It is classified as an *autoimmune* disease because the disease is caused by the immune system attacking the body itself. Symptoms include painful, stiff, and swollen joints, fever, and fatigue. RA is characterized by an

ligaments strong fibrous bands of connective tissue that hold bones together. Injuries can result in sprains.

tendons cords of connective tissue that attach muscle to bone. Injuries can result in strains, ruptures, or inflammation.

joint the location or position where bones are connected to each other. A joint contains synovial fluid and cartilage.

inflammation of the cartilage around the joints that leads to a thickening and hardening of the **synovial fluid**. Eventually, RA attacks the visceral organs, which can cause lung or heart fibrosis, renal amyloidosis, and inflammatory conditions such as endocarditis and pericarditis.

Osteoarthritis

Osteoarthritis is a progressive disease characterized by the breakdown of joint cartilage. Weight-bearing activities, such as marching, running, and jogging, are the main cause of the wear-and-tear breakdown of joints. Such joint erosion may cause the body to identify particles of the worn bone as foreign material in the joint; an immune reaction sends phagocytes to the site, resulting in irritation and inflammation.

synovial fluid liquid that fills the space between the cartilage of each bone; provides smooth movement by lubricating the cartilage.

Workplace Wisdom Osteoarthritis

Reports indicate that as many as 40 million Americans are affected by osteoarthritis.

Workplace Wisdom Knee Joint Pain

Knee joint pain is the most common musculoskeletal complaint that sends people to their doctors. With today's increasingly active society, the number of knee problems is increasing. See Figure 24-6 for an illustration of the knee joint.

Gout

Gout is a painful joint inflammatory disease that was first described in the days of Hippocrates, BCE 400 to 300. Gout is caused by the deposit of uric acid in the joint synovial fluid of the big toes, knees, and elbows, and some soft tissues. Not necessarily localized to the joints, gout is a systemic disease.

Gout is caused by an excess or overproduction of uric acid or by the inability of the kidneys to adequately excrete uric acid from the body. Uric acid is formed every day from the metabolism of nucleic acids. Because humans cannot use uric acid, it is normally secreted into the urine by renal tubules. The condition of having too much uric acid in the blood is called *hyperuricemia*.

An increase in the amount of uric acid in the blood leads to the formation of needle-like uric acid crystals in the joints, which act as an irritant and cause an arthritis-like pain and inflammation that imitates osteoarthritis. When phagocytes (leukocytes) enter the area and attack the uric acid crystals, leading to a decrease in the pH (acidity) of the joint fluid, more uric acid accumulates in the joint, and the destructive cycle begins again if the uric acid levels in the blood remain high. This occurs when uric acid is not filtered or cleared via the glomerulus of the nephrons in the kidneys.

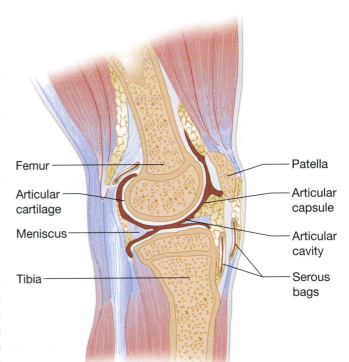

FIGURE 24-6 The knee joint.

Acute gout is the vicious cycle of inflammation that produces edema, redness, and severe pain. Chronic gout is characterized by uric acid slowly depositing in soft tissues, causing *tophi* (the bulging, deformed joints characteristic of gout). Uric acid may also collect in the urinary tract as kidney stones. Calcium pyrophosphate deposits, rather than uric acid crystals, cause *pseudoarthritis,* which is sometimes mistaken for gout.

Workplace Wisdom Gout

As much as 3 percent of the United States population is affected by gout.

An excess of certain fermented alcoholic beverages (wine and beer), and certain foods that are aged and/or contain a high purine content (such as legumes [peas, lentils, beans]; cheeses; anchovies and sardines; scallops, mussels, and other shellfish; organ meats [liver, kidneys, heart]; and red meats) increase the uric acid level of the blood. This may precipitate a gout attack. Medications, including hydrochlorothiazide (a diuretic) and some transplant immunosupressant medications, such as cyclosporine and tacrolimus, can also increase uric acid levels.

Certain disease states and genetic factors can predispose a person to gout. A high incidence has been noted in New Zealanders, Pacific Islanders, and postmenopausal women. However, gout affects men more than women by a ratio of 20:1. Obesity, high blood pressure, kidney disease, and genetics are all risk factors for gout.

Arthritis Treatment

This section describes some common treatments for arthritis.

Disease-Modifying Antirheumatic Drugs

If taken early in the course of the disease, disease-modifying antirheumatic drugs (DMARDs) can help prevent the progression of the disease. DMARDs usually take up to six to eight months to evoke a response and thus are considered slow-acting drugs (remittive). DMARDs are now regarded as a long-term solution to symptom control. Generally, DMARDs are used for RA, but some can also be used for juvenile RA, ankylosing spondylitis, psoriatic arthritis, and lupus. DMARDs are immunosuppressants, and a major adverse reaction is an acquired illness due to the mechanism of action that lowers immune system response. Therefore, the patient must watch for such signs of infection as sore throat, cough, fever, or chills. Furthermore, vaccinations may pose a problem for those taking DMARDs, as DMARDs suppress or lower the immune system enough to make a vaccine a source of infection rather than protection. Table 24-3 lists some commonly prescribed antirheumatic agents.

Gold Compounds

Gold compounds were discovered accidentally by a French physician, Jacques Forrestier, after he injected gold salts into a tuberculosis patient, who coincidentally had arthritis; the arthritis improved. Gold has been used to treat arthritis ever since. The exact mechanism of action is not known, but it is believed that the gold interferes with the functions of the white blood cells that are responsible for joint damage and inflammation. Gold slows destruction, but it cannot cure existing joint deformities. Side effects include an itchy rash on the lower extremities and mouth ulcers, which disappear when the medicine is discontinued; and transitory diarrhea or loose bowel movements. Fifty percent of users discontinue this medication because of the side effects.

Penicillamine

Penicillamine is related to the antibiotic penicillin. However, patients who are allergic to PCN can take penicillamine. Known as a *chelator*, penicillamine binds to heavy metals in the body. It may become more active or potent if combined with copper, which is present naturally in the body. Used since the 1970s for RA, the exact mechanism or mode of action (MOA) of penicillamine is unknown, but it is believed to act like gold, interfering with the functions of the white blood cells that are responsible for joint damage and inflammation. Side effects include skin rashes, mouth sores, loss of taste, and GI upset. Kidney damage may also occur; therefore, the patient must be monitored for protein in the urine.

Sulfasalazines

A combination of salicylate and an antibiotic, originally used to treat inflammatory bowel disease, sulfasalazines have been on the scene since the 1940s. Because sulfasalazine is not as toxic as gold or penicillamine, a renewed interest in usage for RA has developed. Side effects include loss of appetite, nausea and vomiting (N/V), diarrhea, renal problems, and blood dyscrasias. In addition, it may cause severe allergic reactions or anaphylactic shock in those allergic to sulfa drugs.

Table 24-3   Antirheumatic Agents

TRADE NAME	GENERIC NAME	AVAILABLE STRENGTH AND DOSAGE FORM(S)	DOSAGE
Arava®	leflunomide	Tab: 10 mg, 20 mg, 100 mg	100 mg daily × 3 days, then 20 mg daily
Aurolate® Myochrysine®	gold sodium thiomalate (~50% gold)	Inj soln: 50 mg/mL	Weekly doses: 10 mg IM week 1 25 mg IM weeks 2 & 3 50 mg IM subsequent weeks
Azulfidine®	sulfasalazine	Tab: 500 mg	1 gm bid
Cuprimine®	penicillamine	Cap: 125 mg, 250 mg	125–250 mg daily, up to 750 mg daily
Depen®	penicillamine	Tab: 250 mg, titratable	125–250 mg daily, up to 750 mg daily
Plaquenil®	hydroxychloroquine sulfate	Tab: 200 mg	400–600 mg daily
Ridaura®	auranofin (29% gold)	3 mg capsule	6 mg daily or 3 mg bid
Solganal®	aurothioglucose (~50% gold)	Inj susp: 50 mg/mL	Weekly doses: 10 mg IM week 1 25 mg IM weeks 2 & 3 50 mg IM subsequent weeks

Hydroxychloroquine

Originally used to treat malaria and recently lupus, this medication has been around for many years. Hydroxychloroquine is indicated for patients with RA who have not responded well to NSAIDs. It has few side effects and blood test monitoring is not required. Once-a-day dosing is usual, with one rare toxic effect: The drug may deposit in the retina and cause visual impairment. Therefore, an ophthalmologic exam is recommended every six months.

Leflunomide

Leflunomide helps to slow the progression of joint damage caused by RA. Although there is no cure for RA, leflunomide may keep the disease from progressing. It has been shown to inhibit structural damage (as evidenced by X-rays of erosions and joint space narrowing) and improve physical function. Leflunomide is an isoxazole immunomodulatory agent that inhibits an enzyme involved in pyrimidine synthesis. By blocking this enzyme, leflunomide prevents T-cell actions and proliferation that lead to the disabling inflammation of RA. Side effects include dry mouth, insomnia, hair loss, nausea, diarrhea, tiredness, and acne. Signs of toxicity include dark yellow urine, difficulty breathing or shortness of breath, increases in blood pressure, and yellowing of the skin or eyes. Leflunomide has the potential to cause liver damage; therefore, patients must be monitored. Rash, swelling, and difficulty breathing may be signs of a possible allergic reaction and should be reported immediately.

Secondary Lines of Therapy

Nonsteroidal anti-inflammatory drugs (NSAIDs) and other steroidal anti-inflammatory drugs are commonly used for the symptoms of rheumatoid arthritis, but they do not prevent progression of the disease. There is also some research showing that NSAIDs interfere with the bone-rebuilding process.

Treatment of Gout

Colchicine is mainly used only during the first 48 hours of an acute gout attack, as it will cause nausea and vomiting when taken for longer periods. Colchicine alters the ability of the phagocytes to attack the uric acid crystals, which prevents the pH of the joint or synovial fluid from decreasing. Thus, the cycle of deposition of uric acid crystals and acid is broken and the gout attack subsides. If a patient is taking "blood thinners," such as aspirin, dipyridamole, or warfarin, or is prone to ulcers caused by NSAIDs or ASA, colchicines may be the drug of choice. See Table 24-4.

Anti-inflammatory analgesics, such as aspirin and ibuprofen, can be used to reduce the pain and inflammation of acute gout attacks. Indomethacin is most often prescribed for gout inflammation.

Preventive Treatment

Prophylactic therapy is the long-term use of drugs to prevent the reoccurrence of gout attacks and tophi. Two major types of drugs are used for preventive treatment: hypouricemic agents and uricosuric agents.

Hypouricemic agents decrease production of uric acid in the blood. The enzyme xanthine oxidase is necessary to convert hypoxanthine into uric acid. The MOA is inhibition of the enzyme xanthine oxidase, so that hypoxanthine is not made. Therefore, uric acid is not formed, and hypoxanthine is then excreted in the urine.

Table 24-4 Comparative Chart of Drugs Used to Treat Gout

INDICATION	CLASSIFICATION	TRADE NAME	GENERIC NAME	PURPOSE	MOA
Acute Gout Attack	antigout agent	no trade name	colchicine	To stop the cycle of deposition of uric acid crystals and lower pH, during an immediate acute attack, within the first 48 hours	Alters phagocytes' ability to attack uric acid crystals, prevents decrease in the pH of the joint or synovial fluid. Stops the cycle of uric acid crystal formation and high pH.
Acute or Chronic Gout	NSAID	Indocin®	indomethacin	Anti-inflammatory analgesics; reduce pain and swelling	Inhibits/blocks the enzyme COX-2, which starts the reaction of inflammation; prevents prostaglandin synthesis.
Chronic	hypouricemic agent	Zyloprim®	allopurinol	Prophylactic therapy: decreases production of uric acid in the blood	Inhibition of the enzyme xanthine oxidase, stopping production of hypoxanthine and thus preventing formation of uric acid.
	uricosuric agent	Anturane® Benemid®	sulfinpyrazone probenecid	Prophylactic therapy: increases the excretion of uric acid	Blocks renal reabsorption of uric acid, so that uric acid passes into the urine.
	combination drug	Colbenemid®	probenecid + colchicine	Reduces urate blood levels and prevents further gout attacks	MOA is same as for the individual drugs in combination.

Over a period of time, the amount of uric acid in the blood decreases, preventing the future formation of tophi and urate stones in the kidney.

Uricosuric agents increase the excretion of uric acid through urination rather than altering the formation of uric acid. Uricosuric drugs promote the excretion of uric acid via the kidney, which leads to a rapid clearance of uric acid from the blood. These drugs block reabsorption of uric acid in the renal tubules of the kidney, so that uric acid passes into the urine. Uricosuric drugs frequently cause GI distress. It is recommended that these drugs be taken with meals, milk, or antacids.

Some drugs for gout combine prophylactic and maintenance drugs. Often, probenecid is administered in combination with colchicine as Colbenemid®, which reduces urate blood levels and prevents further gout attacks. To reduce the likelihood of developing renal urate stones, it is also recommended that the patient drink plenty of water daily.

Inflammation

Inflammation is a symptom common to bursitis, tendonitis, muscle pain, dysmenorrhea, arthritis, and gout. Inflammation, along with pain, is the most common symptom of all the previously discussed inflammatory diseases. The inflammatory process is a normal response to injury: When tissues are damaged, substances such as histamine, prostaglandins, and serotonin are released. These substances produce vasodilation and increased permeability of the capillary walls. As inflammation increases, the inflamed tissue hits nerves, which causes pain because the pain receptors are stimulated. This occurs while proteins and fluids leak out of the damaged cells. As blood flow to the damaged area increases, leukocytes migrate to the area to destroy harmful substances introduced by the injury. All of this results in the development of the cardinal signs of inflammation:

- redness
- edema
- warmth
- pain
- loss of function or immobilization

INFORMATION

In some instances, the inflammatory process becomes chronic and repeats over a long period of time, often with little or no provocation. When exaggerated or prolonged, it results in further tissue damage. The inflammation itself becomes a disease.

Treatment of Inflammation

There are basically three choices of anti-inflammatory agents to treat inflammation: salicylates, topical corticosteroids, and NSAIDs.

Salicylates

Salicylates relieve inflammation by inhibiting the synthesis of prostaglandin. Along with their anti-inflammatory properties, salicylates are also used as analgesics and antipyretics. Side effects of salicylates include:

- *Nausea and vomiting*—Salicylates directly irritate the stomach mucosal lining and stimulate the chemoreceptor trigger zone (CTZ) in the medulla oblongata located in the brain stem, which directly excites the vomiting center.
- *Hemorrhagic (antiplatelet) effect*—Platelets are the sticky element in the blood necessary for clot formation. The anti-coagulant effect of ASA inhibits the aggregation of platelets and thins out the blood, increasing the risk of hemorrhage and GI ulcer. Therefore, patients can bleed excessively if cut, undergo surgery, or have dental work while taking ASA and salicylamides.

- *Tinnitus*—In low doses, salicylates relieve pain, aches, and fever. Unfortunately, to relieve the pain of arthritis, gout, and rheumatoid arthritis, they must be used in large doses for extensive periods of time. Megadose therapy with ASA or NSAIDs is frequently associated with toxic effects, and may also cause tinnitus by their effect on the inner ear, cochlea, and spiral ganglion.

The dangerous and often fatal reactions to acute salicylate poisoning are respiratory depression and acidosis. Reye's syndrome, a fatal disease affecting the brain and liver in children who take aspirin after or during a viral infection, has been the main reason for the decrease in the use of ASA in children.

Very good documentation supports the fact that ASA blocks the enzyme COX-2, thereby blocking the first step in the inflammatory process and further blocking prostaglandins from being made. In addition, the platelet-aggregating substance thromboxane A2 is also blocked when ASA blocks the production of prostaglandin, thereby preventing further stroke or MI. This is why salicylates are also used for their antiplatelet or anticoagulant effect. If ulcers are not present, continual administration of aspirin may be beneficial to prevent the formation of thromboemboli. Usually, a child's dose of 81 mg is given. In layman's terms, this "thins out" the blood. Although too much aspirin or other salicylates may cause hemorrhage, a small amount on a daily basis for the patient with a potential for stroke or MI will be beneficial. Table 24-5 lists some salicylate drugs.

Corticosteroids

Topical corticosteroids are also used to treat inflammation and most of its causes, including chemical, mechanical, microbiological, and immunological agents. When applied to inflammation, corticosteroids inhibit the movement of macrophages and white blood cells into the area, resulting in a decrease in swelling, redness, and itching.

Nonsteroidal Anti-Inflammatory Drugs

NSAIDs relieve inflammation and pain (see Table 24-6). Some of the many types of arthritis are also associated with infection. An NSAID will reduce the fever, as well as any pain associated with the fever, but will not affect the infection. Therefore, antibiotics are needed to combat the infection directly.

Long-term use of NSAIDs may have a damaging effect on chondrocyte (cartilage) function, which leads to more arthritic symptoms and disease. With chronic use, all anti-inflammatory and salicylate drugs may produce nausea, GI distress, and ulceration.

Table 24-5   Salicylate Drugs

TRADE NAME	GENERIC NAME	STRENGTH AND DOSAGE FORM AVAILABLE	DOSAGE
various trade names	acetylsalicylic acid (ASA); aspirin	various-strength tablets	3.2–6 g/day for RA 325–650 mg q4 hr for minor aches/pain
Arthropan®	choline salicylate	870 mg/5 mL	870–1740 mg up to 4 times daily for RA
Dolobid®	diflunisal	Tab: 250 mg, 500 mg	1 gm 1st dose, then 500 mg q8–12 hr for mild/moderate pain 250–500 mg bid for osteoarthritis & RA
	salsalate (salicylsalicylic acid)	Tab: 500 mg, 750 mg	3,000 mg/day in divided doses
	sodium salicylate	Tab: 325 mg, 650 mg	325–650 mg q4 hr

Table 24-6 Examples of NSAIDs

TRADE NAME	GENERIC NAME	STRENGTH AND DOSAGE FORM AVAILABLE	USUAL ADULT DOSE
Ansaid®	flurbiprofen	50 mg, 100 mg tab	200–300 mg in divided doses 2, 3, or 4 times daily
Cataflam®	diclofenac	50 mg tab	100–200 mg/day in divided doses
Voltaren® Voltaren-XR®		25 mg, 50 mg, 75 mg, 100 mg extended-release (ER) tab	
Celebrex®	celecoxib	100 mg, 200 mg, 400 mg cap	100 mg bid or 200 mg daily
Clinoril®	sulindac	150 mg, 200 mg tab	300–400 mg/day in 2 divided doses
Daypro®	oxaprozin	600 mg cap	1,200 mg daily
Daypro® ALTA		678 mg oxaprozin potassium (equivalent to 600 mg oxaprozin)	Maximum dose: 1,800 mg/day or 26 mg/kg (whichever is lower) in divided doses
Feldene®	piroxicam	10 mg, 20 mg cap	10 mg bid or 20 mg daily
Indocin®	indomethacin	25 mg, 50 mg cap 75 mg SA cap, 50 mg supp 25 mg/5 mL susp	Taper up to 150–200 mg/day in divided doses
Lodine®	etodolac	400 mg, 500 mg tab 200 mg, 300 mg cap 400 mg, 500 mg, 600 mg ER tab	300 mg bid–tid or 400–500 mg bid 400–1,000 mg/day (ER tab)
Meclomen®	meclofenamate	50 mg, 100 mg cap	50–100 mg q4–6 hr, NTE 400 mg/day
Motrin IB® (OTC)	ibuprofen	OTC: 50 mg, 100 mg, 200 mg tab	1.2–3.2 g/day in divided doses tid–qid, NTE 3.2 g/day
Motrin®		200 mg cap 40 mg/mL drops 100 mg/5 mL, 100 mg/2.5 mL susp Rx: 400 mg, 600 mg, 800 mg tab	
Nalfon®	fenoprofen	200 mg, 300 mg cap 600 mg tab	300–600 mg tid–qid
Naprosyn®	naproxen sodium	250 mg, 375 mg, 500 mg tab 375 mg, 500 mg delayed-release tab	250–500 mg bid
Anaprox®		250 mg, 500 mg tab	

Table 24-6 Examples of NSAIDs (*continued*)

TRADE NAME	GENERIC NAME	STRENGTH AND DOSAGE FORM AVAILABLE	USUAL ADULT DOSE
Naprelan®		375 mg, 500 mg continuous-release tab	
Orudis®	ketoprofen	12.5 mg tab 50 mg, 75 mg cap	50 mg qid or 75 mg tid
Oruvail®		100 mg, 150 mg, 200 mg ER cap	200 mg daily (ER)
Relafen®	nabumetone	500 mg, 750 mg tab	1,000 mg daily to start, increasing to 1,500–2,000 mg daily. Can divide doses
Tolectin®	tolmetin	200 mg, 600 mg tab 400 mg cap	400–600 mg tid
Toradol®	ketorolac tromethamine	10 mg tab 15 mg/mL, 30 mg/mL inj	10 mg q4–6 hr, NTE 40 mg/day 15–30 mg q6 hr, NTE 120 mg/day

However, ibuprofen has been reported to produce less gastric distress. Toxic effects of NSAIDs include bone marrow suppression that leads to blood disorders. Therefore, NSAIDs are used more for their anti-inflammatory effect than for their analgesic (pain-relieving) or antipyretic (fever-reducing) effects. If another pain reliever or fever reducer with fewer adverse reactions can be used, it is often preferred over an NSAID.

NSAIDs work by inhibiting or blocking the enzyme that starts the reaction of inflammation by making prostaglandin. This enzyme, called cyclooxygenase II (COX-2), catalyzes arachidonic acid to prostaglandins and leukotrienes. Further, NSAIDs block the action of the synthesis of prostaglandin that promotes inflammation.

The enzyme cyclooxygenase I (COX-1) produces the prostaglandins that cause the building and thickening of the mucosal lining of the stomach, thereby protecting the stomach against acid. The enzyme COX-2 produces the prostaglandins that contribute to inflammation.

When NSAIDs block *all* prostaglandin synthesis, by blocking both COX-1 and COX-2, although the mucosal lining of the GI tract thins out and inflammation is reduced, a patient can then get a GI ulcer. Therefore, COX-2 inhibitors, which block only the cyclooxygenase II that makes PGE-2, contribute less to ulcers while still treating inflammation. With COX-2 inhibitors, only the inflammation process is inhibited; the viscosity of the gastric mucosal lining is not affected.

The COX-2 inhibitors have been successfully marketed on the basis of the belief that the main mechanism by which nonselective NSAIDs cause gastrointestinal ulcers is inhibition of COX-1. According to this hypothesis, selective COX-2 inhibitors will have similar anti-inflammatory activity with less GI toxicity. Short-term clinical studies (CLASS and VIGOR), in which all patients underwent endoscopy, showed fewer cumulative gastroduodenal erosions and ulcers with the COX-2 inhibitors (9–15 percent) than with nonselective NSAIDs (41–46 percent). The FDA authorities judged this outcome as insufficient to prove that selective COX-2 inhibitors were better than nonselective NSAIDs in terms of the life-threatening complications of NSAIDs (namely, ulcers complicated by GI bleeds, perforations, and obstructions). Therefore, the monographs and package inserts of celecoxib (Celecoxib®) and meloxicam (Mobic®) include the same warnings and patient precautions about GI toxicity as all other NSAIDs.

According to the VIGOR and CLASS studies, COX-2 selective inhibitors are associated with an increased incidence of serious adverse events as compared with nonselective NSAIDs. Therefore, more studies are being done to prove or disprove this hypothesis.

A study in Germany shows that the use of leeches in knee arthritis yields a great reduction in swelling and pain. Acetaminophen (trade name, Tylenol®), also known as paracetamol or N-Acetyl P-Aminophenol (APAP), is now thought to selectively block the newly discovered enzyme COX-3 in the brain and spinal cord, thereby reducing pain and fever without unwanted gastrointestinal side effects. Still, APAP has very little or no anti-inflammatory effect.

It is important to emphasize the adverse reactions of NSAIDs. Long-term use of NSAIDs may have a damaging effect on chondrocyte (cartilage) function, which will lead to more arthritic symptoms and disease. Therefore, in the long run, use of NSAIDs may exacerbate any arthritis-related disease.

PROFILES IN PRACTICE

Regina is working as a pharmacy technician in a retail pharmacy. A customer informs Regina that he has been experiencing stomach upset over the past few days. The customer's profile shows that a prescription for piroxicam 10 mg po bid was filled two days earlier.

- Is it possible that the patient's new prescription is causing the stomach upset?
- How can it be alleviated?
- As a technician, what are you able to tell the patient?
- What do you think the pharmacist might tell the patient?

Skeletal Muscle Relaxants

Skeletal muscle relaxants (SMRs) are used to relax specific muscles in the body and relieve the pain, stiffness, and discomfort associated with strains, sprains, or other muscle injuries (see Table 24-7). SMRs may also be used in spastic diseases, such as multiple sclerosis and cerebral palsy, as well as to help relax the patient or a specific part of the body prior to surgery. Drug therapy does not take the place of recommended rest or exercise, nor does it alleviate muscle problems caused by tetanus. Skeletal muscle relaxants act either in the central nervous system (CNS) or directly on the muscle to produce their relaxant effects.

The use of skeletal muscle relaxants can also facilitate surgical and orthopedic procedures and intubations (see Tables 24-7 and 24-8). They may also be used to treat

Table 24-7 Skeletal Muscle Relaxants

TRADE NAME	GENERIC NAME		
Direct-Acting Skeletal Muscle Relaxants			
Dantrium®	dantrolene	Cap: 25 mg, 50 mg, 100 mg	25 mg daily to start, increase to 25 mg bid–qid, then increase up to 100 mg bid–qid; NTE 400 mg/day
		20 mg/vial (0.32 mg after reconstitution)	2.5 mg/kg IV; about 1 hour before anesthesia, infused over 1 hour

Table 24-7   Skeletal Muscle Relaxants (*continued*)

TRADE NAME	GENERIC NAME		
Central-Acting Skeletal Muscle Relaxants			
Lioresal®	baclofen	Tab: 10 mg, 20 mg	Titrate to 40–80 mg/day
Soma®	carisoprodol	Tab: 350 mg	350 mg tid–qid
Parafon Forte DSC®	chlorzoxazone	Tab: 250 mg, 500 mg Cap: 250 mg Caplet: 500 mg	250–750 mg tid–qid
Flexeril®	cyclobenzaprine	Tab: 5 mg, 10 mg	20–40 mg/day in divided doses
Valium®	diazepam	Tab: 2 mg, 5 mg, 10 mg Oral soln: 5 mg/5 mL Conc: 5 mg/mL Inj: 5 mg/mL	2 mg—10 mg tid-qid 2–5 mg tid–qid IM/IV
Skelaxin®	metaxalone	Tab: 800 mg	800 mg tid–qid
Robaxin®	methocarbamol	Tab: 500 mg, 750 mg 100 mg/ml inj	Initial: 1.5 g qid Maintenance: 1 g qid, 750 mg q4 hr or 1.5 g tid IV/IM: NTE 3 g for longer than 3 consecutive days
Norflex®	orphenadrine citrate	Tab:100 mg, 100 mg SR Inj: 30 mg/mL	100 mg qam & qpm 60 mg IV/IM; may repeat q12 hr
Zanaflex®	tizanidine HCl	Tab: 2 mg, 4 mg Cap: 2 mg, 4 mg, 6 mg	Initial: 4 mg q6–8 hr Titrate in 2–4 mg steps, maximum 3 doses/day. NTE 36 mg/day

overexertion of the muscles and injuries accompanied by aches and the pain of sore, stiff, and swollen joints. Other drugs used to treat the soreness associated with overworked muscles are analgesics and anti-inflammatory agents.

Skeletal muscle relaxants that inhibit neuromuscular function are either peripheral acting or central acting. Direct-acting SMRs are a subtype of peripheral-acting skeletal muscle relaxants. The peripheral-acting SMRs block muscle contraction at the neuromuscular junction within the contractile process. The contractile process begins with an electrical impulse originating in the CNS that is conducted via the spinal cord to the somatic, or voluntary, motor neurons. These motor neurons connect to skeletal muscle fibers, creating the neuromuscular junction. Acetylcholine (ACH) forms in the endings of the somatic motor fibers and then travels to the neuromuscular synapse, an area between two neurons. When the ACH attaches to the nicotinic–II (NII) receptors, depolarization occurs, causing the contractile substances of myosin and actin to produce a muscle contraction.

Peripheral-acting SMRs inhibit contraction in two ways: as nondepolarizing agents and as depolarizing agents. Nondepolarizing SMRs block NII receptors, thereby inhibiting depolarization and stopping nerve transmission and muscle contraction.

Table 24-8   Agents for Surgical Procedures That Provide Temporary Muscle Paralysis

TRADE NAME	GENERIC NAME
Nondepolarizing Agents	
Mivacron®	mivacurium chloride
Nimbex®	cisatracurium besylate
Norcuron®	vecuronium bromide
Pavulon®	pancuronium bromide
Tracrium®	atracurium besylate
Zemuron®	rocuronium bromide
Depolarizing Agents	
Quelicin®, Anectine®, Sucostrin®	succinylcholine chloride

Depolarizing SMRs attach to the NII receptors, stimulating them to cause depolarization and consequent contraction; this changes the NII receptors so that they do not respond to the natural ACH neurotransmitter in the future. This one-two punch is called the *neuromuscular blockade*.

The adverse actions of skeletal muscle relaxants vary from mild to major. It is well documented that, to fall asleep, the body and muscles as well as the brain's thoughts and impulses must relax. Therefore, side effects include drowsiness, dizziness, nausea, vomiting, fatigue, and weakness. An overdose will produce toxic effects with possible paralysis of the respiratory muscles; respiratory failure and death may result. The main problem is potentiation of the neuromuscular blocker by any CNS depressant or other muscle relaxant, which can lead to an increased and faster approach to death by respiratory depression. Table 24-9 gives some examples of drugs that interact with muscle relaxants.

Table 24-9   Examples of Drugs That Interact with Muscle Relaxants

CLASSIFICATION	TRADE NAME	GENERIC NAME
alcohol	various	Various (even if in another medication preparation)
antibiotics	Cleocin®	clindamycin
	Pipracil®	piperacillin
		neomycin
	Achromycin V®, Tetracyn®, Sumycin®	tetracycline (TCN)
benzodiazepines and other tranquilizers or sedatives	Halcion®	triazolam
	Valium®	diazepam
	Dalmane®	flurazepam
	Xanax®	alprazolam
antiarrhythmics	Xylocaine®	lidocaine
general anesthetics	Amidate®	etomidate
	Brevital®	methohexital
	Diprivan®	propofol
	Ethrane®	enflurane
	Fluothane®	halothane
	Forane®	isoflurane
	Ketalar®	ketamine
	Penthrane®	methoxyflurane
	Pentothal®	thiopental sodium

> **INFORMATION**
>
> Curare is a natural product produced by South American plants such as *Strychnos toxifera* and *Strychnos castelnaei*, and was originally used as an arrow poison. When prepared and used properly, curare assists in temporary muscle paralysis for surgery.

Spastic Diseases

Spastic diseases are motor diseases characterized by tonic spasms (continued muscular tension) and involuntary, exaggerated muscle contractions coupled with abnormal and automatic reflexes, lack of dexterity, and fatigability. This section briefly discusses two of the most common spastic diseases.

Multiple Sclerosis

More commonly known as MS, multiple sclerosis is characterized by multiple areas of inflammation and scarring of the myelin in the brain and spinal cord. MS is an autoimmune disease in which, for unknown reasons, the body's immune system begins to attack normal body tissue. In the case of MS, the body attacks the cells that make myelin, the tissue that covers and protects the nerve fibers. Nerve communication is thereby disrupted. A person with MS experiences varying degrees of neurological impairment, depending on the location and extent of the scarring. Although there is as yet no known cure for MS, much can be done to make the patient's life easier.

Symptoms of MS may include fatigue, weakness, spasticity, balance problems, bladder and bowel control problems, numbness, vision loss, tremor, and vertigo. Not all symptoms affect all MS patients. Symptoms and signs may be persistent, or the patient may experience periods of remission. Treatment of MS includes the use of steroidal anti-inflammatory agents (synthetic adrenal glucocorticoids) and corticosteroids such as betamethasone, dexamethasone, methylprednisolone, prednisone, and prednisolone.

Cerebral Palsy

Cerebral palsy is a condition in which the affected person has poor control of the brain, muscles, and joints. Cerebral palsy is caused by an injury to the brain before, during, or shortly after birth. Because body movements and muscle coordination are affected, children with cerebral palsy may not be able to walk, talk, eat, or play in the same ways as most other children.

Cerebral palsy is characterized by an inability to fully control motor function, particularly muscle control and coordination, and is manifested by the following symptoms:

- muscle tightness or spasm
- lack of muscle coordination
- disturbance in gait and mobility
- abnormal sensation and perception
- impairment of sight, hearing, or speech
- seizures

Depending on the individual child's needs, physical therapy, occupational therapy, and speech-language therapy are employed to improve posture and movement. Pharmaceutical therapy includes drugs to prevent seizures and spasticity (see Tables 24-10 and 24-11).

Table 24-10 Drugs Used to Treat Seizures Associated with Cerebral Palsy

TRADE NAME	GENERIC NAME
Dilantin®	phenytoin
Luminal®	phenobarbital
Tegretol®	carbamazepine

Table 24-11   Drugs Used to Treat Spasticity Associated with Cerebral Palsy

TRADE NAME	GENERIC NAME
Dantrium®	dantrolene—peripheral direct-acting SMR
Lioresal®	baclofen—muscle relaxant; acts to decrease activity of nerves, blocking nerves within the reticular formation
Valium®	diazepam—benzodiazepine SMR

SUMMARY

The musculoskeletal system, which consists of the bones and skeletal muscles, provides the body with both form and the ability to move. The musculoskeletal system has four main functions: to provide a framework or shape for the body, to protect the internal organs, to allow body movement, and to provide storage for essential minerals. There are 206 bones in the human body. The five classes of bones are long, short, flat, irregular, and sesamoid. Skeletal muscles are classified as skeletal (voluntary muscles attached to the bone to provide body movement), cardiac (involuntary muscle attached to the heart), or smooth muscle (involuntary muscles attached to or lining the internal organs).

The musculoskeletal system is affected by numerous disorders, some of which cause only discomfort and pain, and some of which can completely disable the individual. Osteoporosis, the most prevalent bone disorder in the United States, affects approximately 20 million Americans, and is a major cause of bone fractures. Osteoarthritis, a progressive disease of the joints, affects up to 40 million Americans.

A wide range of pharmaceuticals is used for the treatment of diseases of the musculoskeletal system, though many provide only symptomatic relief. However, intensive research is being done to develop new products that will prevent or retard disease, particularly osteoporosis and osteoarthritis, to provide a cure for the millions of Americans afflicted with these debilitating diseases.

CHAPTER REVIEW QUESTIONS

1. This type of muscle is attached to the heart and is also known as the myocardium.
   a. skeletal muscle
   b. smooth muscle
   c. cardiac muscle
   d. heart muscle

2. A _____ is specialized dense connective tissue that provides the shape and support for the body.
   a. joint
   b. cartilage
   c. ligament
   d. bone

3. An infection inside the bone is known as:
   a. osteoarthritis.
   b. osteoporosis.
   c. osteoclast.
   d. osteomyelitis.

4. This type of muscle is also known as visceral muscle and is considered involuntary muscle.
   a. skeletal muscle
   b. smooth muscle
   c. cardiac muscle
   d. heart muscle

5. A _____ is connective tissue that holds bones together.
   a. joint
   b. bone marrow
   c. tendon
   d. ligament

6. A _____ is connective tissue that attaches muscle to bone.
   a. joint
   b. bone marrow
   c. tendon
   d. ligament

7. Which of the following refers to muscle pain?
   a. bursitis
   b. tendonitis
   c. myalgia
   d. anemia

8. Gout is an inflammatory disease of the:
   a. tendons.
   b. joints.
   c. ligaments.
   d. bones.

9. What type of drug is currently considered a long-term solution to controlling arthritis symptoms?
    a. NSAIDs
    b. DMARDs
    c. SMRs
    d. SERMs

10. Which of the following treats seizures associated with cerebral palsy?
    a. phenytoin
    b. carbamazepine
    c. phenobarbital
    d. all of the above

11. COX-2 inhibitors:
    a. produce prostaglandins that contribute to inflammation.
    b. block the inflammatory effects of the enzyme cyclooxygenase II.
    c. block the actions of NSAIDs.
    d. increase the viscosity of the mucosal lining of the GI tract, thus reducing ulcers.

12. The purpose of bone marrow is to:
    a. produce red, purple, and yellow blood cells for oxygen production.
    b. produce red blood cells, some white blood cells, and platelets.
    c. produce immune cells.
    d. separate the yellow fat cells from the red cells.

13. Which of the following is a direct-acting SMR?
    a. diazepam
    b. cyclobenzaprine
    c. methocarbamol
    d. dantrolene

14. Which of the following is considered a depolarizing agent?
    a. rocuronium
    b. succinylcholine
    c. mivacurium
    d. vecuronium

15. Gout is caused by the overproduction of:
    a. red blood cells.
    b. calcium pyrophosphate.
    c. insulin.
    d. uric acid.

CRITICAL THINKING QUESTIONS

1. What are the advantages and disadvantages of using salicylates rather than NSAIDs to treat inflammation?

2. If you had to choose a course of therapy for osteoporosis in menopause, which therapy would you choose, and why?

3. Explain why a doctor might choose a drug that only blocks COX-2 over a drug that blocks both COX-2 and COX-1.

WEB CHALLENGE

1. Go to http://www.niams.nih.gov/bone/optool/index.asp and complete the survey to determine the health of your bones.

2. Go to http://www.gwc.maricopa.edu/class/bio201/muscle/mustut.htm for a tutorial and to learn more about muscles.

REFERENCES AND RESOURCES

Adams, MP, Josephson, DL, & Holland, LN Jr. *Pharmacology for Nurses—A Pathophysiologic Approach*. Upper Saddle River, NJ: Pearson Education, 2008.

Arthritis Today, 2004 Drug Guide. "DMARDs" (accessed April 8, 2008): http://www.arthritis.org/conditions/DrugGuide/about_dmards.asp

Colbert, B, Ankney, J, & Lee, K. *Anatomy and Physiology for Health Professionals: An Interactive Journey*. Upper Saddle River, NJ: Pearson Education, 2007.

DeNoia, Vicki. "Bisphosphonates For Osteoporosis: A Closer Look At Efficacy And Safety." (accessed 4/12/2008) http://www.arthritispractitioner.com/article/7413

Drug Facts and Comparisons, 2006 ed. St. Louis, MO: Wolters Kluwer Health.

"Functions of the Muscular System." (accessed April 8, 2008) http:// training.seer.cancer.gov/module_anatomy/unit4_1_muscle_functions.html

Holland, N, & Adams, MP. *Core Concepts in Pharmacology*. Upper Saddle River, NJ: Pearson Education, 2007.

The Merck Manual of Diagnosis and Therapy. http://www.merck.com/mrkshared/mmanual/section5/chapter57/57a.jsp

MOA of APAP, News on APAP (accessed April 8, 2008): http://www.pharmweb.net/pwmirror/pwy/paracetamol/pharmwebpicmechs.html

National Institute of Arthritis and Musculoskeletal and Bone Diseases. "Osteoporosis and Medicine: Medications to Treat and Prevent Osteoporosis." (accessed April 7, 2008): http://www.niams.nih.gov/Health_Info/Bone/Osteoporosis/Medicine/default.asp

National Library of Medicine. "A review of SERMs and National Surgical Adjuvant Breast and Bowel Project Clinical Trials" (accessed July 15, 2007): http://www.ncbi.nlm.nih.gov/entrez/query.fcgi?cmd=Retrieve&db=PubMed&listuids=14613021&dopt=Abstract

The Virtual Anesthesia Textbook. "Non-Opioid Analgesics" (accessed July 15, 2007): http://www.virtual-anaesthesia-textbook.com/vat/non_narcotics.html#intro

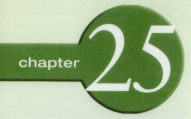

The Respiratory System

LEARNING OBJECTIVES

After completing this chapter, you should be able to:

- Identify and list the basic anatomical and structural parts of the respiratory tract.

- Describe the function or physiology of the individual parts of the respiratory system and the external exchange of oxygen and waste.

- List and define common diseases affecting the respiratory tract and understand the causes, symptoms, and pharmaceutical treatments associated with each disease.

- List the trade and generic names and identify the classification of various drugs used in treatment of diseases and conditions of the respiratory tract.

Introduction

Children commonly hold their breath to find out what it feels like. Adults do so while swimming. It is hard to consciously *not* breathe for very long without giving up. Oxygen is crucial to sustain life, and humans take in oxygen by the act of breathing.

Some people can survive for weeks (50–80 days) without food, for several days (3–14) without water, and a few hours without adequate warmth in cold conditions. However, after several minutes without air, the brain begins to suffer, major organs shut down, and eventually the person dies. The longer the body goes without air, the more damage is done. The respiratory system is what performs the essential action of receiving and exchanging gases, through the lungs, during the process known as breathing or *respiration*.

Function of the Respiratory System

The respiratory system has the following two purposes:

1. Transport of air (gases) to and from the lungs.
2. Exchange of oxygen for carbon dioxide.

The primary function of the respiratory system is to supply oxygen to the blood. The blood, in turn, carries the oxygen to all parts of the body, via the "freeways" of the circulatory system (veins, arteries, and capillaries). The heart is the pump that propels blood to and from the lungs.

Respiration is the mechanism through which gases are exchanged. During breathing, one inhales air containing oxygen and exhales carbon dioxide, a by-product of the use of oxygen in the body. During its journey into the lungs, the air is humidified, warmed, and purified (suspended particles are removed). This exchange of gases is how the respiratory system gets oxygen into the blood. When blood stops moving, oxygen does not get to the body tissues. If a sufficient supply of oxygen does not get to a specific part of the body, that body part will eventually die. Without sufficient oxygen, the whole body will eventually die. The respiratory and circulatory systems work in tandem to accomplish their mutual function of sustaining life.

The lymphatic system also supports respiration by maintaining fluids, providing immunity, and removing inhaled solid materials and microorganisms. For example, the flow of lymph from lung-tissue interstitial spaces into the blood helps to eliminate excess fluid, and the lymphoid tissue of the tonsils protects against infection at the entrance to the respiratory tract.

Anatomy of the Respiratory System

The respiratory system is divided into two parts, the upper respiratory tract and the lower respiratory tract. The upper respiratory tract consists of the nose or nasal cavity, paranasal sinuses, **pharynx**, and larynx (see Figure 25-1). The larynx acts in conjunction with the epiglottis to guard the entrance to the trachea and lower airways. The lower respiratory tract consists of the trachea, two lungs, and two main bronchi; the bronchi then branch into bronchioles, alveolar ducts, and alveoli (see Figure 25-2).

pharynx the part of the throat from the back of the nasal cavity to the larynx.

FIGURE 25-1 The upper respiratory tract.

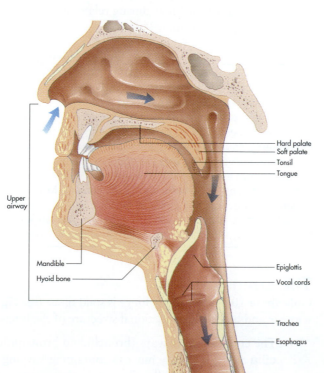

Upper airway

Mandible

Hyoid bone

Hard palate
Soft palate
Tonsil
Tongue

Epiglottis
Vocal cords

Trachea
Esophagus

FIGURE 25-2 The lower respiratory tract.

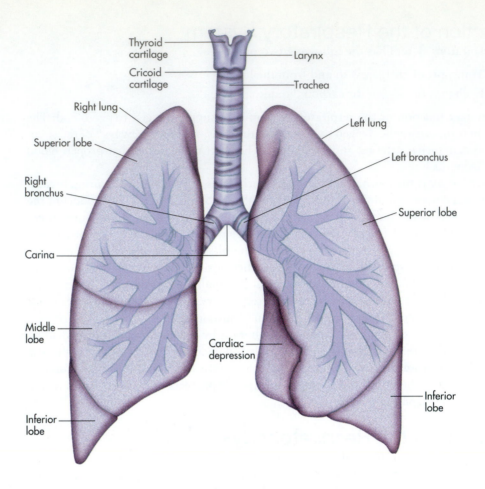

The Diaphragm

The dome-shaped *diaphragm* is a layer or sheet of muscle that lies across the bottom of the chest cavity. Breathing occurs as the diaphragm contracts and relaxes. It pushes carbon dioxide out of the lungs during relaxation and pulls oxygen-containing air into the lungs during contraction.

INFORMATION

What is a hiccup? A hiccup, technically known as a *singultus*, is a diaphragmatic spasm. The diaphragm usually works without a hitch, but sometimes it can become irritated and jerk, causing the breath to be exhaled differently. An irritation or stimulation of the glossopharyngeal area causes this irregular breath. During the jerking motion, the diaphragm contracts involuntarily, causing the person to take a quick breath of air into the lungs. This irregular breath hits the voicebox, and the sound it makes is called the *hiccup*. Things that can irritate the diaphragm are eating or swallowing too quickly, eating too much, an irritation in the stomach or the throat, or nervousness or excitement. Most cases of hiccups last for only a few minutes. However, some cases of hiccups can last beyond a few days, which usually indicates that there is another medical problem. The longest attack of hiccups ever recorded was experienced by an American pig farmer whose hiccups lasted from 1922 to 1987.

The Lungs

Only about 10 percent of the lungs is solid tissue (see Figure 25-3). The remainder is filled with air and blood. The functional structure of the lungs can be divided into two parts:

cilia the tiny hair-like organelles found in the nose and bronchial passageways.

1. The conducting airways (bronchi and bronchioles), which are tubes lined by **cilia** and respiratory mucosa containing varying amounts of muscle and hyaline cartilage in their walls. The conducting airways provide "dead air space" for

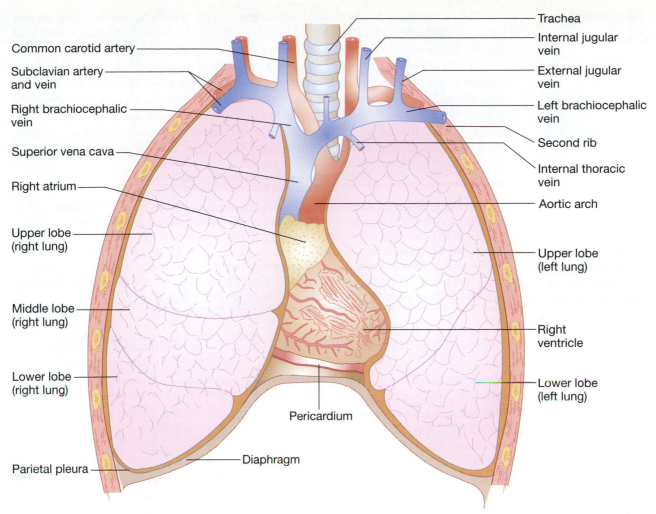

Common carotid artery

Subclavian artery and vein

Right brachiocephalic vein

Superior vena cava

Right atrium

Upper lobe (right lung)

Middle lobe (right lung)

Lower lobe (right lung)

Parietal pleura

Trachea

Internal jugular vein

External jugular vein

Left brachiocephalic vein

Second rib

Internal thoracic vein

Aortic arch

Upper lobe (left lung)

Right ventricle

Lower lobe (left lung)

Pericardium

Diaphragm

FIGURE 25-3 The lungs.

ventilation and gas-exchange areas for perfusion. They move approximately 10,000 liters of inspired (inhaled) air per day.

2. Cartilage, which is a form of protection and cushioning for the bronchi. The bronchi contain hyaline cartilage rings in their walls to keep the airways open. The bronchioles, however, contain little cartilage; instead, they have a thick layer of smooth muscle.

INFORMATION

What is a yawn? Although it is not completely understood, most medical schools teach that a yawn is caused by a lack of oxygen in the alveoli, which makes the lungs stiffen and react to bring in more oxygen.

Respiration

Respiration is achieved through the mouth, nose, trachea, lungs, and diaphragm. Inspiration of air occurs when the pressure inside the lung, known as *intrapulmonary pressure*, becomes lower than the outside or *atmospheric* pressure. This change in pressure allows air to flow into the alveoli of the lungs. During inspiration, the intrapulmonary pressure is less than the atmospheric pressure of 760 mm Hg. Oxygen enters the upper respiratory system through the mouth and the nose, where it is warmed and filtered by cilia.

larynx the voicebox.

trachea the windpipe.

The oxygen then passes through the **larynx** and the **trachea**, then into two smaller tubes called the *bronchi*. Each bronchus splits off into the bronchial tubes, which lead into the lungs and in turn branch off into many *bronchioles*, which connect to alveoli.

Alveoli are often described as grape-like clusters of air sacs; the average adult lungs contain about 600 million of them. Oxygenated air passes into the alveoli and then diffuses through the membranes into the surrounding capillaries. As oxygen travels into the arterial blood, the waste product carried in the blood, carbon dioxide, is released into the alveoli. Carbon dioxide leaves the lungs during exhalation. If this waste gas is not exhaled, the carbon dioxide will accumulate in the blood and cause all body parts to suffocate.

INFORMATION

Do we breathe when we swallow? The esophagus is located at the back of the throat and the windpipe for air is located at the front. When we swallow during ingestion, a flap called the **epiglottis** swings down to cover the windpipe, so that food cannot go down the "wrong pipe." This flap blocks the air coming in for just a second, so for that short moment we are not breathing. Therefore, we do not breathe when we are swallowing. In addition, because smell and breathing are crucial in tasting food, we do not taste our food as we swallow; that has already been done by our taste buds prior to swallowing!

---

epiglottis the small, leaf-shaped cartilage attached to the tongue that prevents substances other than air from entering the trachea.

Diseases and Conditions of the Respiratory Tract

Many diseases and conditions of the respiratory tract can be treated with over-the-counter medications. However, infections and cancer must be treated with specific anti-infectives, antibiotics, and chemotherapeutic drugs. This section explores the common cold, allergies, anaphylactic shock, and chronic obstructive diseases such as emphysema and asthma.

Colds

Colds, caused by viral infections, lead to more absences at work or school each year than any other medical condition. The virus that is responsible for a cold inflames the membranes in the lining of the nose and throat, causing **rhinitis** and sore throat. More than 200 different viruses can cause the common cold. Among the most common are *rhinoviruses*, which thrive in the nasal mucosa, and *coronaviruses*, which cause respiratory, neurological, and enteric infections.

rhinitis inflammation of the nasal passages.

One reason for the increased incidence of colds during the fall and winter months is that people are more often indoors, in heated buildings, and in closer proximity to each other. Also, the lower humidity during colder months makes the nasal passages drier and more vulnerable to infection. Colds usually start two to three days after the virus enters the body, and symptoms last from several days to several weeks. Common cold symptoms may include:

- stuffy nose or congestion
- difficulty breathing
- runny nose (**rhinorrhea**), with either a watery discharge from the nose or a discharge that thickens and turns yellow or green
- sneezing
- sore or scratchy throat
- cough
- headache
- low-grade fever and/or chills
- achy muscles and bones
- fatigue

rhinorrhea runny nose.

Coronaviruses are named for their corona-like or halo-like appearance in electron spectrographs, which is caused by various projections on the surface of the viral envelope.

One of these projections is the E2 glycoprotein, the viral attachment protein that is the target of neutralizing antibodies. These viruses primarily affect adults and are difficult to culture in a laboratory.

Colds can best be prevented by avoiding contact with others who have colds and doing frequent handwashing. Avoid touching your eyes, nose, or mouth when in contact with others who are contaminated with a virus. Using humidifiers and occasionally rinsing the nasal passages with a saline solution may help nasal membranes from becoming overly dry and vulnerable.

How a Cold Virus Causes a Disease

The exact mechanism by which a virus causes a cold is not fully known or understood. The following is the most probable explanation of the sequence of events by which a cold virus becomes a disease. Viruses cause infection by overpowering the immune system. The first line of immunity defense is mucus produced in the nose and throat. Mucus captures inhaled material, such as pollen, dust, pollution, bacteria, and viruses. After a virus contacts a mucous membrane in the nose, ear, eye, or skin, it then enters a cell and takes over protein synthesis in that cell to manufacture new viruses, which, in turn, attack surrounding body cells.

Cold symptoms are most likely a result of the immune response to viral attack. Virus-infected nose cells emit signals that summon white blood cells to the site of the infection. In turn, these cells send out immune system chemicals such as kinins. Kinins lead to the symptoms of the common cold by causing swelling and inflammation of the nasal membranes, leakage of proteins and fluid from capillaries and lymph vessels, and the increased production of mucus. Researchers are examining whether drugs to block kinins and other immune system substances, or the receptors on cells to which they bind, might benefit people with colds.

Table 25-1 compares some common symptoms of colds and virus-caused flu.

Workplace Wisdom Antibiotics and Viral Infections

Antibiotics will not cure a cold or any other viral infection. However, it is possible to develop a secondary bacterial infection, for which antibiotics will most likely be prescribed.

Table 25-1 Comparison of Cold and Flu Symptoms

COLD SYMPTOMS	FLU SYMPTOMS
Low or no fever	High fever
Sometimes a headache	Usually a headache
Stuffy or runny nose	Clear nasal passages
Sneezing	Sometimes sneezing
Mild, hacking cough	Productive cough; may become severe
Slight aches and pains	Often severe aches and pains
Mild fatigue	Severe fatigue; may last for weeks
Sore throat	Usually a sore throat
Normal energy level	Extreme exhaustion
Colds occasionally lead to secondary bacterial infections of the middle ear or sinuses, requiring treatment with antibiotics.	Influenzas occasionally lead to secondary bacterial infections of the lungs (bronchi and bronchioles), or to pneumonia.

Treating the Common Cold with Medication

The treatment of colds is considered symptomatic treatment. OTC drugs and commonsense therapies are available for uncomplicated cases of the common cold. Among them, bed rest, keeping warm, drinking plenty of fluids, gargling with warm salt water, and using petroleum jelly for a rubbed-raw nose are the most accepted. Treatment of colds is done with medications (whether OTC or prescription) in the following classifications:

- antihistamines
- decongestants
- cough suppressants, expectorants, and mucolytics
- analgesics
- antipyretics
- NSAIDs

INFORMATION

To date, there is no conclusive data showing that large doses of vitamin C prevent colds. Although vitamin C megadoses may reduce the severity or duration of symptoms (there is no definitive evidence that it does), it may also change blood and urine glucose test results and cause severe diarrhea (dehydration is a danger for the elderly and children). Combinations of oral anticoagulant drugs and vitamin C can produce abnormal results in blood-clotting tests and affect the coagulation of blood.

Coughs

A cough may be a symptom of a cold, flu, other respiratory problems, or even nonrespiratory tract diseases. Most experts agree that a cough most likely begins with an irritation of nerves in the respiratory tract. The irritation may come from a clump of mucus in the airway, from exposure to an airborne offender (such as a chemical aerosol like paint fumes), or from postnasal drip (PND). PND usually occurs in the patient who has recently had a cold or flu or suffers from allergic rhinitis or acute or chronic sinusitis.

There are, of course, many other causes of coughs. Disease states such as asthma, bronchitis, congestive heart failure, and GERD, as well as side effects of certain drugs (such as ACE inhibitors), can also contribute to cough. A psychogenic or "nervous" cough is emotional or psychological in origin. Cystic fibrosis, an idiopathic pulmonary fibrotic disease, can cause thick mucus to build up that must be expelled or expectorated. Asthma, sinusitis, and GERD are the most frequent causes of chronic cough in children. Serious respiratory complications of GERD include cough, chronic bronchitis, progressively worsening bronchial asthma, and other pulmonary diseases.

Although it goes away in time, postinfectious cough may persist for three or more weeks, usually as the only remaining symptom of an upper respiratory tract viral infection due to persistent inflammation. A persistent acute cough that lasts for three or fewer weeks is usually caused by the common cold, but may be symptomatic of a more serious illness, such as pneumonia or congestive heart failure.

A *chronic cough* is a recurring cough that lasts for three or more weeks at a time. It is sometimes caused by more than one condition. It is most common among tobacco smokers, but also occurs in nonsmokers with postnasal drip syndrome (PNDS), gastroesophageal asthma, and GERD. "Smokers' cough" can mask a more serious condition such as pneumonia or congestive heart failure.

If *pertussis* or whooping cough exists, antibiotic treatment is warranted to fight the bacterial infection, both in the patient and possibly in all persons who were exposed to pertussis. Children usually get pertussis. During this disease, it is difficult for the child to stop coughing and get air. Patients experience coughing spasms with a typical "whooping" sound that follows the cough. This sound indicates that the child is trying to catch his or her breath before the next bout of whooping. Complications that may set in are pneumonia, seizures, brain damage, and death. Children under seven years of age need to be vaccinated with a series of five injections of DPT (diphtheria/pertussis/tetanus) vaccine.

An effective, purposeful cough requires normal nerve pathways in the respiratory tract so that cough can occur when needed. Normal muscle tone of the diaphragm and abdomen (respiratory muscles) are required to create a strong push to the lungs for expiration with normal mucus stickiness and viscosity. Excessive coughing can affect normal muscle tone, hampering the ability of the cough to dislodge mucus or phlegm from bronchial airways.

Mucus is brought up out of the lungs by a productive cough; a nonproductive cough is a dry, hacking cough. A productive cough is purposeful, although sometimes drugs are required to promote the removal of mucus, and may help some patients cough up and expel abnormally thick mucus by thinning it out. It is important to keep the airways free of mucus, to prevent invasion by bacteria that can cause serious disease to the respiratory tract.

A nonproductive cough is usually not purposeful and may persist, becoming as problematic as it is annoying. A nonproductive cough can be exhausting depending on the duration and forcefulness of the cough. Intercostal tissue of the rib cage may tear if the cough persists. Drugs can be given to stop the cough; however, some nonproductive coughs result as a side effect of a medication that is being taken for a different condition or disease.

Cough Medications

There are two types of coughs and two types of treatments (see Table 25-2). Nonproductive cough is treated with a cough *suppressant* or *antitussive* to quiet the cough; these allow the upper respiratory tract to stay moistened (coughing dries it out and further irritates the respiratory tract). *Expectorants* are used to increase the moisture content and decrease the viscosity of mucus, to ease removal of mucus during coughing.

Decongestants

Decongestants thin out the mucus in an inflamed, stuffy nose and clear the nasal passages, allowing easier breathing. Indications for use are nasal and bronchial congestion.

Oral pseudoephedrine and phenylephrine are alpha-adrenergic agonists, which act on alpha-adrenergic receptors in the blood vessels of the nasal mucosa to produce vasoconstriction, resulting in decreased blood flow and shrinkage of tissue in the nasal passages. This effect reduces the vascular inflammation and edema that are associated with congestion.

Pseudoephedrine, like ephedra, creates its effect indirectly by releasing norepinephrine from storage sites in the nerve endings. However, pseudoephedrine can also relax the bronchial smooth muscles by acting directly on beta-2 adrenergic receptors in the mucosa of the respiratory tract. This stimulation produces vasoconstriction, which shrinks swollen nasal mucus membranes; reduces tissue hyperemia (excessive blood), edema, and nasal congestion; and increases the patency (openness) of the nasal airway passages. In addition, it promotes an increase in the drainage of sinus secretions. Obstructed eustachian tubes may also be opened.

Side effects of oral decongestants include irregular heartbeat, palpitations, hypertension, and shortness of breath. CNS toxic effects include convulsions, hallucinations, and stimulation. Those with sulfite sensitivities may have allergic reactions and asthmatic attacks.

Table 25-2 Comparison of Cough Formula for Nonproductive versus Productive Coughs

INDICATIONS—NONPRODUCTIVE COUGH	INDICATIONS—PRODUCTIVE COUGH
Symptoms—Dry, hacking cough that does not produce mucus or phlegm.	Symptoms—A cough in which there is production and removal of phlegm or mucus; sometimes called a "wet" cough.
Purpose—Suppressants (antitussives) are used to suppress the cough centers in the brain and to moisten and lubricate the throat to relieve irritation and quiet the cough.	Purpose—Expectorants are drugs that loosen and clear mucus and phlegm from the respiratory tract, and also moisten and lubricate the throat to relieve irritation.
Generic Ingredient, Nonnarcotic Cough Suppressants—dextromethorphan	Generic Ingredient, Nonnarcotic Expectorant—guaifenesin
Narcotic Cough Suppressants—codeine and hydrocodone	
Trade Names of Nonnarcotic Antitussives: Dimetapp®, Robitussin-DM®, Delsym®, Pertussin®, Drixoral®, Vicks Formula 44®, Triaminic®, Coricidin®	Trade Names of Nonnarcotic Expectorants: Robitussin®, Humibid®, Humibid LA®, Mucinex®, Organidin NR®, Fenesin®
Trade Names of Narcotic Antitussives: Hycodan®, Mycodone®, Tussigon®, Tussionex®	
Mechanism of Action of Dextromethorphan: Works on the CNS to suppress cough centers in the brain (in the medulla oblongata). When coughing is suppressed, the throat does not lose moisture.	Mechanism of Action of Guaifenesin: Thins mucus and lubricates the irritated respiratory tract.
Mechanism of Action of Codeine: Codeine is a centrally acting agent that elevates the threshold for cough in the medulla oblongata. As a result, dry, unproductive coughs become more productive and less frequent. It may be combined with an expectorant.	
Side Effects: Drowsiness or tranquilization, constipation, overdrying of respiratory secretions, upset stomach. At high doses, can cause nausea, itchy skin, visual and auditory hallucinations, loss of motor control, and a feeling of being "stoned" and "out of it."	Side Effects: Rare, but may include vomiting, diarrhea, stomach upset, headache, skin rash, and hives.
Contraindications: Patients with hypertension, kidney problems, diabetes, or glaucoma must seek approval from their doctor; increases the effects of those conditions. Pregnancy. Patients with persistent lingering cough, excessive phlegm, or chronic cough due to bronchitis, smoking, asthma or emphysema.	Contraindications: Pregnancy; patients with persistent lingering cough; excessive phlegm; chronic cough due to bronchitis, smoking, asthma, or emphysema.

Workplace Wisdom Oral Decongestants and MAOIs

Patients must not use pseudoephedrine or phenylephrine if they are currently taking a prescription monoamine oxidase inhibitor (MAOI), or for two weeks after stopping the MAOI drug. MAOIs are used in the treatment of depression, psychiatric, or emotional conditions, and Parkinson's disease. MAOIs potentiate the cardiovascular effects of oral decongestants.

Benefits and disadvantages of oral decongestants, compared with topical nasal inhalation decongestants, are as follows:

- Oral drugs have prolonged decongestant effects, but delayed onset; topicals usually work quickly within five minutes.
- Oral drugs do not cause rebound congestion; topical has a rebound effect. The *rebound effect* occurs with topical decongestants only when more and more

product is needed to produce the same effect. This will increase side effects as well. This happens with prolonged use (more than three to five days) when nasal decongestants lose effectiveness and even cause swelling in the nasal passages. The patient then increases the frequency of the dose. Congestion worsens, and the patient responds by increasing the doses or frequency of doses to as often as every hour. Patients can become dependent on use of topical decongestants. This effect may occur with ophthalmic decongestants as well. Oral drugs are less potent than topicals; topicals have a more direct effect and less systemic effect.

INFORMATION

Pseudoephedrine is an essential chemical used in the production of methamphetamine—"meth," an illegal, highly addictive street stimulant. The Combat Methamphetamine Epidemic Act of 2005 requires that any product containing pseudoephedrine, ephedrine, or phenylpropanolamine be sold from a locked cabinet or from behind the pharmacy counter. The seller must ensure that consumers do not have access to the products prior to sale, and must keep an electronic record ("log") of each sale. The act also puts limits on how much of the drug a person can purchase at one time.

Topical nasal decongestants act as vasoconstrictors, sending edema-causing fluids and blood back to the vessels from which they originally leaked, thereby shrinking the dilated blood vessels. Topical decongestants are used for the temporary relief of nasal congestion or stuffiness caused by hay fever or other allergies, colds, or sinusitis.

Side effects of topical decongestants include burning, dryness, or stinging inside the nose; increase in nasal discharge; and sneezing. Toxic effects of topical decongestants include blurred vision; fast, irregular, or pounding heartbeat; headache; dizziness; drowsiness or lightheadedness; high blood pressure; nervousness; trembling; trouble sleeping, and weakness. One might think that a topical agent is safe for all patients; its simple route of administration fools many people. In fact, there is a long list of contraindications for this simple dosage form of topical (and) nasal sprays and drops. Do not use on patients with the following conditions:

- diabetes mellitus
- excessively dry nasal membranes
- enlarged prostate (difficulty in urinating may worsen)
- glaucoma (mydriasis may worsen)
- heart or blood vessel disease such as CHF or coronary artery disease
- high blood pressure (oxymetazoline in particular may make the condition worse)
- overactive thyroid gland (decongestants may increase tachycardia)

Table 25-3 shows some examples of nasal decongestants.

INFORMATION

After much debate, public hearings that began in 1985, and a controlled case study that began in 1994, phenylpropanolamine (PPA) was removed from the market in November 2000 because it increased the risk of intracranial bleeding associated with hemorrhagic stroke. PPA was used in OTC cough and cold remedies as a decongestant, as well as an appetite suppressant in weight-loss formulas. This bleeding risk was found to be higher in women than in men, mainly because the incidence of stroke occurred more with diet aids than with cold medications, and diet aids are used more by women than men.

Table 25-3 Nasal Decongestants

GENERIC NAME	TRADE NAME
naphazoline HCl	Privine®
oxymetazoline HCl	Afrin®, Dristan® 12-Hr Nasal Spray
phenylephrine HCl	Sudafed® PE (oral), Neo-Synephrine® 4-Hr, 4-Way Fast Acting®, Afrin® Children's Pump Mist
phenylephrine HCl + pheniramine maleate	Dristan® Fast Acting Formula
pseudoephedrine	Sudafed® (oral)
tetrahydrozoline HCl (Rx only)	Tyzine®
xylometazoline HCl	Otrivin®, Natru-Vent®

Note: OTC and topical unless otherwise indicated.

Treatment of Allergies

allergy the result of the immune system's reaction to a foreign substance.

The treatment of **allergies** with respiratory responses includes antihistamines and antitussives to alleviate the symptoms, and mast cell stabilizers to prevent initial allergic reactions and reccurrence.

Antihistamines

Like many drugs, antihistamines have many different uses that are based on their desired effects and side effects. They are used to treat seasonal allergies, to dry up mucous membranes, and as a sleep aid.

allergen a substance capable of causing a hypersensitivity reaction.

If a patient takes an antihistamine before exposure to the **allergen**, such as pollen, the drug will go to the H-1 receptor site. When the person is exposed to the pollen, the mast cells will release histamine-1, which will try to find H-1 receptors. However, because the antihistamine is already bound to the H-1 receptor sites, it blocks or inhibits, the histamine from getting in. Thus, no allergic reaction will occur.

If a patient has been exposed to the allergen or pollen first, the receptor sites are already occupied by histamine. If a person takes antihistamines *after* exposure to the allergen, the drug will wait until the histamine, a protein, degrades and exits the receptor site. Since there are both more histamine and antihistamine molecules waiting to get into open receptor sites while the person is still exposed to the allergen, the antihistamine will race the histamine to get into the receptor site first. Fortunately, antihistamines always win the race! This mechanism of action is known as *competitive inhibition*. Once inside of or attached to the H-1 receptor site, the antihistamine does not fit perfectly, but fits well enough to bind, preventing or blocking the histamine from getting in. This blocking is known as *inhibition*. Because the antihistamine does not fit in the receptor-site "lock" quite as well as the correct histamine "key," the "key" is never "turned," and thus there is no chemical change and no allergic reaction. This is somewhat like a jigsaw puzzle piece that looks like it is the right color, right size, and right shape, but just does not fit exactly and so does not snap into place. Individuals with prostate problems or glaucoma should avoid antihistamines, unless they have authorization from their physicians.

Antihistamines have two mechanisms of action to combat colds and one additional MOA to combat allergies. First-generation antihistamines have the anticholinergic effect of drying the mucous membranes of the nose, mouth, and eyes; they do so by attaching to muscarinic or cholinergic receptors, which blocks the effect of acetylcholine (ACH).

Workplace Wisdom First-Generation Antihistamines

Only first-generation antihistamines work on cholinergic receptors. This MOA helps to combat both the common cold and allergies.

First-generation antihistamines are lipophilic; therefore, they cross the blood-brain barrier and enter the central nervous system, causing sedation. This side effect can be desirable for those with a cold, who may need rest and sleep, but is often undesirable for allergy patients. Side effects of antihistamines can include drowsiness, sleepiness, and overly dry mucous membranes. Some antihistamines also stop nausea, vomiting, and motion sickness. Tables 25-4 to 25-7 include some examples of various antihistamines.

Table 25-4   Examples of OTC Antihistamines (H-1 Antagonists) Used for Cold and Allergy Symptoms

GENERIC NAME	TRADE NAME
chlorpheniramine	Chlor-Trimeton®
clemastine	Tavist-1®
diphenhydramine	Benadryl®, Banophen®, Diphedryl®
loratadine	Alavert®, Claritin®—does not cause drowsiness
loratadine/pseudoephedrine	Claritin-D®—does not cause drowsiness

Note: Formulations cause drowsiness unless otherwise indicated.

Table 25-5   Examples of Prescription Antihistamines (H-1 Antagonists) for Allergy

GENERIC NAME	TRADE NAME
azelastine	Astelin NS®—possible drowsiness
brompheniramine	BroveX CT
cetirizine	Zyrtec®—does not cause drowsiness
cyproheptadine	Periactin®
desloratadine	Clarinex
fexofenadine	Allegra®—does not cause drowsiness
hydroxyzine HCl	Atarax®—also used as an antiemetic
hydroxyzine pamoate	Vistaril®—also used as an antiemetic
phenyltoloxamine citrate, pyrilamine maleate, pheniramine maleate	Poly-Histine® (antihistamine combination)
promethazine HCl	Phenergan®—also used as an antiemetic

Note: Formulations cause drowsiness unless otherwise indicated.

Table 25-6   Examples of Prescription Ophthalmic Antihistamines (H-1 Antagonists)

GENERIC NAME	TRADE NAME
azelastine HCl	Optivar®
emedastine difumarate	Emadine®
epinastine HCl	Elestat®
ketotifen fumarate	Zaditen®
olopatadine HCl	Patanol®

Table 25-7 Comparison of Degree of Sedation of Various Types of Antihistamines

ETHANOLAMINES		ETHYLENEDIAMINES		ALKYLAMINES
clemastine	Greater sedation than —>	pyrilamine	Greater sedation than —>	pheniramine
diphenhydramine		thonzylamine		brompheniramine
doxylamine				
				chlorpheniramine
				triprolidine

Mast Cell Stabilizers

The use of antihistamines is one way to treat allergies, as these drugs stop histamine from entering or binding to cells in the nose, eye, skin, or other body area and thus causing an allergic reaction. *Mast cell stabilizers* prevent the allergen from attaching to the mast cell, thereby preventing the mast cell from releasing histamine. If histamine is not released from the mast cell, it cannot be free to seek the new binding receptor site of a body cell. For example, if no histamine is available to bind to the nose receptor site, the nose will not become itchy, have congestion, or become runny. In other words, mast cell stabilizers act prophylactically to prevent allergic responses. They are considered anti-inflammatory agents. The benefits of mast cell stabilizers are that they:

- stop the allergic response before it begins, without causing drowsiness, irritability, or a decreased ability to think or focus.
- do not reverse allergy symptoms that are already present, but do prevent new exposure to new allergens, thus preventing allergic symptoms.
- can be used for weeks or months at a time without the fear of rebound effects or threat of addiction that decongestants may pose.

Mast cell stabilizers are used most often to prevent asthma attacks, but can be used to prevent allergic rhinitis. Mast cell stabilizers are available for use in the nose, lungs, and GI tract. Other names for mast cell stabilizers are *mast cell inhibitors* and *mediator-release inhibitors* (see Table 25-8).

Side effects are so few, and the drug is so gentle, that cromolyn sodium, the drug of choice, has been used successfully on infants and children and is now an over-the-counter remedy known as Nasalcrom®. A new mast cell stabilizer, Tilade® (nedocromil sodium), has

Table 25-8 Mast Cell Stabilizers

GENERIC NAME	TRADE NAME	DOSAGE FORMS
cromolyn sodium	Intal®	inhalation solution
	Nasalcrom®	aerosol
	Gastrocrom®	oral concentrate
	Crolom®	ophthalmic solution
lodoxamide tromethamine	Alomide®	ophthalmic solution
nedocromil sodium	Tilade®	aerosol
	Alocril®	ophthalmic solution
pemirolast potassium	Alamast®	ophthalmic solution

also been effective, and has a longer duration. Nedocromil may have more anti-inflammatory properties than cromolyn sodium.

- Mast cell stabilizers may reduce renal and hepatic function; therefore, the dosage should be decreased in patients with kidney and liver problems. Due to the propellants in the inhalant canisters, these canisters should be used with caution by patients who have coronary artery disease or a history of cardiac arrhythmias. If a patient develops eosinophilic pneumonia (or pulmonary infiltrates with eosinophilia), this treatment should be discontinued.

Cromolyn sodium and nedocromil inhibit mast cell degranulation and activation by creating a protective barrier around the cells in the nose and respiratory tract, so that pollen, mold, dust, and animal dander cannot bind or attach to them. The exact MOA is not fully understood, but it is believed that cromolyn indirectly inhibits calcium ions from entering the mast cell and triggering release of cellular contents. The mast cell stabilizers inhibit both the early and late phases of bronchoconstriction induced by inhaled antigens. In clinical trials, they have also been shown to be effective in mitigating the response induced by cold air, environmental air pollutants, exercise, sulfur dioxide, and other triggers. It is important to note the following:

- Mast cell stabilizers do not have bronchodilation, anticholinergic, antihistaminic, or glucocorticoid effects.
- Mast cell stabilizers are not used in any acute phase of severe bronchoconstriction.

Cystic Fibrosis

Cystic fibrosis (CF) is a genetic disease in which a defective gene causes the body to produce an abnormally thick, sticky mucus. This disease affects approximately 30,000 children and adults in the United States. The abnormally viscous mucus clogs the lungs, and leads to life-threatening lung infections, breathing difficulty, and digestive problems. These thick secretions also block the pancreas, preventing digestive enzymes from entering the intestines; this in turn prevents the metabolism (the chemical breakdown and absorption) of food nutrients. According to the CF Foundation's National Patient Registry, the median age of survival for a person with CF is 33.4 years, and 95 percent of men with CF are sterile.

CF symptoms include very salty-tasting skin, persistent coughing with or without phlegm, wheezing or shortness of breath, excessive appetite with poor weight gain, and greasy, bulky stools. Symptoms may vary partly because more than 1,000 mutations of the CF gene exist. Treatments include:

- chest percussion physical therapy, a form of airway clearance performed on a routine daily basis that involves vigorous clapping on the back and chest to dislodge the thick mucus from the lungs
- antibiotics to treat infections
- bronchodilator and corticosteroid inhalers
- nutritional supplements
- mucolytic treatment

Mucolytics thin out the sticky, viscous mucus that causes the breathing and digestive problems associated with CF. The viscosity of the mucus depends on the amount of mucoprotein produced. The more mucoprotein there is, the greater the number of disulfide bonds there will be, making the mucus thicker. N-acetylcysteine (the generic name of the active drug in Mucomyst® and Airbron®) breaks the disulfide bonds in mucin, which thins the mucus and makes it more easily dislodged from the lungs by the mucociliary elevator (MCE).

N-acetylcysteine is also used as an antidote in acetaminophen overdose, to prevent or mitigate hepatic injury (damage to the liver). Toxic effects of acetaminophen poisoning are inevitable if not treated in time. These effects include hepatic necrosis, renal tubular necrosis, hypoglycemic coma, and thrombocytopenia, but the potential for severe, irreversible hepatic failure, damage, and necrosis is usually the main concern. Results of hepatic toxicity may not be measurable, clinically or by laboratory tests, until 48 to 72 hours after administration of the initial oral overdose. Signs and symptoms of acute APAP overdose are dose-related, but may include nausea, vomiting, diaphoresis, and general malaise.

Possible adverse effects of acetylcysteine include hemoptysis, stomatitis, nausea, vomiting, and severe rhinorrhea. Interestingly, bronchoconstriction has also been reported with acetylcysteine therapy. The recommended dose of acetylcysteine is 3 to 5 mL of a 20 percent solution diluted with an equal volume of water or saline, or 6 to 10 mL of a 10 percent solution administered three to four times daily.

Another agent, Pulmozyme® (recombinant human deoxyribonuclease I, rhDNase, or dornase alpha) is an enzyme that cleaves DNA left behind by neutrophils in the lungs. When a neutrophil dies, its DNA leaks out, which then comes into contact with mucus, making it very thick. A patient with cystic fibrosis is affected greatly by this natural process. The mechanism of action is one of hydrolysis; when this recombinant human DNA enzyme is inhaled, it hydrolyzes or cuts the neutrophil DNA apart and subsequently thins out the mucus for an easier removal by the MCE. This agent is delivered by inhalation.

Side effects may include chest pain or discomfort, hoarseness, and sore throat. Less common are difficulty breathing; fever; redness, itching, pain, swelling, or other irritation of eyes; runny or stuffy nose; upset stomach; hives or welts; itching; redness of skin; and skin rash.

Asthma

Asthma is a chronic respiratory disease characterized by inflammation of the airways and tightening of the muscles around the airways. *Bronchoconstriction* occurs when the smooth muscles encircling the airways or tubes tighten, causing the airways to spasm. The actual interior wall constricts because the tissue becomes inflamed, and the inflammation further constricts airflow. The narrowing of the bronchi during an asthmatic attack may be fatal if the person cannot get the passageways opened quickly. In addition, more mucus is made, further narrowing the airways. As a result, the patient may feel weak; exhibit wheezing, coughing, and chest tightness or pain; and be short of breath. Albuterol and other bronchodilators are often the drug of choice for quick relief and restoration of airflow.

The exact cause of asthma is unknown, but if a family member has it, you are more likely to develop it. Research suggests that allergic triggers (allergens and irritants), as well as viral infections and exercise, play a large role in triggering airway inflammation and asthma symptoms. If a child has allergies, he or she is more likely to develop asthma. Approximately 17 million people (mostly children) have asthma attacks caused by allergies to airborne pollutants such as dust, mold, mites, pollen, and animal dander.

There are many substances, called *biochemical mediators*, inside each mast cell. These mediators can be released during exposure to allergens. Two of the most common mediators released from the mast cells that cause allergies are leukotrienes and histamine. *Leukotrienes* are potent mediators that are released by mast cells, eosinophils, and basophils. They work to contract airway smooth muscle, increase vascular permeability, increase mucus secretion, and attract and activate inflammatory cells in the air passageways of patients with asthma. Among the many other mediators that are released during respiratory inflammation are eosinophilic chemotactic factor of anaphylaxis (ECF-A), various prostaglandins, cytokines such as tumor necrosis factor (TNF), and interleukins.

One of the most important prostaglandin mediators involved in asthma is the slow-reacting substance of anaphylaxis known as SRS-A. Leukotrienes B, C, D, and E are also released; C, D, and E help to make SRS-A. The effects of SRS-A last longer than histamine, creating mucosal edema and leukocyte infiltration and causing major bronchoconstriction.

" Workplace Wisdom Asthma Statistics

Asthma affects more than 15 million people and is responsible for as many as 1.5 million emergency-room visits and 500,000 hospitalizations each year. "

Diagnosis of asthma may include chest X-ray to rule out other diseases, blood tests, sputum studies, physical exam in which the examiner listens to the sounds and notes symptoms, and spirometry tests. A spirometry breathing test measures the amount of air intake and the rate at which air can pass through the patient's airways. Less air will pass through the airways, and at a lower speed, if they are narrowed because of inflammation. This results in abnormal spirometry values.

Chronic Obstructive Pulmonary Disease

Chronic obstructive pulmonary disease (COPD) is an umbrella term for emphysema and chronic bronchitis. It is a serious respiratory condition that causes breathing difficulty for those affected. COPD is characterized by partially blocked bronchi and bronchioles, which makes it very difficult to get air into and out of the lungs and consequently causes shortness of breath. COPD is the fourth leading cause of death in the United States; more than 120,000 people die of it every year. About 80 to 90 percent of all COPD is related to cigarette smoking.

chronic obstructive pulmonary disease (COPD) a condition resulting from continual blockage of oxygen external exchange in the lungs; an umbrella term for emphysema and chronic bronchitis.

Emphysema

Emphysema affects approximately 3.8 million Americans and is ranked (with COPD) as the fourth leading cause of death in the United States. Forty percent more men than women are affected by emphysema.

Emphysema involves destruction of the alveoli. The external exchange of gases is interrupted when these thin, fragile air sacs become permanently and irreversibly damaged, as a protein called *elastin* is destroyed. The alveoli become less able to transfer oxygen to the blood system. In addition, bronchioles are less able to dilate, and often collapse due to a lack of elastin.

A major symptom is shortness of breath. As alveoli are destroyed, the lungs lose the elasticity needed to keep the airways open. The alveoli stay full of air and carbon dioxide, but are unable to exhale the waste and inhale the much-needed air from which to extract oxygen. Another symptom is great difficulty in exhaling, which leads to the characteristic fully expanded chest, known as a "barrel" chest.

Other symptoms include the inability to perform normal daily activities or exercise. Chronic breathing problems, such as bronchitis and asthma, may also develop before emphysema is diagnosed. The main cause of emphysema is long-term exposure to pollutants that irritate the alveoli, such as tobacco smoke, asbestos, pollution, coal dust, and chemical fumes. Also, it is believed that more than 100,000 Americans have been born with a protein deficiency that can lead to an inherited form of emphysema called alpha 1-antitrypsin (AAT) deficiency-related emphysema.

Chronic Bronchitis

Chronic bronchitis is characterized by inflammation of the airways that lasts for long periods of time or keeps returning. The main cause is exposure to cigarette smoke, both first-hand and second-hand. A person who smokes is more likely to get chronic bronchitis, and the condition will continue to worsen if the person does not quit. Symptoms of chronic bronchitis include shortness of breath, wheezing, fatigue, headaches, lower extremity swelling that affects both sides, and a cough that produces large amounts of mucus (which may contain blood).

Treatment of Asthma and COPD

The autonomic nervous system plays an important role in COPD and especially in asthma. Stimulation of the sympathetic nervous system's beta-2 receptors by epinephrine creates bronchodilation, whereas stimulation of the parasympathetic nervous system, specifically the activation of the vagus nerve by irritants, causes bronchoconstriction. Bronchodilators act to either open airway passages immediately, prevent attachment of the allergen to mast cells, or stop prostaglandin synthesis. Bronchodilators administered orally include ephedrine, albuterol, and terbutaline. Oral epinephrine is unavailable because it is broken down in the digestive system before it can reach the lungs.

Treatments that open up the air passageways are usually stimulant inhalers; treatments for prevention of inflammation are usually anti-inflammatory corticosteroids. The aim of treatment is to reduce inflammation and prevent further injury to the airway. There are also oral medications that can prevent inflammation. There is mounting evidence that, if left untreated, asthma can cause a long-term decline in lung function.

Oral and nasal inhalers used in the treatment of asthma are divided into two groups:

- Treatments used for quick relief, to immediately open the airway passages
- Treatments used for prophylactic maintenance, to decrease and prevent swelling, irritation, and inflammation on a daily basis, and treatments used to prevent the release of histamines and leukotrienes so that asthma attacks will not occur.

Bronchodilators

Beta-adrenergic inhalers act within approximately 15 minutes. One exception is salmeterol, which is a long-acting bronchodilator that is not designed to give an immediate effect. The mechanism of action of these *sympathomimetic* drugs is to mimic or simulate epinephrine stimulation of the beta-2 receptors of the respiratory tract, directly relaxing smooth muscles and causing immediate bronchodilation (see Table 25-9).

Xanthines

The exact mechanism of action of xanthines, which are respiratory smooth muscle relaxants, is unknown. However, the following lists some of the ways in which xanthines are believed to work:

- Increase levels of energy-producing cyclic adenosine monophosphate (cAMP).
- Competitively inhibit phosphodiesterase (PDE), an enzyme that chemically breaks down cAMP.
- Inhibition of PDE results in increased cAMP levels, smooth muscle relaxation, bronchodilation, and airflow through air passages.

The result of these actions is increased CNS and cardiovascular stimulation, force of contraction, kidney secretion, and diuretic effect. Side effects include nausea, vomiting, anorexia, gastroesophageal reflux during sleep, sinus tachycardia, extrasystole, palpitations, ventricular dysrhythmias, and transient tonic/clonic convulsions. Some

Table 25-9 Beta-Adrenergic Bronchodilators

GENERIC NAME	TRADE NAME	STRENGTH/DOSAGE FORM(S) AVAILABLE	AVERAGE ADULT DOSAGE
albuterol	Ventolin, Proventil	Tab: 2 mg, 4 mg	2–4 mg tid–qid
		Syr: 2 mg/5 mL	
		ER tab: 2 mg, 4 mg	8 mg q12 hr
		90 mcg inhaler	2 puffs q4–6 hr
		Inh soln: 0.083%, 0.5%, 0.021%, 0.42%	2.5 mg tid–qid via nebulizer
albuterol + ipratropium bromide	Combivent®	Aerosol	2 puffs qid
	DuoNeb®	Inh soln	3 mL qid with 2 additional doses per day prn
bitolterol	Tornalate®	Inh soln: 0.2%	
epinephrine	Adrenalin	Inh soln:10 mg/mL	0.5 mL no more than q3 hr
		Aerosol: 0.22 mg	
		Inj: 1 mg/mL, 0.1 mg/mL	
fluticasone + salmeterol combination	Advair® Diskus	100 mcg/50 mcg	1 inhalation bid
		250 mcg/50 mcg	
		500 mcg/50 mcg	
formoterol	Foradil®	12 mcg inhaled powder in capsule	12 mcg q12 hr via aerolizer inhaler
isoproterenol	Isuprel®	Inj: 0.2 mg/mL, 0.02 mg/mL	0.2 mg IV; repeat prn
levalbuterol	Xopenex	Inh soln: 0.31 mg/3 mL, 0.63 mg/3 mL, 1.25 mg/3 mL	0.63 mg tid (q6–8 hr) via nebulizer
metaproterenol	Alupent®, Metaprel®	0.65 mg inhaler	2–3 puffs tid–qid; NTE q4 hr
		Inh soln: 0.4%, 0.6%, 5%	
pirbuterol	Maxair®	0.2 mg inhaler	2 puffs q4–6 hr
salmeterol	Serevent®		
salmeterol zinafoate	Serevent® Diskus	50 mcg	50 mcg bid
terbutaline	Bricanyl®, Brethine® (also SQ & PO)	Tab: 2.5 mg, 5 mg	5 mg q6 hr
		Inh: 1 mg/mL	0.25 mg sq; repeat dose in 15–30 min

xanthines, such as theophylline, may cause increased nervousness when used with the herbs St. John's Wort, ma huang, or ephedra.

Anticholinergics

Anticholinergics block the effects of acetylcholine by competing for the ACH receptor site. Bronchoconstriction is prevented and airway-passage dilation is assisted. Possible side effects include dry mouth or throat, gastrointestinal distress, headache, coughing, and anxiety (see Table 25-10).

Table 25-10 Various Treatments for Asthma

GENERIC NAME	TRADE NAME	DOSAGE FORM	ADULT DOSAGE
natural xanthines	caffeine, tea, cocoa, choclolate	PO	100 mg = 1 cup coffee
Methyl Xanthines and Derivatives			
aminophylline (79% theophylline)		Tab: 100 mg, 200 mg	individualized dosing
		Inj: 250 mg/10 mL	
		Supp: 250 mg, 500 mg	
oxtriphylline (64% theophylline)		Tab: 100 mg, 200 mg; 400 mg & 800 mg SR tabs, elixir and pediatric syrup	4.7 mg/kg q8 hr
theophylline	Theodur®, Bronkodyl®, Slo-Bid®	Tab/cap: 100 mg, 125 mg, 200 mg, 300 mg; 100 mg, 200 mg, 300 mg, 400 mg, 450 mg, 600,mg extended- & timed-release tabs/caps	individualized dosing
		Syr: 150 mg/15 mL	
		Elix: 80 mg/15 mL	
Anticholinergics			
albuterol + ipratropium combination	Combivent®	Aerosol	2 puffs qid
	DuoNeb®	Inh soln	3 mL qid with 2 additional doses per day prn
ipratropium bromide	Atrovent®	Inhaler	2 puffs qid
tiotropium bromide	Spiriva®	Powder for inhalation caps	1 capsule daily in the HandiHaler device

Anti-Inflammatory Agents

Corticosteroids are not quick acting, so they are used prophylactically. The result of corticosteroid action is decreased inflammation of the airway passages, which allows the patient to breathe more easily. The mechanism of action is one of inhibition: Glucocorticoids exert their effects by binding to the glucocorticoid receptor (GR), which then inhibits or increases gene transcription through processes known as *transrepression* and *transactivation*, respectively. In this manner they also reduce the immune response (see Table 25-11).

Oral thrush, or *thrush mouth*, is the common term for a yeast infection by *Candida albicans* that occurs in the back of the throat of patients who use corticosteroid inhalers. The main symptom is a white film located at the back of the throat, tongue, and tonsil area. Antifungal mouthwash may be used to treat this infection (all yeast are fungi, but not all fungi are yeast). This common side effect occurs because steroids alter the local bacterial and fungal population of the mouth, enhancing fungal growth. Using a space inhaler or rinsing the mouth very thoroughly after each corticosteroid use will help to prevent it.

Mast Cell Inhibitors

As discussed in the preceding section on allergies, mast cell inhibitors are also known as mast cell stabilizers, mediator-release inhibitors, or prophylactic drugs. Benefits of Intal® (cromolyn sodium) and Tilade® (nedocromil) include reduction in asthma

Table 25-11   Corticosteroids

TRADE NAME	GENERIC NAME	DOSAGE FORM	ADULT DOSE
Inhalers			
Advair Diskus®	fluticasone + salmeterol combination	100 mcg/50 mcg 250 mcg/50 mcg 500 mcg/50 mcg	1 inhalation bid
Aerobid®	flunisolide	MDI, intranasal form for rhinitis	2–3 puffs bid to tid, NTE 12 puffs per day
Azmacort®	triamcinolone	MDI, PO, TOP, SC, ID, IM	2 puffs tid–qid, NTE 16 puffs per day
Flovent®	fluticasone	MDI	2 puffs bid (44 mcg each), NTE 10 puffs per day (440 mcg/day)
Pulmicort®	budesonide	dry powder inhaler (DPI)	1–2 puffs qd (200 mcg/inhalation); NTE 4 puffs per day (800 mcg/day)
QVar®, Beclovent®	beclomethasone	MDI, intranasal form for rhinitis	1–2 puffs tid–qid
Oral			
Deltasone®, Meticorten®	prednisone	PO only	5–10 mg/day; reduction in dose should be gradual to decrease the risk of adrenal insufficiency
Dexone®, Decadron®	dexamethasone	Tab: 0.5 mg, 0.75 mg, 1.5mg, 4 mg	0.75 to 9 mg/day
Medrol®, Medrol DosePak®	methylprednisolone	PO: 2 mg, 4 mg, 6 mg, 8 mg, 16 mg, 24 mg, 32 mg tablets; also available IM, SC for neoplasia and adrenal insufficiency	4–48 mg qd; reduction in dose should be gradual to decrease the risk of adrenal insufficiency
Injectable			
Decadron®	dexamethasone sodium phosphate	Inj: 4 mg dexamethasone phosphate in 1 mL ampoule	For anaphylactic shock: 10–100 mg IV (1 mg/kg) slow IV bolus)
SoluCortef®	hydrocortisone	IV, IM, Infusion sterile powder: 100 mg, 250 mg, 500 mg, 1000 mg Act-O Vial	100–500 mg for 48–72 hrs, over 30 seconds to 10 minutes, q2, 4, or 6 hr; then decreased gradually to a maintenance dose
SoluMedrol®	methylprednisolone	IV, IM, and Infusion sterile powder: 40 mg, 125 mg, 500 mg, 1 gram Act-O Vial	30 mg/kg over 30 min, MR q4–6 hr x 48 hrs at least 30 minutes. Dosage must be discontinued gradually.

symptoms, improved peak expiratory flow rates, and decreased need for short-acting beta-2 agonists.

Antileukotriene Drugs

There are two types of antileukotriene drugs: leukotriene receptor antagonists and leukotriene inhibitors. This is the first new class of asthma-fighting drugs to appear in more than 30 years. Leukotriene inhibitors may be used to reduce the need for low-dose corticosteroid inhaler regimens. The long-term effects of leukotriene inhibitors therapy have yet to be determined. It is speculated that, in the future, IV formulations of these agents may be useful in emergency situations.

Table 25-12 Mast Cell Stabilizers and Antileukotrienes

TRADE NAME	GENERIC NAME	MECHANISM OF ACTION
Mast Cell Stabilizers		
Intal®, Nasalcrom® (OTC)	cromolyn sodium	MDI; 2 puffs of 1 mg each qid; takes 2–4 weeks before results are seen. NTE 8 mg/day
Tilade®	nedocromil	MDI; 2 puffs of 2 mg each qid; NTE 16 mg/day
Leukotriene-Receptor-Blocking Drugs (LTRAs)		
Accolate®	zafirlukast	MOA: selectively blocks receptors of leukotrienes D_4 and E_4. LTD_4 and LTE_4 are components of slow-reacting substance of anaphylaxis (SRS-A).
Singulair®	montelukast	MOA: binds with high affinity and selectivity to the $CysLT_1$ receptor rather than prostanoid, cholinergic, or beta-adrenegic receptors, and inhibits the actions of LTD_4 at the $CysLT_1$ receptor without any agonist activity.
Leukotriene Formation Inhibitors		
Zyflo®	zileuton	MOA: Blocks the synthesis of leukotrienes by specifically inhibiting the enzyme that enables the formation of specific leukotrienes from arachidonic acid.

Leukotrienes are substances released when a trigger, such as animal dander, mold, or dust, starts a series of chemical reactions in the body. Histamine is also released. Leukotrienes attach to the allergen and then to the mast cell, causing inflammation, increased mucus production, and bronchoconstriction. The patient will experience coughing, wheezing, and shortness of breath.

Antileukotriene agents block or inhibit the leukotrienes from attaching to the receptors on the mast cells in the lungs and the basophils in blood circulation. The result is a decrease in neutrophil and leukocyte infiltration to the lungs that decreases inflammation in the lungs, thus mitigating and preventing asthma symptoms. The specific MOAs of these new drugs are further explained in Table 25-12.

Unfortunately, antileukotriene agents do have toxic effects. They may cause liver dysfunction; therefore, liver assessments must continue during therapy with these agents. Side effects of Accolate® and Zyflo® may include headache, dyspepsia, diarrhea, dizziness, and insomnia. The toxic effect is liver dysfunction. Montelukast has fewer side effects and no toxic effects on the liver.

PROFILES IN PRACTICE

Mr. Smith, an elderly patient, is currently on the asthma medications albuterol (2 inhalations 15 minutes prior to exercise) and theophylline (100 mg po bid). While checking out, he asks the pharmacist which of his breathing medications he should take first, as he takes both drugs before going to the gym.

• What would be the most beneficial order to take the medications, and why?

Other Treatments

Another drug, atropine, may also be used to fight allergic reactions and anaphylactic shock, because it has antisecretory properties. It decreases the amount of nasal and respiratory secretions in the body.

There are many medications in many different dosage forms and routes of administration for respiratory diseases. Medications taken orally almost always have a much higher *systemic concentration* (concentration in the entire body and blood system) than inhaled medications. Therefore, an inhaled route is preferred whenever possible. The idea behind an inhaler is that the full dose is delivered to the lungs, where it is immediately absorbed by the lung tissue and can take local effect. Excess drug that may be absorbed by the bloodstream is then distributed to the rest of the body. The lungs receive an immediate, high concentration of the drug, while the rest of the body receives very little drug. One advantage of oral medications is that some are available as time-release formulations, so that the patient takes a tablet only once every 12 hours, whereas the inhaled medication may require dosing every 4 to 6 hours. Keeping track of the number of doses used on an inhaler compared with the number it can deliver is the surest way of telling whether the inhaler is empty. One way to do this is to mark both the beginning date and the date on which the inhaler should be empty if all doses are given.

Products that once relied on chlorinated fluorocarbons (CFCs), such as air-conditioning units, refrigerators, and most aerosol products, have been either totally banned or modified to use alternative chemicals that do not damage the ozone layer. However, metered-dose inhalers (MDIs) have been granted an "essential use" exemption from this ban. This allows the drug manufacturers a few more years to develop new, alternative propellants and devices. The FDA has approved a new non-CFC inhaler, Proventil HFA® (albuterol), which uses hydrofluoralkane instead of CFC propellant.

SUMMARY

The respiratory system is crucial to sustaining life because it is responsible for providing all cells of the body with the oxygen necessary to perform their specific functions. It is the system that performs the intake of oxygen through inhalation, and the excretion of carbon monoxide through exhalation. The respiratory system is divided into two parts, the upper and lower respiratory tracts. The upper respiratory tract consists of the nasal cavity, paranasal sinuses, pharynx, and larynx. The lower respiratory tract is made up of the trachea, two lungs, two main bronchi, secondary and tertiary bronchi, bronchioles, alveolar ducts, and alveoli.

The most common disease of the respiratory system is the common cold. Uncomplicated common colds are generally treated with over-the-counter medications, including antihistamines, decongestants, cough suppressants, analgesics, antipyretics, and anti-inflammatories. The aim of treatment is to provide relief of symptoms.

The pharmacy technician should also be familiar with commonsense treatment measures, such as increased fluid intake, bed rest, gargling with warm salt water, and so on, and be able to assist the pharmacist in advising patients suffering from common colds.

Of course, there are many more serious diseases of the respiratory system, one of which is asthma. Asthma affects more than 15 million people and is responsible for as many as 1.5 million ER visits and 500,000 hospitalizations every year. If left uncontrolled, asthma can cause a long-term decline in lung function.

This chapter also discussed other respiratory diseases, ranging from allergies to life-threatening COPD, and their treatments. Because many respiratory diseases are treated with some form of inhalation therapy, it is important for pharmacy technicians to be able to assist the pharmacist in educating clients in the proper, safe use of inhalation products and devices.

CHAPTER REVIEW QUESTIONS

1. Cetirazine is to _____ as chromolyn sodium is to _____.

   a. Zyrtec®, mast cell stabilizer.
   b. H1 Antagonist, Intal®.
   c. H1 Antagonist, mast cell stabilizer.
   d. Intal®, mast cell stabilizer.

2. The tiny air sacs of the lungs are known as:
   a. bronchial tubes.
   b. capillaries.
   c. lobes.
   d. alveoli.

3. A genetic disease in which a defective gene causes the body to produce an abnormally thick and sticky mucus is known as:
   a. pneumonia.
   b. cystic fibrosis.
   c. bronchitis.
   d. emphysema.

4. Mucomyst® is indicated for cystic fibrosis and:
   a. emphysema.
   b. COPD.
   c. aspirin overdose.
   d. acetaminophen overdose.

5. Singulair® belongs to which of the following classifications?
   a. nasal decongestant
   b. leukotriene-receptor blocking drug
   c. expectorant
   d. antihistamine

6. Which of the following antihistamines is also indicated for nausea and vomiting?
   a. azelastine

b. diphenhydramine
c. promethazine
d. loratadine

7. Zyrtec® is to _____ as _____ is to fexofenadine.
   a. azelastine; Vistaril®
   b. brompheniramine; Clarinex®
   c. cetirizine; Tavist-1®
   d. cetirizine; Allegra®

8. Mucomyst® is classified as what type of drug?
   a. mucolytic
   b. expectorant
   c. antileukotriene
   d. antihistamine

9. Anticholinergic drugs block:
   a. norepinephrine.
   b. epinephrine.
   c. acetylcholine.
   d. mast cells.

10. Flovent® is to _____ as Azmacort® is to _____.
    a. triamcinolone; fluticasone
    b. fluticasone; salmeterol
    c. triamcinolone; albuterol
    d. fluticasone; triamcinolone

CRITICAL THINKING QUESTIONS

1. Discuss the advantages and disadvantages of the different types of treatment for asthma.

2. Which would be a better choice for a person with severe bronchitis, a narcotic or nonnarcotic cough suppressant? Explain your answer.

WEB CHALLENGE

1. Go to the American Lung Association's website at http://www.lungusa.org to learn more about asthma and allergies.

2. A "Methacholine Challenge" test may be given to determine if someone has asthma. See http://

asthmallergy.com/methacholine.htm for a brief description of this test.

REFERENCES AND RESOURCES

"About Air" (accessed April 8, 2008): http://www.engineeringtool box.com

Adams, MP, Josephson, DL, & and Holland, LN Jr. *Pharmacology for Nurses—A Pathophysiologic Approach*. Upper Saddle River, NJ: Pearson Education, 2008.

American Academy of Allergy, Asthma, and Immunology: http://www.aaaai.org/

"Cure for the Common Cold?" (accessed April 8, 2008): http://www.quantumhealth.com/news/articlecold.html

"Diaphragm Development" (accessed April 8, 2008): http://www.breathing.com/articles/diaphragm-development.htm

Drug Facts and Comparisons, 2006 ed. St. Louis: Wolters Kluwer Health.

"Emphysema" (accessed October 10, 2007): http://www.cdc.gov

"Emphysema" (accessed April 6, 2008): http://www.wrongdiagnosis.com/e/emphysema/intro.htm

"End Allergy and Asthma Misery" (accessed April 8, 2008): http://www.acaai.org/powerpoint/online/slide1.html

"Exchange" (accessed April 4, 2008): http://www.mrothery.co.uk/exchange/exchange.htm

"Hiccup" (accessed April 1, 2008): http://www.tipsofallsorts.com/hiccup.html#facts

Holland, N, & Adams, MP. *Core Concepts in Pharmacology.* Upper Saddle River, NJ: Pearson Education, 2007.

"Into the Thorax" (accessed April 8, 2008): http://www.saburchill.com/chapters/chap0020.html

"Legal Requirement for the Sale and Purchase of Drug Products Containing Pseudoephedrine, Ephedrine, and Phenylpropanolamine" (accessed July 15, 2007): http://www.fda.gov

"Little Mystery: Why do we yawn?" (accessed April 8, 2008): http://www.msnbc.com/news/205574.asp?cp1=1

"Molecular mechanism of action of theophylline: Induction of histone deacetylase activity to decrease inflammatory gene expression" (accessed April 8, 2008): http://www.pubmedcentral.nih.gov/articlerender.fcgi?artid=124399

National Emphysema Foundation (accessed October 10, 2007): http://www.emphysemafoundation.org

National Institute of Allergy and Infectious Diseases. "Common Cold" (accessed April 8, 2008): http://www.niaid.nih.gov/factsheets/cold.htm

"Respiratory System—Basic Function" (accessed April 8, 2008): http://www.ama-assn.org/ama/pub/category/7165.html

"Respiratory Tract" (accessed April 8, 2008): http://www.radiation-scott.org/deposition/respiratory.htm

"What allergies do you suffer from?" (accessed April 8, 2008): http://allergies.about.com/

"What Kind of Inhalers Are There?" (accessed April 8, 2008): http://www.radix.net/~mwg/inhalers.html

"What Is Alpha-1 Antitrypsin Deficiency Emphysema?" (accessed October 10, 2007): http://www.lungusa.org

"What is COPD?" (accessed October 13, 2007): http://www.nhlbi.nih.gov

chapter 26

The Cardiovascular, Circulatory, and Lymph Systems

LEARNING OBJECTIVES

After completing this chapter, you should be able to:

- List, identify, and diagram the basic anatomical structure and parts of the heart.
- Explain the function of the heart and the circulation of the blood within the body.
- List and define common diseases affecting the heart, including the causes, symptoms, and pharmaceutical treatment associated with each disease.
- Explain how each class of drugs works to mitigate symptoms of heart diseases.
- Describe the mechanism of action of anticoagulants, indications for use, and antidotes for overdose.
- List a variety of drugs intended to affect the cardiovascular system, their classifications, and the average adult dose.
- List the total cholesterol, LDL, HDL, and triglyceride ranges for an average adult and describe the differences between HDL, LDL, and triglycerides.
- Describe the structure and main functions of the lymphatic system, and explain its relationship to the cardiovascular system.

Introduction

The heart is both an organ and a muscle. Its main purpose is to send oxygenated blood throughout the body by a pumping mechanism. The heart, which is about the size of a fist, is located just to the left of the sternum in the mediastinum, between the two lungs. This unique muscle pumps about 4,300 gallons of blood a day, even though the human body only contains about 5.6 liters of blood.

Coronary artery disease, congestive heart failure, hypertension, and high cholesterol are serious cardiovascular diseases that affect millions of Americans. This chapter discusses the current classifications of cardiovascular drugs and average adult dosages used for treatment of cardiovascular diseases.

Anatomy of the Heart

The *circulatory system* is composed of organs and blood vessels that transport oxygenated blood to all parts of the body. Specifically, the circulatory system is made up of the heart, lungs, veins, arteries, and capillaries.

The *pericardium* is a double layer of serous and fibrous tissue, a fluid-filled sac that surrounds and protects the heart. It also permits free movement of the heart during contraction. The heart sits inside the pericardial cavity. The *endocardium* is the innermost wall layer that covers the inside surface of the heart. The *myocardium* surrounds the heart and causes chamber contractions.

The heart is composed of four chambers. The *septum* divides the heart into the right and left sides (see Figure 26-1). The top two chambers are the *atria* and the bottom two chambers are the *ventricles*. The right atrium receives deoxygenated blood from the body and the left atrium receives oxygenated blood from the lungs. The right ventricle pumps deoxygenated blood to the lungs to pick up oxygen and drop off waste. The left ventricle, the strongest chamber, pumps oxygenated blood to the rest of the body and back to the heart.

Functionality of the heart can be determined by listening to the "lup-dup, lup-dup" sounds of the opening and closing valves. The four heart valves, which direct blood flow forward in a single direction and prevent the backflow of blood, are the:

- Tricuspid valve—located between the right atrium and the right ventricle.
- Pulmonary valve—located between the right ventricle and the pulmonary artery.

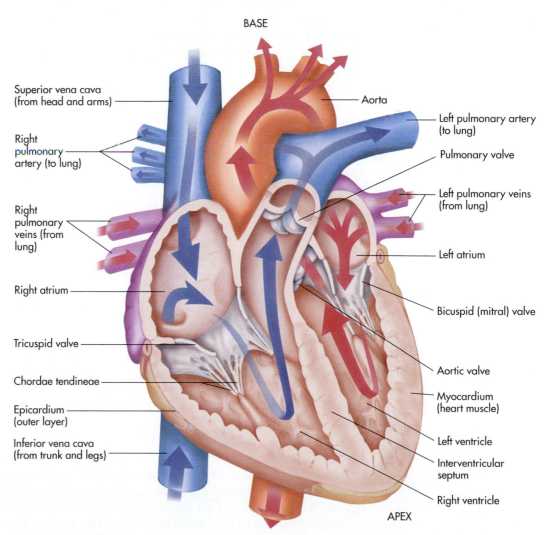

FIGURE 26-1 The heart.

- Mitral or bicuspid valve—located between the left atrium and the left ventricle.
- Aortic valve—located between the left ventricle and the aorta.

Arteries are blood vessels or tubes through which oxygenated blood travels. The largest artery is the *aorta*, which branches off the heart, divides into many smaller arteries, and then divides into the smallest, called **arterioles**. *Veins* carry the deoxygenated blood. Veins take deoxygenated blood back to the heart, then to the lungs to pick up more oxygen. *Capillaries* form a network of tiny blood vessels connecting arterioles and carrying oxygenated blood and nutrients to **venules** (the smallest veins) that carry deoxygenated blood and metabolic waste. During its passage through the many capillaries of the body, blood deposits the materials necessary for growth and nourishment into the tissues; at the same time, it receives from the tissues the waste products resulting from metabolism.

Although blood pulses through the chambers at all times, the heart does not receive its needed oxygen and nutrients from this blood. Instead, it receives its own fresh blood supply via the *coronary arteries*, which branch directly off of the aorta. These arteries feed blood deep into the thick heart muscle. Carbon dioxide and waste are removed through the *coronary veins*.

arterioles the smallest arteries.

venules the smallest veins.

Blood

Blood is a liquid tissue, and is considered the fluid of life, growth, and health. The average adult body contains approximately 5.6 liters of blood, which constitutes about 7 percent of the body mass. Blood carries oxygen, nutrients, hormones, disease-fighting cells, and other substances to all parts of the body and transports waste to the kidneys for filtration and to the lungs for expiration. Blood is composed of erythrocytes, **leukocytes**, platelets, and plasma. A drop of blood contains millions of red blood cells (RBCs), but only 7,000 to 25,000 white blood cells (WBCs). Red blood cells contain a protein chemical called *hemoglobin* that contains the element iron, which makes the blood bright red. As blood passes through the lungs, oxygen molecules attach to the hemoglobin. As the blood passes through the body's tissues and organs, the hemoglobin releases the oxygen to the cells. Immediately, the empty hemoglobin molecules bond with carbon dioxide or other waste gases from the tissues, transporting the waste away.

leukocyte white blood cell.

Function of the Heart

Every cell in the body needs oxygen to live and function properly. The purpose of the heart is to pump or deliver oxygen-rich blood to all body organs, tissues, and cells.

The atria fill with blood at the same time and then contract, pushing the blood through the valves into the ventricles. While relaxed, the ventricles fill with blood; then they contract simultaneously to push the blood out of the heart through the pulmonary valve and aortic valve into the lungs and the rest of the body, respectively. Therefore, the heart beats top to bottom, not right to left or diagonally, with two pumping actions from left to right within one pumping system.

It is important to know the pattern of blood flow to understand the normal circulation of blood within the body (see Figure 26-2). There are two kinds of blood, venous and arterial. *Venous blood* contains waste, primarily carbon dioxide (CO_2), and is dark red and deoxygenated. Veins carry deoxygenated blood to the heart to be sent to the lungs, where the external exchange of gases occurs. Arterial blood contains nutrients and oxygen (O_2), and is bright red and oxygenated. Arteries carry oxygenated blood to the body to feed and nourish all the body tissues. There is, however, one exception to this rule. The pulmonary artery carries deoxygenated blood from the heart to the lungs and the pulmonary vein carries oxygenated blood from the lungs back into the heart.

Venous, deoxygenated blood leaving the lower part of the body enters the right atrium (RA) of the heart via the inferior vena cava; the deoxygenated blood from the upper part of the body enters the RA via the superior vena cava. The blood then flows from the RA through the tricuspid valve to the right ventricle (RV). From the RV,

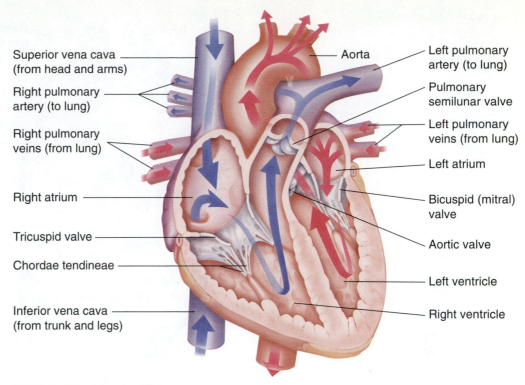

Superior vena cava
(from head and arms)

Right pulmonary
artery (to lung)

Right pulmonary
veins (from lung)

Right atrium

Tricuspid valve

Chordae tendineae

Inferior vena cava
(from trunk and legs)

Aorta

Left pulmonary
artery (to lung)

Pulmonary
semilunar valve

Left pulmonary
veins (from lung)

Left atrium

Bicuspid (mitral)
valve

Aortic valve

Left ventricle

Right ventricle

FIGURE 26-2 Blood flow through the heart.

the blood flows through the semilunar pulmonary valve into the pulmonary artery, which branches and takes the deoxygenated blood to the right and left lungs (see Figure 26-3).

Blood is cleaned in the lungs as the CO_2 waste is dropped off. During respiration, O_2 is picked up and the external exchange occurs. The CO_2 is exhaled out of the body, while the clean, oxygenated blood travels out of the lungs via the pulmonary vein to the left atrium of the heart. The blood then flows through the bicuspid valve to the left ventricle. The oxygenated blood then leaves the heart via the semilunar aortic valve to the aorta.

Oxygenated blood flows from the aortic arch to the arteries, then to the arterioles and capillaries. The oxygenated blood drops off its oxygen and picks up the diffused CO_2 waste in a process called *internal exchange*. The deoxygenated blood then leaves the capillaries, flowing through a succession of widening vessels. From the capillaries, the deoxygenated blood flows through the venules, then the veins, and finally the superior and inferior vena cavas back to the right atrium of the heart, to start the circulation process over again.

The Conduction System

The *conduction system*, or electrical system, of the heart controls the speed of the heartbeat. The spontaneous contractions of the heart muscle cells are coordinated by the sinoatrial (SA) node. This specialized nodal tissue, which provides energy in the form of electricity to the heart, has characteristics of both muscle and nervous tissue. The SA node sends electrical impulses, which, in turn, cause the heart muscle to contract.

This conduction tissue has an unusual characteristic, known as *autorhythmicity,* that allows the heart to generate its own electrical stimulation. The electrical impulse generated within the SA node is known as the *natural pacemaker*. The impulse continues through the atrioventricular (AV) node, known as the *electrical bridge*, into the common bundle of His (AV bundle) through the left and right bundle branches and Purkinje fibers.

This conduction pathway for an electrical impulse results in contraction of the atria immediately followed by contraction of the ventricles. Therefore, coordination

FIGURE 26-3 Pulmonary circulation.

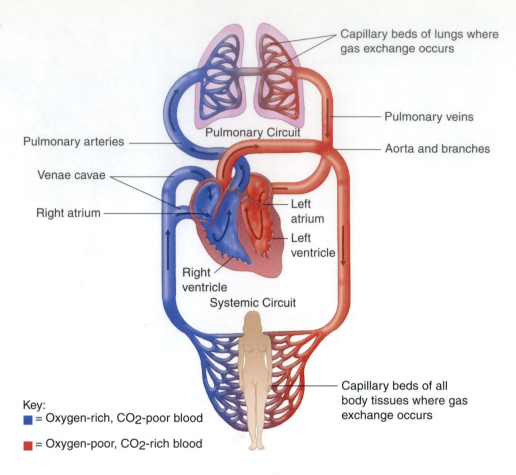

Capillary beds of lungs where gas exchange occurs

Pulmonary veins

Pulmonary Circuit

Pulmonary arteries

Aorta and branches

Venae cavae

Left atrium

Right atrium

Left ventricle

Right ventricle

Systemic Circuit

Capillary beds of all body tissues where gas exchange occurs

Key:
■ = Oxygen-rich, CO$_2$-poor blood

■ = Oxygen-poor, CO$_2$-rich blood

of the contractions of the heart chambers depends on both the SA node and autorhythmicity. In a healthy human, as the electrical impulse moves through the heart, the heart contracts about 60 to 100 times a minute. Known as the *heart rate,* each contraction represents one heartbeat. The atria contract about 1/10 of a second before the ventricles, so that the atrial blood empties into the ventricles before the ventricles contract. This delay occurs when impulses reach the AV node and are then sent down the *AV bundle,* a bundle of fibers that branches off into two bundles. From there, the impulses are carried down the center of the heart to the left and right ventricles, where the atrioventricular bundles divide further into Purkinje fibers. When the impulses reach these fibers, they trigger the muscle fibers in the ventricles to contract.

The *cardiac cycle* is the pattern of events that occur when the heart beats. There are two phases of this cycle:

1. *Diastole,* when the ventricles are relaxed.

2. *Systole,* when the ventricles contract.

During the diastole phase, both the atria and ventricles are relaxed and the **atrioventricular valves** open to allow blood to pass into both ventricles. Deoxygenated blood from the superior and inferior vena cava flows into the right atrium and from the pulmonary vein into the left atrium. The SA node contracts and prompts the atria to contract at the same time. The right atrium empties all its blood into the right ventricle, while the left atrium simultaneously empties its contents into the left ventricle. The atrioventricular valves prevent the blood from flowing back into the atria.

During the systole phase, the right ventricle receives electrical impulses from the Purkinje fibers and contracts simultaneously with the left ventricle. The atrioventricular valves close and the **semilunar valves** open. Deoxygenated blood is pumped into the pulmonary artery and oxygenated blood is pumped into the aorta.

atrioventricular valves include the tricuspid and mitral valves of the heart.

semilunar valves include the aortic and pulmonary valves of the heart.

Diseases of the Heart

There are three common forms of heart disease: hypertension, congestive heart failure, and coronary artery disease. This section explores the complications that can occur and the pharmaceutical treatment for each.

Hypertension

Hypertension (HTN) is the sustained elevation of systemic arterial blood pressure. *Blood pressure (BP)* is the force of the blood against the arterial walls when the heart beats (systole) and when the heart relaxes (diastole). Blood pressure is measured in millimeters of mercury (mm Hg). Hypertension can be a very serious problem, as most people with the condition do not even realize that they have it. However, if blood pressure is extremely high, the person may experience symptoms such as severe headache, chest pain, irregular heartbeat, and fatigue (see Table 26-1).

Risk factors for high blood pressure include:

- obesity
- high-sodium diets
- lack of physical activity
- stress
- excessive alcohol consumption
- genetics
- age (most hypertension occurs in those over 35 years of age)
- race (African-Americans are at higher risk of high blood pressure than other racial groups)

People with hypertension are at greatly increased risk of heart disease, liver failure, heart attack, and stroke.

Workplace Wisdom Heart Failure

Heart failure is responsible for 40,000 deaths each year, as well as 2.9 million doctor visits and 875,000 hospitalizations.

Congestive Heart Failure

In *congestive heart failure (CHF)*, the heart fails to cycle all the blood it receives. CHF is caused by a decreased **contractility** of the myocardium. In other words, the heart receives more blood than it can pump out, because the myocardium is not strong enough to push the blood out of the atria through the valves into the ventricles. This causes a backup of blood in the atria, resulting in congestion as blood accumulates inside the atria, stretching and enlarging the heart. This enlargement weakens the heart muscle, which is trying to move ever-increasing amounts of blood each time it contracts.

contractility the ability to contract; also, the degree of contraction.

Table 26-1 American Heart Association Classes of Blood Pressure Levels

BP CATEGORY	SYSTOLIC (MM HG)		DIASTOLIC (MM HG)
Normal	> 120	and	> 80
Prehypertension	120–139	or	80–89
Stage 1 hypertension	140–159	or	90–99
Stage 2 hypertension	160 or higher	or	100 or higher

With less blood leaving the atria, less blood is available to be sent to the lungs and the rest of the body. Therefore, less CO_2 leaves the lungs and less O_2 enters the blood during external exchange. Less blood throughout the body means less oxygen available to feed the organs and body parts; because of the lack of oxygen, *necrosis* (tissue death) may occur.

Symptoms of CHF include upright posture or leaning forward; anxiety and restlessness; cyanotic (bluish), clammy skin; persistent cough; rapid breathing; fast heart rate; and edema (swelling) of the lower limbs.

Ischemia

Ischemia is a condition in which the oxygen-rich blood is stopped, blocked, or restricted to a specific part of the body. *Cardiac ischemia* refers to lack of blood flow and oxygen to the myocardium. If ischemia is sustained, it can cause a *myocardial infarction (MI)* and can lead to heart tissue damage or death. In most cases, a temporary blood shortage (oxygen deprivation) to the heart causes *angina pectoris* (pain in the chest and heart area).

Myocardial Infarction

The result of ischemia is damage to or death of the tissue that did not receive enough oxygen. If this necrotic tissue is in the heart or cardiac muscle, the necrosis is called an *infarction*. If the tissue within the heart dies, it is a *myocardial infarction* (MI). This tissue death or damage can be fatal if the area of the infarct is large enough, as in a massive MI. Some people can survive two or three MIs, if they are small and do not overlap to create a large area of damage. Tissue that has undergone a myocardial infarction will never heal or return to the status of functional cardiac muscle. Therefore, the functionality of the heart muscle is reduced with each MI.

Arrhythmias

Arrhythmias are irregular patterns in the beating of the heart or a change in the force or speed of the heart's contraction. They can occur in the atrium, the ventricle, or both, at one time or at irregular intervals. Arrhythmias can be due to cardiac diseases, such as CHF, coronary artery disease, HTN, or MI, or to the side effects of some medications. The most serious arrhythmia is *ventricular fibrillation*, which constitutes a medical emergency because the ventricles cannot contract efficiently to maintain adequate blood circulation; this results in MI or death. Slow heartbeats are known as *bradycardia* and fast heartbeats are known as *tachycardia*.

Antiarrhythmic drugs restore normal rhythm patterns but do not cure the cause of the irregular heartbeat. These drugs are grouped into four classes according to their effect on the cardiac cycle (see Table 26-2).

Class I Antiarrhythmic Agents

Class I antiarrhythmic drugs cause local anesthetic effects, slow down the heart rate, slow conduction velocity, prolong the refractory period, and decrease automaticity of the heart. This is accomplished by blocking the influx of sodium ions to excitatory membranes during depolarization and excitation.

Class II Antiarrhythmic Agents

Beta-adrenergic blockers (class II antiarrhythmic agents) slow down the heart rate, slow conduction velocity, prolong the refractory period, and decrease automaticity by blocking both the release of sympathetic neurotransmitters and their activity. Because they antagonize the effects of norepinephrine at beta-1 cardiac receptors, these drugs work particularly well on ventricular myocardium.

Class III Antiarrhythmic Agents

Class II antiarrhythmics block the efflux of potassium (K^+) ions during repolarization phases 1–3, thus prolonging the refractory period and decreasing the frequency of arrhythmias.

Table 26-2 Antiarrhythmic Agents

GENERIC NAME	TRADE NAME	AVAILABLE DOSAGE FORM(S)/ STRENGTH	AVERAGE ADULT DOSE
Class I Antiarrhythmic Agents			
disopyramide	Norpace®	100 mg, 150 mg caps 100 mg, 150 mg extended-release (ER) caps	400 mg–800 mg/day in divided doses (q6 hr for immediate-release forms and q12 hr for ER)
flecainide	Tambocor®	50 mg, 100 mg, 150 mg tabs	50–150 mg q12 hr; not to exceed (NTE) 400 mg/day
mexiletine	Mexitil®	150 mg, 200 mg, 250 mg caps	200–400 mg q8 hr
procainamide	Procanbid®	250 mg, 500 mg, 750 mg ER tabs 250 mg, 375 mg, 500 mg caps	50 mg/kg in divided doses
propafenone	Rhythmol®	150 mg, 225 mg, 300 mg tabs 225 mg, 325 mg, 425 mg ER caps	150–300 mg q8 hr 225–425 mg q12 hr (ER)
quinidine	Quinaglute® Quinadex®	200 mg, 300 mg tabs 300 mg, 324 mg SR tab	200–400 mg tid–qid 300–600 mg q8–12 hr
Class II Antiarrhythmic Agents			
esmolol	Brevibloc®	10 mg/mL, 20 mg/mL, 250 mg/mL	50–200 mcg/min IV
propranolol	Inderal®	10 mg, 20 mg, 40 mg, 60 mg, 80 mg, 90 mg tabs 60 mg, 80 mg, 120 mg, 160 mg ER caps 4 mg/mL, 8 mg/mL soln 80 mg/mL conc soln 1 mg/mL inj	HTN: 120–240 mg/day po in 2 to 3 divided doses 80–160 mg po daily (ER) 1–3 mg IV q4 hr
Class III Antiarrhythmic Agents			
amiodarone	Cordarone®	100 mg, 200 mg, 400 mg tabs	Loading dose: 800–1,600 mg/day Maintenance: 400–600 mg/day
bretylium tosylate		2 mg/mL, 4 mg/mL, 50 mg/mL inj	5–10 mg/kg IV q6 hr
sotalol	Betapace®	80 mg, 120 mg, 160 mg, 240 mg tabs	160–640 mg/day in 2 or 3 divided doses

Table 26-2   Antiarrhythmic Agents (*continued*)

GENERIC NAME	TRADE NAME	AVAILABLE DOSAGE FORM(S)/ STRENGTH	AVERAGE ADULT DOSE
Class IV Antiarrhythmic Agents—Calcium Channel Blockers			
amlodipine	Norvasc®	2.5 mg, 5 mg, 10 mg tabs	2.5–10 mg once daily
bepridil	Vascor®	200 mg, 300 mg tabs	200–400 mg once daily
diltiazem	Cardizem® Dilacor® XR	30 mg, 60 mg, 90 mg, 120 mg tabs	120–360 mg qid
		120 mg, 180 mg, 240 mg, 300 mg, 360 mg, 420 mg ER tabs	180–540 mg once daily (ER tabs)
		60 mg, 80 mg, 120 mg, 180 mg, 240 mg, 300 mg, 360 mg, 420 mg ER caps	180–540 mg once daily or in 2 divided doses (ER caps)
felodipine	Plendil®	2.5 mg, 5 mg, 10 mg ER tabs	2.5–10 mg once daily
isradipine	DynaCirc®	5 mg, 10 mg continuous-release (CR) tabs	5–10 mg once daily (CR)
		2.5 mg, 5 mg caps	2.5–10 mg bid
nicardipine	Cardene®	20 mg, 30 mg caps	20–40 mg tid
		30 mg, 45 mg, 60 mg ER caps	30–60 mg bid (ER)
nifedipine	Procardia®, Adalat®	10 mg, 20 mg caps	10–20 mg tid
		30 mg, 60 mg, 90 mg ER tabs	30–90 mg once daily (ER)
nimodipine	Nimotop®	30 mg cap	60 mg q4 hr x 21 days
nisoldipine	Sular®	10 mg, 20 mg, 30 mg, 40 mg ER tabs	10–60 mg once daily
verapamil	Calan®, Isoptin®	40 mg, 80 mg, 120 mg tabs	240–480 mg/day in 3 or 4 divided doses
		120 mg, 180 mg, 240 mg (ER tabs & caps, SR tabs)	ER & SR: individualize doses
		100 mg, 200 mg, 300 mg ER caps	

Note: Calcium channel blockers are also indicated for hypertension.

Class IV Antiarrhythmic Agents

Calcium channel blockers or antagonists (class IV antiarrhythmic drugs) block the pathways for calcium entry to excitable membranes of the heart and blood vessels that develop action potentials. This action decreases SA node activity, slowing down the heart rate and conduction velocity of the AV node. Supraventricular tachycardia often responds to class IV antiarrhythmic agents.

Workplace Wisdom Quinidine

Quinidine is derived from cinchona bark and is also used in the treatment of malaria. Quinidine may cause cinchonism (poisoning). Overdose causes tinnitus, headache, dizziness, excessive salivation, and hallucinations.

Treatment for Heart Disease

Pharmaceutical treatment of congestive heart failure involves the administration of drugs from various drug classifications. The following drug classes are discussed in this section:

- cardiac glycosides
- diuretics
- vasodilators
- ACE inhibitors
- beta-adrenergic blockers
- phosphodiesterase inhibitors

Cardiac Glycosides

Cardiac glycosides are used to increase the force of myocardial contraction, without causing an increase in the consumption of oxygen. Cardiac glycosides, which are derived from the *digitalis purpurea* or *digitalis lanata* plants, have been used for hundreds of years. Cardiac glycosides increase blood flow and kidney filtration, thereby reducing sodium and other electrolytes that cause fluid retention, a main culprit in CHF. The main mechanism of action is acceleration of calcium cations inside the myocardium by blocking the enzyme adenosine triphosphate (ATP), which in turn shuts off the Na^+/K^+ pump. This pump would normally remove sodium (Na^+) ions from inside the heart muscle. The sodium ions now being brought into the heart muscle will be exchanged for calcium (Ca^{++}) ions.

Workplace Wisdom Cardiac Glycoside or Aminoglycoside?

Be careful not to confuse cardiac glycosides with *aminoglycosides*, which are potent antibiotics.

Calcium ions in the myocardium increase the synthesis of actinomycin and the force of contraction of the heart muscle. With a greater force of contraction, more blood can be pumped out of the heart.

Hypokalemia (low potassium levels in the serum) increases the toxic effects of the glycosides on the heart. Hypokalemia may increase the potential for arrhythmias, ventricular fibrillation, or sudden death. Hyperkalemia (high potassium serum levels) blocks the therapeutic effects of cardiac glycosides. Hypercalcemia (high calcium serum levels) increases the therapeutic effects of cardiac glycosides and can also increase the force of contraction and speed enough to create arrhythmias. A patient taking cardiac glycosides should never consume grapefruit or grapefruit juice, because it decreases absorption rates of these medications.

The most common cardiac glycoside is digoxin. Digoxin doses are highly individualized. Most patients are started on a high dose of digoxin and then maintained on about one-quarter of the original dose. This process, called *digitalization*, is used to produce a rapid high blood level, somewhat like a loading dose, and then deliver an average adult maintenance dose of 0.125–0.5 mg po daily. The trade name for digoxin is Lanoxin®, which is available in the following strengths/forms: 0.5 mg, 0.1 mg, 0.2 mg capsules, 0.125 mg, and 0.25 mg tablets; 0.05 mg/mL pediatric elixir; 0.1 mg/mL and 0.25 mg/mL injection.

Diuretics

Diuretics, commonly called "water pills," are used to eliminate excess sodium and water via the urinary tract. Retention of sodium results in the retention of water and a subsequent increase in blood volume, which causes edema. Both lead to and aggravate the congestion and blood circulation problems associated with CHF.

Less sodium means less water in the blood and a lower blood volume, resulting in less need for contraction force from the heart. Diuretics lower blood pressure because they help to decrease blood volume and the force of the blood against vessel walls.

Because they promote water loss, diuretics are used to treat both HTN and CHF. The layperson's term for a diuretic is a "water pill." Potassium serum levels must be monitored when a patient is taking diuretics. The four main diuretic categories are:

- *Thiazide* diuretics—produce mild to moderate diuretic effects and are the type of diuretic most commonly used for CHF. Thiazides are also indicated for the treatment of edema, hypertension, and renal impairment (see Table 26-3).

- *Loop* diuretics—work in the loop of Henle within the kidneys. These diuretics have a moderate to potent diuretic effect. Used often for acute CHF, loop diuretics are also indicated for edema, hypertension, **pulmonary edema**, and nephrotic syndrome (see Table 26-4).

- *Potassium-sparing* diuretics—allow water loss without loss of the important electrolyte potassium. Low levels of potassium lead to a weak heart muscle that has less ability to contract and to pump, thereby exacerbating the CHF condition. Any diuretic that has some amount of a potassium-sparing diuretic added as a combination drug is considered a potassium-sparing drug in total. Potassium-sparing diuretics are often used in conjunction with thiazide and loop diuretics (see Table 26-5).

- *Carbonic anhydrase inhibitors*—inhibit the enzyme carbonic anhydrase, resulting in a reduction of the amount of aqueous humor and a decrease in intraocular pressure. Carbonic anhydrase inhibitors are used in the treatment of glaucoma and for the prevention or mitigation of acute mountain sickness symptoms (see Table 26-6).

pulmonary edema fluid collection in the pulmonary vessels or lungs.

Table 26-3 Thiazide Diuretics

GENERIC NAME	TRADE NAME	AVAILABLE DOSAGE FORM(S)/ STRENGTH	AVERAGE ADULT DOSE
chlorothiazide	Diuril®	250 mg , 500 mg tab 250 mg/5 mL susp 500 mg inj	500–1,000 mg po daily
chlorthalidone	Hygroton®	25 mg, 50 mg, 100 mg tabs	Edema: 50–100 mg daily HTN: 25–50 mg daily
hydrochlorothiazide (HCTZ)	Hydro-Diuril®	25 mg, 50 mg, 100 mg tabs 12.5 mg cap 50 mg/5 mL soln	Edema: 25–100 mg daily HTN: 12.5–50 mg daily
metolazone	Zaroxolyn®	0.5 mg, 2.5 mg, 5 mg,10 mg tabs	Edema: 5–20 mg daily HTN: 2.5–5 mg daily

Table 26-4 Loop Diuretics

GENERIC NAME	TRADE NAME	AVAILABLE DOSAGE FORM(S)/ STRENGTH	AVERAGE ADULT DOSE
bumetanide	Bumex®	0.5 mg, 1 mg, 2 mg tabs	0.5–2mg po daily
		0.25 mg/mL inj	0.5–1 mg IM or IV; repeat in 2–3 hr. NTE 10 mg
furosemide	Lasix®	20 mg, 40 mg, 80 mg tabs	Edema: 20–80 mg po daily
		10 mg/5 mL, 40 mg/5 mL po soln	20–40 mg IM or IV daily–bid
		10 mg/mL injection	HTN: 40 mg po bid
torsemide	Demadex®	5 mg, 10 mg, 20 mg, 100 mg tablets	ave dose 10 mg– 20 mg po daily

Table 26-5 Potassium Sparing Diuretics

GENERIC NAME	TRADE NAME	AVAILABLE DOSAGE FORM(S)/ STRENGTH	AVERAGE ADULT DOSE
spironolactone	Aldactone®	25 mg, 50 mg, 100 mg tabs	Edema: 25–200 mg daily
			HTN: 50–100 mg daily
spironolactone + HCTZ	Aldactazide®	25 mg spironolactone and 25 mg HCTZ tabs	1–8 tabs daily
		50 mg spironolactone and 50 mg HCTZ tabs	1–4 tabs daily
triamterene	Dyrenium®	50 mg, 100 mg caps	100 mg bid po, NTE 300 mg/day
triamterene + HCTZ	Dyazide®, Maxzide®	37.5 mg triamterene and 25 mg HCTZ	1–2 caps daily

Table 26-6 Carbonic Anhydrase Inhibitors

GENERIC NAME	TRADE NAME	AVAILABLE DOSAGE FORM(S)/ STRENGTH	AVERAGE ADULT DOSE
acetazolamide	Diamox®	125 mg, 250 mg tabs	250–1,000 mg po daily in divided doses
		500 mg SR caps	
		500 mg pwd inj	
methazolamide	Neptazane®	25 mg, 50 mg tabs	50–100 mg bid–tid

Table 26-7   Peripheral Vasodilators

GENERIC NAME	TRADE NAME	AVAILABLE DOSAGE FORM(S)/STRENGTH	AVERAGE ADULT DOSE
hydralazine	Apresoline®	10 mg, 25 mg, 50 mg, 100 mg tabs	10–50 mg po qid
		20 mg/mL inj	20–40 mg IV/IM prn
isoxsuprine HCl	Vasodilan®, Voxsuprine®	10 mg, 20 mg tabs	10–20 mg tid–qid
minoxidil	Loniten®	2.5 mg, 10 mg tabs	10–40 mg/day; can divide
papaverine HCl	Pavabid®	150 mg timed-release (TR) cap	150 mg q12 hr

Vasodilators

By dilating blood vessels, *vasodilators* allow more blood to exit the heart, thereby preventing or mitigating congestion and increasing cardiac output. They have a stronger effect on arteries than they do on veins, but will work on both.

Vasodilators relax the arterioles, causing them to dilate so that more blood can pass from the ventricles to the lungs and from the aorta to the rest of the body. They lower blood pressure which, in turn, decreases the workload and oxygen consumption of the heart so the heart does not have to pump as hard.

Vasodilators can be used alone or in combination with cardiac glycosides and diuretics to treat CHF. Nitro-Bid® relaxes smooth muscle, which causes venous dilation and results in a decreased workload for the heart. It also dilates the arteries leading to the heart, which helps improve oxygen supply.

Peripheral vasodilators (see Table 26-7) work directly on the blood vessels in the arms and legs to treat moderate to severe hypertension; they are often used in conjunction with diuretics and/or other antihypertensive drugs. Coronary vasodilators are used in the treatment of acute angina to stop the pain and promote immediate dilation of the coronary artery, which allows oxygen to the heart muscle; they can be used prophylactically to manage chronic angina. Nitrates, beta blockers, and calcium channel blockers are all coronary vasodilators (see Table 26-8).

ACE Inhibitors

Angiotensin-converting enzyme inhibitors (ACE inhibitors) are now thought to be one of the best treatments for CHF (see Table 26-9). ACE inhibitors are considered the **drug of choice (DOC)** for CHF. They lower high blood pressure and are thought to shrink an enlarged heart, while increasing the vital signs.

The kidneys make renin, which helps to make angiotensin I (AI) in the blood vessels. AI has no effect on blood pressure, but is converted to angiotensin II (AII) by angiotensin-converting enzyme (ACE). AII is a natural vasoconstrictor that commences the synthesis and release of aldosterone, cardiac stimulation, and renal reabsorption of sodium.

When AII binds to the angiotensin I (AT1) receptors in the blood vessels, vasoconstriction occurs, leading to high blood pressure. ACE inhibitors block the conversion of AI to AII by combining with ACE. Because AI is not converted to AII, there is no AII to bind to the AT1 receptors in the blood vessels; therefore, the blood vessels do not constrict and blood pressure does not increase.

Side effects include dizziness, fainting, or lightheadedness and a very annoying dry cough. Many ACE inhibitors have the suffix of "pril" (such as benazepril or captopril) in the generic name.

drug of choice (DOC) the drug preferred for treatment of a particular condition or disease.

Table 26-8 Coronary Vasodilators

GENERIC NAME	TRADE NAME	AVAILABLE DOSAGE FORM(S)/STRENGTH	AVERAGE ADULT DOSE
isosorbide dinitrate	Isordil® Titradose, Isordil®	5 mg, 10 mg, 20 mg, 40 mg tabs	10–40 mg po q6 hr
		2.5 mg, 5 mg, 10 mg SL & chewable tabs	2.5–5 mg SL chewable: 5–titrate upward until relief
isosorbide mononitrate	Monoket®, Imdur®	10 mg, 20 mg tabs	20 mg bid given 7 hours apart
		30 mg, 60 mg, 120 mg ER tabs	30–120 mg po daily (ER tab)
nitroglycerin	Nitrostat®, Nitro-Bid®, Nitro-Dur®	0.3 mg, 0.4 mg, 0.6 mg tabs	1 tab SL q5 min; NTE 3 tabs in 15 min
		2.5mg, 6.5mg, 9mg SR caps	2.5 mg qid up to 26 mg qid; give smallest effective dose
		2% topical oint	1–2 inches q8 hr up to 4–5 inches q4 hr
		0.2 mg/hr, 0.4 mg/hr, 0.6 mg/hr transdermal patches	0.2–0.8mg/hr q24 hr

Table 26-9 Angiotensin-Converting Enzyme Inhibitors

GENERIC NAME	TRADE NAME	AVAILABLE DOSAGE FORM(S)/STRENGTH	AVERAGE ADULT DOSE
benazepril	Lotensin®	5 mg, 10 mg, 20 mg, 40 mg tabs	10–40 mg daily or divided in 2 doses; NTE 80 mg/day
benazepril + amlodipine	Lotrel®	10 mg/2.5 mg 10 mg/5 mg 20 mg/5 mg 20 mg/10 mg	NTE 80 mg benazepril & 20 mg amlodipine/ day
captopril	Capoten®	12.5 mg, 25 mg, 50 mg, 100 mg tabs	25–150 mg bid–tid; NTE 450 mg/day
captopril + HCTZ	Capozide®	50 mg/25 mg 50 mg/15 mg 25 mg/25 mg 25 mg/15 mg	NTE 150 mg captopril & 50 mg HCTZ per day
enalapril	Vasotec®	2.5 mg, 5 mg, 10 mg, 20 mg tabs	10–40 mg daily or in 2 divided doses
enalapril + diltiazem	Teczem®	5 mg/180 mg	NTE 40 mg enalapril & 360 mg diltiazem/day
enalapril + felodipine	Lexxel®	5 mg/2.5 mg 5 mg/5 mg	NTE 40 mg enalapril & 10 mg felodipine/day

Table 26-9   Angiotensin-Converting Enzyme Inhibitors *(continued)*

GENERIC NAME	TRADE NAME	AVAILABLE DOSAGE FORM(S)/STRENGTH	AVERAGE ADULT DOSE
enalapril + HCTZ	Vaseretic®	10 mg/25 mg 5 mg/12.5 mg	
fosinopril	Monopril®	10 mg, 20 mg, 40 mg tabs	20–40 mg/day
lisinopril	Prinivil®, Zestril®	2.5 mg, 5 mg, 10 mg, 20 mg, 30 mg, 40 mg tabs	20–40 mg daily
lisinopril + HCTZ	Prinizide®, Zestoretic®	20 mg/25 mg 20 mg/12.5 mg 10 mg/12.5 mg	NTE 80 mg lisinopril & 50 mg HCTZ/day
moexipril	Univasc®	7.5 mg, 15 mg tabs	3.75–30 mg/day in 1 or 2 divided doses
moexipril + HCTZ	Uniretic®	15 mg/25 mg 15 mg/12.5 mg 7.5 mg/12.5 mg	
perindopril	Aceon®	2 mg, 4 mg, 8 mg	4 mg daily titrated to maximum of 16 mg/day
quinapril	Accupril®	5 mg, 10 mg, 20 mg, 40 mg tabs	10–80 mg/day in 1 or 2 divided doses
ramipril	Altace®	1.25 mg, 2.5 mg, 5 mg, 10 mg caps	2.5–10 mg daily
trandolapril	Mavik®	1 mg, 2 mg, 4 mg	1–4 mg/day
trandolapril + verapamil	Tarka®	1 mg/240 mg 2 mg/180 mg 2 mg/240 mg 4 mg/240 mg	NTE 8 mg trandolapril & 480 mg verapamil/day

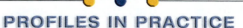

PROFILES IN PRACTICE

Ms. Lopez presents a new prescription for nitroglycerin 0.2 mg/hr transdermal patch—apply 1 patch every 24 hours. Nitroglycerin patches are indicated for the prevention of angina, and work by dilating blood vessels to allow increased blood flow and oxygen to the heart.

- What information about the placement of these transdermal patches should the pharmacist communicate to Ms. Lopez?

Angiotensin II Receptor Blockers

As discussed earlier, once AI is converted to AII by ACE, it binds to AT1 receptors in the blood vessels, causing vasoconstriction and high blood pressure. Angiotensin II receptor blockers (angiotensin receptor antagonists) block AII from getting into the AT1 receptors in the blood vessels (see Table 26-10), by competitive inhibition

Table 26-10   Angiotensin II Receptor Blockers (Angiotensin II Antagonists)

GENERIC NAME	TRADE NAME	AVAILABLE DOSAGE FORM(S)/STRENGTH	AVERAGE ADULT DOSE
candesartan	Atacand®	4 mg, 8 mg, 16 mg, 32 mg tabs	2–32 mg/day in 1 or 2 divided doses
eprosartan	Tevetan®	600 mg tabs	400–800 mg/day in 1 or 2 divided doses
irbesartan	Avapro®	75 mg, 150 mg, 300 mg tabs	150–300 mg daily; NTE 300 mg/day
losartan	Cozaar®	25 mg, 50 mg, 100 mg tabs	25–100 mg daily
losartan + HCTZ	Hyzaar®	50 mg/12.5 mg, 100 mg/12.5 mg, 100 mg/25 mg tabs	25–100 mg losartan daily
olmesartan	Benicar®	5 mg, 20 mg, 40 mg tabs	20–40 mg daily
telmisartan	Micardis®	20 mg, 40 mg, 80 mg tabs	20–80 mg/day
valsartan	Diovan®	40 mg, 80 mg, 160 mg, 320 mg tabs	80–320 mg daily

(competing with AII to get into the AT1 receptors first). In most cases, angiotensin receptor blockers get to the receptor first, but they have been found to increase blood levels of potassium. Rifampin reduces the blood levels of losartan and fluconazole reduces the conversion of losartan to its active form, thus decreasing its effects.

Beta-Adrenergic Blockers

Beta-adrenergic blockers are used to block beta-1 and beta-2 receptors from receiving the sympathetic neurotransmitters norepinephrine (NE) and epinephrine (EPI) (see Tables 26-11 through 26-13). Beta-1 receptors are found in the heart and are stimulated

Table 26-11   Nonselective Beta-Adrenergic Blocking Agents

GENERIC NAME	TRADE NAME	AVAILABLE DOSAGE FORM(S)/STRENGTH	AVERAGE ADULT DOSE
labetolol	Normodyne®	100 mg, 200 mg, 300 mg tabs	100–400 mg bid
nadolol	Corgard®	20 mg, 40 mg, 80 mg, 120 mg, 160 mg tabs	80–240 mg daily
pindolol	Visken®	5 mg, 10 mg tabs	10–60 mg daily in 2 divided doses
propranolol	Inderal®	10 mg, 20 mg, 40 mg, 60 mg, 80 mg, 90 mg tabs	HTN: 120–240 mg/day po in 2 to 3 divided doses
		4 mg/mL, 8 mg/mL soln	
		80 mg/mL conc soln	
		60 mg, 80 mg, 120 mg, 160 mg ER caps	80–160 mg po daily (ER)
		1 mg/mL inj	1–3 mg IV q4 hr
timolol	Blocadren®	5 mg, 10 mg, 20 mg tabs	20–40 mg daily in divided doses

Table 26-12   Selective Beta-Adrenergic Blocking Agents

GENERIC NAME	TRADE NAME	AVAILABLE DOSAGE FORM(S)/STRENGTH	AVERAGE ADULT DOSE
acebutolol	Sectral®	200 mg, 400 mg caps	200–1,200 mg daily in 2 divided doses
atenolol	Tenormin®	25 mg, 50 mg, 100 mg	50–100 mg once daily
bisoprolol	Zebeta®	5 mg, 10 mg tabs	2.5–20 mg once daily
esmolol	Brevibloc®	10 mg/mL, 20 mg/mL, 250 mg/mL inj	50–200 mcg/kg/min IV
metoprolol	Lopressor®	25 mg, 50 mg, 100 mg tabs	100–450 mg daily
		25 mg, 50 mg, 100 mg, 200 mg XL tabs	50–400 mg once daily (XL)

by both NE and EPI. Beta-2 receptors are found in the lungs and are stimulated by EPI, but not by NE. When the heart beta-1 receptor is stimulated, the following changes occur, first in the heart and then in the lungs:

- Heart rate increases
- Pulse rate increases
- Vasoconstriction increases
- Blood pressure increases

Table 26-13   Antiadrenergic Agents

GENERIC NAME	TRADE NAME	AVAILABLE DOSAGE FORM(S)/STRENGTH	AVERAGE ADULT DOSE
clonidine	Catapres®	0.1 mg, 0.2 mg, 0.3 mg tabs	100–600 mcg daily in divided doses
		0.1 mg/24 hr, 0.2 mg/24 hr, 0.3 mg/24 hr transdermal patches	1 patch every 7 days
guanabenz acetate	Wytensin®	4 mg, 8 mg tabs	4–32 mg bid
guanadrel	Hylorel®	10 mg tabs	10–75 mg daily in 2 divided doses
guanethidine	Ismelin®	10 mg, 25 mg tabs	10–50 mg once daily
guanfacine	Tenex®	1 mg, 2 mg tabs	1–2 mg daily at bedtime
methyldopa	Aldomet®	250 mg, 500 mg tabs	250–2,000 mg daily in 2 to 3 divided doses
reserpine		0.1 mg, 0.25 mg tabs	0.5 mg daily for 1–2 weeks, then decrease to 0.1–0.25 mg daily

- Force and contraction rate of the heart increase
- Breathing rate increases
- Bronchodilation increases
- Oxygen consumption increases

Likewise, when beta-2 receptors in the lungs are stimulated by EPI, the following changes occur, first in the lungs and then in the heart:

- Bronchodilation increases
- Breathing rate increases
- Heart rate increases
- Pulse rate increases
- Vasoconstriction increases
- Blood pressure increases
- Force and contraction rate of the heart increase
- Oxygen consumption increases

When the sympathetic neurotransmitters are blocked from the beta-1 and/or beta-2 receptors, the following occurs:

- Heart rate decreases
- Pulse rate decreases
- Vasoconstriction decreases
- Blood pressure decreases
- Force and contraction rate of the heart decrease
- Oxygen consumption decreases (prevents ischemia and angina)
- Breathing rate decreases
- Bronchodilation decreases

If a patient has hypertension, angina, or cardiac arrhythmias, beta-1 blockers will mitigate these conditions. Selective beta blockers that block only beta-1 receptors in the heart are used primarily for HTN. Beta blockers may affect insulin and glucose levels. Inderal® is also indicated in the treatment of migraine headaches, glaucoma, cardiac arrhythmias, and post-MI.

Antiadrenergic Agents

An *antiadrenergic agent* is a centrally or peripherally acting antihypertensive agent. This drug interferes with the manufacture of NE at nerve endings. Because less NE is being made, the antiadrenergic agents are stored as a false transmitter and are released like natural NE when needed. Drowsiness may occur upon initial therapy.

Coronary Artery Disease

Coronary artery disease (CAD) occurs when there is insufficient blood flow to the heart via the right or left coronary artery. The reduced blood flow is usually due to arteriosclerosis and/or atherosclerosis. Over time, CAD can lead to angina, heart attack, arrythmias, stroke, pulmonary embolism, and heart failure. CAD is the most common form of heart disease; the National Heart, Lung, and Blood Institute ranks CAD as the leading cause of death in the United States.

Arteriosclerosis, often referred to as "hardening of the arteries," is the actual stiffening of the arteries themselves. It occurs over a period of many years, during which the arteries thicken and lose elasticity, and develop areas that become hard and brittle. This occurs because of the deposition of calcium in the vessel walls. During exercise the arteries should constrict, and during rest they should dilate. With arteriosclerosis, the arteries will become inflexible and will not constrict or dilate as they should, when they should. A *stenosis*, or narrowing of the lumen, may also occur. A person can have both a hardening and a narrowing of the arteries, or one condition without the other. Arteriosclerosis can lead to hypertension, MI, and stroke. All the organs that are fed by the sclerotic (hardened) arteries can suffer damage and fail to function properly. Causes include genetics, diet, and normal aging.

plaque fatty deposit that is high in cholesterol.

Atherosclerosis, a specific form of arteriosclerosis, is a condition in which **plaque** builds up on the walls of the coronary arteries and hardens them. Atherosclerosis is believed to be initiated by an injury to the artery wall; the injury may have been caused by a diet high in cholesterol, smoking, high blood pressure, or diabetes. Plaque adheres more easily to a damaged wall, and as it builds up (*accretes*), the lumen soon becomes occluded. Blood clots (**thrombi**) can also form because the arterial wall is no longer smooth. Instead, the wall has an irregular surface that platelets stick to easily. This will further impede blood flow and lead to ischemia, which may in turn cause angina, MI, stroke, or pulmonary embolism. The terms *arteriosclerosis* and *atherosclerosis* are often used interchangeably.

thrombi blood clots (singular, *thrombus*).

Treatment of Coronary Artery Disease

Coronary artery disease, especially atherosclerosis, creates a condition in which blood clots form easily. Normal blood contains platelets that help the blood to clot when necessary. As more blood with more sticky platelets runs through the narrowed tunnels of coronary arteries with atherosclerosis, the platelets aggregate (clump together). Blood clots "snowball," getting larger and larger, until the lumen is eventually occluded, causing ischemia and angina. To prevent blood clots from forming or getting bigger, antiplatelet drugs are given to reduce the number of platelets and anticoagulants are given to reduce the stickiness of the platelets. Think of a platelet as a piece of adhesive tape. The more tape there is, the more stickiness there will be. To reduce stickiness, you can either reduce the number of tape pieces or reduce the amount of adhesive on each piece of tape. Doing both achieves the best results, reducing both the number of platelet and their stickiness—and hence reducing blood's ability to clot.

Antiplatelets

Also called *platelet aggregation inhibitors*, antiplatelet drugs (see Tables 26-14 and 26-15) reduce and prevent platelet aggregation by interfering with the extrinsic and intrinsic pathways. Because antiplatelets reduce the ability of the blood to coagulate, the chance of internal and external hemorrhage exists. Side effects include **hematuria**, blood in the feces or tarry stools, and/or heavy menstrual bleeding.

hematuria blood in the urine.

Table 26-14   Antiplatelet Agents

GENERIC NAME	TRADE NAME	AVAILABLE DOSAGE FORM(S)/STRENGTH	AVERAGE ADULT DOSE
anagrelide HCl	Agrylin®	0.5 mg, 1 mg caps	0.5 mg qid or 1 mg bid
cilostazol	Pletal®	50 mg, 100 mg	100 mg bid
clopidogrel	Plavix®	75 mg	75 mg daily
dipyridamole	Persantine®	25 mg, 50 mg, 75 mg	75–100 mg qid with warfarin therapy
dipyridamole + ASA	Aggrenox®	200 mg SR dipyridamole/ 25 mg ASA caps	1 cap bid
ticlopidine	Ticlid®	250 mg	250 mg bid with food

Table 26-15 Comparison of Antiplatelet Agents

FIRST-GENERATION SUBCLASSIFICATION: PLATELET INHIBITORS	SECOND-GENERATION SUBCLASSIFICATION: THIENOPYRIDINES	THIRD-GENERATION SUBCLASSIFICATION: PARENTERAL GLYCOPROTEIN II/IIIA PLATELET INHIBITORS (ANTAGONISTS)
aspirin (acetylsalicylic acid or ASA)	Ticlid® (ticlopidine) Not used as much as Plavix because it causes blood disorders such as thrombocytopenia	ReoPro® (abciximab)
Persantine® (dipyridamole)	Plavix® (clopidogrel)	Centocor® (abciximab) Aggrastat® (tirofiban) Integrilin® (eptifibatide)
Mechanism of Action		
The MOA of ASA is the inhibition of cyclooxygenase, which prevents prostaglandin G2 from forming, which, in turn, prevents the formation of thrombaxane A2, a potent platelet aggregator and vasoconstrictor		Glycoprotein II/IIIa receptor inhibitors/antagonists block certain receptors on the platelets responsible for clumping and therefore block platelet activity
Side Effects		
Bleeding gums, poor healing of scratches or sores, bruises, hematuria or heavy menstrual bleeding, GI upset with external or internal bleeding	Bleeding gums, poor healing of scratches or sores, bruises, hematuria or heavy menstrual bleeding, GI upset with external or internal bleeding	Bleeding gums, poor healing of scratches or sores, bruises, hematuria or heavy menstrual bleeding, GI upset with external or internal bleeding
Toxic Effects		
anemia	rare but serious blood disorders or dyscrasias, thrombocytopenic purpura, anemia, neurological changes, acute onset of altered mental status, renal failure	anemia
Special Considerations and Warnings		
Blood must be monitored to dose patients properly and to avoid anemia or blood disorders	Blood must be monitored to dose patients properly and to avoid anemia or blood disorders (especially with Ticlid®)	Blood must be monitored to dose patients properly and to avoid anemia or blood disorders

The patient's blood-clotting ability, urine, and stools should be monitored. GI upset and bleeding may also lead to GI ulcers. Therefore, platelet inhibitors should be taken on a full stomach and at least two hours apart from antacids. Ticlid® has been known to cause blood **dyscrasias** such as thrombotic thrombocytopenia, neutropenia/agranulocytosis, and thrombotic thrombocytopenic purpura.

dyscrasia an abnormal condition of the body, especially a blood imbalance.

Table 26-16   Anticoagulants

GENERIC NAME	TRADE NAME	AVAILABLE DOSAGE FORM(S)/STRENGTH	OVERDOSE ANTIDOTE
heparin sodium (Na)		1,000 units/mL, 2,000 units/mL, 5,000 units/mL, 10,000 units/mL, 20,000 units/mL, 40,000 units/mL inj	protamine sulfate
warfarin Na	Coumadin®	1 mg, 2 mg, 2.5 mg, 3 mg, 4 mg, 5 mg, 6 mg, 7.5 mg, 10 mg tabs	vitamin K
LMWHs			
dalteparin Na	Fragmin®	2,500 units/mL, 5,000 unit/mL, 7,500 units/mL, 10,000 units/mL, 25,000 units/mL inj	
enoxaparin Na	Lovenox®	30 mg/0.3 mL, 40 mg/0.4 mL, 60 mg/0.6 mL, 80 mg/0.8 mL, 100 mg/1 mL, 120 mg/0.8 mL, 150 mg/1 mL, 300 mg/3 mL inj	
tinzaparin Na	Innohep®	20,000 units/mL	

Note: Doses vary with blood monitoring results.

Anticoagulants

Sometimes erroneously called "blood thinners," anticoagulants do not thin out the blood (see Table 26-16). Instead, they prevent clots from forming or existing clots from getting bigger. However, they *cannot* dissolve existing blood clots. Warfarin is the oral DOC and heparin is the parenteral DOC.

Warfarin is used in the long-term prevention or management of venous thromboembolic disorders, including **deep venous thrombosis**, pulmonary embolism, and clotting associated with atrial fibrillation and prosthetic heart valves. It is also used after MI to prevent reinfarction, venous thromboembolism, and death. It works by preventing the synthesis of clotting factors II, VII, IX, and X. Warfarin dosages are monitored by prothrombin time (PT) values. Signs of bleeding are usual indications for treatment with vitamin K. Warfarin takes several days for onset, with a long duration of two to five days after it is discontinued.

Heparin is a parenterally administered anticoagulant used prophylactically to prevent and treat DVT and pulmonary embolism; to treat **thrombophlebitis**; and to prevent clotting during cardiac and vascular surgery, extracorporeal circulation, hemodialysis, blood transfusions, and in blood samples for laboratory tests. Heparin is a mucopolysaccharide found in bovine (cattle) and porcine (pig) lung and intestinal tissue. Heparin combines with antithrombin III to inactivate clotting factors IX, X, XI, and XII. This inhibits the conversion of prothrombin to thrombin, thus preventing the formation of fibrin, one of the main clotting ingredients of blood, and thereby inhibiting the formation of a clot. Heparin also interferes with platelet aggregation and inhibits thromboplastin so that more thrombin cannot be manufactured. Heparin must be administered parenterally by intravenous or subcutaneous injection or by IV infusion. It is destroyed by gastric juices and cannot be given orally. The onset of action of heparin is immediate when given IV and within 20–30 minutes when given subcutaneously. However, it has a short duration and must be given continuously while needed.

Bioequivalence is still a disputed issue among different manufacturers of warfarin and unfractionated heparin (UFH). It is still considered sound judgment not to switch manufacturers of products during therapy for an individual patient once therapy has begun. Low-molecular-weight heparins (LMWHs) are also not interchangeable. Both UFH and LMWHs inactivate factor Xa by interacting with antithrombin. UFH

deep venous thrombosis (DVT) a blood clot in one of the veins of the legs or other deep veins.

thrombophlebitis inflammation of a vein with a thrombus.

inactivates factors IIa and Xa, whereas LMWHs inhibit factor Xa but only minimally affect thrombin (factor IIa).

Some advantages of LMWHs over UFH are:

- Longer half-life of LMWHs allows less frequent dosing and yields more predictable response.
- Reduce hospital stay times and therefore are cost-efficient.
- UFH has less bioavailability because it binds to more blood components; there is greater variability in patient response to each dose.
- Lower incidence of heparin-induced thrombocytopenia with LMWHs than with UFH.
- LMWHs are smaller molecules, because some mucopolysaccharides have been removed; thus, subcutaneous absorption is better.

The disadvantage of LMWHs is that there is *no* specific antidote, as there is for unfractionated heparin. Protamine sulfate reverses only about 60 percent of the anti-factor Xa activity of low-molecular-weight heparin.

Tissue Plasminogen Activators

Tissue plasminogen activators (t-PAs) and other thrombolytic enzymes chemically break down blood clots by reversing the clotting order and interfering with the synthesis of various clotting factors (see Table 26-17). The main indication for use of these "clot-busting" drugs is in the management of acute, severe thrombolytic disease such as MI, pulmonary embolism, and iliofemoral thrombosis.

Tissue plasminogen activators must be administered by parenteral infusion within a "window of opportunity," to avoid intracranial hemorrhage. This window is usually less than three hours from the onset of symptoms; however, some thrombolytics may be used within six hours of the onset of symptoms. A fatal error occurs if a thrombolytic is given for an MI caused by a stenosis instead of a clot. Therefore, because of their potency and possible adverse reactions, t-PAs are used only in emergency cases for acute myocardial infarctions, acute ischemic stroke, and pulmonary embolism caused by blood clots. Quick, expensive blood testing and electrocardiography must be

Table 26-17 Thrombolytics and Tissue Plasminogen Activators

GENERIC NAME	TRADE NAME	TYPE	AVERAGE ADULT DOSE
alteplase recombinant	Activase®	t-PA, thrombolytic	15 mg IV bolus, then 50 mg over 30 min, then 35 mg over 60 min
anistreplase	Eminase®	thrombolytic	30 units IV over 2–5 min
retiplase recombinant	Retivase®	r-PA, thrombolytic	10 unit IV bolus over 2 min, repeated 30 min later
streptokinase	Strepase®	thrombolytic	1.5 million units IV over 60 min
tenecteplase	Metalyse®	TNKase	30–50 mg IV bolus over 5 sec (based on patient's weight)
urokinase	Abbokinase®	thrombolytic	4,400 units/kg @ 90 mL/hr over 10 min, then 4,400 units/kg @ 15 mL/hr for 12 hr

performed before a thrombolytic can be administered. This takes precious time in the window of opportunity, but it is well worth it. Thrombolytics stimulate the synthesis of fibrinolysin, which breaks down a clot into soluble products.

These drugs are extremely expensive: thousands of dollars just for the product alone, not including diagnosis, the ER personnel who order and administer the drug, and pharmacy preparation of the drug. A recently compounded thrombolytic usually has an expiration time of 8 to 24 hours. Because of the expense and short shelf life of the compounded drug, thrombolytics are usually prepared by the pharmacy just prior to administration.

Contraindications include previous stroke, major surgery, head injury, and history of stomach ulcers or abnormal bleeding problems. Patients who have previously had an injection of streptokinase should not receive a further dose of streptokinase at any time, unless it is within four days of the first dose. Streptokinase stimulates the formation of antibodies that will reduce the effectiveness of a second dose. A second heart attack or clot treatment will require administration of an alternative thrombolytic drug.

Thrombolytics should not be given if the ECG wave pattern shows no ST segment elevation. Possible side effects include nausea and vomiting; bleeding at the injection site, gums, or other areas; and large bruises.

Thrombin Inhibitors

Traditionally, anticoagulant therapy has been used to prevent the production of thrombin or its activity (see Table 26-18). However, new direct thrombin inhibitors inactivate bound thrombin by binding to the enzyme and blocking its interaction with its fibrin substrates. There are two receptor sites on thrombin IIa.

The active-site directed thrombin inhibitor, argatroban, binds to the thrombin without displacing the fibrin, which inactivates the thrombin so that it cannot form a clot. Bivalent direct thrombin inhibitors, such as hirudin and bivalirudin, displace thrombin from fibrin during binding and the inactivation process.

These new agents may have potential advantage over heparin because thrombin inhibitors produce a more predictable anticoagulant response, as they do not bind to plasma proteins like heparin does. Therefore, there is greater capability for maintained and accurate dosing and response with thrombin inhibitors.

Antidotes for Overdose of Antiplatelets or Anticoagulants

Should overdose of antiplatelet or anticoagulant drugs occur, a number of antidotes exist.

Warfarin Overdose

Vitamin K is a natural precursor to the synthesis of some clotting factors. Vitamin K is found in cabbage, cauliflower, spinach, other green leafy vegetables, cereals, soybeans, and egg yolks. It is also made by the bacteria that line the gastrointestinal tract.

Table 26-18   Thrombin Inhibitors

GENERIC NAME	TRADE NAME	AVAILABLE DOSAGE FORM(S)/STRENGTH	AVERAGE ADULT DOSE
argatroban	Novastin®	100 mg/mL inj	2 mcg/kg/min IV
bivalirudin	Angiomax®	250 mg pwd for inj	1 mg/kg IV bolus, followed by a 4-hr infusion of 2.5 mg/kg/hr
desirudin	Iprivask®	15 mg pwd for inj	15 mg SC q12 hr
lepirudin	Refludan®	50 mg pwd for inj	0.4 mg/kg for patients up to 110 kg

Vitamin K may reduce the effectiveness of the oral anticoagulant warfarin. Because of this, Vitamin K may also be used as an antidote to stop hemorrhage when too much warfarin has been given and is causing excessive bleeding. Bleeding may be internal or external. Note the locations and clotting factors on the coagulation pathway where vitamin K is required, particularly factors VII and IX and Prothrombin.

INFORMATION

Here is a note about factor VIII that has little to do with diseases of the heart, but pertains to the subject of clotting factors. Hemophilia A is the most common hereditary disorder affecting blood coagulation (*heme* = blood, *philia* = loving). It is caused by a lack of plasma protein factor VIII.

The disorder is caused by an inherited, sex-linked recessive trait. The defective gene is located on the X chromosome. Because females have two copies of the X chromosome, there is a good chance that there will not be a defective gene on both chromosomes. Males, however, carry only one X chromosome, so if the factor VIII gene on that chromosome is defective, male offspring will be born with the disease. Hemophilia A affects about 1 out of 5,000 men. Females with one defective factor VIII gene are carriers of this trait. All female children of a male hemophiliac are carriers of the trait.

Although some cases of hemophilia go unnoticed until later in life, when trauma, surgery, or injury occurs, many cases show the classic symptoms of severe bleeding. Hemorrhage may be internal or external.

Heparin Overdose

The only antidote for heparin overdose is protamine sulfate, used for the emergency reversal of heparin-induced bleeding. Heparin's clotting ability centers around the clotting factor called factor IXa. Activated partial thromboplastin time (aPTT) of more than 100 seconds may require administration of protamine sulfate.

Thrombolytic Enzyme Overdose

Aminocaproic acid and tranexamic acid can be used to counter a thrombolytic enzyme overdose. The fibrinolysis-inhibitory effects of aminocaproic acid are exerted principally via inhibition of plasminogen activators and to a lesser degree through antiplasmin activity. Tranexamic acid competitively inhibits the activation of plasminogen to plasmin.

Cholesterol

Cholesterol is a waxy fat-like substance that is found in all cells and is needed to make hormones, vitamin D, and digestive substances. The liver may synthesize cholesterol, or may take up all the cholesterol the body needs from circulating lipoproteins or from what is absorbed in the small intestines. However, because it is found in many foods, many people have more cholesterol than the body needs. When there is excess cholesterol and other fats in the blood, the condition is called **hyperlipidemia**. These fats are transported in the blood via larger molecules called *lipoproteins*. The five categories of lipoproteins are:

hyperlipidemia high concentrations of lipids in the blood.

- chylomicrons
- very-low-density lipoproteins (VLDLs)
- intermediate-density lipoproteins (IDLs)
- low-density lipoproteins (LDLs)—"bad" cholesterol
- high-density lipoproteins (HDLs)—"good" cholesterol

Regular screenings for hyperlipidemia are needed because high cholesterol is asymptomatic. The first line of defense in the fight against high cholesterol is diet and exercise. When this fails to bring the LDL and VLDL levels down to normal, or if the amount of HDL decreases, a prescription medication must be employed. Normally HDL carries LDL and VLDL away from artery walls. Hyperlipidemia occurs when there is a higher than normal amount of LDL.

" Workplace Wisdom Cholesterol Levels and Age

Risk for high blood cholesterol increases with age, until the age of 65. **"**

Triglycerides

Triglycerides are a form of energy stored in adipose and muscle tissues. They are gradually released and metabolized between meals as the body's energy needs fluctuate. Lipids are also found in the adipose tissue, the liver, and the blood. Immediately after a meal, triglycerides can be found in the blood. Triglycerides are often measured to depict fat ingestion and metabolism, and the measurements can be used to assess CAD risk factors.

Chylomicrons, which are produced in the intestines, deliver dietary cholesterol and triglycerides. Usually, the fatty acids are removed from the triglycerides, found in the center of the chylomicrons, as they pass through various tissues, particularly adipose and skeletal muscle. The remainder of chylomicron is then delivered to the liver and disappears from the blood within two or three hours. The remaining triglycerides, plus any triglycerides synthesized by the liver, are then secreted into the blood by the liver as VLDL. See Tables 26-19 through 26-22.

Table 26-19   Total Cholesterol Levels

CHOLESTEROL LEVELS	RANGES FOR MOST ADULTS
Optimal cholesterol level—**GOOD**	200 mg/dL or lower
Borderline high cholesterol	200–239 mg/dL
High cholesterol—**AT RISK**	240 mg/dL or higher

Table 26-20   High-Density Lipid (HDL) Levels (Good Cholesterol)

	RANGES FOR MOST ADULTS
High HDL/low HDL—**GOOD**	60 mg/dL or higher
Borderline low HDL	40–59 mg/dL
Low HDL—**AT RISK**	Less than 40 mg/dL

Table 26-21   Low-Density Lipid (LDL) Levels (Bad Cholesterol)

	RANGES FOR MOST ADULTS
Optimal LDL—**GOOD**	Less than 100 mg/dL
Near or above optimal LDL	100–129 mg/dL
Borderline high LDL—**AT RISK**	130–159 mg/dL
High LDL—**AT RISK**	160 mg/dL or higher

Table 26-22   Triglycerides

	RANGES FOR MOST ADULTS
Normal triglycerides—**GOOD**	Less than 150 mg/dL
Borderline high triglycerides	150–199 mg/dL
High triglycerides	200–499 mg/dL
Very high triglycerides—**AT RISK**	500 mg/dL or higher

Antihyperlipidemics

Antihyperlipidemics are drugs that help prevent the progression of coronary artery disease by lowering plasma lipid levels (see Table 26-23). Some are also useful in treating diabetes insipidis and in prevention of stroke and MI. Patients with CAD and high cholesterol are most likely to benefit from treatment with long-term antihyperlipidemic drug therapy.

There are various steps in the synthesis of cholesterol. Therefore, drugs with various mechanisms of action are needed to lower or reverse cholesterol synthesis. The most frequently prescribed drugs, called *statins*, have been found to be highly effective in

Table 26-23   Antihyperlipidemics

GENERIC NAME	TRADE NAME	AVAILABLE DOSAGE FORM(S)/STRENGTH	AVERAGE ADULT DOSE
atorvastatin calcium	Lipitor®	10 mg, 20 mg, 40 mg, 80 mg tabs	10–80 mg once daily
atorvastatin + amlodipine	Caduet®	Antihyperlipidemic/HTN combination—various strengths	individualized dosing
cholestyramine	Questran®	Powder for suspension	4 gm daily or bid
colesevelam	WelChol®	625 mg tab	3 tabs bid or 6 tabs daily
colestipol	Colestid®	1 g tab / 5 g/dose granules	5–30 g daily or in divided doses
ezetimibe	Zetia®	10 mg	10 mg once daily
ezetimibe + simvastatin	Vytorin®	10 mg/10 mg, 10 mg/20 mg, 10 mg/40 mg, 10 mg/80 mg tabs	1 tab daily
fenofibrate	Tricor®	48 mg, 145 mg tabs	48–145 mg/day
fluvastatin sodium	Lescol®	20 mg, 40 mg tabs	20–80 mg/day
	Lescol® XL	80 mg XL tabs	80 mg once daily (XL)
gemfibrozil	Lopid®	600 mg tabs	600 mg 30 min before the morning and evening meal
lovastatin	Mevacor®	10 mg, 20 mg, 40 mg tabs	10–80 mg daily or in 2 divided doses
	Altoprev®	10 mg, 20 mg, 40 mg, 60 mg ER tabs	10–60 mg once daily (ER)
niacin		500 mg tabs	1–2 g bid–tid
		500 mg, 750 mg, 1,000 mg ER tabs	500–2,000 mg daily (ER)
pravastatin sodium	Pravachol®	10 mg, 20 mg, 40 mg, 80 mg tabs	initial dose: 40 mg/day, may increase to 80 mg/day
rosuvastatin calcium	Crestor®	5 mg, 10 mg, 20 mg, 40 mg tabs	5–40 mg once daily
simvastatin	Zocor®	5 mg, 10 mg, 20 mg, 40 mg, 80 mg tabs	55–80 mg/day once a day or in divided doses

lowering LDL cholesterol. The statins are a group of drugs that suppress cholesterol synthesis by inhibiting the enzyme HMG CoA reductase.

Statins decrease the synthesis of cholesterol by the liver, which has two important effects: (1) the up-regulation of LDL receptors by hepatocytes and consequent increased removal of certain lipoproteins from blood circulation; and (2) a reduction in the synthesis and secretion of lipoproteins by the liver. The net effect of statin therapy is to lower plasma concentrations of cholesterol-carrying lipoproteins, the most prominent of which is LDL.

Statins also increase the removal of and reduce the secretion of remnant particles, specifically VLDL and IDL. For patients with elevated LDLs and triglycerides, a statin is one of the therapies of choice, because of its ability to effectively lower LDL and non-high-density lipoprotein cholesterol (non-HDL-C) levels.

A newer antihyperlipidemic drug, ezetimibe, also enables patients to reach their lipid goals, but works in the digestive tract rather than the liver. However, it does not affect fat absorption. Ezetimibe selectively inhibits cholesterol absorption by intestinal microvilli and villi. This prevents cholesterol from entering the blood system, which in turn decreases hepatic storage of cholesterol, and increases clearance from the blood. The cholesterol moves right through the intestinal tract, leaving the body essentially unchanged, and without affecting bowel function or the absorption of fat-soluble vitamins. This distinct mechanism is complementary to that of HMG-CoA reductase inhibitors.

Another alternative is vitamin B3 (niacin), which works indirectly to reduce total cholesterol by reducing the production of building blocks for LDL and increasing production of HDL.

The Lymphatic System

The lymphatic system is a complex system of lymph organs, nodes, ducts, tissues, vessels, and capillaries that transport lymph fluid to the circulatory system. The cardiovascular and lymphatic systems work in tandem and are joined by a capillary system through which lymph and blood move (see Figure 26-4). Blood circulates in the

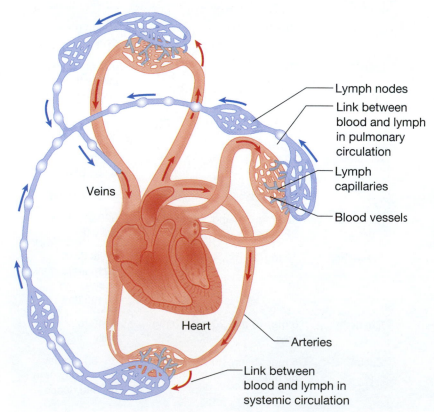

FIGURE 26-4 The lymphatic system and the circulatory system.

closed, revolving circulatory system; in constrast, lymph fluid moves in one direction to eliminate waste such as bacteria, old blood cells, debris, and cancer cells.

Some medical experts consider the lymphatic system to be part of the blood circulatory system, because lymph fluid comes from blood and returns to blood and because the lymphatic ducts are very similar to the blood vessels. Others consider it the main component of the immune system. Throughout the body, wherever blood vessels are located there are also lymph vessels, and the two systems work together.

Lymph fluid is not pumped as the heart pumps blood. The lymphatic system uses the contraction of skeletal muscles to move the fluid through the lymph vessels. Bone marrow produces certain cells called **lymphocytes**, **monocytes**, and leukocytes. *Lymph nodes* are areas where lymphocytes concentrate along the lymphatic veins. The lymphatic system supports the immune system by:

- filtering out organisms that cause disease
- producing specific white blood cells
- manufacturing antibodies
- distributing fluids and nutrients throughout the body
- draining excess fluids and protein so that tissues do not swell or become inflamed

lymphocyte type of white blood cell.

monocyte type of white blood cell.

SUMMARY

The cardiovascular system, often referred to as the circulatory system, is responsible for transporting blood to all parts of the body. It consists of the heart, arteries, arterioles, veins, venules, and capillaries. The arteries are responsible for carrying oxygen-rich blood to the cells; the veins carry deoxygenated blood back to the heart and lungs. The lungs and respiratory system work in tandem with the cardiovascular system to sustain life.

To accomplish its primary purpose of pumping blood to all parts of the body, the heart relies on a conduction system comprised of nodes and nodal tissues that regulate the various aspects of the heartbeat. In addition, the nervous system plays a vital role in regulating heart rate.

The two most common diseases affecting the cardiovascular system are congestive heart failure and coronary artery disease. CHF occurs when the heart pumps out less blood than it receives, resulting in a weakened and enlarged heart, and in less blood being pumped out to feed the body. Complications of CHF include ischemia, myocardial infarction, and cardiac arrhythmias. CHF is responsible for 40,000 deaths each year, as well as for 2.9 million doctor visits and 875,000 hospitalizations.

CAD is characterized by insufficient blood flow to the heart. CAD is the result of atherosclerosis or arteriosclerosis; however, many factors can contribute to CAD, including diet, stress, smoking, normal aging, and genetics. As a pharmacy technician, you need to be aware of lifestyle factors that can lead to the development of CAD.

Hypertension and hyperlipidemia are two additional conditions that affect the cardiovascular system. Hypertension is high blood pressure, for which many pharmaceutical treatments exist, including diuretics, vasodilators, ACE inhibitors, beta blockers, and calcium channel blockers. Hyperlipidemia is high blood cholesterol. Both hypertension and hyperlipidemia often go undetected, as these conditions do not have substantial symptoms.

The lymphatic system and circulatory system work closely together, as blood and lymph fluid move through the same capillary system. Lymph fluid removes wastes and debris from the body and supports the immune system by filtering out pathogens and draining excess fluid from the body.

This chapter contains a thorough discussion of the available treatments for diseases of the cardiovascular system. Keep in mind that although great strides have been made in the ability to treat CHF and CAD, cardiovascular disease remains the leading cause of death in the United States.

CHAPTER REVIEW QUESTIONS

1. Approximately how many gallons of blood are estimated to be pumped by the heart each day?
   a. 4,300
   b. 3,300
   c. 2,300
   d. 1,300

2. The average adult body contains how much blood?
   a. 7.6 L
   b. 6 L
   c. 5.6 L
   d. 5 L

3. Which of the following cholesterol ranges would make the patient "at risk" for hyperlipidemia?
   a. LDL level less than 100 mg/dL
   b. tryglyceride level of less than 150 mg/dL
   c. total cholesterol level of 220 mg/dL
   d. HDL level less than 40 mg/dL

4. Which of the following is considered the "bad" cholesterol?
   a. VLDL
   b. HDL
   c. LDL
   d. both a and c

5. Which of the following drugs is an ACE inhibitor?
   a. captopril
   b. enalapril
   c. ramipril
   d. all of the above

6. Which of the following beta blockers is also used to treat migraine headaches?
   a. timolol
   b. labetalol
   c. esmolol
   d. propranolol

7. _____ is the blood's ability to clot.
   a. Thrombocytopenia
   b. Hematuria
   c. Coagulation
   d. Plasminogen

8. Drugs in the following category are very expensive and are not mixed or prepared until the patient is ready for administration of the drug.
   a. anticoagulants
   b. antiplatelet agents
   c. diuretics
   d. tissue plasminogen activators

9. Which of the following is used as an antidote for heparin overdose?
   a. warfarin
   b. aminocaproic acid
   c. protamine sulfate
   d. tranexamic acid

10. Which of the following drugs is not an antihyper-lipidemic drug?
    a. atorvastatin
    b. lovastatin
    c. colestipol
    d. verapamil

11. Which of the following is a Class II antiarrhythmic agent?
    a. disopyramide
    b. bretyllium
    c. propranolol
    d. diltiazem

12. Antiplatelet agents:
    a. stop the coagulation of blood.
    b. dissolve blood clots.
    c. reduce and prevent platelet aggregation.
    d. both a and c.

13. Which of the following blood pressure readings (in mm Hg) would be indicative of Stage I hypertension?
    a. 160/110
    b. 120/80
    c. 145/95
    d. 110/85

14. Beta-1 receptors are found on the:
    a. heart.
    b. lungs.
    c. liver.
    d. brain.

15. Vasodilators are drugs that are used to:
    a. constrict blood vessels.
    b. relax blood vessels.
    c. treat CHF.
    d. b and c.

CRITICAL THINKING QUESTIONS

1. Diagram the flow of the blood through the body.

2. Explain the process of blood oxygenation and carbon dioxide exchange.

3. Why might a doctor prescribe a diuretic along with an antihypertensive drug for a patient with hypertension?

WEB CHALLENGE

1. To view an animation of how the heart works, go to http://www.smm.org/heart/

2. Find out if your diet is "hurting your heart." Take a cholesterol quiz at http://www.mayoclinic.com/health/cholesterol/QZ00046

3. Find out how much you know about heart disease. Go to http://www.webmd.com/content/tools/1/quiz_heart_disease and take the heart disease quiz.

REFERENCES AND RESOURCES

Adams, MP, Josephson, DL, & and Holland, LN Jr. *Pharmacology for Nurses—A Pathophysiologic Approach.* Upper Saddle River, NJ: Pearson Education, 2008.

"Arteriosclerosis/Atherosclerosis" (accessed July 10, 2007): http://www.mayoclinic.com/health/arteriosclerosis-atherosclerosis/DS00525

"Atherosclerosis" (accessed July 10, 2007): http://www.americanheart.org/presenter.jhtml?identifier=4440

"The cardiac cycle" (accessed April 8, 2008): http://www.jdaross.cwc.net/cardiac_cycle.htm

"Cholesterol" (accessed October 15, 2007): http://www.americanheart.org

"Endocardium and periocardium" (accessed April 8, 2008): http://www.medterms.com/script/main/art.asp?articlekey=3236

"Geriatic Drug Review: Nitrobid" (accessed April 6, 2008): http://agenet.agenet.com/?Url=link.asp?DOC/1339

"The Heart" (accessed April 8, 2008): http://www.leeds.ac.uk/chb/HUMB2040/prac3thor.pdf

Holland, N, & Adams, MP. *Core Concepts in Pharmacology.* Upper Saddle River, NJ: Pearson Education, 2007.

"Hypertension: Symptoms of High Blood Pressure" (accessed July 9, 2007): www.webmd.com

"Lymphatic System" (accessed April 8, 2008): http://www.innerbody.com/image/lympov.html

Maybaum, S. *Medical Treatments for Congestive Heart.* Columbia, NY: New York Presbyterian Hospital and Ainat Beniaminovitz.

"Myofilaments, Sarcoplasmic Reticulum (SR)" (accessed April 1, 2008): www.biology.eku.edu/RITCHISO/301notes3.htm

"Spleen Disorders" (accessed April 1, 2008): http://www.merck.com/mrkshared/mmanual_home2/sec14/ch179/ch179a.jsp

"Thrombophlebitis" (accessed April 8, 2008): http://www.nlm.nih.gov/medlineplus/thrombophlebitis.html

"What is Coronary Artery Disease?" (accessed July 9, 2007): http://www.nhlbi.nih.gov/health/dci/Diseases/Cad/CAD_WhatIs.html

LEARNING OBJECTIVES

After completing this chapter, you should be able to:

- Explain how the body's nonspecific and specific defense mechanisms work to keep the body safe from disease-causing microorganisms.
- Understand the basic relationships between the immune system and the various body systems.
- List and describe the different types of infectious organisms.
- Compare and contrast HIV-1 and HIV-2 and identify the various subgroups of HIV.
- List the five stages of progression of HIV to AIDS.
- Explain how the different classes of HIV drugs work.
- Describe autoimmune disease and identify various types.
- Understand how drug resistance develops and what steps can be taken to stop it.
- List and define common anti-infective drug classifications, their mechanisms of action, and their side effects.
- Describe both tuberculosis and malaria and their causes, treatments, and prevention.
- Identify the different types and uses of vaccines and how they work in the body.

Introduction

The immune system protects the body from foreign invaders that would otherwise destroy it, or parts of it, via infection or cancer. The immune system uses numerous kinds of responses to fend off attacks from these foreign invaders, and is amazingly effective most of the time. Its defensive barriers and mechanisms include the skin, mucus and cilia in the linings of the respiratory and digestive passageways, the blood clotting process, white blood cells and other infection-fighting substances, the thymus gland, and the lymph nodes.

Many different classes of medications affect the immune system. These include drugs for the treatment of HIV/AIDS, tuberculosis, and malaria, as well as for many other immune-related conditions and diseases. It is important for pharmacy technicians to have a clear understanding of what these drugs are and how they work to protect the body.

The Body's Defense Mechanisms

A human body protects itself with nonspecific defense mechanisms, which are considered the first line of defense against disease and infection. Specific defense mechanisms are the body's second line of defense. When these mechanisms fail or are destroyed, and leave a person susceptible to infection, the person is said to be *immunosuppressed* or *immunocompromised*.

Nonspecific Defense Mechanisms

Nonspecific defense mechanisms include physical barriers, natural deterrents (fluids or chemicals and immune cells that prevent or attack invaders), and the inflammatory process. These mechanisms effectively reduce the workload of the immune system by preventing the entry and spread of microorganisms in the body. The body's physical and anatomical barriers against disease and infection include:

- Mucus in the respiratory tract—traps particles and microbes before they can infect the lungs.
- Vertebral column, spinal cord fluid, and the meninges—protect the central nervous system from injury or infection.
- Skin—protects the inside of the body from attack with its hard, dry, dead-skin-cell layer and it salty and somewhat acidic pH. These qualities of skin work together to prevent microorganisms from reproducing and growing.

Natural physiological deterrents to pathogens include:

- Acidic secretions of the vagina—create an environment that prevents the growth of many pathogens.
- Tears—continually flush irritants and microorganisms out of the eyes.
- Lysozyme—an enzyme that breaks down bacterial cell walls and aids in the prevention of microorganism growth. Lysozyme is present in tears, saliva, mucus, blood, sweat, and many other tissue fluids.
- Nonspecific immune system cells, such as **phagocytes** and **macrophages**—can detect, target, track, engulf, and kill invading microorganisms, host cells, and debris.

phagocyte specialized cell that engulfs and ingests other cells.

Blood components act as defense mechanisms in the following ways:

- Clotting factors found in blood cause clotting at the site of injury (scabbing), which can prevent pathogens from entering or invading. This is a type of "perimeter" effect.
- Proteins aid in inflammation and release of phagocytes. Proteins bind to the surface of bacterial or viral host cells and destroy (*lyse*) them. Inflammation can aid in prevention or recognition of invasion; however, uncontrolled inflammation may lead to more tissue damage and even death.

macrophage white blood cell, found primarily in connective tissue and the bloodstream.

The *normal flora* consists of a group of microorganisms that occur naturally in the mouth, skin, and gastrointestinal (GI) tract. These flora do not usually cause disease unless they move outside of their natural environment. Instead, they prevent infection by exogenous microorganisms by competing with them so that the foreign pathogens cannot penetrate, invade, or grow in the human host tissues.

Suppression of the natural endogenous microorganisms of the normal flora ("good" microorganisms) allows opportunistic exogenous ("bad") microorganisms to infect and cause disease. The natural flora may become suppressed during antibiotic treatment, in some females, or in some cancer patients during chemotherapy.

Specific Defense Mechanisms

When the nonspecific mechanisms of defense fail, the body initiates a second, specific, line of defense: the immune system (see Table 27-1). The immune system can create specialized protein molecules and cells that function to fight foreign invaders. Two types of these specialized protein molecules are called *antibodies* and *complement*. In

Table 27-1 Relationships between Body Systems and the Immune System

SYSTEM	THE SYSTEM'S ROLE IN AND EFFECT ON THE IMMUNE SYSTEM	THE IMMUNE SYSTEM'S EFFECTS ON AND ROLE IN THE SYSTEM
Integumentary	1. Provides a physical barrier to microorganisms. 2. Utilizes inflammation as a caution signal. 3. Aids in reduction and prevention of further inflammation.	Provides antibodies found in skin (IgA, IgG, etc.) to assist in immune function of protection.
Digestive	1. Provides important nutrients to the lymph tissues. 2. Digestive acids/enzymes destroy microorganisms.	1. The tonsils destroy infective bacteria and viruses of the mouth and throat. 2. Lymph vessels carry absorbed lipids to the bloodstream.
Musculoskeletal	1. Muscles protect and cushion lymph nodes and vessels. 2. Muscles contract to help push lymphatic fluid through vessels, into the circulatory system, and to elimination. 3. Lymphocytes and other immune cells are produced and stored in bone marrow.	1. Assists in repair after injuries. 2. Assists in repair of bone. 3. Macrophages (phagocytes) fuse to make bone cells.
Respiratory	1. Lung cells present antigens to trigger the immune defense response. 2. Provides essential oxygen and eliminates carbon dioxide, both necessary for optimum immune cell function.	1. Tonsils, which are lymphoid tissue, protect against infection at the entrance to the respiratory tract. 2. Lungs remove inhaled and deposited solid material and microorganisms. 3. Plays a supportive role in maintaining and eliminating fluids.
Circulatory	1. Distributes white blood cells and antibodies. 2. Clotting factors in blood make thrombi to assist as barriers to microorganisms.	1. Fights circulatory and blood vessel infections. 2. Returns interstitial tissue fluid to circulation via veins.

Table 27-1   Relationships between Body Systems and the
Immune System (*continued*)

SYSTEM	THE SYSTEM'S ROLE IN AND EFFECT ON THE IMMUNE SYSTEM	THE IMMUNE SYSTEM'S EFFECTS ON AND ROLE IN THE SYSTEM
Renal	1. Eliminates waste produced by immune cells as a by-product of reproduction, phagocytosis, and attack. 2. Acid pH of urine kills microorganisms.	Fights bladder and kidney infections.
Endocrine	1. Adrenal gland corticosteroid hormones have an anti-inflammatory effect. 2. Thymus hormone, *thymosin*, stimulates the development and maturation of lymphocytes.	Thymus gland secretes thymosin.
Reproductive	1. Certain enzymes (*lysozymes*) and chemicals in vaginal and other body secretions kill bacterial microorganisms. 2. Reproductive hormones have been shown to regulate the immune system. Estrogen has been shown to regulate the expression, distribution, and activity of immune chemicals called *cytokines*.	1. Produces antibodies to assist in immune system function. 2. Through cytokine- and interleukin-mediated pathways, regulates the reproductive system by inducing the release of gonadotropins (luteinizing hormone and follicle-stimulating hormone).
Nervous	Neurons have antigens that stimulate specific immune defense responses—the second line of defense.	Produces *cytokines*, immune hormones that affect the production of other hormones by the hypothalamus.

simple terms, antibodies mark an invading substance as a target; complement destroys the invader.

Antibodies, sometimes called *immunoglobulins*, have a concave area on the surface called a *combining site*. The **epitopes** of antigens fit perfectly into the combining sites of antibodies. When the two combine with or bind to each other, the antigen is inactivated and unable to harm the body. This process makes a toxin nonpoisonous or makes harmful substances stick together (*agglutinate*). Macrophages or phagocytes then consume the disabled foreign invaders. The ability of antibodies to disable or inactivate foreign invaders is called *humoral immunity*.

Complement is a group of normally inactive enzymes that is activated by the antibodies and **antigen** attachment. The antibody-antigen binding changes the shape of the antigen, exposing two complement binding sites. This activates two different complement enzymes, each of which binds to one of the sites. Thus, the antibody "holds" the antigen and makes it vulnerable while the complement enzymes bind to it. The function of complement is to kill invading cells by "drilling" a hole in the cell

antibodies proteins that specifically seek and bind to the surface of pathogens or antigens.

epitope a region on the surface of an antigen that is capable of producing an immune response.

complement a large group of proteins that are activated in sequence when cells are exposed to a foreign substance; activation eventually results in the death or destruction of the substance. In general, complements amplify or enhance the effects of antibodies and inflammation.

antigens specific molecules that trigger an immune response.

membrane wall, which allows body fluid to fill the inside of the invading cell and burst it open. There are about 30 different complement enzymes in the plasma.

pathogen a disease-causing organism.

The specific immune response empowers the body to seek and target specific **pathogens** and the body's own infected cells for destruction. It depends on specialized white blood cells called *lymphocytes*, which include *T-cells* (produced from lymphocytes that matured in the thymus gland) and *B-cells* (produced from lymphocytes that matured in the bone marrow). There are two complementary parts of the specific immune response: the cell-mediated response and the antibody-mediated response.

The *cell-mediated response* involves T-cells and is responsible for:

- destroying body cells that are infected with a virus.
- destroying cancerous cells (mutated cells that grow rapidly).
- activating other immune cells to be more efficient pathogen killers.

The *antibody-mediated response* involves both T-cells and B-cells and is necessary for the destruction of invading pathogens and for the elimination of toxins. After a macrophage engulfs a pathogen, both the cell-mediated and antibody-mediated responses commence. Macrophages digest the pathogen, then exhibit antigens from the pathogen on their surfaces. By this "flagging" or targeting of pathogenic proteins, the macrophages stimulate specific helper T-cells to release signal molecules called *lymphokines*. The lymphokines, in turn, stimulate both the cell-mediated and antibody-mediated responses.

In the cell-mediated response, the lymphokines released from the helper T-cells stimulate killer T-cells and phagocytic cells to help to destroy the pathogen-infected cells. These natural killer T-cells attach themselves to the pathogen-infected cells and destroy them; phagocytic cells produce toxin molecules that directly kill the pathogen.

hematopoietic blood-forming.

In the antibody-mediated response, the lymphokines activate specific B-cells to produce antibodies that act like a "flag" or signal to the phagocytic cells. Other B-cells go on to become *memory B-cells*, which respond by quickly producing more antibodies upon future infection by the same pathogen—even if the reinfection is years later. The memory of healthy B-cells lasts for the person's lifetime. The memory B-cell response is very quick, so the pathogen does not have time to reproduce enough to cause disease before the host's body destroys it. The effectiveness of vaccination is explained by the mechanism of the memory response, which prevents many diseases even at the first encounter.

Lymphocytes

Immune system cells are "on the lookout" for invading cells and other foreign substances that may have entered the body. *Lymphocytes* circulate within the body fluids, especially the blood and lymph, and may reside in the lymph nodes, lymphatic tissue, thymus gland, spleen, or liver. Lymphocytes are made in the bone marrow from primitive cells called **hematopoietic** stem cells. Lymphocytes may be either B-cells or T-cells.

B-cells are produced and mature in the bone marrow. After entering the bloodstream, they are carried to the lymph nodes (see Figure 27-1), where they multiply and divide. If the B-cell attaches to an antigen that fits into its receptor site, it becomes an activated B-cell. These activated B-cells transform into either *plasma cells* or *memory B-cells*. Plasma cells immediately make and secrete hundreds of thousands of antibodies into the blood to attack the antigen,

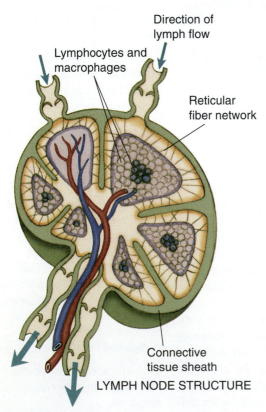

Direction of lymph flow

Lymphocytes and macrophages

Reticular fiber network

Connective tissue sheath

LYMPH NODE STRUCTURE

FIGURE 27-1 Lymph node.

but they have a short life span. The B cells that are not converted to plasma cells transform into memory cells. These memory cells, which "remember" that particular invader, have a much longer life span; therefore, they quickly secrete the appropriate antibodies when the body comes into subsequent contact with the same antigen.

T-cells are first produced by stem cells in the liver, just before and after birth. The T-cells are then carried to the thymus gland, where they undergo the first stage of development; hence the name *T-cell*. A T-cell undergoes a second change when it moves to the lymph node where it will reside. There it develops a binding site, shaped for a specific protein, that will attach to a specific kind of antigen. This binding sensitizes the T-cell and allows it to produce cell-mediated immunity, or resistance to disease organisms.

Some T-cells release a toxin, called *lymphotoxin,* that kills foreign invading cells. Although there are many lymphotoxins, two of the primary ones are *chemotactic factor* and *macrophage activating factor*. Chemotactic factor brings macrophages to invading substances, whereas macrophage activating factor tells the macrophages to destroy the cells by phagocytosis (eating/engulfing them).

INFORMATION

All cells have at least three common structures:

- **Cell membrane**—a selectively permeable phospholipid membrane that allows some material to pass into or out of the cell while preventing other material from doing so.
- **Cytoplasm**—a fluid where cell respiration takes place; usually contains **RNA** (a nucleic acid that enables protein synthesis).
- **DNA**—the genetic code of an organism, floating freely in the cytoplasm of some cells or isolated inside the nucleus of other cells.

RNA ribonucleic acid; a nucleic acid needed for the metabolic processes of protein synthesis. In viruses, RNA may carry the genetic information of the virus.

DNA deoxyribonucleic acid; a nucleic acid that carries genetic information and is capable of self-replication and synthesis of RNA.

Types of Infectious Organisms

Any animal or plant microorganism that causes a disease is called a *pathogen*. Animal pathogens are parasites, bacteria, rickettsia, or viruses. Plant pathogens are fungi or yeasts.

Animal Microorganisms

The differences in pathogens can be observed under a microscope. They vary in shape, size, motility, and other characteristics.

Parasites

Parasites may be bacterial, protozoal, or helminthes. The most common in the United States are pinworms, roundworms, and tapeworms. Transmission usually occurs via ingestion of contaminated food or soil. Some types are large enough to see with the naked eye. Infecting worms can perforate the intestines by burrowing. They can also do this to the muscles, lungs, and liver.

Parasites can damage or block organs by clumping together in balls. These balls are often mistaken for cancer tumors as they travel into the brain, heart, or lungs. These worms rob the host of the crucial vitamins, minerals, and amino acids needed for human digestion and nutrition, leaving some people anemic or drowsy after meals. Some worms give off metabolic waste products that are poisonous to their human hosts (*verminous intoxification*). The toxins are not easily eliminated, and usually are reabsorbed through the intestines. Because it must work harder to counteract these toxins, the immune system becomes overtaxed and suppressed, which leads to further fatigue and leaves the host vulnerable to other illnesses. Symptoms of parasitic infestation are diarrhea, loss of appetite, intense anal itching (worms lay eggs there), and abdominal cramping.

Protozoa

Protozoa are single-celled eukaryotes that play a vital role in controlling the numbers of bacteria. (Note, though, that bacteria are necessary for maintaining soil, plant, and animal and human life.) An example is the protozoan that lives in the mosquito and is transmitted via a mosquito bite, causing malaria. There are four types of protozoa, distinguished by their methods of obtaining food:

- *Ameboids* are protozoa that most often consume algae, bacteria, or other protozoans.
- *Ciliates* have a specialized opening in the outer edge to capture their prey.
- *Zooflagellates* exist in symbiotic relationships, meaning that their co-existence in another living creature has mutual benefits.
- *Sporozoans* are parasites that live inside a host and often cause disease by robbing the host of vital nutrients.

Bacteria

aerobic requires oxygen for life.

anaerobic does not require oxygen for life.

Most bacteria are round (*coccus/cocci*), rod-shaped (*bacillus/bacilli*), or spiral-shaped. These organisms can be **aerobic** or **anaerobic**. Bacteria are unicellular, prokaryotic microorganisms that multiply by dividing or splitting into two parts, in a process called *binary fission. Bacteria* is plural and *bacterium* is singular.

A *coccus* bacterium is spherical, oval, elongated, or flattened on one side, and has an approximate measurement of about 0.5 μm in diameter. After cell replication, division in one plane produces the following:

- *Coccus*—one bacterium.
- *Diplococcus*—two bacteria connected side by side.
- *Streptococcus*—several bacteria aligned in a row or a chain (which may be straight or curved).

Division in two planes produces a *tetrad* arrangement of four bacteria in a square. Division in three planes produces a *sarcina* arrangement, an "eight-pack" cube. Division in random planes produces a *staphylococcus* arrangement, which looks like a bunch of grapes (see Figure 27-2). Examples of the latter are *Staphylococcus aureus*, which causes skin, respiratory, and wound infections; and *Clostridium tetani,* which produces a toxin that can be lethal to humans.

A *bacillus*, or rod-shaped, bacterium has an approximate measurement of 0.5–1 μm in width and from 1–4 μm in length. Bacillus bacteria are found in three possible arrangements:

- *Bacillus*—a single bacterium.
- *Streptobacillus*—a chain or a string of bacilli.
- *Coccobacillus*—an oval bacillus similar to oval cocci.

Spiral or wave-shaped bacteria appear in one of the following arrangements:

- *Vibrio*—comma-shaped or resembling part of a wave.
- *Spirillium*—a rigid spiral wave.
- *Spirochete*—thin and flexible spiral wave.

Rickettsia

Rickettsia is the genus of several parasitic microorganisms, made up of small rod-shaped coccoids, that live in the gut of arthropods such as lice, fleas, ticks, and mites. These bacteria are transmitted to humans and other animals via a bite. The diseases they cause in humans have flu-like symptoms and include typhus, scrub typhus, Q fever, and Rocky Mountain spotted fever.

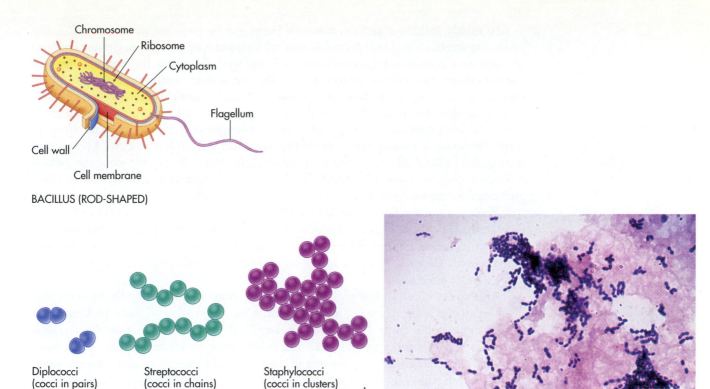

Chromosome
Ribosome
Cytoplasm
Flagellum
Cell wall
Cell membrane

BACILLUS (ROD-SHAPED)

Diplococci
(cocci in pairs)
Di = two

Streptococci
(cocci in chains)
Strept(o) = chain

Staphylococci
(cocci in clusters)
Staphyl(o) = Bunch

COCCI (SPHERICAL)

FIGURE 27-2 Examples of different types of bacteria.

Viruses

A *virus* is an ultramicroscopic infectious pathogen that can replicate only within cells of a living host, by using the DNA and RNA of the host. Viruses consist of nucleic acid covered by protein, although some animal viruses are surrounded by a membrane. Viruses are both nonliving pathogens and intracellular parasites. Very tiny and surrounded by a capsid or protein coating, a basic virus contains only a few genes (DNA and RNA), with which it replicates itself by commandeering the "machinery" inside the host cell. Although most viruses are host-specific, some can cross, or "jump," species. It is thought that HIV, the retrovirus that causes AIDS, jumped species from monkeys to humans. Figure 27-3 shows an illustration of a virus.

There are more than 200 types of viruses that can cause the common cold. Although these parasites only live about three to ten days in a healthy human, in an immunosuppressed patient they can live longer, causing further damage to the body and immune system. Some viruses are damaging or fatal from the start. Viruses are difficult to cure because they mutate constantly and develop different strains that require different drugs for treatment. In addition, because the virus lives inside host cells, attacking the virus usually means attacking the host's own cells. This leads to suppression of (and sometimes damage to) whatever system is affected.

Plant Microorganisms

Fungus is a plant-like, filamentous, or single-celled eukaryotic organism characterized by a lack of chlorophyll, heterotrophic growth, and the production of extracellular enzymes. Fungi include

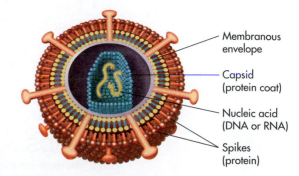

Membranous envelope

Capsid (protein coat)

Nucleic acid (DNA or RNA)

Spikes (protein)

FIGURE 27-3 An illustration of a virus.

yeasts, molds, mildews, and mushrooms. Fungi can be parasitic or saprobic. Canker sores, ringworm, some kinds of molds, and mildews are fungal diseases. Common examples are the *Candida* and *Aspergillus* fungi. Fungi feed themselves by secreting digestive enzymes that release organic molecules from the tree, soil, or organism (human) in which they are living. The fungus then absorbs those released organic molecules. Fungal infections flourish in moisture, heat, and darkness; tropical conditions allow fungi to grow easily. Athlete's foot is an example of growth of fungus in a moist, hot, dark environment: the sneaker. Fungal infections of the blood are the hardest to cure. Many drugs used to fight fungal and yeast infection end in *azole*. Examples are ketoconazole (which has many drug interactions), sulfamethoxazole, fluconazole, and itraconazole. Another antifungal is amphotericin B, which can have many side effects.

Yeast is a microscopic, dehydrated, hydrophilic single-celled organism of the fungus family, which eats sugar and produces alcohol and carbon dioxide as it grows and ferments. *Candida albicans* is a yeast-like fungus that causes vaginal yeast infections (*candidiasis*). *Candida glabrata* is a more resistant yeast that also causes thrush and vaginal yeast infections.

Antibiotics taken to kill pathogenic bacteria may also kill friendly bacteria that are part of the normal flora. These bacteria, such as lactobacilli, help to keep yeast in the vagina under control. Without lactobacilli, the balance of yeast in the vagina is disrupted and *Candida* can take over. Antibiotics have no effect on yeast itself; however, they can change the environment in the vagina just enough to cause a yeast overgrowth or infection (also known as *vaginal thrush*). If the body is weak after an illness such as influenza, or too busy fighting off another infection, the natural yeast in the body may not be adequately "policed," and may take the opportunity to multiply uncontrollably.

INFORMATION

Female diabetics with poor immune systems are prone to yeast infections, as diabetes increases sugar levels in both urine and vaginal secretions. Urine left on the genital area, tight or damp clothing, a change in the normally acidic vaginal environment, and some foods may contribute to vaginal yeast overgrowth. Some practitioners suggest avoiding sugar, dairy products, coffee, tea, and wine, all of which contribute to thrush by increasing urinary sugar content.

The following drugs are antifungals that work in similar ways to break down the cell wall of the *Candida* organism until it disintegrates. They are available as vaginal suppositories (inserts) and topical creams applied with an applicator once at night for three or seven consecutive nights. It takes at least seven days to cure a yeast infection, no matter which adminstration method is used. All of the applications in the specific package must be used.

- Femstat 3® (butoconazole nitrate)
- Gyne-Lotrimin® (clotrimazole)
- Monistat 7® (miconazole)
- Vagistat® (tioconazole)
- Diflucan® (fluconazole), one 150 mg tablet po × 1 dose (approved for yeast infections)

HIV/AIDS

HIV (human immunodeficiency virus) can be categorized as either HIV-1 or HIV-2. Unless specified otherwise, most references here are to HIV-1, the most common worldwide. Both types are transmitted by sexual contact; through blood, semen, and vaginal fluid; and from mother to child. Both types of HIV cause clinically indistinguishable AIDS (acquired immune deficiency syndrome). AIDS is the eventual outcome of HIV infection, as the body's immune system becomes severely suppressed and cannot fight opportunistic infections. People with AIDS often suffer lung, brain, skin, eye, and other organ diseases, along with diarrhea, debilitating weight loss, candidiasis and other fungal infections, toxoplasmosis, dementia, and Kaposi's sarcoma. The presence of HIV antibodies in the blood confirms that an individual has been infected. On March 19, 2004, the FDA approved the first oral fluid-based rapid HIV test kit (OraQuick®), which provides results in 20 minutes with more than 99 percent accuracy.

Five-Stage Progression of HIV to AIDS to Death

- Stage 1—initial transmission and infection with HIV
- Stage 2—infection without presentation of signs or symptoms (may last 10 or more years)
- Stage 3—signs and symptoms of HIV begin to appear
- Stage 4—AIDS opportunistic infections begin; CD4 cell count or level at or below 200 per cubic millimeter of blood
- Stage 5—final stage of wasting and infections; ends in death

HIV/AIDS Drugs

Reverse transcriptase inhibitors block the conversion of the HIV single-strand viral RNA to double-strand viral DNA, thus preventing the synthesis of copies of the viral RNA. There are two types of reverse transcriptase:

- *Nucleoside analogs,* often called "nukes," mimic the building blocks used by reverse transcriptase to make copies of the HIV genetic material. The fake building blocks interrupt or interfere with viral replication.
- *Nonnucleoside* reverse transcriptase inhibitors (NNRTIs) prevent the reverse transcriptase enzyme from working.

Once the new double-strand hybrid DNA is transcribed to a viral RNA, the RNA serves as a **genome** for new HIV viruses. *Protease inhibitors (Pis)* block the protease enzyme, which blocks translation. This means that the HIV makes copies of itself that cannot infect new cells. Studies have proven that PIs can reduce the amount of virus in the blood and increase CD4 cell counts.

Currently, the best way to avoid drug resistance is to stop or reduce production of HIV virus in the body. The less HIV there is in the body, the less chance there will be of creating a virus that is resistant to anti-HIV drugs. It is recommended that protease inhibitors be taken in combination with at least two other anti-HIV drugs (see Table 27-2). This treatment protocol is known as *highly active anti-retroviral therapy,* or *HAART.* The implementation of HAART increases the anti-HIV effect and prevents or overcomes resistance; this is sometimes referred to as *protease boosting.* Drug resistance tests are ordered to determine which combination of drugs to use. The following is an example of one such combination, or "cocktail," given to HIV/AIDS patients:

genome the complete hereditary material or code of an organism.

zidovudine + lamivudine + efavirenz
600 mg/day   300 mg/day   600 mg/day

Table 27-2 Antiretroviral Agents

ANTI-AIDS DRUG CLASSIFICATION	TRADE/GENERIC NAME	POSSIBLE SIDE EFFECTS
Vaccine	in research	—
Attachment inhibitors	in research	—
Fusion (fusion inhibitors)	Fuzeon® (enfuvirtide)	itching, swelling, redness, pain, tenderness, hardened skin and bumps near the injection sites, asthenia, insomnia, depression, myalgia, constipation, pancreas problems, numbness of feet and legs, dyspnea, fever, uremia, peripheral edema (feet)
Reverse Transcriptase Inhibitors		
Nucleoside reverse transcriptase	Combivir® (zidovudine + lamivudine) (AZT + 3TC) Emtriva® (emtricitabine) (FTC) Epivir® (lamivudine) (3TC) Epzicom® (abacavir + lamivudine) (ABC + 3TC) Hivid® (zalcitabine) (ddC) Retrovir® (zidovudine) (AZT or ZDV) Trizivir® (abacavir + zidovudine + lamivudine) (ABC + AZT + 3TC) Truvada® (tenofovir disoproxil fumarate + emtricitabine) (TDF + FTC) Videx® (didanosine, buffered versions); Videx® EC (didanosine, delayed-release capsules) Viread® (tenofovir disoproxil fumarate) (TDF or Bis(POC) PMPA) Zerit® (stavudine) (d4T) Ziagen® (abacavir) (ABC)	Headache Nausea Skin rash and skin discoloration on palms and soles Lactic acidosis Severe hepatomegaly with steatosis Possible redistribution of body fat, peripheral wasting, facial wasting, breast enlargement, and cushingoid appearance
Nonnucleoside reverse transcriptase (NNRTIs)	Viramune® (nevirapine) Rescriptor® (delavirdine mesylate) Sustiva® (efavirenz)	Headache Dizziness Fatigue Nausea, vomiting, diarrhea Rash (may be severe) Liver problems, which can be severe and life-threatening. Regular blood tests may be needed to monitor for liver problems. Insomnia Drowsiness (sedation)
Protease inhibitors	Agenerase® (amprenavir) Lexiva® (fosamprenavir) Crixivan® (indinavir) Kaletra® (lopinavir/ritonavir) Norvir® (ritonavir) Invirase® and Fortovase® (saquinavir) Viracept® (nelfinavir) Zrivada® (atazanavir)	Increased blood pressure Diabetes Lipodystrophy—inability to absorb fat Liver toxicity may worsen hepatitis

Autoimmune Diseases

A person with an autoimmune disease has an immune system that mistakenly targets and attacks the cells, tissues, and organs of its own body. The immune system cells and molecules accumulate at a target site, in a gathering broadly referred to as *inflammation*. Approximately 75 percent of autoimmune diseases affect women.

Some autoimmune diseases are prevalent in specific populations. For example, lupus is more common in Hispanic and African-American women than in Caucasian women of European ancestry. Rheumatoid arthritis and scleroderma affect more residents of some Native American communities than the general population of the United States.

Autoimmune diseases are not contagious and are not related to AIDS or cancer (see Table 27-3). Many are inherited; some are triggered by sunlight (lupus); others are caused by dormant viruses that are reactivated and mistakenly "protected" by the immune system, while the original antibody is attacked (such as in the case of rheumatoid arthritis). Most autoimmune diseases are not curable, but are treatable with appropriate drug therapy to manage daily living.

Table 27-3 Common Autoimmune Diseases

DISEASE	NOTES
Autoimmune Oophoritis and Orchitis	
Site of action: the gonads.	Endocrine System
Treatment includes: no known treatment or cure; hormone replacement therapy is used, but it cannot return fertility.	Patients with oopheritis may have premature menopause before 40 years of age, or the ovaries are destroyed before the first menstruation (no treatment available). Orchitis is an enlargement of the testis, in which infertility antisperm antibody can be detected.
Crohn's Disease	
Site of action: the gut or intestine.	Gastrointestinal System
Treatment includes: Remicade® (infliximab), a monoclonal antibody engineered as an inhibitor of tumor necrosis factor alpha, a protein that promotes inflammation in the body.	Inflammation of the bowel, both in the ileum (lower small intestine) and in the colon (large intestine), possibly caused by a reaction to a virus.
Entocort EC® (budesonide), which uses the high affinity of budesonide for glucocorticosteroid receptors; potent anti-inflammatory effect about 200 times that of cortisol and 15 times that of prednisolone.	
Graves' Disease	
Site of Action: the thyroid.	Endocrine System
Treatment includes: propylthiouracil iodine (radioactive).	Immune cells attack both the eye muscles and the thyroid, leading to dysfunction of both. This may cause hyperthyroidism and increased thyrotoxicosis that produces intolerance of heat, weight loss.
	May have exophthalmy, in which the eyes appear protruded or unusually popped out.
Lupus or Systemic Lupus Erythematosus	
Site of action: affects various tissues and organs; also varies among individuals with the same disease.	Multiple Organs, including the Musculoskeletal System

Table 27-3   Common Autoimmune Diseases (*continued*)

DISEASE	NOTES
Treatment includes: corticosteroids, NSAIDs, immunosuppressant COX-2 inhibitors.	Ultimate damage to specific tissues may be permanent. Example is destruction of insulin-producing cells of the pancreas, resulting in Type 1 diabetes mellitus. Immune cell complexes and inflammatory molecules can block blood flow and ultimately destroy organs such as the kidney. Lupus may be worsened or triggered by sunlight.
Multiple Sclerosis	
Site of action: the brain.	Nervous System
Treatment includes: glatiramer acetate, interferon beta 1-a, interferon beta 1-b.	Patients with MS produce antibodies that attack the white matter in the brain and spinal cord, causing the myelin sheath, or coating of nerve fibers, to become inflamed in the brain and spinal cord, which results in an inability to transmit signals along the nerves.
Myasthenia Gravis	
Site of action: the muscles.	Nervous System
Treatment includes: thymectomy (removal of thymus gland) to improve immune system function.	Autoantibodies attack a part of the nerve that stimulates muscle movement.
Plasmapheresis—abnormal antibodies are removed from the blood.	
High-dose intravenous immune globulin, which temporarily provides the body with normal antibodies from donated blood.	
Pernicious Anemia	
Site of action: the blood.	Circulatory System
Treatment includes: restorative vitamin B12 shots, folic acid.	Pernicious anemia is caused by the inability of the body to absorb vitamin B12 from the digestive tract into the bloodstream; the supply of this vital nutrient to organs and bone marrow is compromised, and eventually results in immune attack on organs such as the liver, spleen, kidneys, heart, and brain.
Psoriasis	
Site of action: the skin.	Integumentary System
Treatment includes: corticosteroids such as Dovonex® (calcipotriene).	Very small areas of skin or the entire body may be covered with a buildup of red and silvery scales called *plaques*; may be painful and unattractive.
Coal tars, Anthra-Derm® (anthralin).	
Topical receptor-selective retinoid—tazarotene (thought to normalize the proliferation of keratinocytes, as well as to decrease cutaneous inflammation).	Epidermal cell kinetics with abnormal activation of immune mechanisms are thought to be the major contributors.
Immunosuppressive dimeric fusion protein—Amevive® (alefacept) primarily blocks the activation of immune system T-cells.	

Table 27-3 Common Autoimmune Diseases (*continued*)

DISEASE	NOTES
Rheumatoid Arthritis	
Site of action: the joints and other tissues and organs. Treatment includes: DMARDs, which slow down the disease process by modifying the immune system in some way other than by inhibition of prostaglandin.	Multiple Organs, including the Musculoskeletal System In rheumatoid arthritis, reactive oxygen intermediate molecules and other toxic molecules are made by overproductive macrophages and neutrophils that invade the joints. The toxic molecules contribute to inflammation, which is observed as warmth and swelling, and participate in damaging the joint.
Scleroderma	
Site of action: the skin and blood vessels. Treatment includes: pallative only; no cure. Immunosupressants—cyclophosphamide. Nifedipine and calcium channel blockers. Antibiotics.	*Cytokines*, proteins that may cause surrounding immune system cells to become activated, grow, or die, may also influence nonimmune system tissues. Some cytokines may contribute to the thickening of the skin and blood vessels that is symptomatic of scleroderma. Systemic sclerosis (scleroderma) is characterized by fibrosis of the skin, vasculature (blood vessels), and internal organs.
Ulcerative Colitis	
Site of action: the large intestine. Treatment includes: anti-inflammatories—aka 5-ASA (mesalamine), Azulfidine® (sulfasalazine), Asacol® (sulfur-free), Pentasa®, Colazal® (balsalazide), Rowasa® enema, corticosteroids. Immunosuppressants—Imuran, 6-MP, cyclosporin. Immune modulators—Remicade® (infliximab).	Gastrointestinal System An irritable bowel disease; inflammation due to ulcers of a part of the large intestine, or the entire colon and rectum, possibly resulting from a weakened immune response to bacteria.
Vitiligo	
Site of action: the skin. Treatment includes: pallative, with cosmetics and self-tanning products.	Integumentary System The body makes antibodies to its own pigment cells or melanocytes, creating patches of lighter skin. Cycles of pigment loss, followed by remission during which the pigment does not change, may continue indefinitely.

Therapeutic agents that slow or suppress immune system response, in an attempt to stop the inflammation during an autoimmune attack, are called *immunosuppressive medications*. These drugs include corticosteroids, azathioprine, cyclosporin, cyclophosphamide, and methotrexate (MTX). Unfortunately, these medications also suppress the ability of the immune system to fight true infections, and they cause potentially serious adverse reactions. The common pharmacotherapeutic goal in the care of patients with autoimmune diseases is to discover treatments that produce remissions, with few side effects. New research for agents that have therapeutic antibodies against specific T-cell molecules may produce drugs with fewer long-term side effects than the chemotherapies currently being used.

Gram Staining

The *Gram stain* is a method of identifying and separating two main types of bacteria. This important technique is named after Hans Christian Gram, a Danish bacteriologist who devised the test in 1844. It is almost always the first test performed for the identification of bacteria in culture and sensitivity (C&S) laboratory tests. The main stain used in Gram staining is crystal violet, although methylene blue is sometimes substituted. The microorganisms that retain the crystal violet–iodine complex appear purple/brown or blue when examined under a microscope. The microorganisms that stain blue or purple are commonly classified as gram-positive (or gram-nonnegative). Other bacteria, not stained by crystal violet but appearing red, are referred to as gram-negative. The theory of Gram staining is based on the ability of the bacteria cell wall to retain the violet dye during a solvent treatment. The cell walls of gram-positive microorganisms have a higher peptidoglycan (a protein) and lower lipid content than gram-negative bacteria, and thus retain the dye.

Methods of Transmission of Pathogens

Pathogens are transmitted by three main routes: ingestion, inhalation, and physical contact. Sexually transmitted diseases are transmitted via physical contact. The most common form of transmission of pathogens is via unwashed hands. Microorganisms can survive on inanimate objects, such as desks, pencils, and doorknobs, for a very long time. Thus, handwashing is the number-one method for preventing the transmission of pathogens, and the most important way in which you can prevent pathogens from contaminating a drug being prepared.

Anti-Infectives

Anti-infective is an umbrella name under which various types of drugs are subclassified (see Table 27-4). Some anti-infectives treat bacteria only (antibacterials), whereas others treat viruses only (antivirals), or fungi only (antifungals). Other anti-infectives treat more than one type of pathogen. Another word for anti-infective is *antimicrobial* (against the growth of a microorganism or microbe).

Table 27-4   Comparison of Various Anti-Infectives

ANTI-INFECTIVE CLASSIFICATION	COMMON SIDE EFFECTS	TOXIC EFFECTS	DRUG, FOOD, AND HERB INTERACTIONS	SPECIAL NOTES AND CROSS-HYPERSENSITIVITY
Antibacterials	Rash GI disturbances Nausea/vomiting/diarrhea (N/V/D) Stomach pain Vaginal itching or discharge	Anaphylactic shock	1. Reduces effect of birth control pills. 2. Avoid taking with hot drinks; the heat from the drink may stop the medicine from working or make it work too fast. 3. Cross-hypersensitivity to a similar drug/classification.	1. Patient who has been taking an antibiotic (AB) must tell doctor or dentist before having surgery with a general anesthetic. 2. ABs may cause incorrect results with some urine sugar tests used by patients with diabetes.

Table 27-4 Comparison of Various Anti-Infectives (*continued*)

ANTI-INFECTIVE CLASSIFI-CATION	COMMON SIDE EFFECTS	TOXIC EFFECTS	DRUG, FOOD, AND HERB INTERACTIONS	SPECIAL NOTES AND CROSS-HYPERSENSITIVITY
Penicillins (PCNs)	Most common side effects, plus allergic reactions	Anaphylactic shock	1. Drugs that reduce the effect of PCNs: chloramphenicol, erythromycin ethyl-succinate (EES), sulfonamides, TCNs, methotrexate (MTX). These drugs also increase chances of side effects.	1. Take PCNs with a full glass of water on an empty stomach (either 1 hour before or 2 hours after meals). 2. May be taken with food or milk to avoid GI upset. PCNs are high in sodium content.
Cephalosporins	Most common side effects, plus joint aches and pain	Anaphylactic shock for PCN cross-hypersensitive patients. Severe or bloody diarrhea and/or black, tarry stools. Chest pain. Chills, cough, fever. Painful or difficult urination. Shortness of breath. Sore throat, sores, ulcers, or white spots on lips or in mouth	1. Drugs that increase chance of bleeding: anticoagulants, dipyridamole sulfin-pyrazone, ticarcillin, valproic acid, heparin, thrombolytic agents, furosemide. These drugs may increase blood levels of cefuroxime. 2. Avoid acidic fruit juices/drinks (e.g., grapefruit juice or orange juice) within 1 hour of taking this medication.	Hypersensitivity to PCN.
Tetracyclines (TCNs)	Most common side effects, plus may cause the teeth to become discolored and/or mottled.	Photosensitivity, which may cause a skin rash, itching, redness, or other discoloration of the skin, or a severe sunburn and thinning of skin, which could lead to skin cancer. Slows down the growth of bones, especially in children	1. Drugs that reduce TCN effects: antacids or calcium supplements, cholestyramine, medicines containing iron and magnesium 2. Antagonistic effect: PCNs decrease TCN effect.	1. Patient who is taking TCN must tell doctor or dentist before having surgery with a general anesthetic. 2. Do not give to children under 8 years of age.
Macrolides	Most common side effects, plus: Stomach upset or cramps. Sore mouth or tongue. Fever. Loss of appetite	Anaphylactic shock (rare)	1. PCN may decrease the effect of EES. 2. May increase blood levels of theophyllin, warfarin, digoxin, dilantin, and tegretol.	Abnormal liver tests or liver dysfunction can also occur with erythromycin.

Table 27-4 Comparison of Various Anti-Infectives (*continued*)

ANTI-INFECTIVE CLASSIFICATION	COMMON SIDE EFFECTS	TOXIC EFFECTS	DRUG, FOOD, AND HERB INTERACTIONS	SPECIAL NOTES AND CROSS-HYPERSENSITIVITY
Quinolones (fluoroquinolones)	Most common side effects, plus: Headache Restlessness	1. Status epilepticus and coma (rare) 2. Anaphylactic shock 3. Loss of consciousness 4. Photosensitivity	1. Do not take with food or drink that contains a lot of calcium, such as milk, yogurt, or cheese. 2. Caffeine or stimulant drugs will increase gamma-aminobutyric acid (GABA) inhibitory effect.	1. Take with a full glass of water on an empty stomach (either 1 hour before or 2 hours after meals). 2. If food must be eaten, avoid calcium. 3. Avoid antacids—take 4 hrs before or after when taking Cipro®; others 2 hrs before or after. 4. Also a GABA inhibitor: contraindicated for patients with preexisting neurological problems or seizures.
Sulfur-containing antibiotics (e.g., trimethoprim-sulfamethoxazole)	Most common side effects, plus: Tiredness Headache Dizziness	Depression Weakness Eye light sensitivity Yellowing of eyes/skin, dark urine Abdominal pain Ringing in the ears Gastrointestinal problems, damage to kidneys, and anemia (rare)	Some diuretics and anticoagulants	Anything containing sulfur: 1. Cross-hypersensitivity to furosemide, birth control pills, acetazolamide, thiazide diuretics, oral antidiabetics, antiglaucoma agents, phenazopyridine (e.g., Pyridium®). 2. Foods with preservatives or dyes.

Antibacterials

This section describes the various types of antibacterials.

Penicillins

Penicillins are divided into four groups of varying spectrum of activity: natural PCNs, penicillinase-resistant PCNs, amino PCNs, and extended-spectrum PCNs (see Tables 27-5 and 27-6). There are four "generations" of penicillins; each newer generation covers a broader spectrum of pathogens. Penicillins work by binding to the proteins in the cell wall of a pathogen, inhibiting them from making the cell wall or continuing to grow. However, the cytoplasm continues to grow, and eventually bursts out of the cell along with the nucleus, destroying the bacterial cell.

There are more allergies to penicillins than to any other drug classification. The usual reaction is a rash or GI disturbance. The worst case is a severe allergy that results in anaphylactic shock; epinephrine must be administered within 5–20 minutes, or the person may die. In an anaphylactic reaction, there is swelling in the airway passages, such as the mouth, tongue, throat, nose/nasal tissue, or in the respiratory bronchi,

Table 27-5   Types of Penicillins

GROUPS OF PENICILLINS	EXAMPLES	SPECTRUM	SPECIFIC INFECTIONS	IMPORTANT NOTES
Natural PCNs: First-generation PCNs	pen G benzathine (Bicillin® IM) pen G potassium IM, IV/IM, IV pen G sodium pen V potassium (Pen V K®, V-Cillin K®, Pen-Vee K®) po	gram + streptococci pneumococci	Ear, throat, gonorrhea, syphilis	The least effective, though still used
Penicillinase-resistant penicillins	cloxacillin (Tegopen®), po dicloxacillin (Dynapen®), po methocillin (Staphcillin®) IM, IV nafcillin (UniPen®, Nafcil®), IM, IV oxacillin (Prostaphlin®) po, IM, IV	Staph (resistant), *Staphylococcus aureus*	Endocarditis, abscesses, difficult-to-treat pneumonia	Effective against PCNase-producing organisms that are difficult to treat and do not respond to other-generation PCNs
Aminopenicillins: second-generation PCNs	ampicillin (Omnipen®), po, IM, IV amoxicillin (Amoxil®) po bacampicillin (Spectrobid®), po	gram + and gram − organisms: *E. coli, Proteus mirabilis, Haemophilus influenzae*	Ear, urinary, and respiratory tract infections	Amoxicillin is well absorbed and causes less or no GI disturbance or diarrhea. Second-generation PCNs are not effective against PCNase-producing organisms
Extended-Spectrum Penicillins				
Third-generation PCNs	carbenicillin (Geocillin®) ticarcillin (Ticar®)	Broader spectrum than second-generation PCNs, with gram + and − coverage: *Pseudomonas aeruginosa, Proteus vulgaris*	Difficult-to-treat respiratory and urinary tract infections	May require additional combination therapy with antibiotics such as aminoglycosides. Not resistant to PCNase
Fourth-generation PCNs	mezlocillin (Mezlin®) IM, IV piperacillin (Pipracil®) IM, IV	Broader than third-generation PCNS, with gram + and − coverage: *Klebsiella pneumoniae, Bacterioides fragilis* (anaerobe), *Pseudomonas aeruginosa, Proteus vulgaris*	Serious infections of skin, urinary tract, and respiratory tract	Made with monosodium salts; reduce sodium intake. Great for CHF, HTN, or diabetic patients. To date, require IV therapy. May require combination therapy

bronchioles, or air sacs. When this happens, oxygen supply is cut off and death may result if the patient is not treated appropriately and very quickly.

Cephalosporins are chemical cousins to penicillins. For this reason, any patient who has a known reaction to penicillin must be monitored if given a cephalosporin, as there is a 5 to 20 percent chance that this patient may also be allergic to these anti-infectives (*cross-sensitivity*). A better choice for the PCN-allergic patient is macrolides, such as erythromycin, tetracyclines, or quinalones.

The best antibacterial to use depends on the culprit pathogen. C&S tests are employed to identify the infecting bacterium, so that drug and pathogen can be matched. Carbapenems may be used on stronger bacteria, but only when PCN is not effective or safe, due to cross-sensitivity to penicillin and the potential for the adverse reactions of pseudomembranous colitis, heart failure, arrhythmias, and kidney or hepatic failure.

Certain enzymes produced by some bacteria provide resistance to specific antibi-otics. These enzymes are produced by both gram-positive and gram-negative bacteria, and are found on both chromosomes and plasmids. These enzymes counter the antibacterial activity of the drugs, so the bacteria survive while the drug is altered and rendered inactive; meanwhile, the patient's infection gets worse.

Scientists were challenged to make a drug that would be impervious to (not affected by) these beta-lactamase enzymes, which are also called *penicillinases*. A drug or agent that destroys or interferes with the action of penicillinase or beta-lactamase is known as a *beta-lactamase inhibitor*.

Beta-lactamases work by hydrolysis of the beta-lactam ring of the basic penicillin structure, which adds a molecule of water (H_2O) to the carbon-nitrogen bond and opens up the ring, thus making the penicillin drug ineffective. Most extended-spectrum beta-lactamase enzymes (ESBLs) remain susceptible to beta-lactamase inhibitors. Currently, there is no oral, broad-spectrum, penicillinase-resistant penicillin; therefore, in some cases combination therapy is required.

Table 27-6 shows some additional antibacterials that are related to penicillins.

Cephalosporins

Discovered in 1948, *cephalosporins* are grouped into four "generations" according to their antimicrobial properties (see Table 27-7). Each newer generation of cephalosporins has significantly greater gram-negative antimicrobial properties than the preceding (earlier) generation. Likewise, older generations have better gram-positive coverage than the newer generations. The first generation is the oldest. The frequency of dosing decreases with increasing generation(s), as does palatability. Cephalosporins are chem-ical cousins to penicillins, and, like PCNs, bind to the proteins in the cell wall of the pathogen, inhibiting them from making the cell wall or growing. The cell wall collapses after the cell contents burst out. The body's natural defenses also continue to fight infection.

Tetracyclines

Tetracyclines are used as systemic agents against acne, bacteria, protozoans, and as antirheumatic agents (see Table 27-8). Some unusual uses are as a diuretic, for the syndrome of inappropriate antidiuretic hormone; and as an intrapleural sclerosing agent. Use of TCNs by patients with diabetes, renal disease, or hepatic disease may make the condition worse. Use of this substance when it is outdated, warm, or changed in taste or appearance may cause *serious side effects*. TCN may be used to treat various systemic diseases, such as Lyme disease, malaria, shigellosis, and pneumothorax.

Tetracyclines are bacteriostatic and therefore slow down the growth and reproduc-tion of bacteria. TCNs enter the bacterial cell, utilizing energy, and bind to a subunit of the ribosome, which blocks protein synthesis of the cell membrane wall. The growth of

Table 27-6 Other Antibacterials Related to Penicillins

CLASSIFICATION	MOA	EXAMPLES	SPECTRUM AND SPECIFIC INDICATIONS	IMPORTANT NOTES
Beta-lactamase inhibitors: clavulanic acid, sulbactam, tazobactam	Block and inactivate the beta-lactamase enzyme, thereby not allowing the molecule to hydrolyze the basic PCN beta-lactam ring.	clavulanic acid + amoxicillin (Augmentin®) clavulanic acid + ticarcillin (Timentin®) sulbactam + ampicillin (Unasyn®) tazobactam + piperacillin (Zosyn®)	Otitis media and acute otitis media caused by PCNase- or beta-lactamase-producing bacteria: strains of *H. influenzae*, *Streptococcus pneumoniae*, *M. catarrhalis*, *Klebsiella pneumoniae*, *E. coli*, *Enterobacter* sp., *S. aureus*, etc.	Used for suspected resistance to PCNase Mainly active against rapidly dividing bacteria
Carbapenems	Similar to PCNs: Interfere with synthesis of cell wall by binding to penicillin protein binding targets.	meropenem (Merrem®) IV imipenem-cilastatin (Primaxin®) IM, IV ertapenem (Invanz®) IM, IV	Complicated intra-abdominal infections due to clostridum, *E. coli*, *Peptostreptococcus*, *Bacterioides fragilis* (anaerobe) Bacterial meningitis due to *S. pneumonaiae*, *N. meningitides*, *H. influenzae*	Structurally related to PCNs. Can be used against PCNase-resistant organisms
Monobactams	Similar to PCNs: Interfere with synthesis of cell wall by binding specifically to protein 3 (PBP 3).	aztreonam (Azactam®)	Skin, urinary, respiratory tract, gynecological, and intra-abdominal infections. Enterococcus and gram-bacteria	Structurally related to PCNs. Can be used against PCNase-resistant organisms. Unlabeled use for PCNase-resistant gonorrhea as an alternative to spectinomycin.

Table 27-7 Cephalosporins

DRUG	ROUTE AND ADULT DOSE
First Generation	
cefadroxil (Duricef®, Ultracef®)	PO; 500 mg–1 g qd–bid (max 2 g/day)
cefazolin sodium (Ancef®, Kefzol®)	IM; 250 mg–2 g tid (max 12 g/day)
cephalexin (Keflex®)	PO; 250–500 mg qid
Second Generation	
cefaclor (Ceclor®)	PO; 250–500 mg tid
cefamandole naftate	IM; 500 mg–1 g tid–qid (max 12 g/day)
cefonicid sodium (Monocid®)	IM; 1 g qd (max 2 g/day)
cefprozil (Cefzil®)	PO; 250–500 mg qd–bid
cefuroxime sodium (Ceftin®, Kefurox®, Zinacef®)	PO; 250–500 mg bid
Third/Fourth Generations	
cefdinir (Omnicef®)	PO; 300 mg bid
cefepime (Maximpime®)	IM; 0.5–1 g bid (max 3 g/day)
cefixime (Suprax®)	PO; 400 mg qd or 200 mg bid
cefotaxime sodium (Claforan®)	IM; 1–2 g bid–tid (max 12 g/day)
ceftriaxone sodium (Rocephin®)	IM; 1–2 g qd–bid (max 4 g/day)

Table 27-8   Tetracyclines

DRUG	ROUTE AND ADULT DOSE
tetracycline hydrochloride (Achromycin®, Panmycin®, Sumycin®)	PO; 250–500 mg bid–qid (max 2 g/day)
demeclocycline hydrochloride (Declomycin®)	PO; 150–300 mg bid–qid (max 2.4 g/day)
doxycycline hyclate (Doryx®, Doxy®, Monodox®, Vibramycin®)	PO; 100 mg on day 1, then 100 mg qd (max 200 mg/day)
minocycline hydrochloride (Dynacin®, Minocin®, Vectrin®)	PO; 200 mg as one dose, followed by 100 mg bid
oxytetracycline (Terramycin®)	PO; 250–500 mg bid–qid

the cell slows down and replication is hindered. The body's immune system then takes over to kill the bacteria.

Macrolides

The antibacterial agents known as macrolides are active against both aerobic and anaerobic gram-positive cocci, with the exception of enterococci (see Table 27-9). They are also active against some gram-negative anaerobes. Macrolides are mainly bacteriostatic. Erythromycin can be bacteriostatic at low doses and bactericidal at high doses; it works by inhibiting the protein synthesis that depends on RNA. Erythromycin has been used orally in combination with an oral aminoglycoside to prepare the bowel before bowel or GI tract surgery.

Aminoglycosides

Aminoglycosides are potent bactericidal antibiotics that act by creating fissures in the outer membrane of the bacterial cell (see Table 27-10). The MOA is to interrupt protein synthesis. They are active against aerobic, gram-negative bacteria and act synergistically against certain gram-positive organisms. Because of their antibacterial activity, spectrum, and toxic effects, they are usually reserved for the treatment of severe infections of the abdomen and urinary tract, endocarditis, and bacteremia. They are given IV only for systemic conditions and topically for ocular infections.

Toxic effects include nephrotoxicity and ototoxicity. Toxic effects result because the body does not metabolize aminoglycosides due to inhibition of certain metabolic enzymes. Renal toxicity is most often documented, and is usually reversible by stopping aminoglycoside treatment. Nephrotoxicity results from renal cortical cumulation that causes tubular cell degeneration and sloughing. Ototoxicity is usually irreversible. Studies in animals have shown that aminoglycoside accumulation in the ear is dose-dependent, but can reach a saturation point at low serum levels. Therefore, toxicity to the cochlear organ of Corti and inner ear is dose-dependent.

Table 27-9   Macrolides

DRUG	ROUTE AND ADULT DOSE
azithromycin (Zithromax®)	PO; 500 mg for one dose, then 250 mg qd for 4 days
clarithromycin (Biaxin®)	PO; 250–500 mg bid
dirithromycin (Dynabac®)	PO; 500 mg qd
erythromycin (E-mycin®, Erythrocin®)	PO; 250–500 mg qid or 333 mg tid

Table 27-10   Aminoglycosides

DRUG	ROUTE
amikacin sulfate (Amikin®)	IM/IV
gentamicin sulfate (Garamycin®, G-mycin®, Jenamicin®)	IM
kanamycin (Kantrex®)	IM/IV/PO
neomycin sulfate (Mycifradin®)	PO
netilmicin sulfate (Netromycin®)	IM
paromomycin sulfate (Humatin®)	PO
streptomycin sulfate	IM
tobramycin sulfate (Nebcin®)	IM, IV

Aminoglycosides are associated with postantibiotic effect. It is believed that after exposure to higher doses of aminoglycosides, leukocytes have enhanced phagocytosis and ability to kill; these effects last for relatively long periods of time after the dose is given. The once-standard dosing of gentamicin 80 mg q8–12 hr is no longer recommended. Correct multiple daily dosing of aminoglycosides often requires pharmacokinetics expertise and close monitoring of drug serum levels and renal function, and is both labor- and lab-intensive. It is now recommended that single daily dosing be used. This method, with high concentrations of aminoglycosides and long dosing intervals of q 24–48 hr, is called *pulse dosing.*

Fluoroquinolones

Fluoroquinolones are used to treat severe infections, such as infections of the bone and joints, skin, urinary tract, serious ear infections, bronchitis, pneumonia, tuberculosis, inflammation of the prostate, some sexually transmitted diseases (STDs) or infections (STIs), and some infections that affect people with AIDS (see Table 27-11). Some fluoroquinolones may weaken the tendons in the shoulder, hand, or heel, making the tendons more likely to tear. Some people feel drowsy, dizzy, lightheaded, or less alert when taking quinolones. Special attention should be paid to patients with renal, hepatic, or CNS disease, or sclerotic cranial arteries, epilepsy, and other seizure disorders. Fluoroquinolones, which are bactericidal, act by inhibiting gyrase, an important enzyme for replication of DNA, during bacterial replication. Because the affected bacteria cannot reproduce, they die off.

Sulfonamides

Antibiotics containing sulfur are called *sulfa drugs* or *sulfonamides.* Sulfonamides (see Table 27-12) are used to treat urinary tract infections, bronchitis, middle ear infections, and traveler's diarrhea. They are also used for the prevention and treatment of

Table 27-11   Fluoroquinolones

DRUG	ROUTE AND ADULT DOSE
ciprofloxacin (Cipro®)	PO; 250–750 mg bid
levofloxacin (Levaquin®)	PO; 250–500 mg/day
ofloxacin (Floxin®)	PO; 200–400 mg bid
sparfloxacin (Zagam®)	PO; 400 mg on day one, then 200 mg daily

Table 27-12　Sulfonamides

DRUG	ROUTE AND ADULT DOSE	NOTES
Gantanol® (sulfamethoxazole)	500 mg tablets: 4 tablets (2 g) initially, then 2 tablets (1 g) three times daily	Must take with plenty of water to prevent crystallization in the kidneys.
Gantrisin® (sulfisoxazole)	500 mg tablets, 4–8 gm in 4–6 divided doses	Must take with plenty of water to prevent crystallization in the kidneys.
Septra®, Bactrim®, Bactrim DS® (sulfamethoxazole + trimethoprim)	Bactrim & Septra - 400 mg/80 mg Dose: 1 tab q6hr or Bactrim DS & Septra DS - 800 mg/160 mg Dose: 1 tab q12hr	Must take with plenty of water to prevent crystallization in the kidneys. May cause photosensitivity.
sulfadiazine (various generics)	500 mg tablets: 2–4 gm in 3–6 divided doses	Must take with plenty of water to prevent crystallization in the kidneys.

Note: All may require a loading dose.

Pneumocystis carinii pneumonia (PCP). Sulfonamides competitively inhibit both para aminobenzoic acid (PABA) and the enzymatic substrate dihydropteroate to block the essential synthesis of folic acid of the bacterial cell.

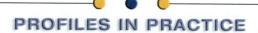

PROFILES IN PRACTICE

A customer mentions to the pharmacy technician that every time she takes an antibiotic for the full course of therapy, she ends ups with diarrhea and vaginitis.

• What could the pharmacist suggest to help alleviate this recurring problem?

Antifungals

The mechanism of action of an antifungal depends on its subclass (see Table 27-13). Imidazoles, such as ketoconazole, interfere with synthesis of ergosterol, the vital, major component of the cell wall membranes of fungi and yeast. The reduced availability of ergosterol increases the permeability of the cell wall, allowing outside material to enter the cell and encouraging leakage of cytoplasm and nucleus to the outside of the fungal cell. This ultimately causes the collapse of the fungal cell and inhibits cell growth.

Triazole antifungals, such as ketoconazole, fluconazole, itraconazole, and voriconazole, also inhibit or interfere with the fungal cell's ability to synthesize ergosterol. Though each drug has a slightly different action, all promote increased permeability, leakage of the cell's inner contents, and collapse of the cell wall, resulting in death of the fungal cell.

In contrast, flucytosine competitively inhibits the cell's production of purine and pyrimadine. Biosynthesis of purine and pyrimadine nucleotides is an essential process in all growing cells, because these molecules are the direct precursors of DNA and RNA. Therefore, by blocking the cell's own production of purine and pyrimadine,

Table 27-13 Antifungal Agents

GENERIC (TRADE) NAME	STRENGTH & DOSAGE FORM(S) AVAILABLE	USUAL ADULT DOSE	NOTES
amphotericin B, desoxy-cholate (Fungizone®)	Powder for injection: 50 mg vials	Depends on weight and diagnosis; 0.25–1.5 mg/kg/day 4 gram max daily dose, given 4–12 weeks	Only used for life-threatening systemic fungal infections, because of drug interactions and toxic effects. Monitor renal patients. May cause respiratory reactions and nephrotoxicity.
amphotericin B, lipid-based (Amphotec®)	Powder for injection: 50 mg single-dose vials	Depends on weight and diagnosis; 3–6 mg/kg/day	Reserved for life-threatening systemic fungal infections. May cause N/V/D, headache, anxiety, asthma, convulsions, MI, anemia, leukemia, more.
fluconazole (Diflucan®)	Tab: 50 mg, 100 mg, 150 mg, 200 mg Powder for PO suspension: 10 mg/1 mL and 40 mg/1 mL when reconstituted Injectable: 2 mg/mL	200 mg day 1, then 100 mg qd For vaginal candidiasis, one 150 mg tablet qd × 7 days	Double the daily dose on day 1 for a loading dose. Caution with renally or hepatically impaired patients. May cause hepatoxicity. Has 26% incidence of adverse reactions associated with 150 mg qd for vaginal candidiasis.
flucytosine (Ancobon®)	Cap: 250 mg, 500 mg	50–150 mg/kg in 4 divided doses, q6 hr	Warning: Monitor renally impaired patients. Usually given with amphotericin B to increase therapeutic action, but combination may also increase toxicity. May cause bone marrow depression.
griseofulvin (Fulvicin®)	Tab: 250 mg, 500 mg	Depends on weight and diagnosis. One tablet daily.	Photosensitivity and lupus-like syndrome.
griseofulvin, ultramicro-size (Fulvicin PG® and Gris-Peg)	Tab: 125 mg, 165 mg, 250 mg, 330 mg		Possible PCN cross-sensitivity.
itraconazole (Sporanox®)	Tab: 100 mg Susp po: 10 mg/mL Pwd for inj: 10 mg/mL	100–200 mg qd. Take capsules whole, with food to increase absorption.	Do not give to CHF patients; may increase CHF symptoms.
ketoconazole (Nizoral®)	Tab: 200 mg	200–400 mg qd	Side effects: headache, dizziness. Toxic effects: May cause anaphylaxis on first dose; hepatoxicity; gastric acidity. Contraindicated with triazolam (may cause CNS depression and psychomotor impairment, or suicidal tendencies).

Table 27-13 Antifungal Agents (*continued*)

GENERIC (TRADE) NAME	STRENGTH & DOSAGE FORM(S) AVAILABLE	USUAL ADULT DOSE	NOTES
			Contraindicated with antacids, which may reduce the effect of ketoconazole; delay administration by 2 hr.
terbinafine (Lamisil®)	Tab: 250 mg	250 mg qd × 6 or 12 weeks	Do not give to patients with liver damage or transplants. May cause renal or hepatic function impairment and Stevens-Johnson syndrome. Inhibits CYP450 enzyme. Caution in use with drugs that also interact with CYP450: MAOIs, TCA, SSRIs, beta blockers.
voriconazole (V-fend®)	Tab: 50 mg, 200 mg (take 1 hour before or 1 hour after meal/empty stomach) Pwd for inj: 200 mg SDV	PO: 50–300 mg q12 hr UAD 200 mg q12 hr	Increase dosage of voriconazole if co-administered with phenytoin.

flucytosine also blocks production of DNA and RNA. In addition, flucytosine metabolizes to 5-fluorouracil (5-FU), which is then incorporated into the RNA of the fungal cell, where it blocks the synthesis of both DNA and RNA, leading to fungal cell death.

Amebicides/Antiprotozoals

Metronidazole is amebicidal, bactericidal, and trichomonacidal. Its selectivity for anaerobic bacteria is a result of these organisms' ability to reduce metronidazole to its active form intracellularly; it then disrupts the helical structure of DNA, inhibiting nucleic acid synthesis by the bacterial cell. This eventually results in bacterial cell death. Metronidazole is equally effective against dividing and nondividing cells. The electron transport proteins necessary for this reaction are found only in anaerobic bacteria. Metronidazole's spectrum of activity includes protozoa and obligate anaerobes, including: *Bacteroides* group (including *B. fragilis*), *Fusobacterium*, *Veillonella*, the *Clostridium* group (including *C. difficile* and *C. perfringens*), *Eubacterium*, *Peptococcus*, and *Peptostreptococcus*. Its protozoan coverage includes *Entamoeba histolytica*, *Giardia lamblia*, and *Trichomonas vaginalis*. It is not effective against the common aerobes, but it combats *Gardnerella (Haemophilus) vaginalis*.

Tables 27-14 and 27-15 list some common antifungal and antiprotozoal agents.

" Workplace Wisdom Metronidazole and Alcohol

If patients who are taking metronidazole drink alcoholic beverages, they may experience disulfiram-like side effects, which include nausea and vomiting, headache, flushing, and abdominal cramps. It is possible for these effects to last two to three weeks after the last dose of metronidazole has been taken. Disulfiram (the generic name for Antabuse®) is used as an anti-alcoholic treatment. Disulfiram also causes cramping with the slightest amount of alcohol, such as that in mouthwash. "

Table 27-14 Common Antifungal Agents

DRUG	USES	BASIC MECHANISM OF ACTION
amphotericin B	Systemic fungal infections	Alters permeability of cell membrane
azoles such as clotrimazole, miconazole, fluconazole	Local candidiasis and dermatological infections	Inhibit sterol synthesis
	Systemic fungal infections	
flucytosine	Serious fungal infections	Competes with uracil

Tuberculosis

Tuberculosis (TB) is caused by a bacterium called *Mycobacterium tuberculosis*, which is very common in Latin America, the Caribbean, Africa, Asia, Eastern Europe, and Russia. These bacteria may attack any part of the body, but usually attack the lungs. Once a leading cause of death in the United States, it was almost eradicated in the 1940s when scientists discovered the drug treatments that are still used today. However, due to complacency and a decrease in funding for TB programs, there has been a resurgence of the illness, and drug-resistant types are appearing.

Despite new programs to combat TB, tens of thousands of cases are still reported in the United States each year. The bacteria are spread by breathing the air that infected people cough or sneeze into. Usually, TB is spread among people in close proximity, who see each other on a day-to-day basis. It is found most commonly in homeless shelters, migrant farm camps, prisons, jails, and some nursing homes in the United States. TB can become active in a person whose immune system is weak and cannot fight it off, or it can be the latent type of TB that stays dormant, alive but inactive, in the body (especially in a person with a strong immune system). Symptoms are different for the two states of TB.

Symptoms include weakness, weight loss, fever, lack of appetite, chills, and sweating at night. Other symptoms of TB disease depend on where the bacteria are growing in the body. If the infection is in the lungs (pulmonary TB), the symptoms may include a bad cough, pain in the chest, and coughing up blood (*hemoptysis*). Those most at risk for developing active TB are patients with the following conditions:

- substance abuse
- diabetes mellitus
- silicosis

Table 27-15 Common Antiprotozoal Agents

DRUG	USES	MECHANISM OF ACTION
chloroquine, quinine	malaria	Inhibits nucleic acid synthesis
imidazoles such as metronidazole, tinidazole	entamoeba, giardia, trichomoniasis	Interferes with several metabolic pathways, disrupts DNA's helical structure
pentamidine	*Pneumonia carinii, Trypanosoma rhodesiense/gambiense*	Inhibits aerobic glycolysis
pyrimethamine	malaria, toxoplasmosis	Inhibits folic acid reduction

- cancer of the head or neck
- leukemia or Hodgkin's disease
- severe kidney disease
- low body weight
- certain medical treatments, such as corticosteroid treatment or organ transplants

Latent TB infection is characterized by having dormant bacteria in the lungs or other parts of the body. Though the dormant pathogens cause no symptoms, the bacteria can become active again whenever the immune system is stressed or weakened. Infected persons in whom the disease is latent can still spread TB to others, and will develop the active form of the disease later in life if they do not receive treatment for the latent infection.

Diagnosis of TB disease usually begins with a positive skin-test reaction. This indicates the presence of TB, but does not necessarily indicate infection. Further diagnostic tests usually include a chest X-ray and sputum test. Because TB bacteria may be found somewhere besides the lungs, blood or urine may also be tested.

The drug of choice for treatment is isoniazid (INH) (see Table 27-16). INH is taken for at least six to nine months, and longer if the patient has a weakened immune system. Compliance is a major problem in the treatment of TB, as many low-income or transient patients do not complete the full course; incomplete treatment builds drug resistance and creates a public health hazard.

A toxic effect is the development of hepatitis. This effect is age-related, with a higher incidence in persons aged 50–64 years. The use of alcohol during treatment can be dangerous and can increase the chances of hepatitis. Precaution statements on the label placed by the pharmacy technician should include a warning that the patient is

Table 27-16   Common Antituberculosis Regimens

REGIMEN 1	REGIMEN 2	REGIMEN 3
Daily INH, rifampin, and pyrazinamide for 8 weeks. Subsequent administration of INH and rifampin daily or 2–3 times weekly for 16 weeks.	Daily INH, rifampin, pyrazinamide, and streptomycin or ethambutol for 2 weeks.	Three times weekly with INH, rifampin, pyrazinamide, and ethambutol or streptomycin for 6 months.
Ethambutol or streptomycin should be added to the initial regimen until sensitivity to INH and rifampin is demonstrated.	Subsequent administration of same drugs twice weekly for 6 weeks.	
Additionally, a fourth drug is optional if the relative prevalence of isoniazid-resistant *Mycobacterium tuberculosis* isolates are present.	Subsequently twice weekly INH and rifampin for 16 more weeks.	

ANTITUBERCULIN DRUGS	USUAL MAXIMUM DAILY DOSE	MAX TWICE WEEKLY DOSE
ethambutol	2.5 g	50 mg/kg
isoniazid	300 mg	900 mg
pyrazinamide	2 g	50–70 mg/kg
rifampin	600 mg	600 mg
streptomycin	1 g (>60 yrs old, 750 mg)	20–30 mg/kg

not to drink alcoholic beverages (wine, beer, or liquor) while taking INH. Side effects should be reported immediately; they may include:

- lack of appetite
- nausea
- vomiting
- jaundice (yellowish skin or eyes)
- fever for three or more days
- abdominal pain
- tingling in the fingers and toes

Workplace Wisdom TB Resistance

Because resistance to TB can develop rapidly, both mycobactericidal or tubercularcidal and tubercularstatic drugs should be given—rifampin and isoniazid/ethambutol, respectively.

Antivirals

The common cold and influenza are discussed in Chapter 26. This chapter investigates antiretrovirals for HIV/AIDS and vaccinations for influenza. Some oral antivirals can be used to prevent the onset of influenza if used within 24 to 48 hours after the onset of signs and symptoms. Amantadine should be continued for 24 to 48 hours after the disappearance of signs and symptoms.

Antivirals change or metabolize to acyclovir triphosphate; acyclovir inhibits the virus-specific DNA polymerase, an enzyme important for viral growth, multiplication, and replication. Replication is interrupted and the viruses die (see Table 27-17).

Table 27-17 Common Antiviral Drugs

DRUG	USES	MECHANISM OF ACTION
acyclovir, famciclovir, valaciclovir	herpes viruses	Nucleoside analogue
amantadine, rimantadine	influenza A	Inhibit virus uncoating and assembly
ganciclovir	cytomegalovirus (group of herpetoviruses that inhabit the salivary glands, causing immunocompromised individuals, such as AIDS and transplant patients, to develop retinitis, pneumonia, colitis, and/or encephalitis)	Nucleoside analogue
ribavirin	respiratory syncytial (RS) virus (common cause of acute bronchitis in small children)	Nucleoside analogue
Antiretrovirals—Used Specifically for HIV		
azidothymidine	HIV	Nucleoside analogue
nevirapine	HIV	Protease inhibitor

" **Workplace Wisdom** Viruses

Because viruses use the host cell's machinery to replicate, they are very difficult to target. The viruses can mutate quickly enough to elude some antiviral drugs. "

Drug Resistance

Resistance is a microorganism's ability to live and grow despite the presence of an anti-infective or antimicrobial drug. Resistance is a result of genetic mutation during the replication or cell division process that causes the pathogen to evade or avoid the mechanism by which a drug destroys the pathogen. A pathogen such as a bacteria, fungus, or virus becomes resistant to a drug; a person does not become resistant to a drug or a pathogen. The ability of the bacterium or pathogen to survive the mechanism of destruction of the antibiotic, or resistance, is promoted by several factors. Basically, though, the process is Darwinian "survival of the fittest" on a small and rapid scale: any pathogens that happen to survive after a patient is treated with a particular drug will reproduce similarly hardy (resistant) cells.

This is one reason it is so important for patients to finish a course of antibiotics. Some patients who are prescribed antibiotics do not take the full dosing regimen; they quit taking the drug when they start to feel better. This often kills off only some of the weaker, nonresistant bacteria, and enhances the resistance ability of the remaining pathogens, which multiply and become stronger. Soon the prescribed antibiotic will no longer work, and a stronger antibiotic will be needed. If the patient again breaks off treatment with the prescribed drug, a stronger antibiotic may not be available, or may not be effective upon a subsequent infection.

Contributing to the problem is the fact that bacteria and other pathogens are remarkably resilient and can develop ways to evade drugs meant to kill or weaken them. The increasing use of antibiotics contributes to this action and is called *antibiotic resistance, antimicrobial resistance,* or *drug resistance.* Research has shown that antibiotics are given to patients more often than recommended by federal guidelines. For example, many patients ask their doctors for antibiotics to treat a cold, cough, or the flu, all of which are viral in etiology and do not respond to antibacterials. Food-producing animals given antibiotic drugs for therapeutic, disease-prevention, or production-enhancement reasons can harbor microbes that become resistant to drugs used to treat human illness. This results in harder-to-treat human infections.

According to the FDA, about 70 percent of *nosocomial* bacteria, which cause infections in hospitals, are resistant to at least one of the most commonly prescribed antibiotics. Some organisms are resistant to all FDA-approved antibiotics and can be treated only with experimental and potentially toxic drugs.

Antibiotic resistance problems must be detected as soon as they emerge, and actions must be taken to contain them; otherwise, the world will be faced with previously treatable diseases that have once again become untreatable. It will be as it was in the days before antibiotics were first discovered and used.

Antibiotic resistance results when bacteria acquire genes conferring resistance in any of the following three ways:

- In spontaneous DNA mutation, bacterial genetic material may change spontaneously to a form that serendipitously resists the action of a drug or drugs. Drug-resistant tuberculosis occurs this way.
- In a type of microbial sex called *transformation,* one bacterium may take up DNA from another bacterium. Penicillin-resistant gonorrhea results from microbial transformation.

- Most powerful is resistance acquired from a small circle of DNA (a plasmid) that can "hop" from one type of bacterium to another. A single plasmid can provide a great number of different resistances. In 1968, 12,500 people in Guatemala died in an epidemic of *shigella* diarrhea because a pathogen harbored a plasmid carrying resistances to four antibiotics.

INFORMATION

Only four years after drug companies began mass-producing penicillin in 1943, penicillin-resistant pathogens began to appear.

1943 — The first bug to battle penicillin was *Staphylococcus aureus,* which caused pneumonia or toxic shock syndrome from infected wounds.

1967 — American military personnel in Southeast Asia were acquiring penicillin-resistant gonorrhea from prostitutes.

1967 — *Streptococcus pneumoniae,* called pneumococcus, surfaced in a village in Papua New Guinea, causing PCN-resistant pneumonia.

1979 to 1987 — According to the Centers for Disease Control and Prevention (CDC), only 0.02 percent of pneumococcus strains are penicillin-resistant.

1983 — A hospital-acquired intestinal infection caused by the bacterium *Enterococcus faecium* appears.

1987 — First vancomycin-resistant enterococcus is reported in England and France.

1989 — Vancomycin-resistant enterococcus is discovered in a New York hospital.

1994 — A full 6.6 percent of pneumococcus strains are resistant.

2002 — The CDC reports a Michigan patient with diabetes, vascular disease, and chronic kidney failure who developed the first *S. aureus* infection completely resistant to vancomycin.

2003 — Epidemiologists report in the *New England Journal of Medicine* that 5 to 10 percent of hospital patients acquire an infection during their stay.

2003 — Study in the *New England Journal of Medicine* found that the incidence of sepsis (blood and tissue infections) almost tripled from 1979 to 2000.

Solutions to Resistance

Pathogens exist in huge numbers. They have short generation times and the ability to swap genes, which makes them flexible and dangerous. Although there may be no ultimate cure for resistance, it can be slowed down.

- Avoid using antibiotics unnecessarily. Use only when bacterial infections warrant such treatment. Do not use for viral or fungal infections.
- Complete any antibacterial regimen; do not have leftover doses.
- Use the most specific antibiotic possible, with the most precise target or narrowest "spectrum." This kills the offending bug without triggering resistance among other bacteria that live in the patient, as broader-spectrum drugs do.
- Use the common antibiotics first; if they work, do not use second-line-of-defense drugs. Reserve these latter drugs for infections on which the first-generation drugs do not work.
- Reduce hospital-transmitted infections by improving infection control in hospitals. This will kill the bugs before they get inside patients.
- Invent new antibiotic drugs that use new mechanisms to kill microbes, and find new drugs that improve the action of existing antibiotics.
- Invent vaccines against common viral diseases to prevent initial infections.
- Reduce the widespread use of antibiotics in animal feeds.

Vaccines

Vaccines were first used by the Chinese, who called it "variolation." They were observed by Lady Mary Wortley Montagu, wife of the British ambassador to Turkey, who brought them back to England in the early 1700s. In the late 1700s, Edward Jenner experienced variolation as a child, survived, and later became a doctor who was told by a milkmaid that she could not catch smallpox because she had already contracted cowpox. In 1796, Jenner infected a boy with cowpox. After the boy's recovery, Jenner injected the pus from a smallpox lesion directly under the boy's skin. The boy never contracted smallpox. Thus the first inoculation was born.

Most of today's immunizations are either inactivated, acellular, or attenuated vaccines (see Table 27-18). *Inactivated* vaccines are composed of killed disease-causing microorganisms. *Acellular* vaccines are taken from the antigenic part of the disease-causing organism, such as the capsule or flagella. These types of vaccines cannot cause disease and therefore can be used in immunocompromised patients. With these vaccine types, booster shots are required every few years. *Attenuated* vaccine contains a live microorganism that has been weakened by aging or altering the viral growth conditions. They are lifelong and do not require booster shots. Although these are the most successful vaccines, they carry a high risk of mutation to virulent strains. Therefore, these types of vaccines should not be used in immunocompromised patients.

Another type of vaccine, called a *toxoid*, is made from viral toxins that have been treated with aluminum salts. Yet another vaccine uses a part of the organism to stimulate a strong immune system response; these are called *subunit* vaccines. They are made

Table 27-18 Types of Vaccines

TYPE OF VACCINE	EXAMPLES	NOTES
Acellular vaccines	*Haemophilus influenzae* B (HIB)	Requires booster shots
Attenuated vaccines	Measles, mumps, and rubella	Highest risk of mutation Lifelong immunization Does not require booster shots
Biotechnology and genetic engineering techniques	Hepatitis B vaccine	Safe for immunocompromised patients
Inactivated or killed vaccines	Typhoid vaccine Salk poliomyelitis vaccine	Organism is killed using formalin
Toxoid vaccines	Diphtheria Tetanus Diphtheria/pertussis (whooping cough)/tetanus (DPT) vaccine	Administered with an *adjuvant*—an agent that increases or enhances the immune response
Use of an organism similar to a lethal organism	BCG vaccine against *Mycobacterium tuberculosis*	

from bacterial or yeast host cells that have had the genome of the infectious agent inserted into them.

The national goal to fully vaccinate 90 percent of 2-year-old children depends on the support of private healthcare providers. The 12 diseases that the Vaccines for Children (VFC) program currently provides protection against are:

- diphtheria
- *Haemophilus influenzae* type B
- hepatitis A
- hepatitis B
- measles
- mumps
- pertussis
- pneumococcal disease
- poliomyelitis
- rubella
- tetanus
- varicella (chickenpox)

Various Infectious Disease States

In addition to varying in appearance, microorganisms vary in the specific disease(s) they cause. Table 27-19 displays some of the most common diseases and their origins.

Malaria

Malaria is a disease transmitted by parasites found in malaria-infected mosquitoes. Malaria is common in large areas of Central and South America, Haiti and the Dominican Republic, Africa, the Indian subcontinent, Southeast Asia, the Middle East, and Oceania. In these areas of risk, about 1 million deaths per year are caused by malaria. The United States sees only a few cases each year.

Malaria can be cured with prescription drugs (see Table 27-20). The type of drugs used and duration of the treatment depend on which type of malaria is diagnosed, where the patient was infected, the patient's age, and the progression of the disease state at the start of treatment. Antimalarial drugs should be taken before, during, and after travel to high-risk areas. One drug in particular is reserved for travelers who cannot take other drugs: Primaquine can cause **lysis** (bursting and destruction) of red blood cells. This occurs in persons who are deficient in glucose-6-phosphate dehydrogenase (G6PD) and can be fatal. Travelers *must* be tested for G6PD deficiency and have a documented G6PD level in the normal range before primaquine is used.

lysis the destruction of cells.

The main focus of treatment is prevention:

- Vaccinations are given four to six weeks before foreign travel, and an antimalarial drug is prescribed. This antimalarial drug must be taken exactly on schedule, without missing doses.
- Prevent mosquito and other insect bites by using DEET insect repellent on exposed skin and flying insect spray in the room where you sleep.
- Protective clothing: Wear long pants and long-sleeved shirts, especially from dusk to dawn, the time when mosquitoes that spread malaria bite.
- Bed nets dipped in permethrin insecticide should be employed if screened or air-conditioned housing is not available.

INFORMATION

Halofantrine (also called Halfan) is widely used overseas to treat malaria. The CDC does *not* recommend the use of Halfan because of serious heart-related side effects, including death.

Table 27-19   Origin of Various Human Infectious Diseases

BACTERIAL ORIGIN	VIRAL ORIGIN	FUNGAL ORIGIN	YEAST ORIGIN	PARASITIC ORIGIN
anthrax	Childhood diseases: mumps, measles, German measles (rubella), chickenpox	athlete's foot (*Tinea pedis*)	vaginal yeast infections (*Candida albicans*, candidiasis, moniliasis)	malaria
cholera	common cold	cryptococcal meningitis	*Cryptococcus neoformans* (opportunistic infection that occurs as a complication of AIDS or use of immunosuppressant drugs)	pediculosis
diphtheria	hepatitis	histoplasmosis (found in bird or bat droppings; when inhaled, causes severe eye disease or blindness)		scabies
dysentery	HIV (progresses to AIDS)	jock itch, thigh area (*Tinea cruris, Trichophyton rubrum*)	Jock itch, inclusive of penis and scrotum (*Candida albicans*)	
meningitis (bacterial, not all)	influenza	ringworm		
pneumonia (bacterial, not all)	meningitis (viral, not all)	sporotrichosis (caused by *Sporothrix schenckii,* found in thorny plants such as roses, hay, sphagnum moss; causes boils and open lesions)		
Rocky Mountain spotted fever (*Rickettsia rickettsii;* bacteria spread by ixodid (hard) ticks	polio (poliomyelitis)	thrush (caused by a yeast-like fungus)		
scarlet fever	pneumonia (viral, not all)	toxoplasmosis		
some STDs: syphilis, gonorrhea, chlamydia	arabies			
tetanus	shingles			
toxic shock syndrome	smallpox			
tuberculosis	warts and genital warts			
typhoid fever (*Salmonella typhi*)				
whooping cough	yellow fever (spread by mosquitoes)			

Table 27-20 Antimalarial Drug Regimens

TRAVEL TO AFRICA, SOUTH AMERICA, THE INDIAN SUBCONTINENT, ASIA, AND THE SOUTH PACIFIC		TRAVEL TO MEXICO, HAITI, DOMINICAN REPUBLIC, AND CERTAIN COUNTRIES IN CENTRAL AMERICA, THE MIDDLE EAST, AND EASTERN EUROPE (THEIR ANTIMALARIAL DRUG IS AVAILABLE AS AN ALTERNATIVE)	
Antimalaria Drug	**Antimalaria Drug Regimen**	**Antimalaria Drug**	**Antimalaria Drug Regimen**
Malarone™—a combination of Mepron® (atovaquone) 250 mg and proguanil 100 mg	Usual adult dose (UAD): 1 adult tablet once a day, with food or milk, same time each day. First dose 1 to 2 days before travel to the malaria-risk area. Last dose once a day for 7 days after leaving the malaria-risk area.	chloroquine (Aralen™)	UAD: 500 mg once a week, same day of the week. Take on a full stomach to lessen the risk of nausea and stomach upset. First dose 1 week before arrival in the malaria-risk area. Last dose 4 weeks after leaving the malaria-risk area.
doxycycline (a type of TCN, various trade names)	UAD: 100 mg once a day, same time each day. First dose 1 or 2 days before arrival in the malaria-risk area. Last dose 4 weeks after leaving the risk area.	hydroxychloroquine sulfate (Plaquenil™)	UAD: 400 mg once a week on the same day of the week. Take on a full stomach to lessen nausea and stomach upset. First dose 1 week before arrival in the malaria-risk area. Last dose 4 weeks after leaving the risk area.
mefloquine (Lariam™)	UAD: 250 mg tablet once a week, on a full stomach with a full glass of liquid. First dose 1 week before arrival in the malaria-risk area; once a week on same day of week thereafter. Last dose 4 weeks after leaving the risk area.		
primaquine (in special circumstances)	UAD: 2 tablets (30 mg base primaquine) once a day. Take the first dose 1–2 days before travel and last dose 7 days after leaving high-risk area.		

Cancer

According to the American Cancer Society (ACS), *cancer* is a group of diseases characterized by the uncontrolled growth and spread of abnormal cells. If the spread is not controlled, it can result in death. It is important to note that increased growth rate alone is not cancer; the cells must be mutated or abnormal to the extent that normal cell function is altered or impaired. As some cells stop functioning normally, they no longer serve a useful or purposeful function, and thus they become cancerous cells.

Normal cells reproduce in a regulated and systematic manner. However, after injury, the cell division and reproduction of normal cells is speeded up until the injury is healed. In comparison, cancer cells divide in a haphazard process. The typical result is that they pile up into a nonstructured mass or *tumor*. When the cancer cells become invasive, they destroy the part of the body where they originated and then spread to other parts of the body. When the cancer spreads, or *metastasizes*, the disease can become life-threatening. Benign growths, in contrast, stay localized and are not cancer, even though the cells may grow or divide fast. The most common types of metastatic cancers include:

- bladder
- breast
- colon and rectal
- endometrial
- kidney (renal cell)
- leukemia
- lung
- melanoma
- non-Hodgkin's lymphoma
- ovarian
- pancreatic
- prostate
- skin (nonmelanoma)

Cancer Treatments

Cancer is treated with a variety of methods. Treatment may include only one method, or use a combination of methods, depending on the type and severity of the cancer.

Surgery is usually the first line of treatment for solid tumors. In early-stage cancer, it may be sufficient to cure the patient by removing all cancerous cells. Benign growths may also be removed by surgery.

Radiation may be used in conjunction with surgery and/or drug treatments. The goal of radiation is to kill the cancer cells by damaging them with direct high-energy beams.

Chemotherapy uses cytotoxic agents—a wide array of drugs—to kill cancer cells. Chemotherapy damages the dividing cancer cells and prevents their further reproduction.

Hormonal treatments prevent cancer cells from receiving the signals necessary for continued growth and division.

Specific inhibitors are a relatively new class of drugs that work by targeting specific proteins and processes used by cancer cells. Inhibition of these proteins and processes prevents cancer cell growth and division.

- *Antibodies* are used to target cancer cells, depriving the cancer cells of necessary growth signals or causing the direct death of the cells. Antibodies may also be called *specific inhibitors*.
- *Biological response modifiers* are naturally occurring, normal proteins that stimulate the body's own defenses against cancer.
- *Vaccines* for cancer also stimulate the body's defenses against cancer, increasing the body's response against the abnormal cancer cells.

Drugs Used to Treat Cancer

Alkylating antineoplastic agents cause the disruption of DNA function and cell death by three methods. Alkylating agents:

- bind or latch alkyl groups to DNA bases, preventing DNA synthesis and RNA transcription from the affected DNA.
- cause a formation of cross-bridges that link two bases together, thus preventing DNA from being separated for synthesis or transcription.

- induce the mispairing of nucleotides, leading to mutations of the cancer cell. (Nucleotide "A" always pairs with "T," and "G" always pairs with "C." Alkylated G bases may erroneously pair with Ts. If this altered pairing is not corrected, it may lead to a permanent mutation—in this case, a fatal mutation is desired).

Antimetabolites inhibit ribonucleotide reductase and DNA polymerase to decrease DNA synthesis. They primarily kill cells undergoing DNA synthesis (S-phase), and under certain conditions block the progression of cells from the G1 phase to the S-phase. Although the mechanism of action is not completely understood, it appears that antimetabolites act through the inhibition of DNA.

Sometimes body misregulation causes overproduction of hormones, such as too much estrogen or testosterone. Prostate cancer is caused by too much testosterone activating cell growth in the prostate. Breast cancer can be caused by too much estrogen activating cell growth in the breast. In some cases, the opposite androgenic hormone is given to suppress the overproduced hormone. For example, estrogen may be given to prostate cancer patients.

Biological response modifiers (BRMs) are substances that help to fight infections; they are found naturally in small amounts in the body. BRMs are produced in the laboratory in large amounts, and then injected into the body to treat cancer. BRMs are sometimes combined with chemotherapy drugs to help to improve the effect of the cytotoxic agents. Unfortunately, BRMs are not effective against most cancers. The following are general types of BRMs: cytokines, monoclonal antibodies, tumor vaccines, and other immunotherapy.

- *Cytokines,* such as interferon, travel into the cells that are affected by a virus or a cancer and stops the virus or cancer from multiplying. Interferon has been used to treat viral infections like hepatitis A, B, C, and D; and cancers such as chronic myelocytic leukemia, melanoma, and breast cancer. Special classes of cytokines are called *colony-stimulating factors (CSFs)*. These agents are used to stimulate the bone marrow to recover after chemotherapy.

- *Monoclonal antibodies* are designed to cause the body to attack a cancerous tumor in the same way that it responds to a viral infection. The antibody can be attached to a medication used in chemotherapy and targeted against a specific cancer or tumor. When the antibody attacks the tumor, the chemotherapy medication is then delivered directly to the tumor.

- *Tumor vaccines* are mostly experimental medications made from bits of tumors. It is hoped and expected that, when the tumor vaccine is administered, the body will attack the tumor—and any similar tumorous tissues—and keep them from growing.

- *Other immunotherapy* includes a bacterium called bacillus Calmette-Guerin (BCG), which is injected into the body to treat certain types of bladder and melanoma cancers. BCG causes the body to mount a general immune response, in the course of which the body also attacks the cancer.

The side effects of most BRMs are similar to flu symptoms. These symptoms include high fever, chills, fatigue, nausea, vomiting, and loss of appetite.

Antitumor *antibiotics* work by binding with DNA to prevent RNA synthesis, thus preventing DNA replication and cell growth. Antitumor antibiotics may also prevent the DNA from mending or reattaching itself, thus again causing cell death. Antibiotics, which are given IV, are used to treat a wide variety of cancers, including testicular cancer and leukemia.

Plant (vinca) alkaloids prevent cell division by binding to tubulin, which prevents the formation of mitotic spindles. During metaphase, mitotic spindles hold the two sets of DNA the cell needs to divide. Cancer cells cannot divide without mitotic spindles. These drugs, which are derived from plants, are used to treat cancers of the lung, breast, and testes.

Table 27-21 lists some common anticancer drugs.

Table 27-21 Anticancer Agents

TRADE/GENERIC NAME	CANCERS OR DISORDERS TREATED	CLASSIFICATION OR TYPE OF ANTINEOPLASTIC AGENTS
Adriamycin PFS®	Variety of cancers	Antibiotic
Adriamycin RDF®; Rubex® (doxorubicin)	In combination with other cytotoxic agents	
Adrucil®, Carac™, Efudex®, Fluoroplex® (fluorouracil)	Variety of cancers	Antimetabolite
Arimidex® (anastrozole)	Breast cancer in post-menopausal females	
Busulfex®, Myleran® (busulfan)	Primary brain cancers, leukemias, and bone marrow disorders	Alkylating agent
Casodex® (bicalutamide)	Prostate cancer	Androgen
Cytosar-U® (cytarabine)	Variety of cancers	Antimetabolite
Cytoxan®, Neosar® (cyclophosphamide)	Variety of cancers	Alkylating agent
	Prevent rejection after organ transplants	
	Treat autoimmune diseases	
Ellence® (epirubicin)	Breast cancer	Anthracycline
Femara® (letrozole)	Breast cancer in post-menopausal women	Aromatase inhibitor, anti-estrogenic agent
Gleevec™ (imatinib)	Chronic myelocytic leukemia	Tyrosine kinase inhibitor
	Specific gastrointestinal cancers	
Hexalen® (altertamine)	Ovarian cancer	Antineoplastic agent, miscellaneous
Imuran® (azathioprine)	Prevents rejection of solid organ transplants and autoimmune diseases	Immunosuppressant agent
Megace® (megestrol acetate)	Endometrial cancer	Progestin
	Breast cancers that have spread	
	Appetite stimulant	
Mylotarg™ (gemtuzumab ozogamicin)	Acute myeloid leukemia (AML)	Natural source (plant)
		Derivative antineoplastic agent
Nolvadex® (tamoxifen)	Breast cancer in women and men	Miscellaneous antineoplastic agent
	Prevention of breast cancer in women at increased risk	
	Induce ovulation	
Navelbine® (vinorelbine)	Variety of cancers	Natural source plant (vinca alkaloids) derivative antineoplastic agent

Table 27-21   Anticancer Agents (*continued*)

TRADE/GENERIC NAME	CANCERS OR DISORDERS TREATED	CLASSIFICATION OR TYPE OF ANTINEOPLASTIC AGENTS
Oncovin®[DSC], Vincasar PFS® (vincristine)	Variety of cancers	Natural source plant (vinca alkaloids) derivative antineoplastic agent
Onxol™ Taxol® (paclitaxel)	Variety of cancers	Natural source plant (vinca alkaloids) derivative antineoplastic agent
Platinol®, Platinol®-AQ (cisplatin)	Variety of cancers	Alkylating agent
Propecia®, Proscar® (finasteride) Avodart® (dutasteride)	Symptoms of benign prostatic hypertrophy (BPH)	Antiandrogen
Rheumatrex®, Trexall™ (methotrexate)	Variety of cancers Psoriasis Arthritis	Antimetabolite
Rituxan® (rituximab)	Non-Hodgkin's lymphoma	Monoclonal antibody
Toposar®, VePesid® (etoposide)	Variety of cancers	Podophyllotoxin derivative
Trelstar™ Depot (triptorelin)	Prostate cancer	Luteinizing hormone releasing hormone analog Antineoplastic agent
Xeloda® (capecitabine)	Breast cancer	Antimetabolite

SUMMARY

The immune system is the body's defense system. Its function is to protect the body from foreign invaders that might otherwise destroy the body or parts of it. These foreign invaders, called pathogens, include parasites, bacteria, viruses, rickettsia, and fungi or yeast. Pharmacotherapeutic treatment of pathogens (with antibacterials, anti-infectives, antifungals, etc.) is an important part of a pharmacy technician's knowledge base.

The body's defense mechanisms are either nonspecific or specific. The nonspecific defense mechanisms include physical barriers, such as the skin and the linings of the respiratory and digestive systems. They also include the lining of the spinal column, clotting factors in the blood, and normal flora (microorganisms) in the digestive tract that compete with invading pathogens so that they cannot penetrate host tissues. Specific defense mechanisms are defined by specialized protein molecules and cells. These include antibodies and their complements, and lymphocytes (B-cells and T-cells).

Sometimes the immune system malfunctions. A person with an autoimmune disease, such as lupus erythematosus or rheumatoid arthritis, has an immune system that mistakenly attacks itself and the body itself. The end result of this misplaced defense reaction is often inflammation. Autoimmune diseases are treated both pharmacologically and nonpharmacologically. The pharmacotherapeutic goal of treatment is to reduce inflammation, or to stop or suppress the inflammatory process.

Many viral diseases are difficult to treat, because of the nature of viral infection. Hence, vaccines play an important part in protecting people from many preventable diseases. Most vaccines are either inactivated, acellular, or attenuated. Some vaccinations last for the lifetime of the person; others require booster shots.

Cancer is the uncontrolled growth of abnormal or mutated cells. Cancer can be treated in a variety of ways, including radiation, surgery, and chemotherapy. Treatments can be given alone or in combination with other treatments. It is important for pharmacy technicians to understand chemotherapy and cancer drug therapy, as well as how to prepare the drugs safely.

CHAPTER REVIEW QUESTIONS

1. Immune system molecules are composed of two types of protein called:
   a. mucus and cilia.
   b. antibodies and antigens.
   c. immunoglobulins and enzymes.
   d. antibodies and complement.

2. The Gram staining technique was developed in:
   a. 1850.
   b. 1844.
   c. 1943.
   d. 1800.

3. _____ are two bacteria connected side by side.
   a. Coccus
   b. Diplococcus
   c. Streptococcus
   d. Staphylococcus

4. In the progression of HIV to AIDS, at which state do signs and symptoms begin to appear?
   a. stage 1
   b. stage 2
   c. stage 3
   d. stage 4

5. Tetanus is an example of which type of vaccine?
   a. inactivated
   b. attenuated
   c. toxoid
   d. accellular

6. Which of the following is an aminoglycoside?
   a. penicillin
   b. cleocin
   c. erythromycin
   d. tobramycin

7. Which of the following is a second-generation cephalosporin?
   a. cefazolin
   b. cefepime
   c. ceftriaxone
   d. cefaclor

8. If a person is allergic to a penicillin drug, what is the chance that he or she will also have cross-sensitivity to cephalosporins?
   a. 1 to 5 percent
   b. 5 to 10 percent
   c. 5 to 20 percent
   d. 10 to 20 percent

9. Which of the following drugs is commonly used to treat the herpes virus?
   a. amantadine
   b. ribivirin
   c. penicillin
   d. acyclovir

10. INH is the drug of choice for the treatment of:
    a. HIV.
    b. TB.
    c. malaria.
    d. otitis media.

11. Which of the following is an attenuated vaccine?
    a. hepatitis B
    b. BCG vaccine
    c. DPT
    d. measles, mumps, and rubella

12. Cytarabine belongs to which of the following chemotherapy drug classifications?
    a. alkylating agent
    b. antibiotic
    c. antimetabolite
    d. plant vinca alkaloid

13. An organism that causes disease is called:
    a. antibiotic
    b. pathogen
    c. bacteria
    d. penicillin

14. Which of the following anti-infective classifications can cause photosensitivity?
    a. penicillins
    b. cephalosporins
    c. macrolides
    d. tetracyclines

15. The duration of therapy for TB is usually:
    a. 1 to 2 weeks.
    b. 1 to 2 months.
    c. 4 to 6 months.
    d. 6 to 9 months.

CRITICAL THINKING QUESTIONS

1. Why do you think some cancer treatments only include one type of therapy, while other treatments combine several different therapies?

2. Why do you think a vaccine for HIV/AIDS has not yet been discovered or developed?

3. Why is the national goal to fully vaccinate 2-year-old children only at 90 percent rather than 100 percent?

WEB CHALLENGE

1. Go to http://www.aids.org to learn more about the disease AIDS and the new treatments that are available.

2. Search the website of the National Institute of Allergies and Infectious Diseases at http://www.niaid.nih.gov/ to learn more about the immune system, infectious diseases, and vaccines.

REFERENCES AND RESOURCES

"About cells" (accessed April 8, 2008): http://staff.jccc.net/pdecell/cells/basiccell.html#introduction

Adams, MP, Josephson, DL, & Holland, LN Jr. *Pharmacology for Nurses—A Pathophysiologic Approach.* Upper Saddle River, NJ: Pearson Education, 2008.

"The Body: An AIDS and HIV Information Resource" (accessed April 8, 2008): http://www.thebody.com/treat/protinh.html

"The Body's Defenses" (accessed April 8, 2008): http://www.langara.bc.ca/biology/mario/Biol1215notes/biol1215chap43.html

"HIV and AIDS Treatments" (accessed April 8, 2008): http://www.hivandhepatitis.com/hiv_and_aids/emtriva.html

Holland, N, & Adams, MP. *Core Concepts in Pharmacology.* Upper Saddle River, NJ: Pearson Education, 2007.

"The Immune System—In More Detail" (accessed October 11, 2007): www.nobelprize.org

"Introduction to Microorganisms" (accessed April 5, 2008): http://www.sparknotes.com/biology/microorganisms/intro/summary.html

McLaughlin Centre, Institute of Population Health, University of Ottawa Health Systems Concerns. "Immune System Fact Sheet" (accessed April 8, 2008): http://www.emcom.ca/health/immune.shtml

The Renal System

LEARNING OBJECTIVES

After completing this chapter, you should be able to:

- List, identify, and diagram the basic parts of the renal system.
- Explain the functions of the nephron, kidney, and bladder.
- List and define common diseases and conditions affecting the renal system and explain the mechanisms of action of each class of drugs used to treat each disease.
- Explain how homeostasis of fluid and electrolytes affects the body.

Introduction

The renal system or urinary system is a fairly simple system with few components; however, its condition has a grave impact on many parts of the body. Genitourinary tract infections, poor kidney filtration, and water imbalance can indicate or cause diabetes, high blood pressure, or dehydration. The proper functioning of the kidneys is essential to maintain life. The drugs most commonly used to treat diseases of the renal system are anti-infectives and diuretics. The use of strong diuretics to remove excess water may also lead to a loss of potassium, which can cause muscle and heart problems. A delicate balance of electrolytes, kidney function, filtration, and waste removal must be maintained at all times, especially during illness and while taking medications that affect or treat the urinary tract.

Anatomy and Physiology of the Renal System

The renal system includes two kidneys, two ureters, one bladder, and the urethra (see Figure 28-1). The filtering system of the kidneys is composed of millions of microscopic kidney cells called *nephrons*. The by-products created as food and drugs are continually metabolized are filtered through the nephrons of the kidneys. The wastes then exit the kidneys as urine via the ureters. The *ureters* are tubes that allow urine to flow into the bladder, where it is stored until it is released. The kidneys, each of which is about the size of a fist, are located in the posterior abdomen just above the waist. The right kidney is slightly lower than the left because of the location of the liver. The kidneys are protected by adipose tissue and the ribcage.

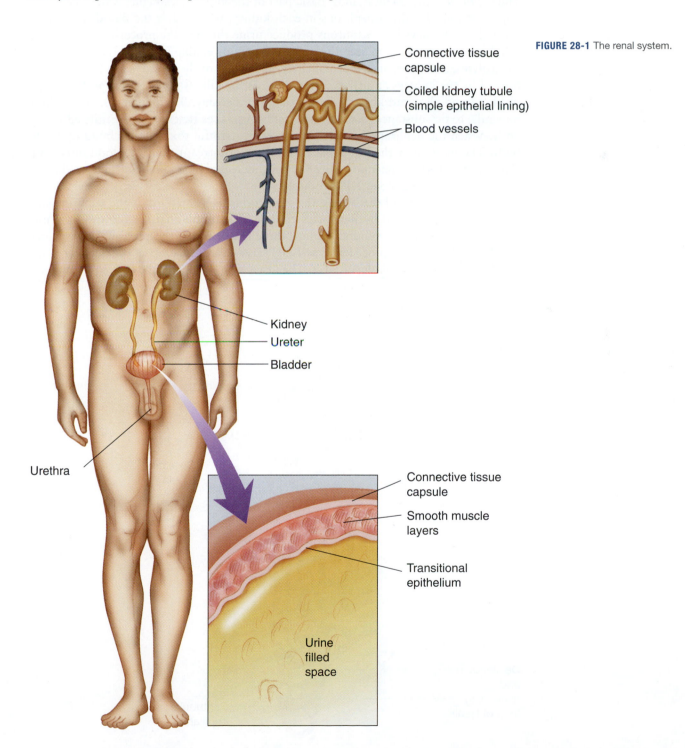

FIGURE 28-1 The renal system.

Connective tissue capsule

Coiled kidney tubule (simple epithelial lining)

Blood vessels

Kidney

Ureter

Bladder

Urethra

Connective tissue capsule

Smooth muscle layers

Transitional epithelium

Urine filled space

The organs of the renal system are responsible for the following life-sustaining processes:

- filtration of waste from the blood
- removal of urine from the body
- maintenance of water balance
- maintenance of electrolyte balance
- maintenance of acid-base balance

The Nephron

The *nephron* is the smallest, most basic part of the kidney (see Figure 28-2). There are approximately 1 million nephrons in each kidney, which filter the blood that passes through the kidneys. The nephrons produce urine through the processes of filtration, tubular reabsorption, and secretion. These functions enable blood to reabsorb water, electrolytes, and nutrients. Approximately 25 percent of the blood in the body is being filtered by the kidneys at any given moment, as the kidneys process about 200 quarts of blood and clear out about 2 quarts of waste per day. Waste includes excess fluid, minerals, toxic substances such as urea, and substances that cannot be utilized by the body. When the nephrons fail to filter correctly, harmful toxic wastes build up in the body. The waste may then flow back into the bloodstream, causing blood infections. This will also result in retention of excess fluid, increased blood pressure, and a reduction in the number of red blood cells produced.

The filter station of the kidney, the *glomerulus*, is located inside the nephrons and is housed and protected by Bowman's capsule. The tubule that the filtrates flow into from the glomerulus is subdivided into three major parts: the proximal convoluted tubule, or PCT; the loop of Henle, or LOH (also called the loop of the nephron); and the distal convoluted tubule, or DCT. The urine then flows into the collecting duct and finally out of the kidney via the ureters.

FIGURE 28-2 The nephron.

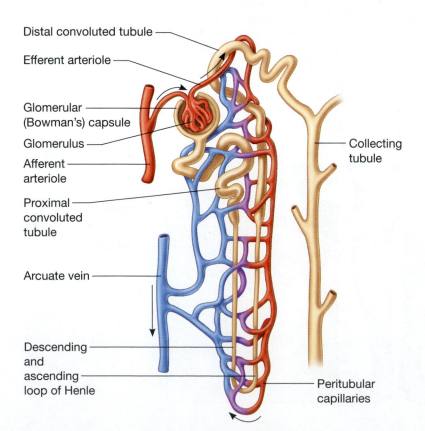

Tubular reabsorption is the means of transporting ions back into the blood. Facilitating the process of transportation and reabsorption is *tubular secretion*, in which ions, acids, and bases are secreted to maintain homeostasis and water balance. Ions are reabsorbed when positively charged sodium (Na^+) cations are exchanged for hydrogen (H^+) cations. The Na^+ returns to the blood; the H^+ cations are secreted in the PCT and the DCT. The mineralocorticoid *aldosterone*, produced by the adrenal cortex, facilitates and regulates the secretion of potassium (K^+) cations in exchange for Na^+ cations in the DCT. When aldosterone gets into the receptors of the distal tubule, it releases K^+ ions which are flushed out of the tubule along with urine into the collecting duct; at this point, Na^+ ions are reabsorbed. This process creates an *osmotic gradient*, in which more sodium ions are in the blood than are in the urine or tubule. This follows the principle that wherever sodium goes, water follows. Therefore, water will follow the sodium ions into the blood, increasing the blood volume. This may exacerbate certain disease states such as congestive heart failure (CHF) or hypertension (HTN).

Tubular secretion serves to eliminate potassium ions, hydrogen ions, weak acids, and weak bases. The carbonic anhydrase system helps to accomplish this and to keep the blood at a proper **pH** (acidity). Carbonic anhydrase (CA) is an enzyme needed to convert carbon dioxide (CO_2) and water (H_2O) into carbonic acid (H_2CO_3), which then rapidly breaks down into hydrogen ions (H^+) and bicarbonate (HCO_3).

pH the measure of acidity or alkalinity of a solution.

When the hydrogen ions are liberated, they become available to acidify urine. This allows the free bicarbonate to be transported or reabsorbed back into the blood, reducing blood acidity by neutralizing the metabolic and toxic wastes. This process raises the blood pH to normal values. Metabolic **acidosis** can occur when CA is blocked. Table 28-1 displays some of the substances found in the nephron and their mechanisms of action.

acidosis excessive acid in the body fluids.

The Bladder and Urine

The capacity of the average adult bladder is approximately 350 mL to 550 mL of urine; about 250 mL triggers a sensation of needing to **void**. Increased volume in the urinary bladder stretches the bladder wall and activates the micturition reflex. After voiding, it is normal to have about 50 mL left in the bladder.

void empty the bladder.

Table 28-1   Actions of Selected Substances in the Nephron

SUBSTANCE	MECHANISM	COMMENTS
water	Reabsorbed by PCT and collecting ducts	Creates osmotic gradient
sodium ions (Na^+)	Reabsorbed by PCT and DCT	Cation exchange for H^+
hydrogen ions (H^+)	Secreted by PCT and DCT	Na^+ and HCO_3 go back into the blood; acidifies urine to less than pH 7
potassium ions (K^+)	Secreted by DCT	Cation exchange for Na^+, when aldosterone receptors are filled with aldosterone
chloride ions (Cl^-)	Reabsorbed by loop of Henle	Na^+ ions follow Cl^- ions
antidiuretic hormone	Released by pituitary gland; opens the pores of the collecting ducts. Water immediately flows toward sodium and is reabsorbed	Decreases the amount of water in urine

Normal urine may vary in color from colorless to dark yellow. Some foods and medications can produce great variations in urine color:

- red—produced by beets, blackberries, rifampin, and some anticoagulants
- orange—produced by phenazopyridine
- green or blue-green—produced by amitriptyline and vitamin B complex
- brown/black—produced by levodopa and iron products

specific gravity a measure of the density of a substance as compared to water; the specific gravity of water is 1.

The **specific gravity** of urine ranges between 1.006 and 1.03. The higher the specific gravity, the higher the concentration of the urine. The specific gravity value will vary, depending on the time of day, amount of food and liquids consumed, and the amount of recent exercise.

The pH of urine is influenced by a number of factors. Generally, a normal urine pH range is from 4.6 to 8, with an average of 6. Usually, there is no detectable urine glucose, urine **ketones**, or urine protein, unless various disease states—notably diabetes—exist. Usually, no red blood cells, white blood cells, hemoglobin, or nitrites are present in urine. Although there may be a trace of **urobilinogen** in the urine, **bilirubin** is normally not detected in the urine.

ketone a by-product of fat metabolism.

urobilinogen substance produced by the breakdown of bilirubin.

bilirubin substance produced by the breakdown of hemoglobin.

Diseases, Conditions, and Treatments of the Urinary System

The urge to urinate varies depending on how much liquid has been consumed and the capacity of the bladder. The first signal occurs when the bladder is about half full. The average person should empty the bladder every three to six hours or four to six times a day. Frequency of urination will vary as a person ages. Usually, the first signal/urge will subside if urination is postponed. As the bladder gets fuller and urination is further delayed, the signal or sensation becomes stronger.

Urinary Incontinence

Certain conditions may cause a person not to be able to hold even half of the bladder's capacity, or not hold the urine long enough to reach a toilet. The inability to hold urine is called *incontinence*; the majority of incontinence occurs in females. There are seven types of incontinence:

- *Stress incontinence*—leakage occurs during exercise, coughing, or laughing.
- *Urge incontinence*—also known as "overactive bladder"; the person has little bladder control, especially when hearing running water, drinking, or sleeping.
- *Overflow incontinence*—occurs when a person cannot completely empty the bladder and there is constant leakage.
- *Functional incontinence*—occurs when a person is not able to get to the toilet in time because of mobility limitations. Functional is the most common form of incontinence in elderly patients.
- *Mixed incontinence*—when a person has more than one form of incontinence, which may or may not be related.
- *Anatomic incontinence*—occurs when a person has a physical abnormality.
- *Temporary incontinence*—may be due to urinary infection or severe constipation, or occur as a side effect of certain medications.

Common causes of incontinence include:

- childbirth, if supportive muscles and nerves of the urethra are damaged
- obesity
- hysterectomy (increases risk of incontinence by 30–40 percent)
- recurrent bladder infections
- medical condition or illness, such as diabetes, lung disease, or stroke

Table 28-2 Drugs Used in the Treatment of Incontinence

GENERIC NAME	TRADE NAME	STRENGTH/DOSAGE FORM(S) AVAILABLE	AVERAGE ADULT DOSAGE
darifenacin hydrobromide	Enablex®	7.5 mg, 15 mg ER tabs	7.5–15 mg once daily
flavoxate HCl	Urispas®	100 mg tab	100–200 mg tid–qid
oxybutynin	Ditropan®	5 mg tab, 5 mg/5mL syrup	5 mg bid–tid
	Ditropan® XL	5 mg, 10 mg, 15 mg tabs	5–30 mg once daily
	Oxytrol®	3.9 mg/day transdermal	1 patch twice weekly
solifenacin succinate	Vesicare®	5 mg, 10 mg tabs	5–10 mg once daily
tolterodine tartrate	Detrol®	1 mg, 2 mg tabs	1–2 mg bid
	Detrol® XL	2 mg, 4 mg XL caps	2–4 mg once daily
trospium chloride	Sanctura®	20 mg tabs	20 mg bid

- drugs, which can relax the bladder too much and permit involuntary urine flow (for example, first-generation, drowsy-formula antihistamines, such as diphenhydramine and chlorpheniramine, as well as some older antidepressants)

Treatment for incontinence will depend on the cause. **Kegel exercises** may be beneficial in controlling urine leakage. Kegel exercises strengthen the muscles of the pelvic floor, thereby improving the urethral sphincter tone and function. Surgery is also available. Medications used to treat stress incontinence are aimed at increasing the contractility of the urethral sphincter muscle.

Kegel exercises pelvic muscle training and toning exercises.

Treatment with medications tends to be most successful in patients with mild to moderate stress incontinence (see Table 28-2). Alpha-adrenergic agonist drugs, such as pseudoephedrine, found in common over-the-counter decongestants, may be used to treat stress incontinence. They work by increasing the strength of the urethral sphincter; in about 50 percent of patients, symptoms improve with this treatment. The tricyclic antidepressant imipramine has similar properties, so it too may be used to treat stress incontinence. Estrogen replacement therapy (ERT) can decrease urinary frequency, urgency, and burning in postmenopausal women. ERT has also been shown to increase the tone of and blood supply to the urethral sphincter muscles. However, the use of estrogen as a treatment for stress incontinence is controversial.

PROFILES IN PRACTICE

A customer arrives at the window of an independent retail pharmacy and explains to the pharmacist that her urine has recently taken on a brownish color. The pharmacist checks the patient's profile and observes that the patient has not gotten any new prescriptions filled. When asked what OTC meds she might be on, the patient states that she is currently taking 81 mg of aspirin, a psyllium laxative, and a multivitamin every day, but also says that she has been taking these medications for quite some time with no problems. However, she recently changed the brand of her multivitamin.

- Could this change account for the discoloration? Why or why not?

Urinary Retention

An inability to urinate is more common in men than in women. When approximately 200–300 mL of urine has collected in the bladder, a signal is sent via nerves in the spinal cord to the brain. The brain then returns a signal that starts contractions or spasms in the bladder wall. At this same moment, the internal sphincter muscle relaxes. With urinary retention, the bladder is not able to release the urine, even though the urge exists. Common causes of urinary retention include:

- Blockage or obstruction of the urethra. The most common cause of urethral blockage in men is enlargement of the prostate gland, called *benign prostatic hypertrophy (BPH)*. The enlarged prostate gland presses against the urethra, blocking the outflow or passage of urine.
- Disruption or damage to the delicate and complex system of nerves that connects the urinary tract with the brain. Common causes include spinal cord injury, spinal cord tumor, herniated disk in the back, or an infection or blood clot that places pressure on the spinal cord.
- Infection in the pelvic area, such as herpes, chlamydia, or pelvic inflammatory disease. The inflammation and swelling that accompany infection can interfere with nerves in the area and/or compress the urethra. Infections of the spinal cord place pressure on the cord, leading to retention because nerve signal transmission is hampered.
- Anesthetic effects during or after surgery. This is a relatively common and temporary cause.
- Other drugs that act to tighten the ureters and block or restrict the flow of urine. These drugs include the ephedrine and pseudoephedrine found in nasal decongestants.

Functional urinary retention is treated with the insertion of a Foley catheter and possibly antibiotics to avoid or treat urinary tract infection. Urinary cholinergics (bethanechol and neostigmine methylsufate) can be used to treat nonfunctional incontinence in postoperative and postpartum patients.

Urinary Tract Infections

Urinary tract infections (UTIs) are bacterial infections of the urinary system. UTIs are most common among women because the distance from the urethra to the anus is shorter in women. UTI symptoms include a frequent urge to void, a burning sensation during voiding, cloudy or strong-smelling urine, and blood in the urine. Two of the most common UTIs are cystitis and pyelonephritis.

Cystitis is an inflammation of the bladder, caused in most cases by *E. coli* and staphylococcus bacteria.

Pyelonephritis is an inflammation of the kidney and upper urinary tract that is usually caused by a bacterial infection of the bladder or cystitis. The backflow of infected urine from the bladder goes up into the ureters and then into the kidney and nephrons.

Pyelonephritis may occur when urine becomes stagnant. In most cases, urine stagnates because of an obstruction of urinary flow caused by a blockage, such as kidney stones, tumors, congenital deformities, or loss of bladder function from nerve disease. When no obstruction is present, the *E. coli* bacterium, normally found in the feces, is the cause of about 80 to 90 percent of acute bladder and kidney infections. Other bacteria that may cause both cystitis and pyelonephritis are *Klebsiella, Enterobacter, Proteus, Pseudomonas,* and *Mycoplasma.*

Symptoms of acute pyelonephritis include sudden onset of fever and chills, burning or frequent urination, aching pain on one or both sides of the lower back or abdomen, nausea and vomiting, cloudy or bloody urine, and fatigue. The flank pain may be extreme. The symptoms of chronic pyelonephritis include HTN, anemia, and protein and blood in the urine.

Approximately 30 percent of all women will experience a urinary tract infection in their lifetimes, as compared with 3 percent of all males. The most common causes of UTI in the male are prostatic enlargement and diabetes. The incidence of UTI in men nears the incidence of UTI in women only in men over 60 years of age. There is evidence that circumcised male neonates have more UTIs than noncircumcised (intact) male neonates.

If left untreated, both cystitis and pyelonephritis can progress to a chronic condition that lasts for months or years and may lead to scarring and possible loss of kidney function. In one study, researchers found that a substance in cranberry juice keeps infection-causing bacteria from attaching to the walls of the urethra. Cranberry juice also makes the urine more acidic.

In addition to treating the infection, phenazopyridine (200 mg tid po) can be used to manage the symptoms of a burning and itching urethra. Treatment of a UTI with phenazopyridine should not exceed two days because there is little or no evidence that the co-administration of phenazopyridine HCl and an antibacterial provides greater benefit than administration of the antibacterial alone after two days. Table 28-3 shows some anti-infectives used to treat UTIs.

Table 28-3 Anti-Infectives for Urinary Tract Infections

GENERIC NAME	TRADE NAME	STRENGTH/DOSAGE FORM(S) AVAILABLE	AVERAGE ADULT DOSE
amoxicillin	Amoxil®, Trimox®	875 mg tabs 250 mg, 500 mg caps 50 mg/mL, 125 mg/5 mL, 200 mg/5 mL, 250 mg/5 mL, 400 mg/5 mL pwd for po susp 200 mg, 400 mg tabs for po susp	500–875 mg q12 hr or 250–500 mg q8 hr
amoxicillin + potassium clavulanate	Augmentin®	250 mg/125 mg, 500 mg/125 mg, 875 mg/125 mg tabs 125 mg/31.25 mg, 200 mg/28.5 mg, 250 mg/62.5 mg, 400 mg/57 mg chew tabs 200 mg/28.5 mg per 5 mL, 250 mg/62.5 mg per 5 mL, 400 mg/57 mg per 5mL powder for oral susp	250–875 mg po q12 hr (based on amoxicillin strength)
	Augmentin® XR	1,000 mg/62.5 mg ER tabs	
	Augmentin® ES-600	600 mg/42.9 mg per 5 mL powder for oral susp	
ampicillin	Principen®	250 mg, 500 mg caps 125 mg/5 mL, 250 mg/5 mL pwd for oral susp	500 mg po q6 hr
		250 mg, 500 mg, 1 g, 2 g pwd for inj	500 mg IV/IM q6 hr
cefaclor	Ceclor®	250, 500 mg caps 125 mg/5 mL, 187 mg/5 mL, 250 mg/5 mL, 375 mg/5 mL pwd for oral susp	250–500 mg q8 hr
	Raniclor®	375 mg, 500 mg ER tabs 125 mg, 187 mg, 250 mg, 375 mg tabs	

Table 28-3   Anti-Infectives for Urinary Tract Infections (*continued*)

GENERIC NAME	TRADE NAME	STRENGTH/DOSAGE FORM(S) AVAILABLE	AVERAGE ADULT DOSE
cefadroxil	Duricef®	500 mg caps 1 g tabs 125 mg/5 mL, 250 mg/5 mL, 500 mg/5 mL pwd for po susp	1–2 g once daily or in 2 divided doses
cephalexin	Keflex®	250 mg, 500 mg caps 250 mg, 500 mg tabs 125 mg/5 mL, 250 mg/5 mL pwd for oral susp	1–4 g daily in divided doses
cephradine	Velosef®	250 mg, 500 mg caps 125 mg/5 mL, 250 mg/5 mL pwd for oral susp	500 mg q12 hr Severe UTI: 500 mg q6 hr or 1,000 mg q12 hr
cepodoxime proxetil	Vantin®	100 mg, 200 mg tabs 50 mg/5 mL, 100 mg/5 mL granules for oral susp	100 mg po q12 hr × 7 days
ciprofloxacin	Cipro®	100 mg, 250 mg, 500 mg, 750 mg tabs 250 mg/5 mL, 500 mg/5 mL pwd for oral susp	100–500 mg po q12 hr × 3 to 14 days
	Cipro® XR	500 mg, 1,000 mg XR tabs	500–1,000 mg q12 hr × 3 to 14 days (XR)
	Cipro® I.V.	200 mg, 400 mg inj	200–1,000 mg IV q12 hr × 7 to 14 days
cinoxacin		250 mg, 500 mg caps	1 g daily in 2 or 4 divided doses for 7 to 14 days
demeclocycline	Declomycin®	150 mg, 300 mg tabs	150 mg qid or 300 mg bid
doxycycline hyclate	Vibra-Tabs® Vibramycin® Doryx®	100 mg tabs 50 mg, 75 mg, 100 mg caps	100 mg bid for at least 7 days
gatifloxacin	Tequin®	200 mg, 400 mg tabs 200 mg/5 mL pwd for po susp 400 mg inj	200–400 mg po or IV once daily for 7 to 10 days
levofloxacin	Levaquin®	250 mg, 500 mg, 750 mg tabs 25 mg/mL oral soln 25 mg/mL inj	250 mg q24 hr po or IV for 3 to 10 days
lomefloxacin	Maxaquin®	400 mg tabs	400 mg daily × 3 to 14 days
nalidixic acid	NegGram®	500 mg caps 250 mg/5 mL susp	1 g qid × 1 to 2 weeks
norfloxacin	Noroxin®	400 mg tabs	400 mg q12 hr × 3 to 28 days, depending on severity
ofloxacin	Floxin®	200 mg, 300 mg, 400 mg tabs	200 mg q12 hr × 3 to 10 days
tetracycline	Sumycin®	250 mg, 500 mg caps 125 mg/5 mL oral susp	500 mg qid for at least 7 days

Table 28-3   Anti-Infectives for Urinary Tract Infections (*continued*)

GENERIC NAME	TRADE NAME	STRENGTH/DOSAGE FORM(S) AVAILABLE	AVERAGE ADULT DOSE
trimethoprim (TMP) + sulfamethoxazole (SMZ)	Bactrim®, Septra®	80 mg/400 mg tabs 160 mg/800 mg DS tabs 40 mg/200 mg per 5 mL susp 16 mg/80 mg per 5mL, 80 mg/400 mg per 5mL inj	160 mg TMP/800 mg SMZ po q12 hr × 10 to 14 days 8–10 mg/kg/day IV (based on TMP strength) in 2 to 4 doses every 6, 8, or 12 hours × 10–14 days

" Workplace Wisdom Common Abbreviations

The abbreviation for sulfamethoxazole is SMZ and the abbreviation for trimethoprim is TMP. "

Other Signs and Symptoms of Renal System Conditions

A person may have many indicators that he or she has a renal system problem; signs and symptoms may include:

- *Anuria*—production or excretion of less than 100 mL of urine per day. If wastes are not eliminated from the body, the person may die from toxemia or septicemia.
- *Dysuria*—difficult or painful urination.
- *Hematuria*—blood in the urine, possibly from an injured kidney or infection.
- *Nephritis*—inflammation of the nephron that causes the tissue of the whole kidney to become inflamed; usually due to infection.
- *Oliguria*—decreased urine production (100–400 mL/day).
- *Pyuria*—pus or bacteria in the urine.
- *Uremia*—urine in the blood.

Kidney Stones

Kidney stones (*urolithiasis*) is a common and painful urinary tract disorder in which solid mineral deposits accumulate in the urinary tract. In addition to possibly obstructing urinary flow, urolithiasis may also lead to UTIs. The pain of "passing" such a blockage or stone is considered excruciating. The mineral masses develop when waste is not completely dissolved in the urine. A microscopic, hard crystal that remains in the kidney is called a *calculus*. The waste substances most commonly found in kidney stones are calcium, oxalate, phosphate, and uric acid.

It is also possible to have solids in the urine because the body does not produce enough water in the urine to dissolve them. In addition, there may be a deficiency of certain chemicals that are normally present in the urine that help break down and dissolve the waste solids. These "helpers" are citrate, magnesium, and pyrophosphate. If calculi obstruct one of the ureters, they can cause the urinary tract to go into a spasm, causing great pain. Large calculi can cause organ damage and even renal failure.

Caucasian males between 30 and 60 years old are the most prone to urolithiasis. Diet plays an important role, as diets high in animal protein increase uric acid levels in the body and can lead to gout and kidney stones. The routine intake of rhubarb, spinach, pepper, cocoa, nuts, or tea can result in excess oxalate in people who have a high level of risk. Dehydration and diarrhea contribute to a lack of water available to dissolve the stones. The following chemical imbalances can contribute to the formation of kidney stones: hypercalcemia, hypernatremia, and hypocitraturia. Also, people who have been diagnosed with hyperthyroidism or hyperparathyroidism are at higher risk, because both conditions allow excess calcium to combine with phosphate or oxalate in the kidneys, resulting in the formation of calculi.

palliative reducing the severity of symptoms.

Treatment of urolithiasis is **palliative**, with pain management, and preventive, with diet consisting of mineral and vitamin supplements and increased fluid intake. Most calculi measure less than $\frac{1}{4}$ inch (4 mm) and spontaneously pass in the urine without need for any treatment. Stones that measure 5 to 7 millimeters can be passed without intervention in about 50 percent of cases. When a stone exceeds 7 millimeters in diameter, however, some form of intervention is usually required.

Pain management depends on the degree of pain. Oral analgesics for mild to moderate pain include diclofenac, acetaminophen with codeine, and propoxyphene HCl. Severe pain requires injections of narcotics such as morphine or meperidine. Because narcotics can cause nausea, vomiting, and diarrhea, it is important not to let the patient get dehydrated if this side effect should occur.

Collection and analysis of the stones can allow the physician to make specific diet and medication recommendations, such as avoiding high-protein and high-fat foods, taking the anti-gout drug allopurinol, increasing fluid intake, and using calcium citrate, magnesium, and cholestyramine to reduce oxalate levels. Taking a potassium citrate supplement or eating citrus fruits increases citrate levels and helps dissolve waste. Taking vitamin B6 supplements helps fight high levels of oxalate. Taking thiazide diuretics may reduce high urinary calcium levels. The patient should avoid decreasing calcium in the diet, as this may lead to the formation of calcium calculi.

Edema and Hypertension

Kidney damage can lead to hypertension, which can then lead to kidney failure. Consistently elevated blood pressure levels can lead to damage of the arteries, in particular, the kidney arteries, which become thickened and narrowed with prolonged high blood pressure. When this happens, less blood gets to the kidneys, resulting in a reduced oxygen supply. Kidney failure can lead to an excess of fluid in the body, peripheral edema, and ascites. This excess fluid places an excessive workload on the heart, raising blood pressure and possibly leading to heart failure or myocardial infarction. Diuretics play an important role in reducing high blood pressure because they reduce the volume of fluid in the body and in the blood. Certain disease states, such as CHF, also require less blood volume.

Diabetes Mellitus and the Kidneys

Diabetes affects many organs of the body, including the eyes, kidneys, and blood vessels. Kidney damage, bladder problems, and UTIs are long-term complications affecting people with diabetes and can lead to renal failure. Diabetic kidney disease (*diabetic nephropathy*) and *end-stage renal disease (ESRD)* require the diabetic person to have either **dialysis** or a kidney transplant. Native Americans and African-Americans are at even higher risk for developing ESRD than diabetics. The warning sign of protein in the urine can trigger early diagnosis and treatment. Familial ESRD, diet, high blood pressure, high blood glucose, and noncompliance are a few of the factors that lead to diabetic nephropathy.

dialysis a medical procedure that removes waste from the blood of patients with renal failure.

Health goals for the diabetic patient include:

- Blood sugar less than 126 mg/dL
- Hemoglobin A1C less than 7
- Blood pressure less than 130/80 mm Hg
- Yearly microalbumin tests to check for protein in the urine

When the glucose in the blood becomes high, the body tries to get rid of the excess sugar by trying to eliminate it in urine. This leads to dehydration and is the reason why diabetics are usually excessively thirsty and urinate frequently. The effects of dehydration depend on the degree of water loss:

- 2% body weight loss reduces performance significantly.
- 5% body weight loss causes heat exhaustion.
- 7% to 10% body weight loss results in heat stroke or death.

Diuretics

Diuretics increase urine output in various ways. Most diuretics inhibit or block sodium absorption by the blood system in the nephron, thus promoting the secretion of sodium. Recall that wherever sodium goes, water follows. Chloride also follows the sodium. The diuresis increases as sodium levels in the tubule increase. See Chapter 26 for a more in-depth look at diuretics.

SUMMARY

The renal system is fairly simple, yet its proper functioning is essential to maintain life. The renal system consists of two kidneys, two ureters, the bladder, and the urethra. The functions of the renal system are to filter waste from the blood and remove it from the body, maintain water and electrolyte balance, and maintain acid-base balance. Any dysfunction of the renal system can have grave impacts on many parts of the body. Kidney damage can lead to hypertension, muscle problems, and serious cardiac disorders.

Common diseases of the renal system include urinary retention or urinary incontinence, kidney stones, and urinary tract infections. Approximately 30 percent of all women will experience a UTI in their lifetimes.

The two drugs most commonly used to treat diseases of the renal system are anti-infectives and diuretics. This chapter contains a thorough discussion of the importance of the renal system in maintaining homeostasis, the incidence of diseases of the urinary tract, and the drug therapies available to treat these conditions.

CHAPTER REVIEW QUESTIONS

1. The main function of the urinary system is to:
   a. remove urine from the body.
   b. filter waste from the body.
   c. maintain water balance.
   d. all of the above.

2. The filter station of the kidney is the:
   a. nephrons.
   b. glomerulus.
   c. loop of Henle.
   d. distal convoluted tubule.

3. Urinary tract infections can be treated with:
   a. amoxicillin.
   b. sulfamethoxazole and trimethoprim.
   c. cephalexin.
   d. all of the above.

4. An inflammation of the kidney is:
   a. nephritis.
   b. pyelonephritis.
   c. cystitis.
   d. urolithiasis.

5. _____ is a condition of blood in the urine.
   a. Uremia
   b. Pyuria
   c. Dysuria
   d. Hematuria

6. An inflammation of the bladder is:
   a. nephritis.
   b. pyelonephritis.
   c. cystitis.
   d. urolithiasis.

7. Kidney stones are also known as:
   a. phlebitis.
   b. pyelonephritis.
   c. cystitis.
   d. urolithiasis.

8. _____ is a condition of urine in the blood.
   a. Uremia
   b. Pyuria
   c. Dysuria
   d. Hematuria

9. A patient with urolithiasis should:
   a. avoid high-fat foods.
   b. increase fluid intake.
   c. avoid a high-protein diet.
   d. all of the above.

10. Uremia is:
    a. painful urination.
    b. blood in the urine.
    c. urine in the blood.
    d. decreased production of urine.

11. Which of the following is used to treat urinary incontinence?
    a. furosemide
    b. chlorthalidone
    c. tolterodine
    d. bumetanide

12. The abbreviation for sulfamethoxazole is:
    a. SMZ.
    b. SMT.
    c. SMX.
    d. SMO.

13. Hematuria is:
    a. painful urination.
    b. blood in the urine.
    c. urine in the blood.
    d. decreased production of urine.

14. Which of the following is also known as "overactive bladder"?
    a. functional incontinence
    b. stress incontinence
    c. urge incontinence
    d. mixed incontinence

15. Which of the following groups is more likely to develop urolithiasis?
    a. African-American females
    b. African-American males
    c. Caucasian females
    d. Caucasian males

CRITICAL THINKING QUESTIONS

1. Explain why women are much more likely than men to develop urinary tract infections.

2. Explain why it is so important to the body that the kidneys work properly. What can happen if the kidneys are not working properly?

3. What causes (other than those listed in this chapter) can contribute to incontinence?

WEB CHALLENGE

1. Go to http://kidney.niddk.nih.gov/kudiseases/pubs/yoururinary/index.htm to learn more about how the kidneys work.

2. Choose one of the conditions discussed in this chapter. Go online and research alternative methods of treatment for the condition.

REFERENCES AND RESOURCES

Adams, MP, Josephson, DL, & and Holland, LN Jr. *Pharmacology for Nurses—A Pathophysiologic Approach*. Upper Saddle River, NJ: Pearson Education, 2008.

"Circumcision and Urinary Tract Infection" (accessed April 8, 2008): http://www.cirp.org/library/disease/UTI

"Control of the hydrogen ion activity (pH) in the body" (accessed April 8, 2008): http://www.usyd.edu.au/su/anaes/lectures/acidbase_mjb/control.html

Drug Facts and Comparisons, 2006 ed. St. Louis: Wolters Kluwer Health.

Health Ask the Doctor BBC (accessed April 8, 2008): http:// www.bbc.co.uk/health/ask_doctor/cystitis_cranberry.shtml

Holland, N, & Adams, MP. *Core Concepts in Pharmacology*. Upper Saddle River, NJ: Pearson Education, 2007.

National Institute of Diabetes and Digestive and Kidney Diseases (NIDDK), NIH: http://diabetes.niddk.nih.gov/

"Types of Urinary Incontinence" (accessed July 24, 2007): www.mayoclinic.org

Whorton, JC. *Nature Cures: The History of Alternative Medicine in America*. New York: Oxford University Press, 2004.

The Endocrine System

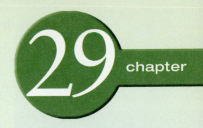

29 chapter

LEARNING OBJECTIVES

After completing this chapter, you should be able to:

- Identify and describe the glands of the endocrine system.
- Describe the functions of the hypothalamus and pituitary gland, and list other body parts that are affected by these glands.
- List and define the hormones of the endocrine system and know which gland or organ secretes each hormone.
- Describe male and female hormones and some products used for replacement in cases of deficiency of these hormones.
- Identify and describe the major diseases and conditions that affect the endocrine system.
- Compare and contrast diabetes mellitus and diabetes insipidus.
- Understand the effects of anabolic steroid use.

Introduction

The endocrine system is a collection of glands that produce hormones to help regulate the body's growth, metabolism, and sexual development and function. In fact, hormones, which are transported to tissues and organs throughout the body, influence every cell in some way. Because the glands of the endocrine system are ductless, the hormones they secrete are released directly into the bloodstream, and travel through the circulatory system to reach the specific target organs where they exert their primary effects.

The nervous system is considered the mass communicator of the human body, and hormones are the chemicals that do the communicating. *Endocrinology* is the study of the chemical communication system that controls a large number of physiologic processes. It is also the study of hormones, their receptors, and the intracellular signaling pathways that they follow and call upon. As mentioned, all cell types, organs, and processes are influenced by hormone signaling, though some more strongly than others. Growth from birth to adulthood involves the endocrine system, critical growth hormones, and other contributing hormones.

Anatomy of the Endocrine System

The endocrine system (see Figure 29-1) is an internal "communication" system that consists of the hypothalamus, pituitary gland, other hormone-producing cells and glands, hormones, and receptors. The major driving forces of the endocrine system are the hypothalamus and the pituitary gland. The pituitary gland controls the thyroid, parathyroid, pancreas, adrenal glands, and gonads. During pregnancy, the placenta also acts as an endocrine gland.

The *hypothalamus*, part of the brain stem, controls the activity of the pituitary gland. Also known as the *hypophysis*, the *pituitary gland* is only about the size of a large pea, but it is called the "master gland" because it controls many of the other glands. Attached to the base of the hypothalamus in the brain, the pituitary gland is composed of an anterior lobe and a posterior lobe. Each lobe contains a number of hormones, which may be released into the general blood circulation.

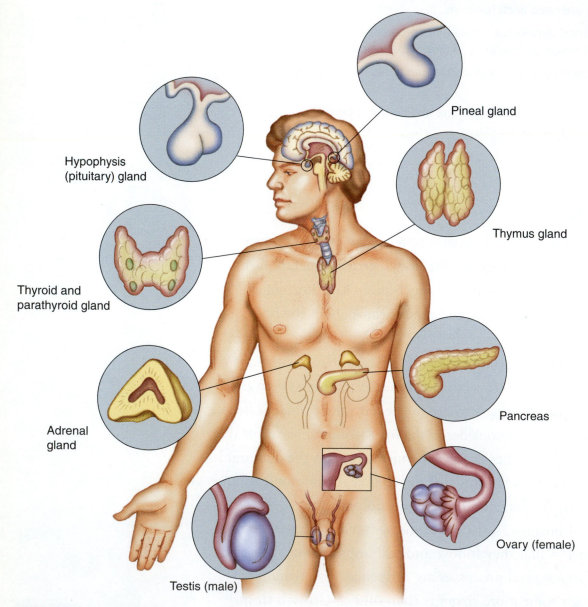

Pineal gland

Hypophysis
(pituitary) gland

Thymus gland

Thyroid and
parathyroid gland

Adrenal
gland

Pancreas

Testis (male)

Ovary (female)

FIGURE 29-1 The endocrine glands.

Some parts of the endocrine system also secrete substances other than hormones. The pancreas, for example, secretes digestive enzymes. The testes and ovaries secrete ova and sperm. Organs such as the stomach, heart, and intestines are involved in hormone production, too, but this is not their primary function.

Hormones

Hormones are the chemicals that take "messages" to the cells through the bloodstream. Hormones transfer information and instructions from one set of cells to another. Each hormone affects only the cells that are genetically programmed to receive and respond to its message. Many factors can affect the level of hormones in the body at any given time. Age, stress, infection, and changes in the balance of fluid and minerals in blood are only a few examples.

hormone a chemical substance, produced by an organ or gland, that travels through the bloodstream to regulate certain bodily functions and/or the activity of other organs and glands.

Hormones are divided into two groups according to their structure:

1. Steroids
   - slow-acting
   - long-lasting
   - names usually end in "rone" (e.g., testosterone, progesterone)
2. Peptides and amines
   - made of proteins
   - fast-acting
   - short-lived
   - include insulin and ADH, among others

Hormone production is controlled by feedback. *Feedback control* depends on a monitoring of supply and demand. When the level of hormone is low, the gland secretes the hormone until the level rises again. When there is a large supply of the hormone, the gland stops making it.

The Endocrine Glands

This section briefly describes each of the glands in the endocrine system.

Hypothalamus

The *hypothalamus* controls many body functions, especially a number important to the female menstrual cycle, pregnancy, birth, and lactation. With regard to the nervous system, the hypothalamus mainly functions to keep the body in **homeostasis**. Dynamic vital statistics such as blood pressure, body temperature, fluid and electrolyte balance, and body weight are held to a given, predetermined value called the *set point*. Although this set point can change over time, from day to day it is generally fixed.

homeostasis a stable and constant environment.

One of the functions of the hypothalamus in achieving and maintaining homeostasis is to control the activity of the pituitary gland. The hypothalamus produces hormones known as *releasing factors*. These are sent to the pituitary gland via small blood vessels, which connect the hypothalamus to the anterior lobe of the pituitary gland. The releasing factors stimulate the release of hormones that are produced in the anterior lobe.

The hormones of the anterior lobe are known as *tropic hormones*. *Tropic* means "growth." The tropic hormones are released into the general blood circulation to control the activities of the other endocrine glands. Sometimes these hormones are called *stimulating hormones* because they stimulate other glands either to produce other hormones or to perform an activity.

The hypothalamus also produces oxytocin and antidiuretic hormone (ADH), two hormones that are stored in the posterior lobe of the pituitary gland. The posterior lobe, also known as the *neurohypophysis*, sits behind the anterior lobe and is actually a continuation of the hypothalamus.

negative feedback the process by which the body is able to return to homeostasis.

The mechanism that controls the release of tropic or stimulating hormones from the anterior pituitary gland is known as **negative feedback**. For example, the thyroid-releasing factor stimulates the release of thyroid-stimulating hormone (TSH), which in turn stimulates the thyroid gland to release the hormone thyroxine (also known as thyroid hormone). As a result, the concentration of thyroxine in the blood increases. When the thyroid hormone concentration rises above normal, this signals the hypothalamus to stop sending releasing factor. Because no releasing factor is sent to the pituitary gland, the pituitary gland does not send out any more TSH and the thyroid gland does not produce more thyroxine. Therefore, these mechanisms are *inhibited*.

Here is another example of the mechanism of negative feedback: After receiving a releasing factor from the hypothalamus, the anterior pituitary gland releases follicle-stimulating hormone (FSH) in response. This FSH from the anterior pituitary gland stimulates the maturation of an egg in the ovary. When the egg has matured, the ovary releases negative feedback to the hypothalamus, telling the brain that the activity has been completed. The hypothalamus responds by *not* sending any more releasing factor to the anterior pituitary gland. In turn, the inhibition of the releasing factor causes the anterior pituitary gland to stop sending FSH to the ovary.

In short, the hypothalamus sends out releasing factors, or releasing hormones (RHs), to the pituitary gland, which responds by sending out tropic, or stimulating, hormones (TH). Some of the important pairings are:

1. Thyroid releasing hormone (TRH) stimulates thyroid-stimulating hormone (TSH).
2. Corticotropin releasing hormone (CRH) stimulates adrenocorticotropin (ACTH).
3. Growth hormone releasing hormone (GHRH) stimulates growth hormone (GH).
4. Somatostatin inhibits GH.
5. Gonadotropin releasing hormone (GNRH) stimulates both luteinizing hormone (LH) and follicle-stimulating hormone (FSH).

Pituitary Gland

The anterior pituitary gland secretes hormones that regulate the activities of the other endocrine glands (see Figure 29-2). All of the hormones stimulate a specific endocrine gland, except the growth hormone (GH), or *somatotropin,* which regulates the growth and maintenance of all body tissues. An excess of GH in a child results in gigantism; a lack or deficiency results in pituitary dwarfism. *Acromegaly* results when the lack of growth hormone occurs in an adult. If this happens, parts of the body grow to be unusually large, such as the head, hands, feet, jaw, arms, and legs.

The pituitary gland sends a signal to the respective gland or body part to initiate its glandular functions:

1. TSH stimulates the thyroid gland (thyroid hormone production).
2. FSH/LH stimulate the gonads (gametogenesis and steroid production).
3. Growth hormone is sent to all body parts for linear growth and intermediate metabolism.
4. ACTH is sent to the adrenal glands to cause growth of the adrenal cortex and synthesis and secretion of cortisol.
5. Prolactin stimulates the mammary glands to produce milk during and after pregnancy.

Classes of pituitary hormones and their other, more technical names are as follows:

1. Somatomammotrophs
   a. Somatotrophs—GH or somatotropin
   b. Mammotrophs—also called lactotrophs, PRL

2. Glycoproteins
   a. Thyrotrophs—TSH or thyrotropin
   b. Gonadotrophs—LH and FSH
   c. Corticotrophs—ACTH or corticotropin
   d. Pro-opiomelanocortin (POMC)—ACTH,
      LPH, endorphins (not described in this book)

Thyroid and Parathyroid

The *thyroid* is a small gland, weighing less than one ounce, located in the front of the neck. It is made up of two lobes that lie along the windpipe and are joined together by a narrow band of tissue called the *isthmus*. The thyroid is directly regulated by the anterior pituitary gland and indirectly regulated by the hypothalamus.

Two types of cells make up the thyroid tissue: follicular cells and parafollicular cells. The majority of the thyroid tissue consists of the *follicular cells*, which secrete iodine-containing hormones called thyroxine (T4) and triiodothyronine (T3). The *parafollicular cells* secrete the hormone calcitonin.

The normal thyroid gland produces about 80 percent T4 and about 20 percent T3; however, T3 possesses about four times the hormone "strength" of T4. When the level of thyroid hormones drops too low, the pituitary gland produces thyroid-stimulating hormone (TSH), which stimulates the thyroid gland to produce more hormones.

The thyroid gland needs iodine to produce these hormones. Thyroid cells are the only cells in the body that can absorb iodine. The richest sources of iodine are seafood and seaweed (especially kelp). In the United States, the primary source of iodine is iodized salt. Thyroid cells combine iodine and the amino acid tyrosine to make T3 and T4. T3 and T4 are then released into the bloodstream and are transported throughout the body, where they control metabolism. Every cell in the body depends on thyroid hormones for regulation of metabolism. The thyroid gland is also responsible for the enhancement of growth and development and for nervous system maturation in children.

The thyroid is a very important gland that affects parts of the body and functions that regulate growth, such as:

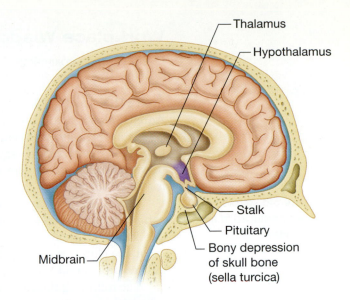

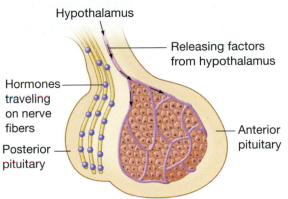

FIGURE 29-2 The pituitary gland.

- Thermogenesis—T4 and T3 produce heat by increasing the body's oxidative metabolism. This is accomplished by the synthesis of Na$^+$/K$^+$ ATPase.

- Growth and development—T4 and T3 are essential for growth in childhood. T4 and T3 stimulate growth by exerting a direct effect on tissue and a permissive effect on growth hormone action.

- Nervous system—in childhood, T4 and T3 are essential for normal myelination and development of the nervous system. Thyroid deficiency in childhood causes mental retardation. In adults, T4 and T3 deficiency causes lethargy and blunting of intellect. T4 and T3 excess causes restlessness and hypersensitivity.

- Heart—excess T4 and T3 can increase heart stroke volume and heart rate by increasing the heart's sensitivity to catecholamines. A deficiency of T4 and T3 has the opposite effect.

Adrenal Glands

Adrenal glands are located on the upper part of each kidney (see Figure 29-3). These glands have an inner or center part known as the *adrenal medulla* and an outer part known as the *adrenal cortex*. The adrenal medulla, which is part of the sympathetic nervous system, secretes epinephrine (EPI) during sympathetic activation. Epinephrine is a catecholamine.

corticosteroid steroidal hormones produced in the adrenal cortex.

The adrenal cortex secretes two types of **corticosteroids** or hormones: *gluco-corticoids* and *mineralocorticoids*. The hormones of the adrenal cortex, the adrenocorticosteroids, are generally referred to as *corticosteroids* or simply *steroids*. As a pharmacological agent, the glucocorticoids, or glucocorticosteroids, are used frequently in the treatment of inflammatory or allergic conditions, such as arthritis or bee sting.

The following three factors induce the hypothalamus to secrete the releasing factor called *adrenocorticotropin (ACTH)*:

- Sleep-wake cycle—larger amounts of adrenocorticotropin (from the anterior pituitary gland) and cortisol (a glucocorticoid from the adrenal gland) are secreted while a person is awake. Smaller amounts of these hormones are present during sleep. During the wake period, cortisol requires body metabolism to meet the requirements of this active period. Cortisol is a natural anti-inflammatory substance.

- Stress—occurs when the body is subjected to increased demands of physical or mental exertion. Stress may be induced by cold weather, exercise, infections, burns, surgery, and anxiety. Stress produces an increase in ACTH, which stimulates the adrenal gland to increase secretion of cortisol. High amounts of cortisol increase the body's ability to cope with the demands of stress.

- Negative feedback—the releasing factor and ACTH stimulate the secretion and return of cortisol into the bloodstream. When the level of cortisol rises above normal, negative feedback begins, which stops the secretion of releasing factors from the hypothalamus to the anterior pituitary gland, which in turn stops further release of ACTH. This in turn stops the signal to the adrenal gland to release cortisol. The end result is that cortisol secretion is inhibited.

Glucocorticoids

The glucocorticoids regulate the metabolism of carbohydrates and proteins, especially during stress. Metabolism is a chemical breakdown. Carbohydrates are sugars and starches, which are metabolized into simple sugars (monosaccharides). During periods of stress involving body injury, trauma, surgery, or wound healing, there is an increased requirement for glucose. Healing wounds and tissues in need of repair use more glucose than normal, and use glucose almost exclusively during repair stages.

Inflammation is considered the first step in the process of wound healing, as immune system mediators come to the rescue after an injury. However, sometimes the normal inflammatory response gets overworked, as in an acute inflammatory reaction; or it becomes continual or is prolonged, as in a chronic inflammatory reaction. In

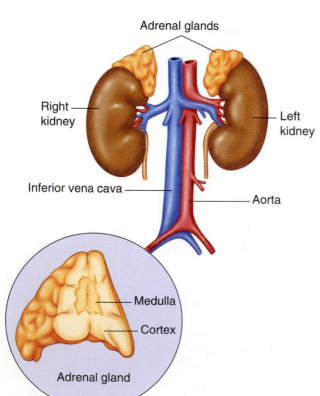

Adrenal glands

Right kidney

Left kidney

Inferior vena cava

Aorta

Medulla

Cortex

Adrenal gland

FIGURE 29-3 The adrenal glands.

this situation, inflammation becomes a disease in itself. Inflammation is also present in various types of allergic reactions, asthma, and anaphylactic shock. Therefore, the glucocorticoids are useful in treating these conditions. The glucocorticoids have potent anti-inflammatory effects. The synthetic glucocorticoids are frequently used to treat inflammatory and allergic conditions because they have a longer duration of action than naturally occurring adrenocorticosteroids.

Although some topical steroids are available over the counter, the higher strengths (all po forms) are available by prescription only. The topical preparations are specifically labeled for temporary relief. They can be used for relief of minor skin irritations, itching, dermatitis, rashes, eczema, insect bites, poison ivy, reactions to cosmetics (perfumes) and detergents, and itching in the anal and genital regions. Glucocorticoids are also given via the IM and IV routes.

Mineralocorticoids

The main function and purpose of mineralocorticoids is to regulate the *electrolyte*, or salt and fluid, balance of the body. Mineralocorticoids are essential for life. Therefore, a deficiency requires replacement therapy so that the patient will not dehydrate, to maintain pH balance in the body, and to assist the electrical functions and processes in the body.

The most important mineralocorticoid is *aldosterone*. The site of action of aldosterone is in the distal tubules of the nephrons in the kidneys (refer to Figure 28-2 for an illustration of the nephron). Nephrons are the smallest working unit (cell) of the kidneys. The hormone aldosterone increases the reabsorption of sodium ions. *Reabsorption* means that the sodium leaves the tubule and returns to the blood supply. During this process, there is an exchange of potassium ions for sodium ions. The potassium cations are led into the nephron tubule and transported into the urine.

Water also is reabsorbed with sodium. Consequently, normal sodium and water levels are maintained in the blood and other body tissues, which are **isotonic**.

Table 29-1 gives examples of glucocorticoids and mineralocorticoids.

isotonic having the same salt concentration as that of blood.

> ## Workplace Wisdom Fludrocortisone
>
> Fludrocortisone is a therapeutic gonadal hormone used to treat Addison's disease and salt-losing adrenogenital syndrome.

Gonads

Gonadotropin releasing hormone (GnRH) is the hormone released by the hypothalamus that precipitates the onset of sexual maturity in both males and females. GnRH is needed for both sexual maturity and normal reproduction. It acts by stimulating the release of luteinizing hormone (LH) and follicle-stimulating hormone (FSH) from the anterior

Table 29-1 Examples of Glucocorticoids and Mineralocorticoids

TRADE NAME	GENERIC NAME
Glucocorticoids	
Aristocort®, Kenalog®	triamcinolone
Celestone®	betamethasone
Cortef®, Hydrocortone®, Corticaine®	hydrocortisone
Decadron®, Hexadrol®	dexamethasone
Deltasone®, Destasone®, Orasone®	prednisone
Medrol®, Solu-Medrol® (inj)	methylprednisolone
Mineralocorticoids	
Florinef®	fludrocortisone

gonads testes and ovaries.

pituitary. LH and FSH act by stimulating the production of sex hormones in the **gonads**, known as *testes* in males and *ovaries* in females.

Both LH and FSH are responsible for the development and secretion of sex hormones and the development of sex organs and secondary sex characteristics. *Secondary sex characteristics* are physical features that start to develop at puberty and serve to distinguish males from females. The primary sex characteristics are the genitals.

Female Sex Hormones

The sex hormones of the female are estrogen and progesterone. *Estrogen* is responsible for the development of secondary sex characteristics, as well as the formation of osteoblasts, inhibition of osteoclasts, and bone loss. *Progesterone* prepares the lining of the uterus for the implantation of a fertilized egg (ovum).

Two additional pituitary hormones are involved in childbirth. *Oxytocin,* secreted by the posterior pituitary gland, but made by the hypothalamus, stimulates the uterus to start contracting at the beginning of labor. *Prolactin* signals the mammary glands to start producing milk.

Male Sex Hormones

Male sex hormones, or *androgens,* are also known as the *masculinizing hormones.* The main sex hormone of the male, *testosterone,* is produced in the testes. The major functions of testosterone are to stimulate the development of male sex organs and to maintain the secondary sex characteristics of the male.

Men also require *progesterone,* produced in the adrenal gland and testes. This hormone plays an integral part in maintaining a healthy prostate.

Table 29-2 is a list of the endocrine glands, the hormones each gland secretes, and the main function of each hormone.

Estrogen Replacement Therapy and Menopause

After menopause, estrone is the most active circulating estrogen; at that point, it is made in the adrenal glands only. Estrogen replacement therapy is, literally, the replacement of estrogen for postmenopausal women (see Table 29-3). It is prescribed for symptomatic treatment of the common symptoms associated with menopause, such as hot flashes and vaginal dryness; the prevention of bone fractures associated with osteoporosis; reduction of the risk of heart attacks and strokes; and to treat excessive and painful uterine bleeding. Topical or vaginal estrogen creams are prescribed for vaginal or vulvar atrophy associated with menopause.

Estrogens reduce LDL cholesterol and increase HDL cholesterol in the blood. When taken alone or in combination with a progestin (synthetic progesterone), estrogens have been shown to reduce the risk of myocardial infarction and stroke by 40–50 percent. In addition, they have bone-promoting effects, which means that they reduce the risk for hip and knee fracture from osteoporosis by 20–30 percent.

However, estrogens used in replacement therapy have also been associated with an increased risk of liver disease, through an unknown mechanism, in patients receiving dantrolene. Women over 35 years of age and those with a history of liver disease are especially at risk. Estrogens increase the liver's ability to manufacture clotting factors, and those taking warfarin must have blood monitored for reduction of the blood-thinning effect. Blood clots are occasional, but serious, side effects of estrogen therapy and are dose-related; that is, they occur more frequently in patients taking higher doses. Cigarette smokers are at higher risk than nonsmokers. Therefore, patients requiring estrogen therapy are *strongly* encouraged to quit smoking.

Estrogens can cause a buildup of the uterine lining (*endometrial hyperplasia*) and increase the risk of endometrial carcinoma. The addition of a progestin to estrogen therapy has been shown to prevent endometrial cancer from developing. There are conflicting data regarding an association between estrogen and breast cancer. It is not known at this time if the addition of a progestin to ERT reduces the risk of breast cancer, as it does for uterine cancer. There is no evidence that estrogens are effective for nervous symptoms

Table 29-2 Endocrine Glands and Secreted Hormones

ENDOCRINE GLAND	HORMONE SECRETED	HORMONE FUNCTION
Adrenal (cortex)		
	aldosterone	Maintains sodium and water balance
	cortisol	Increases blood glucose levels
	gonadocorticoids (androgens & estrogens)	Develops gender characteristics
Adrenal (medulla)		
	epinephrine, norepinephrine	Prepares body for action in emergencies
Ovaries		
	estrogen	Develops female sex/ reproductive characteristics
	progesterone	Prepares uterine lining for pregnancy
Pancreas		
	glucagon	Raises blood sugar level
	insulin	Lowers blood sugar level
Parathyroid		
	parathyroid hormone	Increases blood calcium levels
Pineal		
	melatonin	Affects daily physiologic cycles & reproductive development
Pituitary (anterior lobe)		
	growth hormone	Stimulates the growth of muscles, bones, and organs; influences height
	thyroid stimulating hormone (TSH)	Stimulates thyroid to secrete thyroid hormones
	adrenocorticotropic hormone (ACTH, corticotropin)	Stimulates secretion of cortical hormones of the adrenal gland
	gonadotropic hormones	Regulate the development of the gonads
	prolactin	Initiates and maintains milk production
	follicle-stimulating hormone (FSH)	Stimulates the growth of ovary follicles
	luteinizing hormone (LH)	Stimulates ovulation
Pituitary (posterior lobe)		
	antidiuretic hormone (ADH)	Promotes reabsorption of water in kidneys
	oxytocin	Stimulates contraction of uterus and release of breast milk
Testes		
	testosterone	Develops male sex/ reproductive characteristics

Table 29-2 Endocrine Glands and Secreted Hormones (*continued*)

ENDOCRINE GLAND	HORMONE SECRETED	HORMONE FUNCTION
Thyroid		
	thyroid hormone	Affects growth, maturation, and metabolism
	calcitonin	Reduces blood calcium levels
Other Organs with Hormone Secretion		
Gastric Mucosa		
	gastrin	Stimulates the production of gastrin and hydrochloric acid
Heart		
	atriopeptin	Involved in homeostasis of body water, sodium, and fat
Placenta		
	human chorionic gonadotropin	Signals ovaries to secrete hormones to maintain uterine lining
Small Intestine Mucosa		
	secretin	Regulates pH levels
	cholecystokinin	Stimulates contraction of gallbladder
Thymus Gland		
	thymosin	Involved in immune system development

or depression that might occur during menopause. Estrogens increase the incidence of gallbladder disease and abnormal blood clotting. Indications for estrogen include:

- moderate to severe vasomotor symptoms associated with menopause
- atrophic vaginitis
- kraurosis vulvae—atrophy and shrinkage of the skin of the vagina and vulva
- female hypogonadism
- hysterectomy
- primary ovarian failure
- breast cancer, for palliative therapy only in appropriately selected women and men with metastatic disease
- prostatic carcinoma (palliative therapy of advanced disease)

Estrogen is contraindicated in women with:

- undiagnosed abnormal genital bleeding
- known, suspected, or history of cancer of the breast, except in appropriately selected patients being treated for metastatic disease
- known or suspected estrogen-dependent neoplasia
- history of deep vein thrombosis or pulmonary embolism
- active or recent (within the past year) arterial thromboembolic disease, such as stroke or MI
- liver dysfunction or disease
- known hypersensitivity to ingredients of the particular estrogenic formula
- known or suspected pregnancy

Table 29-3   Replacement Therapy Choices

	TRADE NAME	DOSAGE	COMMENTS
From Natural Sources			
Animal-derived estrogen replacements have been considered more natural than plant-derived estrogens.	Premarin® (conjugated animal estrogen)	0.3 mg, 0.625 mg, 1.25 mg, and 2.5 mg tabs—1 qd; NTE 2.4 mg per day	Extracted from pregnant mares' urine; contains a mixture of different estrogens
		Vaginal cream: 1 app of 0.5 g to 1 g per day	Cream for short-term use for atrophic vaginitis or kraurosis vulvae
		Inj: 25 mg q6 hr prn hemorrhage	Injection for abnormal interuterine bleeding
From Plant Sources			
Plant-derived estrogens are chemically identical to animal estrogen made by the ovaries.	Estrace®		Estradiol is the most potent form of estrogen in premenopausal women
	Estrasorb®	Apply two 1.74 mg packets to calf or thigh/day	Topical estradiol emulsion
	Estrogel®	Applied once daily on one arm from wrist to shoulder	Estradiol gel avoids first-pass metabolism in the liver and minimizes application-site skin irritation; gel dries in as little as 2 to 5 min
	ESTRING® (estradiol)	Soft, flexible vaginal ring with 2 mg estradiol delivery system; placed in the upper third of the vagina by the physician or the patient; worn continuously for 90 days, then removed and replaced if therapy is to be continued	Discontinue during treatment for vaginal infection with vaginal antimicrobial therapy. May not be suitable for women with narrow, short, or stenosed (constricted) vaginas, and prolapse (who are more prone to irritation from a tight-fitting ring), or those with symptoms of vaginal irritation.
	Alora® (estradiol transdermal system)	Apply 0.025 mg/day twice a week to hips, abdomen, or thigh, NTE 1 mg/day twice a week	Continuous delivery for twice-weekly dosing; applied to abdomen, hips, and thigh: 6.5, 12.5, 18.75, and 25.0 cm^2
	Climara® TDP (transdermal patch)	Apply 1 TDP q week to abdomen, buttocks, inner thigh, upper arm, or hips as directed	
Plant-derived progesterones are chemically identical to animal progestins made by the ovaries.	Prometrium® (progesterone)		
Lab-Modified Estrogens			
Plant-derived estrogens that have been chemically modified in a laboratory and are therefore not truly "natural."	Cenestin®	0.625 mg tabs, NTE 1.25 mg qd	Conjugated plant estrogens Treatment of vasomotor symptoms due to menopause. Dosages for other conditions may vary.
	Ogen® Ortho-est®	1 0.625 mg (0.75 mg estropipate) tablet to 2 × 2.5 mg tabs daily	Estrone estropipate
	Estratab®	Avail: 0.3–1.25 mg tabs, 1 tab qd, NTE 1.25 mg/day	Esterified estrogens: Dosage varies per patient and condition/indication
	Menest®		Given cyclically for short-term use only

Table 29-3 Replacement Therapy Choices (*continued*)

	TRADE NAME	DOSAGE	COMMENTS
Synthetic progesterones are known as progestins.	Aygestin® (norethindrone acetate)	5 mg tab	Lab-created progestins: Dosing varies per indication: amenorrhea, uterine cancer, endometriosis
	Provera®, Depo-Provera® (medroxyprogesterone acetate (MPA)	2.5 mg, 5 mg, 10 mg tabs Contraceptive inj: 1 mL × 150 mg/90 days	Contraceptive injection
	Cycrin® (MPA)	2.5 mg, 5 mg, 10 mg tabs	
Combination synthetic progesterone and animal estrogens	Prempro®	1 tab qd	Combines norethindrone acetate or MPA with Premarin®.
	Premphase®	1 maroon tab qd days 1–14, then 1 blue tab days 15–28	Dosage varies with indications: postmenopausal vasomotor symptoms, prevention of osteoporosis
Combination synthetic progesterone and plant estrogens	Activella® (estradiol/norethindrone acetate)	1 tablet daily (1 mg/0.5 mg)	Prevention of osteoporosis, vasomotor menopausal symptoms

━━━━━ INFORMATION ━━━━━

In conjunction with their physician, each patient must weigh the risks and benefits before starting hormone replacement therapy.

- Risks: Estrogen increases the risk of blood clots, gallbladder disease, uterine cancers, and breast cancer.
- Benefits: Relief from frequent hot flashes is achieved with estrogen hormonal treatment. *Hot flashes* are sudden episodes of increased uncomfortable warmth, skin flushing, and sweating, which occur in about 70 percent of women during menopause. These hot flashes are sometimes severe enough to cause insomnia, fatigue, and irritability.

Testosterone Hormonal Replacement

Testosterone also produces an anabolic effect that promotes the synthesis and retention of proteins, for muscle and bone, in the body. The more testosterone there is, the easier it is for the body to build muscle, and the more muscle can be built. In some diseases, muscle will atrophy or become weak. Pharmaceutical anabolic steroids can help the patient with such a disease to rebuild muscle tissue; in addition, they promote weight gain after surgery, trauma, or serious infection (see Table 29-4). Unfortunately, overuse of the steroids (as evidenced by illegal use for athletic performance enhancement) can cause some irreversible effects.

The FDA has approved pharmaceutical steroids for the following uses:

- weight gain for chronic nutritional deficiencies or wasting syndromes, such as those in cancer or AIDS patients
- relief of bone pain associated with osteoporosis
- corticosteroid-induced catabolism
- hereditary angioedema
- severe antimetastatic breast cancer in women
- hypogonadism (hormonal replacement for hormonal deficiency states in males)
- to stimulate the beginning of puberty in certain boys who are late starting puberty naturally
- cryptorchidism (failure of one or both testicles to descend)

Table 29-4   Androgens

TRADE NAME	GENERIC NAME
Androderm®, Testoderm TTS®	testosterone; transdermal patches (abdomen, back, thigh, and arm)
Androgel®, Testim®	testosterone; topical gel applied to shoulders, upper arms, and/or abdomen
Delatestryl®	testosterone (parenteral) for testosterone replacement therapy
Halotestin®	fluoxymesterone (oral tablets)
Oreton®	methyltestosterone (oral capsules)
Oxandrin®	oxandrolone for AIDS wasting syndrome (oral tablets); for bone pain, weight gain, postsurgery/ trauma, corticosteroid-induced protein catabolism
Testoderm®	testosterone; transdermal patches (scrotal)
Winstrol®	stanozolol (oral tablets); anabolic androgen for angioedema

Angioedema is an autosomal-dominant disorder characterized by recurring episodes of swelling of the face, extremities, genitalia, bowel wall, and upper respiratory tract. It is caused by deficient or nonfunctional C1 esterase inhibitor (C1 INH). Stanozolol cannot stop, but can prevent, slow the frequency of, and control the severity of attacks of angioedema and can increase blood serum levels of C1 INH and C4.

Anemia caused by the administration of myelotoxic drugs, as well as acquired aplastic anemia, congenital aplastic anemia, and myelofibrosis, may respond to androgens. Oxymetholone enhances the production and excretion of erythropoietin in patients with anemias caused by bone marrow failure and often stimulates erythropoiesis in anemias stemming from deficient red cell production.

Oral testosterone or testosterone derivatives are contraindicated in male patients who have prostate or breast cancer and in females with hypercalcemia or breast cancer.

Workplace Wisdom AndroGel® Warning

AndroGel® can be passed to another person through unwashed clothing or skin-to-skin contact. Any persons who come in direct contact with clothing or skin that has had the drug applied to it should immediately wash the area of contact with soap and water.

Side Effects of Anabolic Steroids

Too much testosterone or anabolic steroids signals the pituitary gland to stop producing the hormone *gonadotropin*. This fact is the basis for research into a male contraceptive, as gonadotropin is necessary for spermatogenesis. When excessive amounts of anabolic steroids are used, a domino effect occurs, causing testicular atrophy, decreased size and function of the testicles and testes, lowered sperm count, reversible sterility, **priapism**, prostate enlargement, and frequent or continuing erections. Upon cessation of steroid use, the natural ability to produce testosterone may remain completely shut down, possibly leading to a permanent imbalance of the hormone.

Side effects of anabolic steroids in both men and women include:

- edema and weight gain due to sodium and water retention
- jaundice, due to an increased concentration of bilirubin in the liver
- hepatic carcinoma after prolonged steroid use
- high cholesterol and associated diseases
- increased or decreased libido

priapism painful, extended-duration erection.

- chills
- decreased glucose tolerance
- increased serum levels of LDLs and decreased levels of HDLs
- increased excretion of creatine and creatinine

In women, the following effects of masculinization are reversible if the drug is discontinued in time, except as noted:

- acne
- hirsutism (growth of facial hair)
- increases in body hair (permanent)
- deepening of the voice (permanent)
- amenorrhea or other menstrual irregularities
- enlargement of the clitoris (permanent)
- uterine atrophy
- shrinkage of breast size
- masculinization of female fetuses in pregnant women

In men, the following side effects have been documented:

- infertility
- impotence (after as little as 25 mg of testosterone a day for 6 weeks; spermatogenesis declines; androgens will cause the same effect even after drug withdrawal)
- increased frequency of erections
- prepuberty penis enlargement
- testicular atrophy (shrinkage)
- decline in testicular function and decrease in spermatogenesis
- decrease in seminal volume
- chronic priapism
- epididymitis
- bladder irritability and decrease in seminal fluid volume
- gynecomastia (enlarged breast) and nipple tenderness

Workplace Wisdom Federal Regulation of Anabolic Steroids

Because of widespread abuse, the Anabolic Steroids Control Act of 1990 was passed, making anabolic steroids a Schedule III controlled substance. This means that the drugs may be kept under lock and key in the pharmacy.

Androgen Precautions

Although the newer topical testosterone gels have fewer side effects than oral or injectable testosterone, without protection and contact precautions these drugs may contaminate other partners and family members and cause severe side effects. For example, anabolic steroids may cause suppression of clotting factors II, V, VII, and X, and an increase in prothrombin time.

Glandular Disease States

Some cancers, especially those involving the breast, uterus, and prostate gland, are dependent on the presence of sex hormones. The use of sex hormones opposing those found in the cancerous tissue receptors most often appears to antagonize or inhibit tumor growth. Endocrine therapy is palliative (soothing) only.

The following are examples of conditions that benefit from endocrine therapy:

- *Breast cancer*—Breast tissue has estrogen receptors. In breast cancer, estrogen "feeds" the cancer cells. Therefore, adding more estrogen exogenously causes more breast cancer, or enhances the growth of cancer that is already present. Obese men have higher levels of estrogen in their bodies because fat cells produce estrogen from other hormones; these patients may also produce fewer androgens. Taking an androgen as an antiestrogenic therapy will lower the amount of endogenous estrogen; this sort of therapy is used in females, although (as noted) there may be significant side effects. Androgens (and possibly progesterone) exert a protective influence, are used to treat breast cancer in males, and include the drugs tamoxifen (Nolvadex®) and megestrol (Megace®). Tamoxifen, an antiestrogen, works by blocking estrogen in the breast, thus slowing the growth and reproduction of breast cancer cells that depend on estrogen for survival. Megestrol, an antiandrogen, blocks the effect of androgen (a male hormone) on breast cancer cells. Researchers do not know for certain why blocking androgen in the breast helps treat male breast cancer.

- *Polycystic ovary syndrome (PCOS)*—PCOS involves enlarged ovaries containing many fluid-filled sacs. Female PCOS patients exhibit high levels of male hormones (androgens, testosterone). More testosterone would only exacerbate the problem. Therefore, giving these female patients estrogen increases their estrogen levels and helps lower the levels of male hormones.

- *Prostate cancer*—Researchers have found that small amounts of estrogen help reduce the amount of bone loss caused by a common prostate cancer treatment. If the estrogen level in the body is high, the body does not make as much testosterone, so the cancer cannot feed on it. Estrogens actually block prostate cancer growth, but only to a point.

- *Endometrial cancer*—This cancer is dependent on estrogen. Certain stages may be treated with estrogen antagonists such as aromatase inhibitors.

Endocrine System Disorders
Following are some of the abnormalities caused by defects of the endocrine system.

Pituitary Gigantism
Gigantism results from excessive secretion of growth hormone in childhood, and is usually caused by a nonmalignant tumor of the pituitary gland. The affected child grows excessively and is bigger in all areas of the body: height, weight, and size. The size is, however, proportionate. Treatment may include surgical removal or radiation therapy of the pituitary tumor. Medications include somatostatin analogs, such as octreotide or long-acting lanreotide, which reduce secretion of GH. Also used, but less effective, are dopamine agonists, such as bromocriptine mesylate and cabergoline.

Pituitary Dwarfism
Pituitary dwarfism results from a lack of GH. The affected individual may be somewhat short at birth, but in most cases the child's growth in height and weight is normal from birth up to 6 to 12 months of age. At that point, it may become apparent that the child is not growing normally; large amounts of exogenous growth hormone are needed.

The person may have hypoglycemia or low blood sugar because GH is not present to counter insulin. Patients with pituitary dwarfism may have an exaggerated "puppet" or "baby-doll" face, and may be proportionately short, with a chubby body build, because both the height and the growth of all other structures are decreased. Each case differs: there may be an unusually high deficiency of GH, or the person may produce no GH at all. It has been shown that patients with the form of isolated growth hormone deficiency develop anti-GH antibodies when growth hormone replacement therapy is administered (using exogenous GH). Thus, treatment may not be possible or effective for some patients.

The parents' stature may or may not be relevant to the child's dwarfism. Some syndromes are caused by genetic mutations at the moment of conception. Other syndromes are caused by the random combination of two recessive genes that may have been dormant for generations. (The child must receive one recessive gene from each parent to show the trait.) The main course of therapy is growth hormone replacement therapy, with growth hormone (somatotropin), when there is lack of growth hormone in the body. Somatrem®, Protropin®, and Humatrope®, among others, may be used.

A pediatric endocrinologist usually administers this type of therapy before a child's growth plates have fused (joined together). GH replacement therapy is rarely effective after the growth plates have joined, which usually occurs before the child reaches the age of 17. When therapy is effective, height may increase by as much as 4–6 inches (10–15 cm) in the first year of treatment.

Acromegaly

Acromegaly results from an excessive secretion of GH during the adult years. It is characterized by enlarged bones of the cheek, hands, feet, and jaws; the patient will have a predominant forehead and a large nose. The arms, legs, and hands are disproportionately large compared to the rest of the body, but the person will have slender arms, sometimes exacerbated by atrophy of the muscles. There is often a curvature of the spine associated with a deformity of the chest. The lower part of the sternum may project forward because the bones of the chest are increased in size. Ultimately, the person with acromegaly will suffer considerable disability, with joint pain, cardiovascular disease, hypertension, insulin resistance, visual impairment, and severe headaches.

The cause is usually a tumor on the pituitary gland, called a *pituitary adenoma*. Too much growth hormone after the age of 17 will lead to acromegaly, but seldom to gigantism, because the long bones of the limbs have fused and cannot grow any more. Treatment includes surgical removal of the tumor. Medications that may decrease the secretion of GH and reduce the size of the tumor include:

- somatostatin—a brain hormone that inhibits GH release
- octreotide (Sandostatin®)—a synthetic form of somatostatin
- lanreotide (Somatuline LA®)—a synthetic, long-acting form of somatostatin

Diabetes

It is estimated that approximately 6.6 percent of the U.S. population has diabetes, with about one-third of that number unaware of their serious medical condition. Diabetes mellitus is a disease in which the body does not produce or properly use insulin, a hormone that is needed to convert sugar, starches, and other food into the energy necessary for daily life. The cause of diabetes is not certain, but both genetics and environmental factors, such as obesity and lack of exercise, appear to play roles. Some cases appear to be caused by autoimmune reactions.

Diabetes can be categorized as:

- *Type 1*—results from the body's failure to produce insulin. It is estimated that 5–10 percent of Americans who are diagnosed with diabetes have type 1 diabetes.
- *Type 2*—results from *insulin resistance* (a condition in which the body fails to properly use insulin) combined with relative insulin deficiency. Most Americans who are diagnosed with diabetes have type 2 diabetes.
- *Gestational*—affects about 4 percent of all pregnant women (135,000 cases) in the United States each year.
- *Pre-diabetes*—a condition in which a person's blood glucose levels are higher than normal, but not high enough for a diagnosis of type 2 diabetes.

Many people remain undiagnosed because many of the diabetes symptoms seem harmless. Studies indicate that the early detection of diabetes symptoms and treatment can decrease the chances of developing the complications of diabetes.

Diabetes symptoms include:

- frequent urination (**polyuria**)
- excessive thirst (**polydipsia**)
- extreme hunger (**polyphagia**)
- unusual weight loss
- increased fatigue
- irritability
- blurry vision

polyuria excessive urination.

polydipsia ingestion of abnormally large amounts of fluids.

polyphagia excessive hunger or eating.

Type 2 diabetes may be delayed, or even prevented from developing, through diet and exercise. Most people with diabetes have high risk factors for other conditions, such as high blood pressure and cholesterol, which increase their risk for heart disease and stroke. It is estimated that more than 65 percent of people with diabetes die from heart disease or stroke. With diabetes, heart attacks occur earlier in life and often result in death.

Diabetes should not be taken lightly. Anyone can assess their individual risk through pre-diabetes screening. Diabetes is a major chronic disease that causes significant morbidity and mortality from heart and circulatory conditions, renal failure, and blindness. By managing diabetes, high blood pressure, and cholesterol, people with diabetes can greatly reduce their risk of complications. Treatment may include proper diet and exercise, oral hypoglycemics, insulin, or a combination of therapies. Many of the oral hypoglycemics listed in Table 29-5 are available as combination drugs.

Insulin

For some diabetic patients who are insulin dependent (type 1), an array of injectable insulins is available. Which insulin is best for which patient is assessed by the health-care provider. Available insulins include:

- *Lente (L)*—Humulin® L, Novolin® L
- *NPH*—Humulin® N, Novolin® N
- *Peakless/Basal Action*—Lantus® (glargine)
- *Premixed*—Humulin® 70/30, Novolin® 70/30, Humulin® 50/50

Table 29-5   Oral Hypoglycemic Agents

CLASS	EXAMPLE(S)	PRIMARY SITE OF ACTION	MECHANISM OF ACTION
Alpha-glucosidase inhibitors	Precose® (acarbose) Glyset® (miglitol)	intestine	Slow digestion of carbohydrates
Biguanides	Glucophage® (metformin)	liver	Reduce glucose release
Meglitinides	Prandin® (repaglinide) Starlix® (nateglinide)	pancreas	Increase insulin release
Sulfonylureas	Glucotrol® (glipizide) Amaryl® (glimeprimide) Diabeta®, Micronase® (glyburide)	pancreas	Increase insulin release
Thiazolidinediones	Avandia® (rosiglitazone) Actos® (pioglitazone)	muscle	Increase insulin sensitivity

Source: Today's Technician. 5(1).

- *Rapid-acting*—Humalog® (lispro), Novolog® (aspart)
- *Regular*—Novolin® R, Velosulin® BR, Humulin® R
- *Ultralente*—Humulin® U

As with the oral medications, some combination insulins are now available, and others are being developed. Research continues on insulin with the following considerations:

- rapid-acting insulins
- short-acting insulins
- intermediate-acting insulins
- long-acting insulins
- ultra-long-acting insulins
- insulin mixtures

Insulin delivery technology has developed the following innovations:

- insulin injection
- insulin pens (injectors that are about the size and shape of a fountain pen)
- insulin jet injectors
- external insulin pumps
- implantable insulin pumps
- transdermal insulin
- oral spray insulin
- inhaled insulin

Diabetes Insipidus

Diabetes insipidus is a condition that results from a decrease in or hyposecretion of ADH, the antidiuretic hormone. The primary symptom of DI is the same as for diabetes mellitus (DM): high amount of sugar in the blood. Other symptoms include:

- polyuria
- polydipsia
- polyphagia

The lack of antidiuretic hormone in patients with DI is caused by kidneys that do not concentrate urine well. Because the urine is more diluted, the patient must urinate more often, frequently getting up two or three times in the night. People with diabetes insipidus are thirsty all the time and may often want to drink liquids every hour. Excessive urination may cause DI patients to become dehydrated, making them feel lethargic and thirsty. When people feel tired or lethargic, they sometimes interpret the feeling as meaning that they need to eat; weight gain and poor metabolism of food just exacerbate the problem.

Two things are known to cause diabetes insipidus. In the first case, the hypothalamus does not make enough ADH. In the second case, the kidneys do not respond to ADH the way they should. Most people with diabetes insipidus acquire it after a head injury or after brain surgery, or it may be caused by a brain tumor. DI can also be congenital and run in families. DI can be drug-induced, such as by lithium, which is used to treat bipolar disorder. About 25 percent of the time, however, the cause is unknown. Treatment for pituitary DI is with DDAVP nasal spray, which contains a substance much like the body's natural ADH, *vasopressin*. If a person taking DDAVP takes in too much liquid, the body will get overloaded with fluids, making the patient feel weak, dizzy, or generally bad all over.

Table 29-6 compares diabetes insipidus with diabetes mellitus.

Table 29-6 Comparison of Diabetes Insipidus and Diabetes Mellitus

FACTORS	DIABETES INSIPIDUS	DIABETES MELLITUS TYPE I	DIABETES MELLITUS TYPE II
Onset	Birth	Birth; may show up in childhood or adolescence; currently also being seen in older adults.	Adult onset, usually after 40 years of age; current trend of development in younger, overweight children.
Mechanism of the Disease	Lack of ADH or vasopressin secreted by posterior pituitary gland	Beta cells of islets of Langerhans do not manufacture insulin; patient is unable to transport sugar from the bloodstream into cells.	Beta cells of islets of Langerhans do not manufacture enough insulin, or the muscles do not utilize insulin properly; creates inability to transport sugar from the bloodstream into cells.
Other Names	Neurogenic, hypothalamic, pituitary, water diabetes	DM Type A, insulin-dependent diabetes, IDDM, juvenile-onset diabetes, sugar diabetes	DM Type B, non-insulin-dependent diabetes, NIDDM, adult-onset diabetes, sugar diabetes
Subtypes	Gestational Dipsogenic	—	—
Causes	Destruction of posterior pituitary; tumors, infections, head injuries, infiltrations; various inheritable defects	Familial, congenital, acquired	Familial, acquired
Symptoms	Polydipsia, polyuria, polyphagia	Polydipsia, polyuria, polyphagia, weight loss, tiredness/fatigue	Polydipsia, polyuria, polyphagia, weight gain; sometimes asymptomatic
Notes	Rare	Accounts for 10% of DM	Most common; 90% of all DM
Danger	Dehydration, rapid heart rate, fatigue, headache, muscle pain, dry mucous membranes	Too much glucose in the bloodstream and not enough glucose within the cells themselves. Result: cells attempt to derive energy from fat breakdown. Excessive breakdown causes production of harmful by-products called *ketones*. The accumulation of ketones causes the body's pH to become acidic (*ketoacidosis*), which makes the cellular environment inhospitable for normal metabolic functions. This condition can ultimately become life-threatening; requires aggressive medical therapy.	Too much glucose in the bloodstream and not enough glucose within the cells themselves. Result: cells attempt to derive energy from fat breakdown. Excessive breakdown causes production of harmful by-products called *ketones*. The accumulation of ketones causes the body's pH to become acidic (*ketoacidosis*), which makes the cellular environment inhospitable for normal metabolic functions. This condition can ultimately become life-threatening; requires aggressive medical therapy.
Treatment	DDVAP (desmopressin) Pitressin® (vasopressin) Diapid® (lypressin)	Insulin injections	Diet, exercise, oral hypoglycemics; insulin injections as a last resort
Complications	Dehydration, electrolyte imbalance, rapid heart rate, high blood pressure, weight loss, dry skin, muscle pain	Diabetic retinopathy, glaucoma, HTN, renal impairment, neuropathy, heart disease	Diabetic retinopathy, glaucoma, HTN, renal impairment, neuropathy, heart disease

Abnormalities of the Adrenal Gland

The following are common disorders that can occur with abnormalities of the adrenal gland. See Table 29-7 for a summary of endocrine disorders and conditions.

Table 29-7 Endocrine System Disorders

DISORDER	HORMONAL CHANGE	CHARACTERISTICS	TREATMENT
Acromegaly	Increased GH in adults	Enlargement of extremities and certain parts of the body, such as hands, feet, legs, arms, chin, head	Somatostatin analogs such as Somatuline LA® (long-acting lanreotide) or Auto-gel SC® Octreotide® (synthetic somatostatin) Sandostatin® (octreotide) LAR® IM injection (a longer-acting, slow-release form of octreotide)
Addison's disease	Decreased cortisol OR decreased aldosterone	Weight loss, muscle weakness, fatigue, low blood pressure	Synthetic cortisol replacement: oral hydrocortisone tablets, qd or bid Aldosterone replacement with an oral mineralocorticoid qd: Florinef® (fludrocortisone)
Cushing's disease	Increased ACTH	May have a moon face, buffalo hump, obese torso	Surgical removal of pituitary tumor; possibly cortisol inhibitors such as mitotane, aminoglutethimide, metyrapone, trilostane, and ketoconazole
Cushing's syndrome	Increased ACTH	May have a moon face, buffalo hump, obese torso	Treatment varies by cause: Synthetic cortisol; cortisol inhibitors such as mitotane, aminoglutethimide, metyrapone, trilostane, and ketoconazole
Diabetes insipidus	Decreased ADH	HTN, high blood glucose, polydipsia, polyphagia, polyuria	DDVAP® (desmopressin), Pitressin® (vasopressin), Diapid® (lypressin)
Diabetes mellitus	Decreased insulin	High blood glucose, polydipsia, polyuria, polyphagia; may have HTN	Type 1—insulin injections Type 2—diet modification, weight control, regular exercise, oral hypoglycemic agents Sulfonylureas stimulate the beta cells to secrete more insulin: Orinase® (tolbutamide), Diabinese® (chlorpropamide) Meglitinides: Prandin® (repaglinide) Biguanides decrease hepatic glucose output, reducing insulin resistance and lowering blood glucose: Glucophage® (metformin) Thiazolidinediones reduce insulin resistance and improve insulin sensitivity

Table 29-7   Endocrine System Disorders (*continued*)

DISORDER	HORMONAL CHANGE	CHARACTERISTICS	TREATMENT
			Alpha-glucosidase inhibitors block the breakdown of complex carbohydrates and delay the absorption of monosaccharides from the GI tract: Precose® (acarbose), Glyset® (miglitol)
Gigantism	Increased GH in child	Large stature, proportional	Somatostatin analogs, such as Sandostatin® (octreotide) or Somatuline LA® (long-acting lanreotide)
			Auto-gel SC® reduces growth hormone secretion
			Also treated, less effectively, with dopamine agonists, such as bromocriptine mesylate and cabergoline
Goiter	Decreased iodine	Enlargement of the thyroid gland in neck	Add iodine to diet
Graves' disease	Increased TH in adult	Weight loss; feels hot or warm	Propacil® (propylthiouracil [PTU])
Hirsutism	Increased androgens OR increased testosterone	Facial hair on females, unrelated to menopause	Vaniqa™® (eflornithine cream applied 5 minutes after hair removal)
Hypothyroidism/cretinism	Decreased TH in child; also caused by decreased iodine in the fetus	Small stature, not proportional; short limbs, may be overweight; dry skin, thick tongue, and large nose	Post-birth: Immediate treatment with synthetic thyroid hormone is imperative. Treat child with synthetic thyroid hormone or iodine replacement.
Myxedema	Decreased TH in adult	Weight gain, cold	Treat with synthetic thyroid hormones:
			Synthroid®, Levoxyl® (T_4, L-thyroxine, levothroid, levothyroxine)
			Cytomel® (triiodothyronine, liothyronine)
			Armour Thyroid® (synthetic desiccated animal thyroid hormones)
Peripheral edema	Increased ADH	Water and sodium retention, bloating	Exercise, elevate legs and ankles, mild potassium-sparing diuretics such as spironolactone
Pituitary dwarfism	Decreased GH in child	Small stature, proportional	Growth hormone such as Protopin® (somatrem) or Humatrope® (somatropin)

Cushing's Syndrome

Also known as *hypercortisolism* or *hyperadrenocortism*, *Cushing's syndrome* occurs when the body is exposed to high levels of the hormone cortisol for long periods of time. This may occur during long-term or high-stress situations; long-term therapy with glucocorticoid hormones, such as prednisone, for asthma, rheumatoid arthritis, lupus, and other inflammatory diseases; or from immunosuppression after transplantation and overproduction of natural cortisol. Cortisol performs vital tasks in the body by maintaining blood pressure and cardiovascular function; reducing the immune system's inflammatory response; balancing the effects of insulin in breaking down sugar for energy; and regulating the metabolism of proteins, carbohydrates, and fats. One of cortisol's most important jobs is to help the body respond to stress of all kinds.

Considered rare, Cushing's syndrome most commonly affects adults aged 20 to 50, but only affects 10 to 15 people out of every 1 million people each year. People at risk are those suffering from depression, alcoholism, malnutrition, and panic disorders who have increased cortisol levels. Symptoms vary, but may include upper body obesity, rounded face, increased fat around the neck, and thinning arms and legs. Children with this syndrome tend to be obese, with slowed growth rates. Purplish-pink stretch marks may appear on the abdomen, thighs, buttocks, arms, and breasts. There may be weakened bones that fracture easily, fatigue, weak muscles, high blood pressure, and high blood sugar. Irritability, anxiety, and depression are common. Women may experience excess hair growth on the face and body, and have irregular menstrual cycles or absence of menstruation. Men have decreased fertility with diminished or absent libido.

Treatment of Cushing's syndrome varies, depending on the cause, and ranges from surgery to use of synthetic cortisol to maintain and balance the amount needed in the body. Cortisol inhibitors, such as mitotane, aminoglutethimide, metyrapone, trilostane, and ketoconazole are also used.

Addison's Disease

Also called *hypocortisolism*, *Addison's disease* occurs in 1 out of 100,000 people. In this disease, the adrenal glands do not produce enough of the hormone cortisol and, in some cases, also underproduce the hormone aldosterone. For this reason, the disease is sometimes called *chronic adrenal insufficiency*. The disease is characterized by weight loss, muscle weakness, fatigue, low blood pressure, and sometimes darkening of the skin. Causes of cortisol deficiency are a lack of ACTH from gradual destruction of the adrenal cortex (the outer layer of the adrenal glands) by the body's own immune system, as seen with an autoimmune disease. This in turn may cause polyendocrine deficiency syndrome, in which many glands are affected. A secondary cause may be long-term or overuse of glucocorticoids, such as prednisone, for asthma, ulcerative colitis, and rheumatoid arthritis.

PROFILES IN PRACTICE

Mr. Hill, a diabetic and a regular customer at the pharmacy, presents a new prescription for a loop diuretic.

- What important information should the pharmacy technician provide to Mr. Hill regarding his preexisting condition and his new medication?

The addition of exogenous cortisol sends negative feedback to the hypothalamus, causing it to stop making releasing factor CRH; because there is no releasing factor, ACTH is not sent to the adrenal glands. This can happen when someone suddenly stops taking glucocorticoids or abruptly interrupts long-term therapy. Another cause is removal of a tumor of, or injury to, the pituitary gland. Symptoms may include darkening of the skin; penetrating pain in the lower back, abdomen, or legs; severe vomiting and diarrhea, followed by dehydration; low blood pressure; and loss of consciousness. Left untreated, an Addison's disease crisis can be fatal. Treatment is by synthetic cortisol replacement with oral hydrocortisone tablets, taken once or twice a day. If aldosterone is also deficient, it is replaced with oral doses of the mineralocorticoid fludrocortisone acetate.

Cretinism

An underactive thyroid gland, or *congenital hypothyroidism*, is caused by a lack of fetal or childhood thyroid hormone secretion. *Cretinism* may also be due to lack of iodine in the diet of the expectant mother, and therefore in the fetus. The result is babies who are born with, or children who later develop, mental retardation and a type of dwarfism. Other symptoms include coarse, dry skin and a slightly swollen tongue. Immediate treatment with synthetic thyroid hormone is imperative.

Myxedema (Secondary Hypothyroidism)

Myxedema may also be caused by a deficiency of thyroid hormone (TH), due to a lack of secretion of TSH by the pituitary gland, or lack of TRH from the hypothalamus in an adult. It is common among women. Usual symptoms are a coarse thickening of the skin and roughness that may be open with sores. Treatment is with synthetic thyroid hormone.

Graves' Disease

Graves' disease is also known as *thyroid eye disease* or *thyroid orbitopathy*. Characterized by *proptosis* (protruding eye) and swollen and congested eye muscles, it makes the affected eye appear larger than the other eye (see Figure 29-4). The cause is *not* an overactive thyroid gland, as is commonly believed; those with Graves' disease often do have an overactive thyroid gland, but not always. Rather, Graves' disease is an autoimmune disorder, in which immune cells attack both the eye muscles and the thyroid, leading to dysfunction of both. Treatment of Graves' disease depends on the severity of signs and symptoms. Dry eye due to exposure requires the use of nonpreserved, lubricating eye drops. Acute episodes of inflammation result in double vision and optic nerve compression, and corticosteroids such as prednisone are used in these instances.

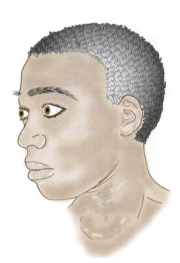

FIGURE 29-4 Eye characteristics of Graves' disease.

Radiation therapy is also used to treat optic nerve compression, to preserve vision, but unfortunately it may result in radiation retinopathy. Only when the disease is under control should surgical orbital decompression be employed to decrease proptosis or strabismus surgery be used to realign the eyes. Of course, the complication of hyperactive thyroid should be addressed with propylthiouracil (PTU), marketed under the trade name Propacil®.

SUMMARY

The endocrine system is a collection of glands that secrete hormones directly into the bloodstream to be distributed to specific target cells. This very complex system interacts with many other body systems via the release of hormones, which act as "messengers" between sets of cells. Some of the main functions of the endocrine system are regulation of the body's growth, metabolism, and sexual development and function.

The primary drivers of the endocrine system are the hypothalamus, located in the brain stem; and the pituitary gland, which is attached to the base of the hypothalamus. The hypothalamus directs the pituitary gland which, in turn, controls the thyroid, parathyroid, pancreas, adrenal glands, and gonads. A complete review of these glands, their secretions, and their effects on body systems illustrates how important the endocrine system is to the proper functioning of the body. For example, every cell in the body depends on thyroid hormone for regulating metabolism.

For the most part, the release of hormones is a self-regulating feedback mechanism that acts according to a simple "supply and demand" model. However, many outside factors can influence the amount of hormones in the body at any given time. Such factors include age, stress, infection, and changes in fluid or mineral balance in the blood, to name a few.

Many of the diseases, disorders, and conditions of the endocrine system discussed in this chapter are very common and familiar to most people (e.g., menopause and diabetes). This chapter also discussed less common disorders, such as Graves' disease, Cushing's syndrome, and Addison's disease, along with the various treatment modalities used to treat disorders of the endocrine system.

CHAPTER REVIEW QUESTIONS

1. The enlargement of extremities, hands, feet, and head is known as:
   a. pituitary dwarfism.
   b. diabetes insipidus.
   c. acromegaly.
   d. gigantism.

2. In the pituitary gland, TRH stimulates which of the following?
   a. ACTH
   b. GH
   c. LH
   d. TSH

3. Which of the following secretions is produced in the stomach?
   a. PTH
   b. gastrin
   c. oxytocin
   d. melatonin

4. Which of the following is often considered the body's "master gland"?
   a. hypothalamus
   b. thyroid
   c. thymus
   d. pituitary

5. Which of the following hormones is not produced in the pituitary gland?
   a. insulin
   b. GH
   c. TSH
   d. LH

6. Which of the following glands is located in the front of the neck?
   a. pituitary
   b. hypothalamus
   c. thymus
   d. thyroid

7. A decreased amount of GH in a child can result in which of the following condiditons?
   a. acromegaly
   b. gigantism
   c. pituitary dwarfism
   d. peripheral edema

8. FSH and LH stimulate which of the following?
   a. gonads
   b. pituitary gland
   c. adrenal gland
   d. mammary glands

9. Diabetes can be treated with:

    a. testosterone.

    b. anabolic steroids.

    c. hydrocortisone.

    d. glipizide.

10. Which of the following diseases is characterized by protruding eyes and swollen/congested eye muscles?

    a. cretinism

    b. myxedema

    c. Graves' disease

    d. Cushing's syndrome

11. Which of the following insulins is considered a mixed insulin?

    a. Humulin® N

    b. Novolin® L

    c. Humulin® 70/30

    d. Humulin® R

12. Which type of diabetes is treated with insulin?

    a. type I

    b. type II

    c. gestational

    d. pre-diabetes

13. Which type of diabetes is usually adult-onset in males?

    a. type I

    b. type II

    c. gestational

    d. pre-diabetes

14. The generic name for Delatestryl® is:

    a. progesterone.

    b. estrogen.

    c. testosterone.

    d. stanozolol.

15. Which of the following is a mineralocorticoid drug?

    a. hydrocortisone

    b. dexamethasone

    c. betamethasone

    d. fludrocortisone

CRITICAL THINKING QUESTIONS

1. Why do you think anabolic steroids are now classified as a controlled substance (C-III)?

2. Why is the pituitary gland considered the "master gland"?

3. Why do you think most people with diabetes do not know that they have the disease?

WEB CHALLENGE

1. Go to www.youtube.com, conduct a search for endocrine system, and watch videos on how the system works.

2. Go to http://www.vivo.colostate.edu/hbooks/path-phys/endocrine/index.html to learn more about the endocrine system. Describe what you learn about the "diffuse endocrine system" and some of the hormones these organs secrete.

REFERENCES AND RESOURCES

"Acromegaly and Gigantism: A Historical Portrait of a Disease" (accessed April 8, 2008): http://www.cladonia.co.uk/acromegaly/ampc.html

Adams, MP, Josephson, DL, & Holland, LN Jr. *Pharmacology for Nurses—A Pathophysiologic Approach*. Upper Saddle River, NJ: Pearson Education, 2008.

"Carbohydrates: Fuel for Your Brain and Body" (accessed April 8, 2008): http://www.iemily.com/Article.cfm?ArtID=274

"Endocrine Glands and Their Hormones" (accessed October 17, 2007): http://training.seer.cancer.gov

"Endometrial Cancer Hormonal Therapy: Prolactin." January 3, 2003 (accessed April 8, 2008): http://sharedjourney.com/define/prolactin .html

Hitner, N. *Pharmacology—An Introduction* (5th ed.). New York: McGraw-Hill, 2005.

Holland, N, & Adams, MP. *Core Concepts in Pharmacology*. Upper Saddle River, NJ: Pearson Education, 2007.

Interpersonal testosterone transfer after topical application of a newly developed testosterone gel preparation. *Clinical Endocrinology*. 2002;56:637–641; http://www.fsdinfo.org/pdf/Interpersonal_testosterone_transfer.pdf

"Medical Supervision of Individuals Using Anabolic-Androgenic Steroid (AAS) for Muscle Growth" (accessed April 8, 2008): http://www.mesomorphosis.com/articles/haycock/medically-supervised-steroid-use-02.htm

Medline Pulse. "Diabetes Insipidus" (accessed April 5, 2008): http://www.nlm.nih.gov/medlineplus/ency/article/000377.htm

"Pituitary Dwarfism" (accessed April 8, 2008): http://www.ecureme.com/emyhealth/Pediatrics/Pituitary_Dwarfism.asp

Unimed package insert online (accessed April 2, 2008): http://www.unimed.com/pdfs/Anadrol.pdf

Zaccardi, N. "Anabolic Steroids" (University of Massachusetts, Amherst, MA) (accessed April 8, 2008): http://www.wellnessmd.com/anabolics.html

The Reproductive System

30 chapter

LEARNING OBJECTIVES

After completing this chapter, you should be able to:

- List, identify, and diagram the basic anatomical structures and parts of the male and female reproductive systems.
- Describe the functions and physiology of the male and female reproductive systems and the hormones that govern them.
- List and define common diseases affecting the male and female reproductive systems and understand the causes, symptoms, and pharmaceutical treatments associated with each disease or condition.
- Describe the indications for use and mechanisms of action of various contraceptives.

Introduction

At the onset of sexual maturity, in both males and females, the hypothalamus secretes gonadotropin releasing hormone, or GnRH. It is needed for both sexual maturation and normal reproduction and acts by stimulating the release of luteinizing hormone (LH) and follicle-stimulating hormone (FSH) from the anterior pituitary. LH and FSH act by stimulating the production of sex hormones in the gonads (the testes and ovaries).

This chapter discusses both the female and male reproductive systems, as well as conditions that affect these systems, such as sexually transmitted diseases and infertility. Different methods of contraception are also introduced, including oral and topical contraceptives and intrauterine and barrier devices.

The Female Reproductive System

The female reproductive system includes the organs and hormones that allow females to reproduce and give them their gender characteristics. This section discusses female reproductive anatomy, contraception, and conditions and diseases (including infertility and sexually transmitted diseases).

Anatomy

ovaries the female reproductive organs that produce eggs.

The female reproductive system is composed of internal organs and external genitals. The internal reproductive organs are two **ovaries**, two fallopian tubes, the uterus, and the vagina (see Figure 30-1). The external genitals are known together as the *vulva*. The vulva consists of the labia minora, labia majora, and clitoris.

Reproductive Cycle

oocyte an immature egg.

ovum a mature egg.

The menstrual cycle consists of two stages: ovulation and menstruation. Females are born with about 2 million **oocytes**. By the time of puberty, only about 400,000 oocytes remain. At the beginning of each monthly cycle, FSH causes one of the many underdeveloped ovarian follicles to fully develop and mature. Within an ovary, an **ovum** (egg) matures about 11 to 17 days before the woman's next menstrual period, or approximately once every 28 to 30 days. As the follicle gets larger, cells that are dedicated to producing the estrogenic hormones estriol, estrone, and estradiol become active.

Estradiol is the most abundant and active of the estrogens. Its main function is to stimulate the development of the uterine lining and the mammary glands to ready the body for pregnancy. The estrogens are known as *feminizing hormones* because they are responsible for the female secondary sex characteristics, such as a higher voice, breast development, curvaceous body shape, and less bulky muscle. Estradiol is the most potent form of estrogen in premenopausal women. Estrone, which accounts for most estrogen in postmenopausal women, is made only in very small quantities by the ovaries; the majority is converted from another hormone, androstenedione, in fat and other body tissues. Estriol, a weaker estrogen, is formed when estradiol and estrone are metabolized.

FIGURE 30-1 The female reproductive system.

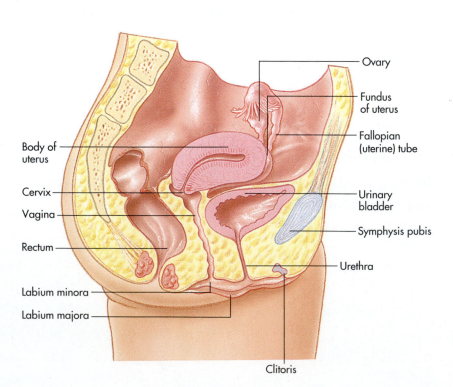

Progesterone, the second major type of female sex hormone made in the ovaries, develops the **endometrium** and the mammary ducts for lactation. Progesterone also maintains the uterine lining if egg implantation occurs. Progesterone literally means "hormone for life."

If the female reproductive cycle is considered on average a 28-day cycle, during the first 12 days, estrogen has little effect. After that, it has a positive effect on the production of gonadotropins, causing a large increase in LH and a small increase in FSH. Midway through the cycle, after approximately 14 days of development, the sudden increase in LH causes the mature follicle to rupture, releasing the ovum. This generally occurs 12 to 14 days before a woman's next period. The mature egg is released from the ovary, passes into a fallopian tube, and is swept by tiny cilia and smooth muscle action into the uterus. It takes about five days before the egg reaches the uterus. This "trip" is known as **ovulation**. If a woman has a cycle shorter or longer than 28 days, ovulation may occur on a different day (day 7 or day 20), but generally takes place 12 to 14 days before she has a menstrual period.

After ovulation, the ruptured ovarian follicle (which remained in the ovary) undergoes a change. LH transforms the follicle into a corpus luteum, which continues to produce estrogen and begins to produce progesterone to prepare the uterine lining for possible implantation. A woman is most fertile around the time she is ovulating. Some women can tell when they are ovulating by watching for changes in vaginal discharge or body temperature. Some women feel pain when the egg is released.

If implantation of the egg does occur, the high levels of estrogen and progesterone will be maintained; these exert a negative feedback effect on the secretion of gonadotropins by the anterior pituitary gland, and pregnancy continues. If implantation does not occur, there is no need for progesterone, so production of that hormone stops.

At the end of the ovarian cycle, the corpus luteum will disintegrate if fertilization of the egg has not occurred; production of the female hormones estrogen and progesterone also stops. The unfertilized egg dissolves, and the absence of the two hormones causes the endometrium (uterine lining) to be shed. This shedding begins what is known as *menstruation*. Simultaneously, a new follicle in the ovary begins to develop, and the cycle repeats again. Somewhere roughly between the ages of 40 and 55, a woman's ovaries stop producing estrogen and progesterone and monthly menstruation ceases. One year from the last menstrual cycle is known as *menopause*.

If pregnancy does occur, the corpus luteum continues to produce estrogen and progesterone until the placenta is developed, around day 12 (see Figure 30-2). The placenta, acting as an endocrine gland, then assumes the role of producing these hormones. The critical transitional time usually occurs and is completed between the second and third month of pregnancy. If the corpus luteum disintegrates before the placenta can maintain the correct hormone level, the uterine lining, along with a fetus, will rupture and shed. This rupture causes hemorrhage, and the end result is a miscarriage.

About 75 percent of postpubescent women experience a mild to moderate condition called *premenstrual syndrome (PMS)*, which occurs during the phase before

endometrium the lining of the uterus.

ovulation the process in which the ovarian follicle ruptures and releases the egg.

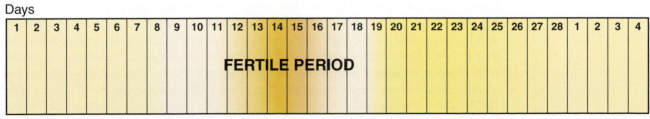

Days

| 1 | 2 | 3 | 4 | 5 | 6 | 7 | 8 | 9 | 10 | 11 | 12 | 13 | 14 | 15 | 16 | 17 | 18 | 19 | 20 | 21 | 22 | 23 | 24 | 25 | 26 | 27 | 28 | 1 | 2 | 3 | 4 |

FERTILE PERIOD

FIGURE 30-2 Fertility and the menstrual cycle.

menstruation begins. Some women have both PMS and uncomfortable periods. Symptoms of PMS include:

- pain or cramping before and during periods
- weight gain before and during periods, due to water retention
- moody or irritable feeling before or during periods
- breakout of acne or pimples before period is due
- diarrhea, constipation, or upset stomach during periods

About 8 percent of menstruating women experience a more severe form of PMS called *premenstrual dysphoric disorder (PMDD)*. In addition to PMS symptoms, women experiencing PMDD may also experience:

- fatigue
- depression
- anxiety
- anger or irritability
- changes in sleep patterns
- changes in appetite

Therapy for PMDD focuses on prevention and mitigation of symptoms. Treatments may include:

- nonsteroidal anti-inflammatory drugs for pain and swelling
- antidepressants
- oral **contraception** to help even out hormone levels
- diet and lifestyle changes, such as exercise, reductions in caffeine intake, and eating more carbohydrates

contraception birth control.

Hormone Contraception

During pregnancy, the levels of estrogen and progesterone are high. The constant high levels of estrogen and progesterone continue to inhibit the release of FSH and LH. Therefore, during pregnancy no other follicle can develop. The mechanism of action of hormone contraception is to maintain a high level of hormone in the blood. A hormonal contraceptive prevents the release of FSH by imitating what happens during pregnancy, thus preventing the development of another follicle or follicles so that no egg is available for fertilization.

There are several types of hormone contraceptives: estrogen and progesterone combinations, and progesterone only (see Table 30-1). Prefertilization and postfertilization are two main mechanisms of action of contraceptives.

- *Prefertilization* mechanisms of action include (1) prevention of ovulation and (2) thickening of cervical mucus to act as a barrier to sperm, reducing the likelihood of implantation.
- *Postfertilization* mechanisms of action include changing the lining of the uterus to block implantation of the embryo.

Although most people define *conception* as the conjoining of an egg and sperm, the blocking of implantation after the conjoining of the egg and sperm is considered an interference with conception. The low-dose progestins or progestin-only (POPs) contraceptives used to prevent pregnancy are also called *minipills*. Progestins can prevent fertilization by preventing the egg from fully developing and by thickening the cervical mucus so that it slows down the flagellation of the sperm (tail movement), preventing the sperm from entering the uterus. Simply put, the sperm cannot "swim" through the thick mucus, so they cannot reach the uterus or fallopian tubes to fertilize the egg. Birth control pills (BCPs) also lower the midcycle LH and FSH peaks. Progestin-only pills are about 93 percent effective; that is, 7 out of 100 women taking a POP will become pregnant each year.

Table 30-1 Examples of Hormone Contraception

TYPE OF CONTRACEPTIVE	TRADE NAME	SPECIAL NOTES
Progestin-Only		
estradiol cypionate/ medroxyprogesterone acetate injection	Lunelle®	Given monthly, injected into the arm, thigh, or buttock.
levonorgestrel subdermal implant	Norplant®	
medroxyprogesterone injection	Depo-Provera®	Given every 13 weeks (3 months).
norethindrone tablets	Ortho-Micronor®	Can be given during lactation.
norgestrel tablets	Ovrette®	Used normally as birth control pills (BCPs). As an emergency contraceptive, 20 tablets are given within 72 hours and repeated within 12 hours.
Emergency Pregnancy Prevention		
levonorgestrel tablets	Plan B®	Used following unprotected intercourse or a suspected contraceptive failure.
levonorgestrel/ethynyl estradiol	Preven®	The first tablet should be taken as soon as possible within 72 hours of intercourse. The second tablet must be taken 12 hours later.
Combination Progestin and Estrogen		
estrogen and progestin (varying strengths of each)	Alesse®, Levlen®, Lo/Ovral®, Nordette®, OrthoCyclen®, Ortho-Novum 7/7/7®, OrthoTri-Cyclen Lo®, Seasonale®, Triphasil-28®, Trivora®, Yasmin®	Seasonale®, a new type of BCP, changes the menstrual cycle to only 4 periods per year. The active pills are taken 84 days in a row, followed by 7 days of nonhormonal pills. The woman has her period while taking the nonhormonal pills.
etonogestrel 120 mcg and ethinyl estradiol 15 mcg vaginal ring	NuvaRing®	A small (about 2 inches in diameter), flexible, colorless ring, inserted at home by patient. Releases a continuous low dose of hormones to prevent pregnancy for that month. Used for 3 weeks per month for continuous contraception. The fourth week, the ring is removed so that the woman can have a menstrual period. The exact position of the ring in the vagina is not critical for it to work.
norelgestromin 150 mcg and ethinyl estradiol 20 mcg transdermal patch	Ortho Evra Patch®	Each small adhesive patch lasts 7 days.

Workplace Wisdom Patient Package Inserts

Federal law requires that all drugs containing estrogen *must* be dispensed with a patient package insert (PPI). Therefore, a pharmacy technician must know which drugs contain estrogen. These drugs are usually birth control and hormone replacement therapy agents. Examples are Lo/Ovral®, Ortho Evra Patch®, NuvaRing®, PremPro®, and Premarin®.

Drug-Drug and Drug-Herb Interactions with Hormone Contraception

Antibiotic, antifungal, antiepileptic, and anticonvulsant drugs may interfere with the active ingredients of birth control agents. The drugs and herbs in Table 30-2 prevent birth control drugs from working well, and the patient may become pregnant.

Workplace Wisdom Contraception Interactions

If a woman must take drugs or herbs that interact with chemical contraception, another method of birth control should be used along with the birth control pills. Condoms with spermicide are a good alternative. If the drugs or herbs are to be used over the long term, she should consult a physician.

Side Effects of Hormone Contraceptives

Side effects may include:

- weight gain
- mild headaches
- breast tenderness
- nausea and vomiting
- hypertension
- decrease of libido
- vaginitis, vaginal skin irritation, and vaginal discharge

Table 30-2 Drugs and Herbs That Interact with Oral Birth Control

CLASSIFICATION	EXAMPLES
Antibiotics	nitrofurantoin (Macrodantin®)
	penicillins (PCNs)
	rifampin
	sulfa drugs
	tetracyclines (TCNs)
Anticonvulsants	carbamazepine (Tegretol®)
	ethosuximide (Zarontin®)
	phenobarbital
	phenytoin (Dilantin®)
	primidone (Mysoline)®
Antifungals	fluconazole (Diflucan®)
Herbs	St. John's Wort (some studies suggest that St. John's Wort may reduce the effectiveness of birth control)

Toxic effects can include:

- shortness of breath (SOB)
- chest pain
- stomach or intestinal pain
- severe lingering headache
- changes in vision (blurred, flashing lights, or diminished vision)
- infertility for 3–12 months after discontinuation
- blood clots (lung, brain/stroke)
- liver tumors
- gallbladder disease

Contraindications apply to women who:

- are over age 35 and who smoke
- are pregnant or suspect pregnancy
- are breastfeeding
- experience unexplained vaginal bleeding
- experience migraine headaches
- have active liver disease (hepatitis) or a history of liver tumors
- have breast cancer or a history of breast cancer or of cancer of any reproductive organs
- have a history of heart disease, stroke, or high blood pressure; blood clotting problems; or diabetes

Topical Contraceptives

Spermicides are topical forms of contraception that are available in various dosage forms, including creams, foams, gels, suppositories, and vaginal films. The active ingredient in most spermicides is nonoxynol-9. Nonoxynol-9 has been reported to cause the lining of the vaginal wall to thin or erode faster, and when used often may actually help bacteria and viruses to enter the flesh faster. Apply and reapply spermicides before sexual intercourse, no earlier than the time stated in the directions, which varies from 20 minutes to 1 hour. It is important for the female to prevent the spermicide from dripping out of the vagina after intercourse so that it can be effective. Although the use of a panty liner may help, lying down for 4–8 hours will better enhance the effectiveness of such products. Also, women should not douche for at least 8 hours after intercourse, because douching may interfere with the effectiveness of the spermicide.

Workplace Wisdom Nonoxynol-9

Studies indicate that nonoxynol-9 spermicides irritate vaginal and rectal linings, increasing the recipient's exposure risk to HIV or a sexually transmitted infection. Anyone using a product containing nonoxynol-9 who notices any genital irritation should discontinue use.

Spermicidal foam, the most effective spermicide, helps prevent pregnancy in two ways:

1. By forming a physical barrier to the entry of sperm into the cervix.
2. By immobilizing and killing the sperm.

Simple skin irritations and allergies to ingredients other than the active ingredient can deter use. Gels must be reapplied if not used within 20 minutes before intercourse. Vaginal filmstrips are good for one hour after insertion.

● ● ●

PROFILES IN PRACTICE

Mary, a pharmacy technician, is entering demographic data into the computer system for Mrs. Dalton, a new customer. During the conversation, Mrs. Dalton reveals to Mary that she is 3 months pregnant.

- Why is it important for Mary to include Mrs. Dalton's pregnancy in her patient profile?

Contraceptive Devices

Oral contraception, in tablet form, is not the only birth control option. Many alternatives are available, such as barrier devices, diaphragms, cervical caps, and intrauterine devices.

Barrier Devices—Male Condoms

Lamb intestine condoms do not provide protection from sexually transmitted diseases or infections (STDs). Latex condoms are the most effective protection against transmission of bacterial and viral infections. The main drawback of these is allergic reactions by either the female or the male. Polyurethane condoms should be used if either partner is allergic to latex. Some condoms also contain a spermicide.

Condoms should never be used with greasy or oily substances, such as Vaseline, because these substances will cause the condom to weaken and burst. Personal water-based lubricants, such as K-Y Jelly, are made for this purpose.

Barrier Devices—Female Condoms

A polyurethane tube or sheath approximately 6.5 inches long, with an inner ring at the closed end that loosely lines the vagina, provides protection from unintended pregnancy and the transmission of STDs. This material does not cause allergies and need not be removed immediately after ejaculation, though it should be taken out before the woman stands up to avoid the semen spilling out. Upon removal, the outer ring should be twisted to seal the condom, so that no semen leaks out. Current standard directions indicate that a female condom should be used only once. However, it can be used with either oil- or water-based lubricants. The simultaneous use of both a male and a female condom is contraindicated because the condoms may create friction, resulting in either or both condoms slipping or tearing and/or the outer ring of the female condom being pushed inside the vagina. Table 30-3 compares male and female condoms.

Table 30-3   Male and Female Condom Comparison

MALE CONDOM	FEMALE CONDOM
Brands: Durex®, Lifestyles®, Magnum®, Trojan®	Brands: Dominique®, Femidom®, Femy®, Myfemy®, Reality®
Nickname: rubber	Nickname: FC
Rolled on the man's penis, fits snugly on the penis	Inserted into the woman's vagina, loosely lines the vagina
Lubricant:	*Lubricant:*
• Can include spermicide	• Can include spermicide
• Can be water-based only; cannot be oil-based	• Can be water-based or oil-based
• Located on the outside of the condom	• Located on both the inside and the outside of the condom

Table 30-3   Male and Female Condom Comparison (*continued*)

MALE CONDOM	FEMALE CONDOM
Requires erect penis	Can be inserted prior to sexual intercourse; not dependent on erect penis
Must be removed immediately after ejaculation	Need not be removed immediately after ejaculation; must be removed before the female stands
Covers most of the penis and protects the woman's internal genitalia	Provides broader protection by covering both the internal and external genitalia of the woman and the base of the man's penis.
Latex condoms can decay if not stored properly	Polyurethane is not susceptible to deterioration from temperature or humidity
Can be used *only* once; is then discarded	Recommended as one-time-use product
Disadvantage: must interrupt foreplay to use	Can be inserted before foreplay, and intercourse occurs without interrupting foreplay
Easy placement	Disadvantage: Takes a while for the female to learn how to use it confidently. Takes practice. Makes a noise that can be silenced with use of more lubricant.

Diaphragms and Cervical Caps

A *diaphragm* is a latex or silicon cervical barrier form of birth control. When properly inserted, the diaphragm forms a seal against the vaginal wall which prevents sperm from entering. Only a trained healthcare provider can fit a woman for these devices. The size of the diaphragm must match the distance from the pubic bone to the posterior fornix of the vagina (or the largest size that is comfortable for the client).

A *cervical cap* is similar to a diaphragm except that it fits over the cervix to prevent sperm form entering the uterus. Cervical caps come in four sizes. A cap that is too small can injure the cervix; one that is too large can slip off during intercourse. A woman may need to have these devices refit if she undergoes any of the following changes:

- gains or loses weight
- has a baby
- has a second- or third-trimester abortion

Both the diaphragm and the cervical cap should be used with spermicides. Diaphragms must be worn for at least six hours after intercourse. Because rubber deteriorates, the devices should be periodically checked for small holes and replaced as needed.

INFORMATION

The Femcap® is a new device, similar to a cervical cap, that is made of silicone rubber, which is being developed for diaphragms in place of the latex to which increasing numbers of people are allergic. The Femcap® can be worn for 48 hours, and may be effective without spermicides. Alternatively, it can be worn continuously, with applications of spermicide before sexual intercourse. It is removed for cleaning and during menstrual periods.

Intrauterine Devices

Intrauterine devices (IUDs) are small, flexible devices made of metal and/or plastic. These devices are inserted into a woman's uterus through her vagina; the procedure is done by a healthcare provider during an office visit. Approximately 15 percent of women of reproductive age currently use IUDs. These devices work to prevent pregnancy by a combination of mechanisms. They inhibit sperm migration in the upper female genital tract, which in turn inhibits ovum transport and stimulates endometrial changes that will not support implantation. Most are unmedicated, but some IUDs are progestin-releasing (levonorgestrel or progesterone). IUDs are safe for 5–10 years, but have the drawback of tending to cause heavy menstrual bleeding. IUDs are 97 to 99.6 percent effective.

PROFILES IN PRACTICE

Jesse is working at an independent retail pharmacy. A woman comes into the pharmacy for Plan B tablets. Both Jesse and his pharmacist have a moral objection to this form of emergency contraception.

- As pharmacy professionals, how should they handle this situation?

Mammary Glands and Childbirth

During the fourth or fifth month of gestation, the pituitary gland secretes prolactin, which causes the mammary glands to produce breast milk even before the baby is born. Postpartum (after birth), the action of sucking on the nipple stimulates the pituitary gland to continue to secrete more prolactin, thus stimulating the production of more milk.

Oxytocin, secreted by the posterior pituitary gland, causes labor contractions. Immediately after the baby leaves the birth canal, oxytocin allows the milk that has been made, according to the prolactin signal, to be secreted. After the birth, sucking also causes oxytocin to be secreted by the posterior pituitary gland; the oxytocin causes the milk ducts in the breast to contract and relax, pushing the milk toward the nipple. Therefore, prolactin causes milk production, while oxytocin enables milk secretion. Many other hormones, such as FSH, LH, and human placental lactogen (HPL), also play vital roles in milk production. When dopamine, a prolactin-inhibitory factor, inhibits prolactin, milk is no longer produced or secreted.

Research shows that oxytocin may also be responsible for the "bonding" attraction between mother and child, as well as between life partners. Injectable oxytocin is available under the trade name Pitocin®. Figure 30-3 shows the relationship between oxytocin and breastfeeding.

Female Infertility

Infertility is defined as failure to conceive after one year of regular, unprotected intercourse. Infertility may occur as a result of a problem in either partner or because of a combination of problems in both partners.

Causes of Female Infertility

About 35 percent of all cases of infertility stem from problems in the man's system; another 35 percent arise from abnormalities in the woman's system; about 20 percent of the time, both the man and the woman have fertility problems. In about 10 percent of cases, no cause can be found. It is known, however, that age often increases the risk of infertility.

Pelvic inflammatory disease (PID) is the major cause of infertility worldwide. PID is an infection of the pelvis or one or more of the female reproductive organs that causes scarring, abscess formation, and tubal damage. It may spread to the appendix or to the entire pelvic area. PID is commonly caused by the same bacteria that cause sexually transmitted diseases or infections, such as gonorrhea or chlamydia. (Chlamydia

FIGURE 30-3 The relationship between oxytocin and breastfeeding.

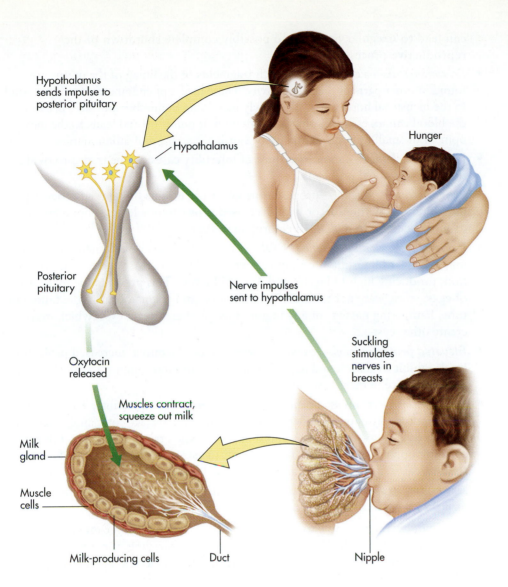

Hypothalamus sends impulse to posterior pituitary

Hypothalamus

Hunger

Posterior pituitary

Nerve impulses sent to hypothalamus

Suckling stimulates nerves in breasts

Oxytocin released

Muscles contract, squeeze out milk

Milk gland

Muscle cells

Milk-producing cells

Duct

Nipple

causes 75 percent of fallopian tube infections.) PID may also develop from infection by the bacteria that thrive during abortion, hysterectomy, childbirth, sexual intercourse, use of an intrauterine contraceptive device, or a ruptured appendix.

Many factors other than PID can lead to infertility, including exposure to high levels of chemicals, toxic substances, high temperatures, and radiation; persistent stress; smoking cigarettes and/or marijuana; and using caffeine and/or other drugs. Other risk factors for infertility include:

- *Age*—a woman's age (more accurately, the age of her eggs) can contribute to infertility. At age 25, the chance of getting pregnant within the first 6 months of trying to conceive is 75 percent. By the time the woman is 40 years old, her chances are lowered to only 22 percent. This decrease in fertility appears to be caused by a higher rate of chromosomal abnormalities occurring in the eggs as the woman ages.

- *Weight*—Fat cells make 30 percent of estrogen. However, overweight patients have an overload of estrogen that throws off the reproductive cycle. Conversely, strict vegetarians, athletes, and dancers who lack sufficient body fat may not produce enough estrogen; these women may also have difficulties because of a lack of vitamin B12, zinc, iron, and folic acid. These deficiencies can lead to irregular periods and possibly complete shutdown of the reproductive process.

- *Endometriosis*—a condition in which fragments of the lining of the uterus are found in other parts of the pelvic cavity. These pieces of endometrium still respond to the menstrual hormonal cycle, slowly increasing in number and size. Because the blood cannot escape during menstruation, it builds up and leads to the development of small or large painful cysts, causing scarring and inflammation.

- *Hormonal changes*—about one-third of infertility cases can be traced to ovulation and hormonal problems.

- *Progesterone deficiency*—progesterone keeps the uterine lining ready to accept implantation. Without it, or with decreased progesterone levels, implantation cannot occur, or an implanted embryo may abort.

- *Polycystic ovarian syndrome (PCO)*—occurs in 6 percent of women and is the major cause of infertility in American women. PCO increases androgen production, producing high LH levels and low FSH levels. This prevents the maturation of eggs, so eggs are not released. Inflammation and edema occur in the fallopian tube, hampering passage of any matured ova and creating a cyst (which may create other cysts).

- *Elevated prolactin levels*—in women who are not lactating, increased prolactin levels inhibit ovulation and may also indicate a pituitary tumor. Parlodel® is the drug of choice in these cases.

- *Medications*—certain medications can cause temporary infertility. These include prescription antibiotics, antidepressants, hormones, and narcotic analgesics, and OTC medications such as ASA and ibuprofen (when taken midcycle). Taking acetaminophen regularly may reduce levels of estrogen and luteinizing hormone. In most cases, once the drugs are discontinued, fertility is restored.

- *Antibodies to sperm*—some women have antibodies to sperm, that attack sperm as if they were harmful foreign bodies or substances.

Sometimes a woman is able to conceive, but the fertilized ovum cannot implant or the endometrial lining sheds despite implantation, carrying the ovum with it. *Spontaneous abortion* has been associated with use of an electric blanket during the month of conception.

Pharmaceutical Treatment of Infertility in Women

Persistent infertility, if untreated, often has damaging psychological effects, creating feelings of guilt or depression in either or both partners and breaking down communication between a couple. Having to have intercourse at specific times of the menstrual cycle, and times at which the female has a specific basal temperature, can add more stress. Therefore, persons who wish to conceive often turn to pharmaceutical treatment to help increase fertility. An example of an antiestrogenic drug is the fertility drug clomiphene (Clomid®, Serophene®). Clomiphene tricks the brain and pituitary gland into "thinking" that there is less estrogen available in the female's body. This stimulates pituitary production of FSH and LH, boosting follicle growth and the release of mature eggs.

Side effects include hot flashes, breast tenderness, mood swings, visual problems, thick cervical mucus, and luteal phase deficiency. The time from ovulation to onset of the next period is known as the *luteal phase*, during which the corpus luteum makes progesterone. Progesterone prepares the uterine lining for embryo implantation. A luteal phase deficiency or a short luteal phase results from a lack of progesterone production by the corpus luteum, or poor response of the endometrium to normal progesterone levels. This lack of progesterone or response to it may cause or exacerbate infertility.

Toxic effects of fertility drugs include long-term safety risks. Use for more than a year may increase the risk of ovarian cancer. The risk of multiple births and low birth weight also increases with the use of fertility drugs.

The Male Reproductive System

The male reproductive system includes the organs and hormones that allow males to reproduce and gives them their gender characteristics. This section discusses male anatomy and some conditions and diseases of the male reproductive system, including infertility, erectile dysfunction, benign prostatic hyperplasia, and sexually transmitted diseases.

Anatomy

The prostate gland is situated at the base of the bladder and encircles the urethra. The organ is roughly the size and shape of a large walnut, with an average normal weight of 20–30 g. Secretions produced in the prostatic glands empty into the urethra during ejaculation, via the prostatic ducts, to make up a sizable volume of the ejaculate. Although the function of this fluid is not fully understood, it is speculated that it neutralizes the acidic environment of the vagina and possibly provides nutrition for the spermatids (young sperm cells). Though not absolutely necessary for fertilization, prostate solutions increase the chances of fertilization.

The **testes**, a pair of organs located in the scrotum and surrounded by a thin mesothelial membrane, are responsible for the production of sperm, as well as the production of androgens. The testes are made up of thousands of tiny tubules supported by fibrous septae, and the entire gland is surrounded by a thick fibrous capsule called the *tunica albuginea*. Mature sperm are stored in the *epididymis*. During ejaculation, the sperm are propelled along the vas deferens into the urethra (see Figure 30-4).

testes The male reproductive organs that produce sperm.

Male Infertility

Fertility in the male begins with the production of gonadotropin-releasing hormone in the hypothalamus, which instructs the pituitary gland to manufacture FSH and LH. FSH causes sperm production and LH stimulates production of the male hormone testosterone. Both sperm and testosterone production occur in the testes. The life cycle of sperm is about 70–75 days. The ability of a sperm to move straight forward rapidly is determined by its *flagellum* (tail), and is probably the most important factor that

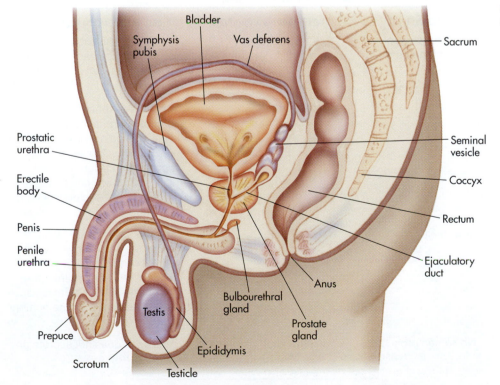

FIGURE 30-4 The male reproductive system.

determines male fertility. During sexual excitement, nerves stimulate the muscles in the epididymis to contract, forcing the sperm into the vas deferens and then through the penis. The *seminal vesicles*, clusters of tissue, contribute seminal fluid to the sperm. The vas deferens also collects fluid from the nearby prostate gland. The mixture of the fluids from the seminal vesicles, the secretions from the prostate gland, and the sperm is called *semen*. The two vas deferens join together to form the ejaculatory duct, which conducts the semen through to the urethra. The urethra is the same pathway in the penis through which urine passes. During orgasm in a healthy male, the prostate closes off the bladder so that urine cannot enter the urethra. The semen is forced through the urethra during *ejaculation*, the final stage of orgasm. Of the 100 to 300 million sperm that are in the ejaculate, about 400 survive the acidic environment of the vagina, and only about 40 reach the egg.

Activities that increase a male's risk for infertility (see Table 30-4) include:

- Smoking, which impairs sperm motility and reduces sperm lifespan.
- Poor nutrition, especially deficiency of vitamin C, selenium, zinc, and/or folate.
- Bicycling. Pressure from a bike seat may damage the blood vessels and nerves that are responsible for erections. Biking exposes the perineum to extreme shock and vibrations, increasing the risk of injuries to the scrotum.
- Oxygen-free radicals (oxidants). Unstable particles called *free radicals* are released as a by-product of many natural chemical processes in the body, such as infection. These oxidants negatively affect the DNA in the sperm.
- Exposure to chemicals such as pesticides, the phylates used to soften plastics, and hydrocarbons (benzene, ethylbenzene toluene, and xylene). Sperm quality may be affected by exposure to heavy metals such as lead, cadmium, or arsenic.
- Hypogonadism, a severe deficiency in GnRH, the hormone that signals the release of testosterone and other important reproductive hormones. Low levels of testosterone may result in defective sperm production. Tumors of the pituitary gland may also affect GnRH, FSH, or LSH levels.

Table 30-4   Categories of Male Infertility

CATEGORY	MEDICAL NAME	DESCRIPTION/COMMENT
Low sperm count (most common cause)	oligospermia	Sperm count is less than 10 million sperm/mL of semen. Numerous and varied causes of temporary and permanent low sperm count.
No sperm	azoospermia	Complete absence of sperm. Relatively rare, affecting less than 1% of all men and 10% to 15% of infertile men. Causes: Obstruction or production failure of sperm in the testes, which can be caused by mumps, genetic disorders, radiation, or exposure to chemicals.
Low-quality sperm	dysspermia	Quality is determined by sperm motility (ability to move), which depends on its flagella or its morphology (shape and structure). The quality of the sperm is usually more significant than the number of sperm (count).
No semen production	aspermia	Ejaculation does not secrete any semen.

- Autoantibodies caused by infections or injury. Sometimes the body reacts to sperm as if they were invading foreign bodies, and creates antibodies to destroy them.
- Retrograde ejaculation, which occurs when the muscles of the urethra do not propel the semen properly during orgasm. The sperm are forced backward into the bladder instead of forward out of the urethra. Retrograde ejaculation may be caused by several conditions, including diabetes, HTN, MS, spinal cord injury, tranquilizers, and HTN medication.
- Cryptorchidism, associated with mild to severely impaired sperm production, is a failure of the testes to descend from the abdomen into the scrotum during fetal development. The testes are exposed to the higher degree of internal body heat, which kills sperm.
- Medications. Anabolic steroids severely impair sperm production. Other drugs that affect male fertility include:
  - cimetidine (Tagamet®)
  - sulfasalazine (Azulfidine®)
  - methadone (Dolophine®)
  - methotrexate (Folex®)
  - phenytoin (Dilantin®)
  - spironolactone (Aldactone®)
  - thioridazine (Mellaril®)
  - calcium channel blockers
  - colchicine
  - corticosteroids

Drugs that can treat male infertility caused by hormonal changes include:

- Antibiotics—to treat infections that interfere with infertility.
- Antihistamines—studies report that "nondrowsy" antihistamines that block mast cells may be beneficial in some cases of low sperm count. Mast cells release inflammatory immune factors that may reduce sperm quality. Overseas studies report improved pregnancy rates with two agents, ebastine and tranilast. Similar antihistamines in the United States are cetirizine (Zyrtec®), fexofenadine (Allegra®), and loratadine (Claritin®).
- Anti-erectile dysfunction agents—drugs such as sildenafil (Viagra®), vardenafil (Levitra®), and tadalafil (Cilalis®) may enhance fertility by increasing sperm motion and *capacitation* (the explosive energy release in the sperm that aids the act of fertilization).
- Bromocriptine (Parlodel®)—used to reduce excess prolactin manufactured by the pituitary in some infertile men.
- Gonadotropin-releasing hormone—beneficial for men with gonadotropin deficiency and hypogonadism, and helps to restore sperm production after chemotherapy.

Erectile Dysfunction

Male sexual *impotence* is defined as the inability to sustain an erection for penetration. Impotence has many causes. A specific sequence of events (such as nerve impulses in the brain, spinal column, and area around the penis, and response in muscles, fibrous tissues, veins, and arteries in and near the corpora cavernosa) must take place, in the proper order, for an erection to occur. It is much like a domino effect, and can be interrupted at many different points in the sequence by various factors and agents. Diseases, such as diabetes, kidney disease, chronic alcoholism, multiple sclerosis, atherosclerosis, vascular disease, and neurologic disease, account for about 70 percent of ED cases. Damage that these conditions cause to nerves, arteries, smooth muscles, and fibrous tissues is the most common cause of *erectile dysfunction (ED)*.

Researchers believe that psychological factors such as stress, anxiety, guilt, depression, low self-esteem, and fear of sexual failure cause 10 to 20 percent of ED cases. Men with an organic physical cause may also experience psychological factors. Smoking, which restricts blood flow in veins and arteries and reduces hormonal (testosterone) secretions, can contribute to ED.

Levitra® (vardenafil), Cialis® (tadalafil), and Viagra® (sildenafil) are used in the treatment of ED. Early tests showed that Cialis® does not affect blood pressure as much as Viagra®. Following sexual stimulation, Cialis® works by helping the blood vessels in the penis to relax, allowing the flow of blood into the penis. Cialis® will not improve sexual performance if the male does not have erectile dysfunction. Levitra® works within 16 minutes, with physical stimulation; Viagra® takes longer, up to one hour. Levitra® is to be taken from 30 minutes to 4.5 hours before desired intercourse. Levitra® can be taken with food, but Viagra® should not.

Levitra® and Cialis® cause no vision or heart side effects. Viagra® helps maintain an erection by blocking the action of an enzyme called phosphodiesterase type 5 in penile tissue. Researchers believe that nonselective blockade of other forms of phosphodiesterase enzymes may trigger some of the drug's adverse side effects, especially facial flushing and visual disturbances (seeing blue).

Benign Prostatic Hyperplasia

Because of their close physical placement, the urethra is susceptible to pressure from hyperplastic enlargement of the prostate. The prostate actually has two anatomical zones: the central zone and the peripheral zone. The central zones are prone to **hyperplasia**; the peripheral zone is much more frequently affected by carcinoma.

As men get older, the prostate gland enlarges. Such an enlargement is called *benign prostatic hyperplasia (BPH)*. This noncancerous growth is the most common benign tumor in men over the age of 50. The enlargement causes the following problems:

- difficult urination
- urinary blockage, urinary retention, or the inability to urinate
- urinary frequency
- a feeling of incomplete voiding (the sensation of incomplete bladder emptying)

Other symptoms include hesitancy or slow initiation of urination (slow start), decreased force of the urinary stream (weak stream), and intermittence (stopping and starting) of the urinary stream. A variety of other symptoms may also occur, including frequent nocturia (nighttime urination) and urgency to urinate.

Changes caused by prostate enlargement are gradual and may often be ignored by the patient. It is thought that from 20 to 30 percent of men will need medical or surgical treatment of BPH before they reach the age of 80.

Pharmaceutical Treatment of BPH

Drugs such as finasteride (Proscar®) and dutasteride (Avodart™), which are 5-alpha reductase inhibitors, prevent the conversion of testosterone to the hormone dihydrotestosterone (DHT). A treatment period of six months may be necessary before one can tell if the therapy is going to work. Finasteride is available in tablet form and dutasteride is available as soft gelatin capsules. These are taken orally once a day. Patients should see their physicians regularly to monitor side effects and adjust the dosage, if necessary.

Side effects include reduced libido, impotence, breast tenderness and enlargement, and reduced sperm count. Long-term risks and benefits have not been studied.

Women who are pregnant or may be pregnant must avoid handling dutasteride capsules and broken or crushed finasteride tablets, as exposure to these drugs may cause serious side effects to a male fetus. To prevent pregnant women from being exposed to the drug and causing teratogenic effects through blood transfusion, patients should wait at least six months after treatment with a 5-alpha reductase inhibitor to donate blood.

hyperplasia the reproduction of cells within an organ at an increased rate.

Table 30-5   Alpha-Adrenergic Blockers

GENERIC NAME	TRADE NAME	STRENGTH/ DOSAGE FORM AVAILABLE	AVERAGE ADULT DOSE
alfuzosin	Uroxatral®	10 mg extended-release (ER) tabs	BPH: 10 mg once daily
doxazosin mesylate	Cardura®	1 mg, 2 mg, 4 mg, 8 mg	BPH: 1–8 mg once daily HTN: 1–16 mg once daily
prazosin	Minipress®	1 mg, 2 mg, 5 mg caps	HTN: 3–20 mg/day in divided doses
tamsulosin	Flomax®	0.4 mg ER caps	BPH: 10 mg once daily
terazosin	Hytrin®	1 mg, 2 mg, 5 mg, 10 mg tabs and caps	BPH: 1–10mg once daily HTN: 1–20 mg once daily

Alpha-adrenergic blockers relax smooth muscle tissue in the bladder neck and prostate, thereby increasing urinary flow. They typically are taken orally, once or twice a day (see Table 30-5).

Side effects of alpha-adrenergic blockers include:

- headache
- dizziness
- low blood pressure
- fatigue
- weakness
- difficulty breathing

Sexually Transmitted Diseases

A **sexually transmitted disease (STD)** is a disease caused by a pathogen (virus, bacterium, parasite, or fungus) that is spread from person to person through sexual contact. STDs may also be referred to as **sexually transmitted infections (STIs)**. STDs can be painful, irritating, debilitating, and sometimes life-threatening. More than 20 sexually transmitted diseases have been identified.

STDs occur most commonly in sexually active teenagers and young adults, but are found among men and women of all economic classes. The risk of contracting an STD increases in those who engage in sex with multiple partners. It is estimated that approximately 200 to 400 million people worldwide are infected with a STD. Examples of STDs are:

- bacterial vaginosis (change in the normal bacteria of the vagina)
- *Chlamydia trachomatis* (bacterium that can cause an STI)
- genital warts (wart-like bumps)
- gonorrhea (bacterium that can cause an STI)
- hepatitis B and hepatitis C (liver diseases)
- herpes (virus)
- HIV/AIDS (acquired immune deficiency syndrome)
- lice and crabs (parasites)
- molluscum (viral infection)
- syphilis (bacterial infection)
- trichomonas (parasite)
- vaginal yeast (fungal infection)

sexually transmitted disease (STD) a disease caused by a pathogen (virus, bacterium, parasite, or fungus) that is spread from person to person through sexual contact.

sexually transmitted infection (STI) a sexually transmitted disease.

INFORMATION

Microbicide products are being developed for use either vaginally or rectally to reduce the transmission of HIV and/or other STDs. Microbicides decrease the ability of a microbe to cause an infection. They may become available in many forms, including gels, creams, suppositories, films, sponges, or vaginal rings. Some microbicides will also offer contraceptive benefits. Microbicides are not currently available, but the demand is great, so it is hoped that the public can expect to find them on the market soon.

Many STDs do not cause much harm or severe symptoms. However, some produce persistent asymptomatic or minimally symptomatic disease. Some people may carry a disease for days, weeks, or even longer. During this time, the infected individual, or *carrier*, can spread disease even if he or she is asymptomatic. Complications of STD infection include the following conditions:

- pelvic inflammatory disease
- inflammation of the cervix (*cervicitis*) in women
- inflammation of the urethra (*urethritis*)
- inflammation of the prostate (*prostatitis*) in men
- fertility and reproductive system problems in both sexes
- damage to an infant infected while in the womb or during birth; consequences include stillbirth, blindness, and permanent neurological damage

A person infected with an STD is more likely to become infected with HIV and a person infected with both HIV and another STD is more likely to transmit HIV.

Treatment and Prevention of STDs

The only sure way to avoid becoming infected with an STD is to practice abstinence or practice monogamy with an uninfected partner. The symptoms of viral STDs, such as genital herpes (HSV) and human immunodeficiency virus (HIV), can be managed with medication, but the infections cannot be cured. Bacterial STDs, such as gonorrhea and chlamydia, can be cured with antibiotics. Fungal and parasitic diseases can be cured with antifungal and anthelminthic agents, respectively. Early diagnosis and treatment increase the chances for cure.

SUMMARY

The reproductive system is made up of internal reproductive organs, associated ducts, and external genitalia. Its primary function is the reproductive process. Sex hormones are produced in the gonads (in males, the testes; in females, the ovaries).

Although many diseases can affect the reproductive system, a pharmacy technician will most frequently encounter conditions involving contraception, infertility, STDs, and BPH. It is important that a pharmacy technician be well informed regarding the different types of contraceptives, including their side effects and contraindications.

CHAPTER REVIEW QUESTIONS

1. The most fertile time during the female reproductive cycle is:
   a. day 1–14.
   b. day 20.
   c. midcycle, usually day 12–14.
   d. end of cycle.

2. The main function of estradiol is:
   a. to stimulate development of the uterine lining and the mammary glands.
   b. to maintain the uterine lining if implantation occurs.
   c. to start menstruation.
   d. to give feminine features.

3. The main function of progesterone is:
   a. to stimulate development of the uterine lining and the mammary glands.
   b. to maintain the uterine lining if implantation occurs.
   c. to start menstruation.
   d. to give feminine features.

4. Azoospermia is a condition characterized by:
   a. low sperm count.
   b. low-quality sperm.
   c. no sperm production.
   d. no semen production.

5. What occurs in BPH?
   a. the prostate gland enlarges
   b. the neck of the bladder narrows
   c. frequent urination, nocturia, and urination hesitancy
   d. all of the above

6. BPH can be treated with:
   a. cardiac stents.
   b. beta blockers.
   c. calcium channel blockers.
   d. alpha-adrenergic blockers.

7. The main risk factor for BPH is:
   a. race.
   b. HTN.
   c. diabetes.
   d. age.

8. Which of the following is a contraindication for women who are taking oral contraceptives?
   a. over 35 years of age
   b. smoking
   c. history of breast cancer
   d. all of the above

9. Which of the following contraceptive agents is a subdermal implant?
   a. Lunelle®
   b. Plan B®
   c. Ovrette®
   d. Norplant®

10. Which of the following is *not* a mechanism of action for oral contraceptives?
    a. prevent ovulation
    b. reduce likelihood of implantation
    c. block implantation
    d. prevent sperm from entering vaginal canal

CRITICAL THINKING QUESTIONS

1. A pregnant women comes into your pharmacy to pick up her husband's Avodart® prescription. What potential complications might arise? What can you do to help to prevent them?

2. Why is a person with an STD more likely to become infected with HIV?

WEB CHALLENGE

1. See an interactive demonstration on the female reproductive cycle and how an oral contraceptive works at: http://www.cnn.com/2000/HEALTH/women/12/14/contraceptives.ap/

2. Research microbicide products to find the latest information on their development. Write a one-page summary of your findings. For example, you might discuss safety issues of whether microbicides protect against all STDs.

REFERENCES AND RESOURCES

Adams, MP, Josephson, DL, & Holland, LN Jr. *Pharmacology for Nurses—A Pathophysiologic Approach*. Upper Saddle River, NJ: Pearson Education, 2008.

CDC Statement on Study Results of Product Containing Nonoxynol-9 (released at the XIII International AIDS Conference held in Durban, South Africa, July 9–14, 2000): http://www.cdc.gov/mmwr/preview/mmwrhtml/mm4931a4.htm

Drug Facts and Comparisons, 2006 ed. St. Louis: Wolters Kluwer Health.

FDA dockets of noncontraceptive, estrogen-containing drugs (accessed April 14, 2008): http://www.fda.gov/OHRMS/DOCKETS/98fr/092799d.txt and http://a257.g.akamaitech.net/7 /257/2422/14mar20010800/edocket.access.gpo.gov /cfr_2002/aprqtr/pdf/21cfr310.517.pdf

FindLaw on estrogen and package inserts: http://caselaw.lp.findlaw.com/scripts/getcase.pl?court=ny&vol=i99&invol=0168

Holland, N, & Adams, MP. *Core Concepts in Pharmacology*. Upper Saddle River, NJ: Pearson Education, 2007.

"Hormone involved in reproduction may have role in the maintenance of relationships" (accessed April 14, 2008): http://www.oxytocin.org/oxytoc/

"Premenstrual Dysphoric Disorder" (accessed October 17, 2007): www.mayoclinic.com

Shands at the University of Florida: http://www.shands.org/professional/drugs/bulletins/0601.pdf

31 The Nervous System

LEARNING OBJECTIVES

After completing this chapter, you should be able to:

- Explain the functions of the nervous system and its division into the central and peripheral nervous systems.
- Compare and contrast the sympathetic and parasympathetic nervous systems.
- Describe the function or physiology of neurons and nerve transmission and the various neurotransmitters.
- Explain the relationship of the nervous system to the other body systems.
- Explain the functions of the blood-brain barrier and describe what types of substances will and will not cross it.
- List and define common diseases affecting the nervous system and discuss the causes, symptoms, and pharmaceutical treatments associated with each disease.
- Identify the common drugs used to treat diseases and conditions of the nervous system.

Introduction

The endocrine and nervous systems work together to maintain homeostasis in the body. The endocrine system communicates relatively slowly, via hormones secreted by ductless glands into the circulatory system and carried by the blood to muscles, glands, and various other parts of the body. By contrast, the nervous system communicates messages very quickly, through nerve impulses conducted from one part of the body to another using the transmission of neurotransmitter chemicals from one nerve cell to another. The nervous system is complex and one of the least understood parts of the body.

At its core, the brain has billions of individual connecting pieces and makes trillions of connections. The specific function of these pieces, known as nerve cells or neurons, is to allow learning, reasoning, and remembering. The brain works on electrochemical energy, allowing you to read this book, smile at a friend, remember a computer password, and decide between eating apples or oranges.

The brain also controls emotions, sex drive, heart rate, breathing and respiration, appetite, and sleep.

The brain requires energy in the form of glucose, a sugar. Essential substances, such as vitamins and minerals, as well as sources of dietary carbohydrate energy, help the brain to function properly. The brain cannot turn off like a computer or radio. While you are asleep, your brain is still active, as if on automatic pilot. This is when you digest and metabolize most of your food; you also continue breathing, but at a much slower rate.

The nervous system is tied into every other system in the body. It interacts with every system to ensure homeostasis. Therefore, diseases and disorders of the nervous system may have far-reaching effects and be difficult to diagnose and treat.

Anatomy of the Nervous System

As shown in Figure 31-1, the nervous system is made up of the brain, spinal cord, nerves, and sensory organs (skin, eyes, and ears). The *neuron* is the basic cell of the nervous system. The nervous system is divided into two parts called the **central nervous system (CNS)** and the peripheral nervous system (PNS). Like the central processing unit (CPU) of a computer that controls other devices, the CNS is the main area that controls all other nervous system functions, some directly and others indirectly via the peripheral nervous system.

The CNS includes the brain and spinal cord; the peripheral nervous system consists of all other nerves and sensory organs. The PNS is divided into two parts, the somatic and the autonomic nervous systems.

The *autonomic nervous system (ANS)* is further divided into two more parts, called the sympathetic and the parasympathetic nervous systems. Many drugs directly affect these two systems, whether beneficially or adversely. Therefore, comparing and contrasting these two subdivisions is critical to understanding how the nervous system works.

central nervous system (CNS) the part of the nervous system made up of the brain and spinal cord.

Functions of the Nervous System

The nervous system has the following three basic functions (see Table 31-1):

1. *Sensory* or **afferent**. This function sends impulses from muscles and other parts of the body toward the CNS. It senses or recognizes external changes in the environment, such as cold or heat; and internal changes in the body, such as a decrease in potassium or calcium.
2. *Integrative*. This function processes perceived information about the sensory changes and interprets or explains them in the external and internal environments.
3. *Motor* or **efferent**. This function sends impulses away from the CNS to muscles and other parts of the body. The efferent system responds to the brain's interpretation of afferent signals and integrates the external and internal environments by making muscles move, groups of muscles interact, and glands secrete hormones or other chemicals into the bloodstream.

afferent sending an impulse toward the CNS.

efferent sending impulses away from the CNS.

The Neuron

About 10 microns in width, the smallest unit of the nervous system is a nerve cell called the *neuron* (see Figure 31-2). The brain is made up of approximately 100 billion neurons. Neurons are similar to other cells, as they are surrounded by a membrane wall; have a nucleus that contains genes; and contain cytoplasm, mitochondria, and other organelles.

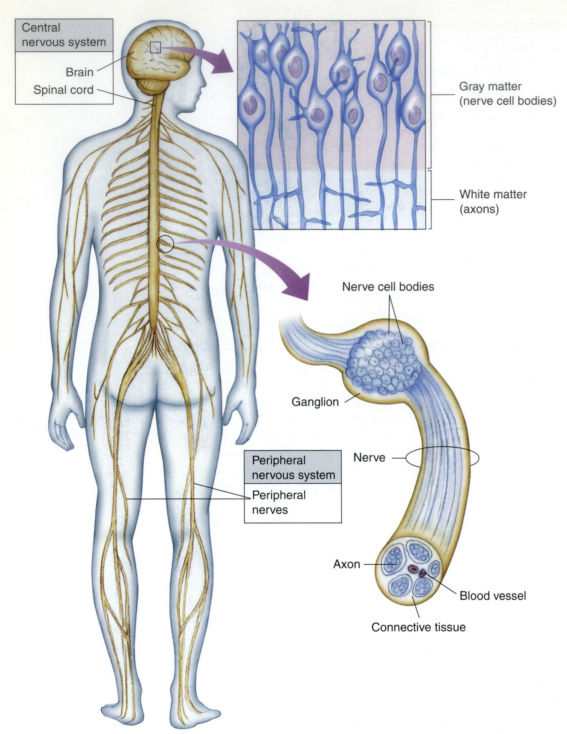

Central nervous system
Brain
Spinal cord

Gray matter (nerve cell bodies)

White matter (axons)

Nerve cell bodies

Ganglion

Peripheral nervous system
Peripheral nerves

Nerve

Axon

Blood vessel

Connective tissue

FIGURE 31-1 The nervous system.

However, neurons differ from other cells in that they have projections called *dendrites* and *axons*. These projections have the following specialized functions:

- Dendrites bring information to the cell body from the CNS.
- Axons take information away from the cell body to the CNS.

Nervous system cells communicate with each other through an electrochemical process, which can be compared to the way a computer sends electrical signals through its wires. The brain sends electrical signals, but does so through neurons. Neurons transfer information to other neurons to control glands, organs, or muscles. Electrochemical hormones called *neurotransmitters* are produced by neurons and stored in the ends of the nerve cells. These neurotransmitters, such as acetylcholine (ACh), are then released

Table 31-1   The Nervous System and Its Relationship with the Body

INTERACTIVE SYSTEM	NERVOUS SYSTEM
Cardiovascular (heart)	Endothelial cells maintain the blood-brain barrier, protecting the brain from harmful substances.
	Baroreceptors send information to the brain about blood pressure. The brain responds by regulating vasodilation, thereby changing heart rate and blood pressure.
	Cerebrospinal fluid drains into the venous blood supply, removing harmful waste from the brain.
Digestive	Digestion of food provides the building blocks of the hormones and neurotransmitters.
	The autonomic nervous system controls the tone of the digestive tract via peristalsis. The nervous system (NS) controls the smooth muscles for peristalsis to allow eating and elimination of food.
	The nervous system (NS) responds to thirst and hunger and controls drinking and feeding.
Endocrine	The hypothalamus controls all other endocrine glands by controlling the pituitary gland.
	Reproductive hormones affect the development of the NS.
	Hormonal feedback to the brain affects the processing and integration of neuronal information.
Integumentary	Receptors in the skin send sensory information to the brain, which then regulates peripheral blood flow and sweat glands.
	Nerves control muscles that connect to hair follicles (arrector pili).
Lymphatic/Immune	The brain stimulates the mechanisms of defense against infection.
Muscular	Muscle receptors send the brain information about body position and movement.
	The brain controls the contraction of skeletal muscle.
	The NS regulates heart rate (myocardial contractions) and the speed at which food moves through the digestive tract (peristalsis).
Renal or Urinary	The bladder sends sensory information to the brain, which controls urination and, therefore, hydration and thirst.
Respiratory	The brain monitors respiratory volume and blood gas levels.
	The brain responds by regulating the respiratory rate.
Skeletal	Bones provide essential calcium for the proper functioning of the NS.
	The skull and vertebrae protect the brain and spinal cord from injury.
	Sensory receptors in bone joints send signals about body position to the brain.
	The brain regulates the position of bones by controlling muscles.

from the end of the neuron and cross the space between neurons, called a *synapse*, to a different neuron. This crossing of the synapse is also part of transmission of a nerve impulse. The neurotransmitters travel across synapses to reach a receiving neuron, where they attach themselves to special structures called *receptors*.

The attachment results in a small electrical response within the receiving neuron. This response may be the "end" or terminal message, or transmission may be continued

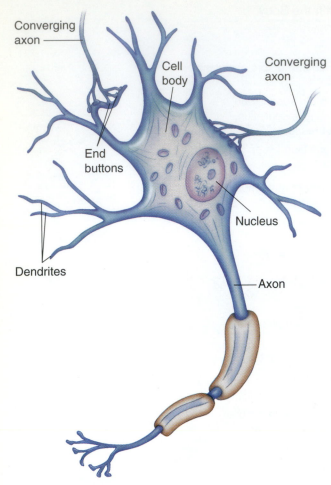

Converging axon

Cell body

Converging axon

End buttons

Nucleus

Dendrites

Axon

FIGURE 31-2 The neuron.

by the second, receiving neuron sending out neurotransmitter messengers of its own. However, this small response does not mean that the message will result in an action by the gland, organ, or muscle. Only when the total signal from all of the synapses involved exceeds a certain level will a large signal, called an *action potential*, be generated and the message be continued.

Neuronal studies can encompass the function of groups of neurons or nerve cells, the role of neurotransmitters, what happens at ion channels on a neuronal and cell membrane, reproduction, or the genetic basis of neuronal function. The nervous system uses neuronal circuits throughout the brain to store memory and undergoes continual modification so that a person can learn new things. The brain can actually "rewire" itself when necessary. After some kinds of brain injuries, undamaged brain tissue can take over functions previously performed by the injured area.

The changes in the environment that set off the nerve impulse to communicate with another neuron are called *stimuli*. The action of the impulse that triggers the release of a neurotransmitter to another neuron is called the *firing of neurons,* and is both electrical and chemical in nature. There are about 50 different neurotransmitters in the brain. These are made of amino acids by the body, with the help of other proteins called *enzymes,* and are stored in the neuron vesicles. Adding a substance that mimics natural neurotransmitters may help the body, or it may cause certain conditions or disease states. Most addictive drugs change the effect of neurotransmitters on neurons.

Neurotransmission and Receptors

A name for the constant exchange of chemical messages between neurons, or firing of neurons, is *neurotransmission*. It is achieved by three basic steps:

1. Neurons release neurotransmitters. When a neuron is excited, it fires, releasing a neurotransmitter.

2. Neurotransmitters bind to receptors. The released neurotransmitters "swim" across the synapse until they "land," or meet the dendrites of the next neuron. This is called *uptake*. The neurotransmitters recognize molecules/sites on the neighboring neuron that are waiting to receive them; these are called *receptors*. Neurotransmitters "dock," or attach, to these specific receptors via a chemical reaction, in a process called *binding*. The neurotransmitters are then released by the receptors. Several things can happen next:

   - Some neurotransmitters may be broken down or destroyed by enzymes.

   - Carrying proteins may transport the neurotransmitters back to the axon from which they originally came, a process called *reuptake*.

   - Neurotransmitters may be used again, in a type of recycling of chemical messengers.

3. Binding passes on or continues (*transduces*) the neurotransmitter's message. The binding itself causes a set of chemical reactions within the receiving neuron. The same kind of impulse that was fired by the sending neuron continues along the nerve pathway from neuron to neuron until it reaches its

terminal destination of a muscle, gland, or organ. The result of this can be a change in the way we respond, behave, think, feel, or react physically.

The Peripheral Nervous System

As noted earlier, the nervous system is divided into two parts, the central nervous system and the peripheral nervous system. The **peripheral nervous system (PNS)** includes all nerves that are not located in the brain and spinal cord. The PNS is further divided into the somatic and the autonomic nervous systems. The somatic nervous system consists of the nerves that connect to the skeletal muscles, and controls voluntary movement of the whole body. The ANS controls the nerves that connect to smooth and cardiac muscles, and thus regulates involuntary movement to perform intricate functions without conscious or voluntary direction. The ANS is further subdivided into two nervous systems called the sympathetic and the parasympathetic.

The sympathetic nervous system (SNS) is governed by the neurotransmitter norepinephrine (NE); the parasympathetic nervous system (PSNS) is governed by acetylcholine (ACh).

The SNS prepares the body for energetic tasks, handles stressful situations, and controls the "fight or flight" response. When NE is inside the receptors of the heart, lungs, and blood vessels, it stimulates or "revs them up." Heart rate, breathing rate, blood pressure, and vasoconstriction increase; gastrointestinal and genitourinary functions decrease temporarily.

The PSNS readies the body for sleep in nonstressful periods and effects the "rest and relaxation" response. When NE is not present inside the receptors of the heart, lungs, or blood vessels, or if ACh is high, the organs are depressed, or slowed down. Heart rate, breathing rate, blood pressure, and vasoconstriction decrease; gastrointestinal and genitourinary functions increase.

peripheral nervous system (PNS) all parts of the nervous system excluding the brain and spinal cord.

" Workplace Wisdom ANS Neurotransmitters

Understanding what each neurotransmitter does to each branch of the ANS is essential to understanding disease states and how they are treated. "

The Central Nervous System

The central nervous system includes the brain and spinal cord. The human brain weighs approximately 1.3 to 1.4 kilograms (2.8 to 3 pounds), as compared to the brain of an elephant (6 kg) or the brain of a rhesus monkey (1 kg). The spinal cord is the main pathway for information connecting the brain to the peripheral nervous system.

Spinal Cord

The spinal cord has 31 paired nerves:

- 8 cervical
- 12 thoracic
- 5 lumbar
- 5 sacral
- 1 coccygeal

The spinal cord is considered to be divided into five main regions:

- skull
- cervical vertebrae
- thoracic vertebrae
- lumbar vertebrae
- sacral vertebrae (sacrum)

cerebrospinal fluid (CSF)
the fluid surrounding the
brain and spinal cord.

The spinal cord is protected from injury by **cerebrospinal fluid (CSF)**, which is contained within a system of fluid-filled cavities called *ventricles*. Receptors in the skin send information to the spinal cord through the spinal nerves. The main functions of CSF are:

- Protection—CSF protects the brain from damage by acting like a cushion to absorb energy and lessen the impact in the event of a blow to the head.
- Excretion of waste products—the one-way flow of CSF into the blood takes harmful metabolites of drugs and other toxic substances away from the brain.
- Endocrine communication—CSF serves as the vehicle to transport hormones to other areas of the brain. Hormones released into the CSF can be carried to remote sites of the brain.

Brain

The head or cephalic region of the body has a bony structure, the *skull*, to protect the brain from injury. Further protection is provided by the three layers of meninges that cover the brain: dura mater, arachnoid, and pia mater (see Figure 31-3). The outermost,

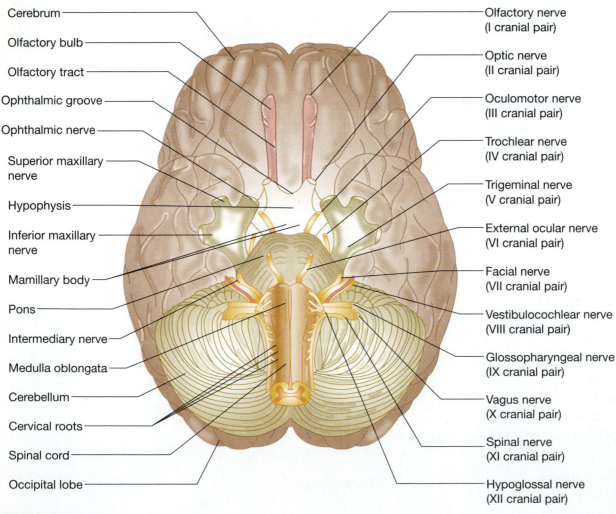

Cerebrum

Olfactory bulb

Olfactory tract

Ophthalmic groove

Ophthalmic nerve

Superior maxillary nerve

Hypophysis

Inferior maxillary nerve

Mamillary body

Pons

Intermediary nerve

Medulla oblongata

Cerebellum

Cervical roots

Spinal cord

Occipital lobe

Olfactory nerve (I cranial pair)

Optic nerve (II cranial pair)

Oculomotor nerve (III cranial pair)

Trochlear nerve (IV cranial pair)

Trigeminal nerve (V cranial pair)

External ocular nerve (VI cranial pair)

Facial nerve (VII cranial pair)

Vestibulocochlear nerve (VIII cranial pair)

Glossopharyngeal nerve (IX cranial pair)

Vagus nerve (X cranial pair)

Spinal nerve (XI cranial pair)

Hypoglossal nerve (XII cranial pair)

FIGURE 31-3 The brain.

hardest layer is the dura mater. The arachnoid has spaces in it that resemble a cobweb and are filled with CSF for further protection.

The brain can be divided down the middle, lengthwise, into two halves called the *cerebral hemispheres*. Each hemisphere (left or right) of the cerebral cortex is divided into the following four lobes:

- **Frontal Lobe.** The frontal lobe is concerned with higher intellect or reasoning, problem solving, parts of speech, movement or motor cortex, and emotion.
- **Parietal Lobe.** The parietal lobe is involved in the stimuli and perception of touch, pressure, temperature, and pain.
- **Temporal Lobe.** The temporal lobe processes perception and recognition of auditory stimuli for hearing and memory (involving the hippocampus).
- **Occipital Lobe.** The occipital lobe is involved with stimuli pertaining to vision.

For the purposes of this overview, we can consider the brain as consisting of three main parts: the cerebellum, the cerebrum, and the brainstem.

Cerebellum

The cerebellum is located behind the brainstem and below the cerebrum. The main purposes of the cerebellum are to coordinate the movement of the body and to maintain equilibrium and balance. Some drugs, such as alcohol, can depress the cerebellum, resulting in a decrease in body coordination and reaction or response time.

Cerebrum

The cerebrum is divided into two main parts:

- **Cerebral Cortex.** The cerebral cortex contains **gray matter** made up of the neurons that control voluntary action. The cerebral cortex is tied in with the somatic part of the peripheral nervous system.
- **Cerebral Medulla.** The cerebra medulla contains **white matter** made up of the myelinated axons of neurons, which conduct nerve impulses to and from different areas of the nervous system. The cerebral medulla also contains more gray matter, known as the *basal ganglia*. The basal ganglia regulate motor activity or movement. Damage to the basal ganglia may result in disorders like Parkinson's disease.

gray matter a major component of the nervous system, composed of nonmyelinated nerve tissue with a gray-brown color.

white matter a major component of the CNS, composed of myelinated nerve tissue that is white in color.

Brainstem

The brainstem, an extension of the spinal cord, is divided into four main parts:

- Thalamus—sits at the top of the brainstem; regulates and evaluates the sensory impulses of pain, hot, cold, and touch. The thalamus directs the sensory information to the correct part of the cerebral cortex or regulates the response.
- Hypothalamus—located just below the thalamus; controls body functions such as water balance, body temperature, sleep, hunger and appetite, sex drive, the autonomic nervous system, and some emotional and behavioral responses.
- Pons—located below the hypothalamus; regulates respiration. The pons is considered the "relay" station for nerve fibers that travel to other parts of the brain.
- Medulla oblongata—located at the base of the brainstem and the top of the spine. The medulla oblongata contains the three vital centers that keep the body alive and functioning: cardiac (heart), respiratory (breathing), and vasomotor (blood vessels). Injury to this area of the brain usually results in death. The reflexes for gagging, swallowing, coughing, and vomiting are regulated by the medulla oblongata.

Reticular Formation

Located throughout the brainstem and cerebrum, a network of nerve fibers known as the *reticular formation* affects the degree of alertness. It is made up of two types of fibers:

- Excitatory fibers—when stimulated by external stimuli such as noises, bright lights, or danger, the degree of alertness is increased. Certain stimulant drugs, such as Ritalin® and caffeine, can increase the activity in the reticular formation, and thus affect the degree of alertness.

- Inhibitory fibers—an absence of external stimuli causes the inhibitory fibers to become more active, which in turn decreases the activity of the excitatory fibers and therefore the degree of alertness. Inhibitory fibers are usually more active during sleep or rest. Certain drugs, such as alcohol, hypnotics, and barbiturates, can decrease the activity of the reticular formation.

Limbic System

One of the least understood areas of the brain is the *limbic system*, a collection of nerve cells in various areas of the brain, especially the hypothalamus, that form a specific neural pathway. The limbic system is associated with such emotional and behavioral responses as sexual behavior, anger, rage, fear, anxiety, reward, and punishment.

Blood-Brain Barrier

The *blood-brain barrier (BBB)* is a semipermeable membrane that allows some substances to cross and reach the brain, but prevents others from getting through. The following are the general properties of the BBB:

- Water-soluble or low-lipid/low-fat-soluble molecules do not penetrate into the brain. Highly lipid/fat-soluble molecules, such as barbiturates, rapidly cross the BBB into the brain.
- Large molecules do not easily pass through the BBB.
- Highly electrically charged molecules are slowed down by the BBB.

The functions of the BBB are to:

- Protect the brain from foreign invaders, or substances in the blood that could injure the brain.
- Protect the brain from hormones and neurotransmitters in the rest of the body.
- Maintain a constant, homeostatic environment for the brain.

The BBB can be broken down. The following disease states can compromise the barrier:

- Hypertension (high blood pressure) can open up the BBB.
- Infectious agents can open up the BBB.
- Hyperosmolarity—a high concentration of a substance in the blood can cause the BBB to open up.

The following physical changes can also break down the BBB:

- When a particular developmental stage is interrupted, the BBB is not fully formed at birth, and thus remains open.
- Exposure to microwaves can open up the BBB.
- Exposure to radiation can open up the BBB.
- Injury to the brain can open up the BBB. Examples include trauma, ischemia, inflammation, and pressure.

Diseases Affecting the Central Nervous System

Mental illness is the most common disorder of the CNS. Mental illness can range from mild and temporary to serious and long-lasting. Pharmacotherapeutics has empowered many people with mental disorders to enhance their lives and reach their fullest potential. The first antipsychotic drug, chlorpromazine, was introduced in the 1950s. Psychotherapy and counseling can be more effective when combined with the use of psychotherapeutic agents. For example, people who were once too depressed to talk to a psychiatrist often begin to respond after a few weeks of treatment with psychotherapeutic drugs.

The following mental disorders may be treated psychotherapeutically: psychosis, depression, anxiety, obsessive-compulsive disorder, and panic disorder. Although there is no cure for mental illness, these drugs will help the patient to have a better experience in daily living and to function more effectively. The National Institute of Mental Health established the following four classifications of psychotherapeutic agents: antianxiety, antidepressant, antimanic, and antipsychotic medications.

Anxiety

Anxiety is associated with the following risk factors: genetics, brain chemistry, life events, and personality. Fewer than one-third of all those suffering from anxiety seek medical treatment, yet it is a most treatable condition. There are many forms of anxiety, categorized: generalized anxiety disorder (GAD), obsessive-compulsive disorder (OCD), panic disorder or panic attack, posttraumatic stress disorder (PTSD), social anxiety disorder (SAD), and specific phobias. Anxiety can strike anyone at any time, but is usually slowly progressive. Some anxiety occurs as a result of a traumatic or childhood event. Specific symptoms or behaviors interfere with work, social situations, or everyday tasks. Table 31-2 describes different types of anxiety.

anxiety an uncomfortable emotional state of apprehension, worry, and fearfulness.

Workplace Wisdom Anxiety Statistics

More than 19 million Americans report experiencing anxiety each year. Among the leading causes are phobia, posttraumatic stress, generalized anxiety, obsessive compulsions, and panic.

A lack of a certain neurotransmitter, *gamma-aminobutyric acid (GABA)*, is associated with anxiety. The more GABA there is, the less anxiety there will be. Conversely, the less GABA there is, the more anxiety there will be. The drug used to treat anxiety depends on the type of anxiety (the cause) and the symptoms. Cognitive and behavioral therapy should be utilized in the treatment of anxiety, along with psychotherapeutic drugs, for the greatest and most beneficial effect.

Anxiety is normally pharmaceutically treated with benzodiazepines, but may also be treated with antidepressant drugs, such as selective serotonin reuptake inhibitors (SSRIs), tricyclic antidepressants (TCAs), monoamine oxidase inhibitors (MAOIs), beta blockers, or any combination of them. Barbiturates are not used as often for anxiety as they once were, because they are highly addictive (C-II) and currently better alternatives are available.

An inability to fall asleep or stay asleep is a common symptom because the person has obsessive thoughts of anticipated or previously experienced events. Serotonin receptors have long been associated with sleep. One antidepressant, Effexor® XR, inhibits the reuptake of both serotonin and norepinephrine.

Table 31-2 Types of Anxiety

TYPE OF ANXIETY AND CAUSE	DESCRIPTION	SYMPTOMS
GAD—The person has unrealistic focus on or chronic worry about everyday living issues, such as health, money, or work/career.	Uncontrollable worry about things that occur in daily living usually is considered GAD if it persists for 6 months or longer; focus may shift from issue to issue.	Trembling, muscular aches, insomnia, abdominal upsets, dizziness, irritability, easy fatigability, trouble sleeping.
OCD—The person has continuous and recurring thoughts (*obsessions*) that reflect exaggerated anxiety or fears. Obsessions can lead to performing a ritual or routine (*compulsions*), which may be repeated many times.	Typical obsessions/compulsions: Fear of germs (washes hands) Fear of improper performance or behavior (repeats phrases that are "magical") Persistent doubts that everything is in order, and thus checks things over and over again (is the iron shut off?)	Symptoms are the compulsions that are manifested to relieve the anxiety: constant cleaning; checking and rechecking if things are all right (doors locked); repeating phrases/words; spending time organizing; hoarding unnecessary items such as junk mail or old bills; unable to part with old, useless items (rooms may get literally filled and dangerous).
Panic attack—An abrupt or sudden onset of fear or discomfort.	Usually accompanied by fear of having a panic attack in the future after experiencing the first one. Usually has at least four symptoms. Most predominant feeling is one of impending doom.	Physical: palpitations, sweating, trembling, nausea or GI disturbances, chest pain or discomfort, tingling sensations, chills or hot flushes, dizziness, and lightheadedness. Emotional: a feeling of imminent danger or doom; a feeling of choking, creating a need to escape; sense of things being unreal or surreal; depersonalization; fear of going crazy; fear of death.
PTSD—Experience of or witnessing a traumatic event, such as criminal assault, a serious accident, a natural disaster, or a death.	The aftereffects of exposure to a traumatic experience impede normal functions of everyday living. Is accompanied by intense fear, helplessness, and/or horror.	Relives the trauma; has recurrent dreams or nightmares; loses interest in things/people previously enjoyed; has excessive response to being startled; becomes irritable or angry.
SAD—Extreme fear of being judged or ridiculed by others.	Extreme fear of social or performance situations and embarrassment that may potentially occur. Fear that others will think poorly of them. Usually have anxiety in anticipation of a feared event.	Heart palpitations, faintness, blushing, profuse sweating, diarrhea, or panic attack; leads to avoidance behavior.
Specific phobias—Usually caused by an event in early childhood.	An extreme fear of, or an intense reaction to, a specific object or situation, such as spiders, heights, being outdoors, being among people.	Fear that may produce panic attacks, which lead to avoidance of everyday situations such as work, intimacy.

The beta-adrenegic blockers, such as propranolol, reduce the autonomic symptoms of anxiety (including changes in breathing rate, heart palpitations, tremors, sweating, and shaking). Non-benzodiazepine hypnotics, such as Ambien® (zolpidem) and Sonata® (zaleplon), selectively bind only to omega-1 or benzodiazepine-1 (BZ-1) receptors affecting the GABA-A receptor, and therefore do not produce an anticonvulsant or muscle relaxant effect. However, an off-label use of these drugs is for anxiety, as they help the person who worries at bedtime and cannot fall asleep. The non-benzodiazepine Buspar® (buspirone) has an anti-anxiety effect without marked sedation or euphoria. As an antagonist, it binds to the serotonin 5-HT1A receptor at postsynaptic sites. As an agonist, it binds at 5-HT1A presynaptic receptors. It has no direct effect on the GABA system.

Depression

Neurotransmitters are generally monoamines, which can be destroyed in the synaptic cleft by enzymes called *monoamine oxidases* (see Table 31-3). Another cause of depression is the excessive reuptake of neurotransmitters or reabsorption into the proximal nerve. Either event leads to a lack of the neurotransmitters serotonin, norepinephrine, and dopamine, and the result is *depression*. Thus, it is hypothesized that clinical depression is related to decreases in concentration of the neurotransmitters. For this reason, pharmaceutical research and current drug therapy are centered around

Table 31-3 Anti-Anxiety Drugs

TRADE/GENERIC NAME	STRENGTH AND DOSAGE FORM(S) AVAILABLE	USUAL ADULT DOSE
Benzodiazepines		
Ativan® (lorazepam) (C-IV); used for GAD, pre-op medication	Tab: 0.05 mg, 0.25 mg, 1 mg, 2 mg Prefilled syringes: 2 mg, 4 mg Concentrated oral soln: 2 mg/1 mL	GAD—Initial dose: 2–6 mg/day given bid or tid Usual range: 2–6 mg/day Largest dose at bedtime
Librium® (chlordiazepoxide) (C-IV); used for GAD	Tab: 5 mg, 10 mg, 25 mg Pwd for inj: 100 mg	Mild anxiety—5–10 mg tid or qid Severe anxiety—20–25 mg tid or qid
Serax® (oxazepam) (C-IV); used for GAD and alcohol withdrawal	Cap: 10 mg, 15 mg, 20 mg	Mild to moderate anxiety—10–15 mg, tid or qid Moderate to severe—15–30 mg
Tranxene® (clorazepate) (C-IV); used for GAD and alcohol withdrawal	Tranxene-T Tablets: 3.75 mg, 7.5 mg, 15 mg Tranxene-SD Tablets: 22.5 mg Tranxene-SD Half-Strength Tablets: 11.25 mg	Tranxene-T: 15–60 mg po daily in divided doses Average daily dose 30 mg Tranxene-SD and SD Half-Strength are given single dose qd
Valium® (diazepam) (C-IV); used for GAD, pre-op medication	Tab: 2 mg, 5 mg, 10 mg Inj: 5 mg/mL (IV or IM) Oral soln: 5 mg/5 mL, 5 mg/mL	2–10 mg po bid, tid or qid 2–20 mg IV or IM injection
Xanax® (alprazolam) (C-IV); used for GAD and panic disorder (PD)	Tab: 0.05 mg, 0.25 mg, 1 mg, 2 mg Intensol oral soln: 1 mg/1 mL	GAD—Initial dose: 0.25 to 0.5 mg given 3 times daily, NTE 4 mg/day PD—NTE 10 mg/day (average dose is 5–6 mg/day)
Non-Benzodiazepines		
Ambien® (zolpidem) (C-IV)	Tab: 5 mg, 10 mg	10 mg HS
Buspar® (buspirone)	Tab: 5 mg, 10 mg, 15 mg, 30 mg	Initial dose: 5 mg tid 15 mg/day Average dose 20–30 mg/day in tid dosing, range 15–60 mg/day NTE 60 mg/day
Sonata® (zaleplon) (C-IV)	Cap: 5 mg, 10 mg	10 mg HS Range 5–20 mg HS
Antidepressants—TCAs		
Anafril® (clomipramine); used for OCD	Cap: 25 mg, 50 mg, 75 mg	Initial po dose: 25 mg/day NTE 250 mg/day
Tofranil® (imipramine), used in panic disorder	Tab: 10 mg, 25 mg, 50 mg	Panic disorder—150–300 mg Depression—50–150 mg/day

Table 31-3 Anti-Anxiety Drugs (*continued*)

TRADE/GENERIC NAME	STRENGTH AND DOSAGE FORM(S) AVAILABLE	USUAL ADULT DOSE
Antidepressants—SSRIs		
Celexa® (citalopram); unlabeled use for SAD	Tab: 10 mg, 20 mg, 40 mg Oral soln: 10 mg/5 mL	Initial dose: 20 mg/day; NTE 60 mg/day
Luvox® (fluvoxamine); used for OCD	Tab: 25 mg, 50 mg, 100 mg	50 mg initial dose, range 50–300 mg/day Doses greater than 100 mg/day to be given in divided doses; NTE 300 mg/day
Paxil® (paroxetine); used for OCD, SAD, and panic disorder	Tab: 10 mg, 20 mg, 30 mg, 40 mg Controlled-release (CR) cap: 12.5 mg, 25 mg, 37.5 mg Oral susp: 10 mg/5 mL	OCD and SAD—20 mg/day initial dose Average range for OCD and SAD: 20–60 mg Recommended for OCD is 40 mg/day; NTE 60 mg/day Panic disorder—initial dose 10 mg, target dose 40 mg/day Controlled-release for panic disorder: 12.5–75 mg/day; NTE 75 mg/day
Prozac® (fluoxetine); used for OCD	Pulvules: 10 mg, 20 mg, 40 mg Tab: 10 mg Oral soln: 20 mg/5 mL	20 mg qAM 20 mg/day in qd or bid dosing (morning and noon) Recommended 20–60 mg/day NTE 80 mg/day
Zoloft® (sertraline); used for OCD, PTSD, and panic disorder	Tab: 25 mg, 50 mg, 100 mg Oral concentrate: 20 mg/mL	OCD—25–200 mg qd PTSD and panic disorder—25–50 mg qd; NTE 200 mg/day
Antidepressants—Other		
Cymbalta® (duloxetine)	Cap: 20 mg, 30 mg, 60 mg	40–60 mg/day in 1 or 2 divided doses
Effexor® (venlafaxine) Effexor XR used for GAD (only XR caps are used after initial dosing)	Tab: 25 mg, 37.5 mg, 50 mg, 75 mg, 100 mg Extended-release (XR) cap: 37.5 mg, 75 mg, 100 mg	Initial dose: 37.5–75 mg (XR caps) Usual range 75–300 mg (XR caps) 225 mg/day (XR caps)
Serzone® (nefazodone); unlabeled use for GAD; may cause hepatic failure	Tab: 50 mg, 100 mg, 150 mg, 200 mg, 250 mg	Initial dose: 50 mg Usual range: 300–550 mg
Beta-adrenergic Blocker of Cardiac Arrhythmias Associated Panic Attacks and Performance Anxiety		
Inderal® (propranolol); unlabeled use for panic disorder	Tab: 10 mg, 20 mg, 30 mg, 40 mg, 60 mg, 80 mg, 90 mg Sustained-release cap: 60 mg, 80 mg, 120 mg, 160 mg Oral soln: 4 mg/1 mL Oral concentrate: 80 mg/1 mL Inj: 1 mg/1 mL	10–20 mg initial dose 10–160 mg/day in divided doses (tid and qid)
Tenormin® (atenolol); unlabeled use for panic disorder	Tab: 25 mg, 50 mg, 100 mg	Initial dose: 25–50 mg/day Range: 25–100 mg/day

drugs that can either block the reuptake of neurotransmitters (for example, cyclic anti-depressants and newer selective serotonin reuptake inhibitors) or interfere with the breakdown of the monoamines within the synaptic cleft (monoamine oxidase inhibitors).

There are many types of depression, including seasonal major depression (seasonal affective disorder), postpartum depression, bipolar disorder, and dysthymia (mild depression on most days of the year). Depression is very treatable. People with depression have symptoms that include a feeling of a "black curtain" of despair coming down over their lives, lack of energy and inability to concentrate, and feeling irritable for no apparent reason. If the symptoms occur for more than two weeks to six months and are interfering with daily life, the person may be clinically depressed. Depressed patients will show behavior changes including:

- constant feelings of sadness, worthlessness, hopelessness, or guilt
- irritability or tension
- decreased interest or pleasure in usual activities or hobbies
- changes in appetite (increase or decrease) with significant weight loss or weight gain
- change in sleeping patterns (increase or decrease) such as difficulty sleeping, early morning awakening, or sleeping too much
- restlessness, fidgeting, or feeling slowed down
- decreased ability to make decisions or concentrate
- thoughts of suicide or death

There is no one specific known cause of depression; rather, it results from a combination of factors. Risk factors for becoming depressed include:

- Genetics—plays an important part in predisposition to depression.
- Trauma and stress—negative issues like financial problems, the breakup of a relationship or the death of a loved one can bring on depression; however, it can also be caused by positive situations or after such life changes as starting a new job, getting married, or graduating from school.
- Pessimistic personality, low self-esteem, or a negative outlook—can contribute to clinical depression; dysthymia can actually have the same characteristics.
- Physical conditions—serious medical conditions or diseases such as cancer, HIV, heart disease, and infertility can contribute to depression, partly because of the physical weakness and stress they bring on. Depression can worsen medical conditions because it weakens the immune system and can make pain more intense. Depression can be induced as a side effect by medications used to treat medical conditions.
- Other psychological disorders—anxiety disorders; schizophrenia; anorexia, bulimia, or compulsive eating disorders; and substance abuse often are masked by or appear with depression.

Depression can make a person feel afraid, alone, and hopeless. It can change how the patient thinks and feels and affect social behavior as it depletes the sense of physical well-being. Depression can affect anyone, of any age, at any time.

Once the illness is identified, most people diagnosed with depression are successfully treated. Psychotherapy and medication are the two primary treatment approaches. Antidepressant medications can enhance psychotherapy for some people; but they cannot cure depression. Antidepressants are not stimulants, like coffee or amphetamines, but they do remove or reduce the symptoms of depression, helping depressed persons feel the way they did before the onset of depression. Antidepressants are also used for anxiety disorders, mainly to block the physical symptoms of panic: rapid heartbeat, nausea, terror, dizziness, chest pains, and breathing problems. They can also be used to treat some phobias, which are also a type of anxiety (see Table 31-4).

Bipolar disorder (BD), which is discussed in more detail in a later section, is characterized by bouts of oscillating high and low moods. Therefore, the depression

Table 31-4   Antidepressant Comparative Chart

TYPE/TRADE/ GENERIC NAME	INDICATION	MECHANISM OF ACTION	SIDE EFFECTS AND TOXIC EFFECTS	USUAL ADULT DAILY DOSE
SSRIs	Mild to major depression, some anxiety disorders	Selectively block the reuptake of serotonin; weak effects on NE and dopamine reuptake. SSRIs have also been studied in the treatment of attention-deficit/hyperactivity disorder (ADHD).	Side effects, mild: headache, nausea and vomiting (N/V), insomnia, tremor, dry mouth. Toxic effects: anemia, hives, skin rash, seizures. Wait at least 14 days when switching to an MAOI. Contraindications: SSRIs should not be used in combination with MAOIs. SSRIs should be avoided by those with a history of seizure disorder as well as in debilitated patients or those taking multiple medications, because of the possibility of drug-induced seizure. SSRIs should only be used with caution in those with a history of liver problems. Use of SSRIs in breast-feeding women is not generally recommended as SSRIs appear in breast milk.	Varies; see specific drug
Celexa™ (citalopram HBr)	Mild to major depression	Same as SSRIs, although its chemical structure is unrelated to other SSRIs.	Common side effects same as SSRIs. Toxic effects: amenorrhea, polyuria, aggravated depression, suicide attempt, confusion. Contraindication: azole antifungals may increase plasma level of citalopram.	Start 20 mg qd, increase to 40 mg/day
Luvox® (fluvoxamine)	Depression, OCD	Same as SSRIs.	Common side effects same as SSRIs. Toxic effects: breathing difficulties, coma, convulsions, arrhythmia, N/V. Monitor liver and kidney functions.	100–200 mg/day
Paxil® (paroxetine), Paxil CR	Depression, panic disorder	Same as SSRIs.	Common side effects same as SSRIs. Toxic effects: blurred vision, dizziness, hypomania, headache, palpitations, weakness, rash, sweating, taste disorders, tingling in hands. Monitor liver and kidney functions.	20–40 mg/day 10–40 mg/day for patients with renal and hepatic problems

Table 31-4   Antidepressant Comparative Chart (*continued*)

TYPE/TRADE/ GENERIC NAME	INDICATION	MECHANISM OF ACTION	SIDE EFFECTS AND TOXIC EFFECTS	USUAL ADULT DAILY DOSE
Prozac® (fluoxetine)	Depression, OCD	Same as SSRIs.	Common side effects same as SSRIs. Toxic effects: abnormal sweating, anxiety, change in appetite, headache, N/V, seizure, nervousness, stomach, rash, cramps, trouble sleeping.	20–40 mg/day
Zoloft® (sertraline)	Depression, panic disorder, social phobia, obesity, OCD	Same as SSRIs.	Common side effects same as SSRIs. Toxic effects: seizures, heart attack, kidney or hepatic disease, Parkinson's disease.	100–150 mg/day, 50 mg tid
Miscellaneous Atypical Antidepressants				
Desyrel® (trazodone)	Depression	Selectively blocks reuptake of serotonin and potentiates the behavioral changes induced by the serotonin precursor 5-hydroxytryptophan.	Side effects: sedation, hypotension.	Initial dose: 150 mg/day in divided doses; NTE 600 mg/day
Effexor® (venlafaxine)	Major depression	Inhibits serotonin and norepinephrine reuptake and weakly inhibits dopamine reuptake.	Common side effects same as SSRIs. Toxic effects: suicide attempts.	Start 75 mg/day, in 2 or 3 divided doses. Increase to 150 or 225 mg/day taken with food
Serzone® (nefazodone)	Depression, GAD	Occupies central 5-HT$_2$ receptors, inhibiting reuptake of serotonin and norepinephrine.	Side effects: sedation, hypotension.	Initial dose: 100 mg bid Target dose: 300–600 mg/day in bid dosing
Wellbutrin®, Wellbutrin SR®, Wellbutrin XL (bupropion); used for GAD	Depression, GAD	Blocks more norepinephrine and dopamine than serotonin.	No weight gain or sexual dysfunction. Contraindication: cannot be used by persons with risk of seizures, bulimia, or anorexia nervosa.	Immediate-release tabs: 300 mg/day, given tid dosing Sustained-release tabs: 150 mg bid
Zyban® (bupropion), 150 mg sustained-release tablets	Nonnicotine aid to smoking cessation; used to treat depression associated with smoking withdrawal	Weakly blocks neuronal uptake of serotonin and norepinephrine. Also inhibits neuronal reuptake of dopamine to some extent.	Common side effects same as SSRIs.	Sustained-release tabs: 150 mg bid
TCAs	Severe depression; depression that occurs with anxiety. Some TCAs have broad anti-obsessional and antipanic effects	Strongly block reuptake of serotonin and norepinephrine, while weakly blocking effects of dopamine.	Common side effects: anticholinergic effects of dry mouth, blurred vision, constipation, and difficulty in urination; postural hypotension; tachycardia, loss of sex drive; erectile failure; photosensitivity; weight gain; sedation; increased sweating.	Usually given in a single daily dose. Begin at lower doses to avoid jitteriness and insomnia. Titrate up to maximum dose. After improvement, may taper off gradually.

Table 31-4 Antidepressant Comparative Chart (*continued*)

TYPE/TRADE/ GENERIC NAME	INDICATION	MECHANISM OF ACTION	SIDE EFFECTS AND TOXIC EFFECTS	USUAL ADULT DAILY DOSE
TCAs (*continued*)			Uncommon side effects: jitteriness, irritation, unusual energy, insomnia. Delayed onset of action from 2–12 weeks. May need to administer an amphetamine for first few weeks. Patient may experience more general anxiety during the first few days, up to three weeks.	
Anafranil® (clomipramine)	Helps control OCD by reducing duration and intensity of symptoms and anxiety. May help as much as imipramine for panic attacks. Relieves depression.	Same as TCAs.	Common side effects same as TCAs. Contraindications: Avoid administering to patients with certain abnormal electrocardiograms, narrow-angle glaucoma, or enlarged prostate.	Start: 25 mg qd; UAD 150–300 mg qd. Taper off slowly over 3–4-week period.
Elavil® (amitriptyline)	Panic attacks, depression	Same as TCAs.	Common side effects same as TCAs, except less potential for insomnia. May be used for patients who are having trouble sleeping, because of its sedating effects; however, sedating side effects can limit productivity and concentration during the day.	Start: 25–75 mg qHS. Increase over 2 weeks to average of 200 mg and maximum of 300 mg. Taper off gradually.
Norpramin® (desipramine)	Depression, panic attacks	Same as TCAs.	Common side effects same as TCAs, except causes little or no drowsiness.	25–300 mg qd. Taper off gradually.
Pamelor®, Aventyl® (nortriptyline)	Depression, panic attacks	Same as TCAs.	Common side effects same as TCAs.	Start: 10–25 mg qd; UAD 50–75 mg qd. May be as high as 150 mg qd, based on blood level. Taper off slowly.
Tofranil® (imipramine)	Panic attacks	Same as TCAs.	Common side effects same as TCAs.	Start: 10 mg qd; titrate up to 250 mg qd.
Tetracyclic Agents	Major depression	Two different actions for these two drugs in same classification.	See specific drug.	Start low, titrate up slowly, and taper off slowly.
Ludiomil® (maprotiline)	Major depression, manic-depressive disorders	Blocks NE at nerve endings.	Side effects: Anticholinergic effects. Contraindications: Do not give to patients with acute phase MI or recent MI; may cause seizures. Do not give within 2 weeks of MAOIs. May cause leukocytopenia or neutropenia.	Start: 25–75 mg qd; UAD 150 mg qd

Table 31-4 Antidepressant Comparative Chart (*continued*)

TYPE/TRADE/ GENERIC NAME	INDICATION	MECHANISM OF ACTION	SIDE EFFECTS AND TOXIC EFFECTS	USUAL ADULT DAILY DOSE
Remeron® (mirtazapine)	Major depression	Potent antagonist of 5-HT$_2$ and 5-HT$_3$ receptors and a moderate peripheral alpha$_1$-adrenergic antagonist.	Sleepiness, dizziness, weight gain, flu-like symptoms, inability to focus, GI upset, tachycardia in some patients. Contraindication: hypersensitivity to mirtazapine. Do not give with Ludiomil or alcohol.	Start: Tablets 15 mg/day, increase up to 15–45 mg/day
MAOIs	Major depression	Blocks the enzyme monoamine oxidase from destroying the monoamines serotonin, norepinephrine, and dopamine.	Dietary restrictions: interacts with tyramine-containing foods, leading to HTN crisis or stroke. Avoid beer, wine, herring, certain aged cheeses. Adverse effects: hypotension, ED, blurred vision, urinary retention, constipation, dry mouth.	See specific drug.
Marplan® (isocarboxazid)	Major depression	Isocarboxazid is a nonselective hydrazine MAOI.	Common side effects same as other MAOIs, plus orthostatic hypotension.	Start: 10 mg; increase to 40 mg/day
Nardil® (phenelzine)	Depression; atypical, nonendogenous or neurotic depression	Potent MAOI.	Common side effects same as other MAOIs, plus leukopenia, ataxia, shock-like coma.	15 mg tid
Parnate® (tranylcypromine)	Major depressive episode without melancholia	Nonhydrazine MAOI.	Common side effects same as other MAOIs, plus anemia, leukopenia, agranulocytosis, thrombocytopenia	Start 30 mg/day; increase to 60 mg/day
Eldepryl® (selegiline)	Specifically for Parkinson's disease (levorotatory acetylenic derivative of phenethylamine)	MOA #1—Inhibition of monoamine oxidase, type B. MOA #2—may increase dopaminergic activity.	Common side effects same as other MAOIs, plus orthostatic hypotension.	5 mg bid

phase of BD may require the use of an antidepressant. There are many types of antidepressants, among them selective serotonin reuptake inhibitors. Tricyclic antidepressants, once the most commonly used, have many drug interactions. Monoamine oxidase inhibitors were often used for atypical depressions that have symptoms of oversleeping, anxiety, panic attacks, and phobias. However, they have some major side effects and drug-food interactions. Both TCAs and MAOIs take two to four weeks to begin working. SSRIs have successfully replaced the use of MAOIs, except in some cases.

A major depressive episode is categorized as a DSM-IV episode by the American Psychiatric Association's *Diagnostic and Statistical Manual for Mental Disorders* (currently in its fourth revision; hence DSM-IV). This type of depressive episode is characterized by an observable and relatively persistent dysphoric mood that is present almost every day for at least two weeks, that usually interferes with daily living or functioning, and includes at least five of the following nine symptoms: depressed mood, insomnia or hypersomnia, loss of interest in usual activities, significant change in weight and/or appetite, psychomotor agitation or retardation, increased fatigue, feelings of guilt or worthlessness, slowed thinking or impaired concentration, and a suicide attempt or suicidal ideation.

Bipolar Disorder

Manic-depressive disorder, now called *bipolar disorder (BD)*, is characterized by peaks and valleys of severe highs (*mania*) and lows (*depression*). Episodes referred to as *mood swings* can be spread over hours, days, months, or years. In the manic state, the patient is overactive and overtalkative, displays a great deal of energy, and sleeps less. Manic patients cannot speak fast enough to catch up with their thoughts. They will have unrealistic thoughts; they may present an angry or irritable state, with false ideas about their importance to others or in the world at large. During a manic high, the patient uses poor judgment in business dealings and may plan and carry out careless romantic encounters or "flings." If left untreated, mania may worsen, developing into a psychotic disorder. As discussed earlier, in the depressive cycle the patient presents with difficulty in concentration, lack of energy, lethargy, slow thinking and moving, more sleeping and eating. The patient has feelings of hopelessness, helplessness, despair, sadness, worthlessness, and guilt. This may be accompanied by thoughts of suicide.

The biological causes of mania are an excess of the neurotransmitter norepinephrine (NE), and possibly other neurotransmitters as well; the depression is caused by a deficiency of monoamines (neurotransmitters) such as serotonin, NE, or dopamine. Lithium (Li+) interferes with sodium-ion-potentiated conduction of nerve impulses.

In mania, an excessive amount of lithium ions help the reuptake of NE and dopamine. Lithium also appears to reduce the release of NE and dopamine from the neurons. Someone who does not have enough lithium, or has too much sodium, will exhibit hyperexcitability of the nerves and signs of mania. Therefore, lithium, a mood-stabilizing drug, is given to reduce the hyperexcitability and hyperactivity (see Table 31-5). This allows the patient to form slower and more realistic thoughts. Sometimes, antidepressant drugs are also given to the patient to manage the lows.

Side effects of lithium include drowsiness, weakness, nausea, fatigue, hand tremor, and increased thirst and urination. Too much lithium contributes to complications in the thyroid, kidney, heart, and brain. Lithium increases the risk of congenital malformations in babies. Too much lithium may be toxic, and too little may not be effective. The difference between the two amounts is very small; this is called a *narrow therapeutic index*. Therefore, blood levels must be monitored. Decreased salt intake or increased output may cause a lithium buildup that could lead to toxicity. Dehydration, fever, vomiting, and diuretics (coffee or tea) can contribute to a decrease in sodium and resultant lithium toxicity. Signs of lithium toxicity include drowsiness, mental dullness, slurred speech, blurred vision, confusion, muscle twitching, irregular heartbeat, and seizures. A lithium overdose can be life-threatening. Lorazepam or clonazepam (2 to 4 mg tid IM or po) can be given in conjunction with lithium for acute management. These agents boost the effects of the antipsychotic lithium so that high doses can be reduced, diminishing the possibility of toxicity.

Because of the toxicity associated with lithium, doctors are prescribing alternative anticonvulsant drugs. Anticonvulsants are also prescribed when lithium does not prove effective. Equally effective for nonrapid-cycling bipolar disorder, and superior to lithium in rapid-cycling bipolar disorder, is valproic acid (Depakote®, divalproex sodium).

Table 31-5   Lithium Carbonate

GENERIC NAME	BRAND NAME	USUAL DOSAGE	HALF-LIFE (HOURS)
Lithium carbonate	Lithobid®	Acute episode	8–35
	Eskalith®	900–2,400 mg/day	
	Lithotabs®	Maintenance 300 mg po bid or tid (blood level of 0.8 to 1.2 mEq/L)	

Adverse side effects include gastrointestinal symptoms, headache, dizziness, double vision, anxiety, and confusion. Valproic acid has caused liver dysfunction in some cases; therefore, liver function tests should be performed before therapy and at frequent intervals after therapy begins. Research shows that anticonvulsant therapy is more effective for acute mania than for long-term management of bipolar disorder. Other anticonvulsants may also be used, although they lack formal FDA approval for treatment of bipolar disorder; see Table 31-6.

Table 31-6 Anticonvulsants Used in Bipolar Therapy

TRADE/ GENERIC NAME	USUAL DOSAGE FORM(S)	USUAL DAILY ADULT DOSE	ADVERSE ACTIONS AND SPECIAL NOTES	HALF-LIFE (HOURS)
Depakote® (divalproex sodium, valproic acid)	Delayed-release tab: 125 mg, 250 mg, 500 mg ER tab: 500 mg Sprinkle cap: 125 mg	750 mg initial dose; increased to effective dose (blood level: 40–40 mg/L) NTE 60 mg/kg/day FDA approved for mania associated with BD	Toxic effect: hepatic failure; liver function must be monitored. Teratogenic effect: spina bifida	6–16
Klonopin® (clonazepam; Class IV benzodiazepine)	K-shaped perforated tab: 0.5 mg, 1 mg, 2 mg	0.75–16 mg/day; NTE 20 mg/day Off-label use for acute mania associated with BD	Side effects: drowsiness, ataxia	18–50
Lamictal® (lamotrigine)	Tab: 25 mg, 100 mg, 150 mg, 200 mg Chewable dispersible tab: 2 mg, 5 mg, 25 mg Also available in special starter kits for those *not* taking enzyme-inducing drugs or valproic acid; for BD patients *only*	NTE 200 mg/day po as monotherapy (used for depressive phase of BD called BD-1) NTE 100 mg/day in combination with valproic acid or 400 mg/day with carbamazepine	Side effects: headache (25%), rash (11%), dizziness (10%), diarrhea (8%), pruritus (6%). Toxic effects: serious rashes or Stevens-Johnson syndrome (0.8%), epidermal necrolysis	Depends on dosing
Neurontin® (gabapentin)	Cap: 100 mg, 300 mg, 400 mg Tab: 600 mg, 800 mg Soln: 250 mg/5 mL	100–1,200 mg/day, usually in tid dosing; NTE 3,600 mg/day Off-label use for BD, migraines, MS, and tremors	Side effects: dizziness, somnolence, peripheral edema	5–7
Tegretol® (carbamazepine)	Tab and chew tab: 100 mg ER tab: 200 mg, 400 mg ER cap: 300 mg Susp: 100 mg/5 mL	400–1,200 mg (blood level: 6 to 12 mg/L) Off-label use for BD (use for acute mania)	May cause aplastic anemia agranulocytosis; requires blood monitoring	25–65
Topamax® (topiramate)	Tab: 25 mg, 50 mg, 100 mg, 200 mg Sprinkle cap: 15 mg, 25 mg	Begin with low doses: target 600 mg/day, NTE 1,600 mg/day Off-label use for rapid-cycling and mixed bipolar states	Side effects: fatigue, somnolence, dizziness, nausea, abdominal pain	21

Psychosis

A person who is out of touch with reality is considered *psychotic*. Symptoms of a particular psychosis, schizophrenia, include:

- illogical thoughts or paranoia, such as the certain "knowledge" of being followed by someone all the time
- hearing someone else's thoughts
- hearing disembodied voices
- seeing people, events, and things that are not there (hallucinations)
- belief that one is someone else, usually of extreme importance or celebrity.

Patients with schizophrenia or other psychoses may also have poor hygiene, spend much time alone, and pass the time at night awake, but sleep during the day. The patient may exhibit delusions of grandeur, but also a lack of insight and poor judgment.

Early antipsychotic drugs caused muscle stiffness, tremor, and abnormal movements. An irreversible adverse reaction called *tardive dyskinesia (TD)*, characterized by involuntary movements, affected about 5 percent of the patients using the older antipsychotics over a long term.

Newer drugs developed in the 1990s, called *atypical antipsychotics*, have lessened the side effects and improved compliance. The most common side effects are drowsiness, rapid heartbeat, dizziness upon moving from one position to another, weight gain, and decreased sexual function or libido.

The degree of effectiveness and the side effects of these drugs vary from patient to patient. In most cases, the drugs take effect within two to six weeks, and improvement can be noticed after a few days, up to several months. Antipsychotic drugs interact with many other drugs, including antihypertensive agents, antiepileptics, anticonvulsants, and anti-Parkinson drugs.

Workplace Wisdom Psychosis Statistic

More than 2.5 million Americans suffer from psychosis.

Mechanism of Action of Antipsychotic Drugs

One of the well-documented causes of psychosis is an increase in dopamine. Antipsychotic drugs attach to the dopamine D2 receptor, blocking its action and thereby decreasing dopamine activity. Conventional or traditional (typical) antipsychotics do this too, but also induce involuntary movements and elevate serum prolactin.

When given within the accepted clinical effective ranges, atypical antipsychotics do not cause these adverse reactions. To understand how these drugs work, it is important to examine the mechanism of action of atypical antipsychotics and how it differs from that of the more typical drugs. The key difference is a physical one: The atypical antipsychotics bind more loosely than dopamine to the dopamine D2 receptor. They also have dissociation constants higher than that of dopamine; in contrast, the conventional antipsychotics bind more tightly than dopamine itself to the dopamine D2 receptor, with dissociation constants that are lower than that of dopamine. (Dissociation measures how easily a molecule is released or unbinds from the receptor.) It is also postulated that atypical drugs block receptors for serotonin, another neurotransmitter, at the same time they block dopamine receptors and that this serotonin-dopamine balance somehow keeps prolactin levels normal, spares cognition, and does not promote involuntary movement.

Clozaril®, the first atypical antipsychotic, has helped 25–50 percent of patients who did not respond to conventional antipsychotics. Unfortunately, Clozaril® is associated with a 2 percent risk of agranulocytosis, which is a deficiency of a specific white blood cell. Agranulocytosis is potentially fatal, but reversible if diagnosed early. When affected by agranulocytosis, the immune system function is decreased, rendering the patient susceptible to infection. Patients using Clorazil® must have their blood checked regularly. Doctors now recommend that Clozaril® be used only after at least two other, safer antipsychotics have been tried without success. It should be noted that patients who take the drug and those who prescribe the drug must be registered with the Clozaril® National Registry (CNR).

Conventional antipsychotics are becoming obsolete because of their serious side effects. Experts usually recommend using a newer, atypical antipsychotic rather than a conventional one unless the patient is already doing well on the older treatment. If the person is noncompliant with multiple daily dosing, the once-a-day dosing of Haldol® or Prolixin® may be more suitable.

Conventional, traditional, or typical antipsychotic drugs include:

- Haldol® (haloperidol)
- Stelazine® (trifluoperazine)
- Mellaril® (thioridazine)
- Thorazine® (chlorpromazine)
- Navane® (thiothixene)
- Trilafon® (perphenazine)
- Prolixin®, Permitil® (fluphenazine)

Newer, atypical antipsychotic drugs are being prescribed more often to reduce side effects, thus improving the quality of life for patients with psychosis (see Table 31-7).

Table 31-7 Atypical Antipsychotic Drugs

TRADE/GENERIC NAME	STRENGTH AND DOSAGE FORM(S) AVAILABLE	DOSAGE
Abilify® (aripiprazole)	Tab: 2 mg, 5 mg, 10 mg, 15 mg, 20 mg, 30 mg	1 tab qd (nrtm*)
Clozaril® (clozapine); given only when two other atypical antipsychotic drugs have not shown improvement or effectiveness	Tab: 25 mg, 100 mg	Initial dose: 12.5 mg (half of a 25 mg tab) qd or bid Target dose: 350–400 mg/day with tid dosing NTE 900 mg/day
Geodon®, Zeldox® (ziprasidone)	Cap: 20 mg, 40 mg, 60 mg, 80 mg	Initial dose: 20 mg bid w/food NTE 80 mg bid
Risperdal® (risperidone)	Tab: 0.5 mg, 1 mg, 2 mg, 3 mg, 4 mg M-Tab (disintegrating) R0.5, R1, and R2 1 mg/mL po solution in 30 mL bottles	1 mg qd or bid initially NTE 16 mg/day
Seroquel® (quetiapine)	Tab: 25 mg, 50 mg, 100 mg, 200 mg, 300 mg and 400 mg	25 mg bid initial dose, with 300–400 mg daily dose in tid dosing as a target of day 4. NTE 800 mg/day in tid dosing
Zyprexa® (olanzapine)	Tab: 5 mg, 10 mg, 15 mg, 20 mg	5–10 mg qd initial dose NTE 20 mg qd

*nrtm means no regard to meals, may be taken with or without food.

Insomnia

Each individual's requirement for sleep varies, as do feelings of satisfaction from sleep. *Insomnia* is described as an individual's complaint of inadequate or poor-quality sleep. Insomnia is characterized by one or more of the following complaints:

- difficulty falling asleep
- difficulty returning to sleep if awakened during the night
- waking up frequently during the night
- waking up too early in the morning
- poor energy or not feeling refreshed in the morning, as if there had been no sleep at all

Insomnia may cause problematic symptoms such as a lack of energy, tiredness, daytime sleepiness, difficulty in focus or concentration, impaired performance, irritability, and a tendency to feel anger. People most likely to experience insomnia include:

- Elderly. People over 60 years of age are most likely to have sleep problems. It has been incorrectly stated that the need for sleep decreases with age; in fact, it is the *ability* to sleep that decreases with age.
- Females, especially after menopause.
- People with a history of depression.

Certain risk factors contribute to the increased likelihood of insomnia:

- anxiety
- stress
- medications
- certain foods and drinks
- sleep–wake scheduling problems
- interruptions, such as jet lag or a change in work shift schedules or nighttime activity
- change in physical surroundings
- change in the environment, such as noise, light, climate, or temperature alterations

Chronic insomnia is multifaceted and results from a combination of factors. Common causes are physical or mental disorders, especially depression, arthritis, kidney disease, diabetes, hyperthyroidism, congestive heart failure, asthma, restless legs syndrome, sleep apnea, fibromyalgia, and narcolepsy.

To overcome insomnia, patients can make changes to their environment, schedules, medications, and diet (such as eliminating caffeine). Also, playing soft music, reading a book, taking a warm bath, and drinking warm milk are good evening habits. Light exercise, yoga, hypnosis, relaxation techniques, and sleep restriction therapy may all work. In some cases, an over-the-counter sleep aid, such as Nytol® (diphenhydramine 25 mg), Sominex® (diphenhydramine 50 mg), or Unisom® (doxylamine 25 mg), which are antihistamines, can help. Recall that the side effects of some OTC antihistamines are drowsiness and sleepiness. The antihistamine ingredient most commonly used is diphenhydramine, although some combination products include analgesics as well. When all else fails, prescription sedatives and hypnotics are available.

Workplace Wisdom Insomnia Statistics

As much as one-third of the global population experiences trouble sleeping during part of the year. Insomnia is reported to be more prevalent in women than in men.

Hypnotics, Sedatives, and Barbiturates

A *hypnotic* is a drug that causes drowsiness, induces sleep onset, and/or maintains sleep. A *sedative* or *tranquilizer* is a drug that calms and relaxes a person. Pharmacologically speaking, a hypnotic and a sedative may have the same active ingredients, varying only in amounts to vary the degree of response. For example, a higher dose of a hypnotic would put patients to sleep very quickly, whereas a smaller dose of the same drug would merely calm them down, reducing nervous tension. Both hypnotics and sedatives decrease mental activity and nervous system function; that is, the nervous system is depressed. By this action, these agents can reduce anxiety, stress, irritability, and excitement. Because relaxation is essential to falling asleep—that is, the muscles and mind must relax—sedatives may cause a person to fall asleep by merely relaxing or calming the mind or loosening the muscles. Because of this, when patients take a sedative close to bedtime to "calm their nerves," they will more than likely fall asleep rather than stay calmly awake.

Barbiturates are very addictive, as they, along with hypnotics and sedatives, are depressants. The pupils become constricted, the vision is blurred, and breathing is shallow. Large doses of barbiturates can cause respiratory depression, coma, and death.

Barbiturates, hypnotics, and sedatives are used when the cause of insomnia is any emotional disturbance other than depression. Tolerance and addiction can result from long-term use. Therefore, all patients should be counseled to use hypnotics only over a short term (two to four weeks) or episodically (no more than a few times a week). Because depressed patients may be prone to suicide, they should be prescribed small quantities requiring frequent refills, rather than supplying them with large amounts, to reduce the opportunity for suicide attempts.

INFORMATION

Patients with depression are commonly prescribed a sedating tricyclic antidepressant such as Elavil® (amitriptyline), Tofranil® (imipramine), or Anafranil® (clomipramine), to be taken about one hour before bedtime. In general, these drugs are prescribed at the lowest dose and for the shortest duration needed to relieve the symptoms of insomnia. Some drugs should be tapered off gradually as the medicine is discontinued, because the insomnia may recur if they are stopped abruptly.

Benzodiazepines

Because benzodiazepines bind to all three BZ receptors, they can relax the muscles, which can lead to a feeling of total relaxation and sleepiness. They are used as hypnotics and sedatives in higher doses, and in lower doses when used as **anxiolytics**. Proper dosing is important so that antianxiety drugs can be given during the day to prevent anxiety episodes and avoid sleepiness. These drugs are also used as anticonvulsants and antiepileptics.

anxiolytic a drug used in the treatment of anxiety.

Benzodiazepines are used to treat many disorders other than anxiety, due to their sedative and hypnotic effects. Benzodiazepines can be used for:

- insomnia
- epilepsy
- muscle spasticity
- anesthesia, as pre-anesthetic or presurgery medication
- alcohol withdrawal
- various psychiatric diagnoses

Side effects are related to dosing and co-administration with drugs or alcohol. High doses taken with alcohol produce lethal effects. Benzodiazepines may cause dependence with long-term use, and are therefore classified as Class IV controlled substances. Because of this, it is now recommended that prescriptions for these drugs be only for short-term use. Research is currently underway to make more selective anxiolytic compounds, such as partial agonists at the benzodiazepine receptor.

Mechanism of Action of Benzodiazepines

Benzodiazepine drugs bind to the GABA-A receptors and *potentiate* (increase) the actions of GABA. When there is a lack of GABA, they act like GABA; when GABA cannot cross the synapse, they facilitate the crossing and binding of GABA into the GABA-A receptors.

Management of Benzodiazepine Overdose

The primary use of Romazicon® (flumazenil) is as a benzodiazepine antagonist in the event of overdose. Romazicon® competitively antagonizes the binding and allosteric effects of benzodiazepines at the BZ GABA-A receptors. An additional use is in the reduction of benzodiazepine effects in general anesthesia or diagnostic procedures. Flumazenil is available only for intravenous administration because it has a high first-pass effect (hepatic/liver). The physician must be certain of the cause of overdose because flumazenil may increase the risk of seizures in patients who are comatose because of alcohol intoxication or overdose of tricyclic antidepressant agents.

Non-Benzodiazepine Drugs

The characteristics of non-benzodiazepines, a miscellaneous group of drugs, vary depending on the specific agent. Conventional benzodiazepines, such as triazolam and flurazepam (the treatment of choice for short-term insomnia for many years), are associated with adverse effects such as rebound insomnia, withdrawal, and dependency. The newer *hypnosedatives*, sometimes called the "Z" drugs, include zolpidem, zaleplon, and zopiclone. These agents are starting to be preferred over conventional benzodiazepines to treat short-term insomnia because they are considered less likely to cause significant rebound insomnia, or tolerance, and are just as efficacious as the conventional benzodiazepines.

Ambien® (zolpidem), an imidazopyridine, acts by increasing GABA potential, but is not useful for anticonvulsant therapy or skeletal muscle relaxation. It is used mainly as a hypnotic for short-term therapy, usually for 7 to 10 days, but extendable up to 28 days. Zolpidem selectively binds to omega-1 BZ receptors and causes little next-morning residual sleepiness or decreased psychomotor function. Sonata® (zaleplon) belongs to the pyrazolopyrimidine class of hypnotics and has the same selective binding as zolpidem. Tables 31-8 and 31-9 show some MOAs of sedative and hypnotic drugs.

PROFILES IN PRACTICE

While ringing up Ms. Carlyle's phenobarbital prescription, the pharmacy technician notices that she is also purchasing OTC Benadryl®.

- Why should the pharmacy technician bring Ms. Carlyle's OTC purchase to the attention of the pharmacist on duty?

Stimulants

narcolepsy a condition characterized by frequent and uncontrolled periods of deep sleep.

Stimulants are a class of drugs that enhance brain activity and increase alertness, attention, and energy. They speed up the physiological and metabolic activity of the body. In addition, they elevate blood pressure and increase respiration and heart rate. Therefore, they are used to treat **narcolepsy**, attention deficit hyperactivity disorder (ADHD), attention deficit disorder (ADD), and depression that has not responded to other treatments. They may also be used as appetite suppressants for short-term treatment of obesity, and for patients with asthma to increase breathing rate. Because of their potential for abuse and addiction, prescription stimulants are usually classified as controlled substance Schedule II drugs and reserved for treatment of only a few diseases or conditions.

Table 31-8   Sedative and Hypnotic Drugs

CLASSIFICATION TYPE	SITE AND MECHANISM OF ACTION	SIDE AND TOXIC EFFECTS/SPECIAL NOTES	DRUG INTERACTIONS
Barbiturate	SOA: Reticular formation and cerebral cortex MOA #1—Low doses increase GABA, causing relaxation. MOA #2—High doses cause sleep and depression of CNS.	Dry mouth, lethargy, drowsiness. Overdose: Cardiovascular and CNS depression, kidney failure, low blood pressure, death. No known antidote.	Increased effect with other CNS depressants and alcohol.
Non-Barbiturates	SOA and MOA vary. Zolpidem and zaleplon selectively bind to omega-1 BZ receptor, potentiating GABA. Eszopiclone mildly binds to omega-1.	Produces less tolerance and addiction. Exception: "Z" drugs produce more dependence in patients with preexisting substance-related addictions. Zolpidem: GI and CNS disturbances; rare—delirium, nightmares, hallucinations; may reduce memory or psychomotor function within first 2 hours after administration of single oral dose. Zaleplon: does not impair memory or psychomotor function, but may cause side-effect headache.	Rifampin induces metabolism of newer hypnosedatives and decreases sedative effects. Ketoconazole, erythromycin, and cimetidine also induce metabolism.
Benzodiazepines	SOA: Reticular formation MOA #1—Low doses increase GABA, causing relaxation. MOA #2—High doses cause sleep and depression of CNS.	Do not cause REM rebound when discontinued. Less addictive than barbiturates; may be used a few weeks longer before tolerance builds up. Halcion® may cause rebound insomnia, nightmares, and daytime anxiety.	Decreased effect with cimetidine. Increased effect with other CNS depressants and alcohol.

Stimulants have chemical structures similar to the monoamine neurotransmitters found in the brain, including norepinephrine and dopamine. Stimulants act like these compounds, increase the amount of them, or promote the synthesis or production of these chemicals in the brain. The results of stimulation of the sympathetic nervous system include:

- increase in blood pressure and heart rate
- constriction of the blood vessels
- increase in blood glucose
- dilation of the respiratory system pathways for easier breathing

In addition, the increase in dopamine is associated with a sense of euphoria that can accompany the use of these drugs. Cocaine is a stimulant that can produce this euphoric effect. Other C-II stimulants are amphetamines such as Ritalin® (methylphenidate), used for ADD/ADHD; and Dexedrine® (dextroamphetamine), a synthetically altered amphetamine used for weight loss, narcolepsy, and ADD/ADHD.

Table 31-9   Dosing of Hypnotic and Sedative Drugs

CLASSIFICATION AND/OR TYPE	TRADE/ GENERIC NAME	CONTROLLED SUBSTANCE SCHEDULE	DOSING
Barbiturates			
	Luminol® (phenobarbital)	C-IV	30–120 mg/day
	Nembutal® (pentobarbital)	C-II	Sedative: 20 mg tid or qid
			Hypnotic: 100 mg HS
	Amytal® (amobarbital)	C-II	Sedative: 50–300 mg
			Hypnotic: 100–200 mg
	Seconal® (secobarbital)	C-II	Hypnotic: 100 mg HS
			Pre-op: 200–300 mg 1 hour before surgery
Benzodiazepines (used as hypnotics)			
	Dalmane® (flurazepam)	C-IV	15–30 mg before bedtime
	Doral® (quazepam)	C-IV	7.5–15 mg before bedtime
	Halcion® (triazolam)	C-IV	0.125–0.5 mg before bedtime
	ProSom® (estazolam)	C-IV	1–2 mg at bedtime
Non-Benzodiazepines			
	Ambien® (zolpidem)	C-IV	10 mg before bedtime
	Lunesta® (eszopiclone)	C-IV	1–3 mg before bedtime
	Sonata® (zaleplon)	C-IV	5–10 mg at bedtime
Miscellaneous Sedatives/Hypnotics			
	Noctec® (chloral hydrate)	C-IV	Sedative: 250 mg tid
			Hypnotic: 500 mg–1 g 30 min before bedtime or surgery
	Rozerem® (ramelteon)	Not a controlled substance	Hypnotic: 8 mg within 30 minutes of going to bed

Over-the-counter pharmacological stimulants include pseudoephedrine (in some cough and cold remedies), caffeine (analgesics), and weight-loss products. Guarana is an example of an herbal stimulant that is used in weight-loss products and Brazilian soda drinks.

Adverse Actions of Stimulants

High doses of some stimulants, taken repeatedly over a short period of time, may lead to feelings of paranoia, anger, or hostility. Other detrimental outcomes are fatally high body temperatures, seizures, arrhythmias, and cardiovascular (CV) failure. Less serious side effects include headache, dizziness, diarrhea or constipation, restlessness, tremor, nervousness, anxiety, insomnia, dry mouth, unpleasant taste in the mouth, erectile dysfunction, changes in libido, GI disturbances, and weight loss.

Contraindications

Because stimulation of the sympathetic nervous system can exacerbate glaucoma, hypertension, coronary artery disease, or an overactive thyroid gland, patients with these conditions should not take stimulant prescriptions or over-the-counter stimulant products. Stimulants cause a fatally acute rise in blood pressure when taken within two weeks of taking an MAOI antidepressant (such as Nardil® or Parnate®). Therefore, patients must be warned and counseled on these drug contraindications. Stimulants should not be given to those with agitation or anxiety.

Withdrawal Treatment

Addiction to prescription stimulants may first be treated with a tapering-off of the drug. Withdrawal treatment may include antidepressants to help manage the symptoms of depression that occur during the early phase of abstinence from stimulants. Detoxification involves behavioral and cognitive psychotherapy. Recovery support or 12-step groups may also be effectively employed in conjunction with psychotherapy.

ADHD and ADD

Attention deficit hyperactivity disorder (ADHD) is a condition in which a person (child or adult) has a very short attention span and is easily distracted, excessively active, and possibly overly emotional or highly impulsive. *Attention deficit disorder* (ADD) does not present the excessive movement or activity (*hyperkinesia*) associated with ADHD. Treatment should include psychological, educational, and pharmacological approaches.

Stimulants Used in the Treatment of ADHD and ADD

- Ritalin® (methylphenidate) is a *mild* central nervous system stimulant.
- Dexedrine® (dextroamphetamine) is a strong CNS stimulant, much more potent than methylphenidate.
- Adderall® (dextroamphetamine sulfate, dextroamphetamine saccharate, amphetamine aspartate, amphetamine sulphate) is a combination drug used to treat ADD/ADHD and narcolepsy. Amphetamine is more potent than dextroamphetamine and amphetamine sulfate is a widely abused street drug. Adderall XR® is an extended-release, once-daily dosage form of Adderall®. Adderall® and Adderall XR® may be better choices than methylphenidate or Dexedrine®, as they last longer and are more powerful. Because the "speed rush" is brought about more gradually, the patient "comes down" more easily and gradually. Most people on Dexedrine® experience a "crash" in which they may sleep for many hours after the drug wears off.
- Concerta® (methylphenidate) is the first once-daily treatment for ADD/ADHD with a 12-hour time-release formula. Medical studies have demonstrated that Concerta® can help children with ADHD improve focus in the classroom and even perform better on math tests. It has a lower incidence of side effects than the immediate-release form of methylphenidate. Taking immediate-release methylphenidate, dextroamphetamine alone, or dextroamphetamine plus an amphetamine usually produces weight loss in patients. In contrast, only 4 percent of patients taking Concerta® reported any loss of appetite or sleep. Sustained-release methylphenidate can be taken with or without food.

Once-a-day dosing is preferable for convenience and patient compliance. It also allows the parent to do the medication administration from home, and eliminates worry about a school nurse or official administering the medication and the stigma to the child associated with being medicated at school.

Nonstimulants Used in the Treatment of ADHD and ADD

Strattera® (atomoxetine), a serotonin/norepinephrine reuptake inhibitor, is a nonstimulant used in the treatment of ADHD and ADD. It is the first nonstimulant drug that has been FDA-approved for attention deficit disorder. It is not a controlled substance and is not addictive. Strattera® is an oral capsule for once- or twice-a-day dosing. Strattera® is the only ADHD medication approved for adults by the FDA.

In addition to those mentioned for stimulants, Strattera® has the following side effects:

- mood swings
- ear infections
- influenza

Because this drug has been tested and is also used on adults with ADD and ADHD, sexual side effects in adults have been reported, including:

- decreased libido
- difficulty in ejaculation
- erectile dysfunction
- urination problems
- painful menstrual cycles

Although rare, potentially serious allergic reactions (anaphylaxis) may occur with use of Strattera®. In addition to having the *same* contraindications as stimulants, Strattera® should not be given to patients with epilepsy or seizure disorders, or liver disease or kidney disease.

Convulsions, Seizures, and Epilepsy

Epilepsy is a disorder of the central nervous system in which the patient may have convulsions or seizures. *Convulsions* are physical/muscular manifestations of the disorder; a *seizure* is irregular electrical activity in the brain, which may cause convulsions. A sudden onset of violent, uncontrollable, and involuntary contractions of the muscles, possible uncontrollable shaking, and twitching of arms or legs, characterizes convulsive seizures. The patient may fall on the ground and lose bladder and bowel control.

Seizures occur due to an abnormal electrical discharge of neurons, in which they fire uncontrollably. The nerve cells in this state are said to be *hyperexcitable*. The seizure causes a sudden break in the stream of thought and activity and may include loss of consciousness. Brain seizures may cause a temporary lack of memory or fainting spells. The presence of the two together is more severe than the seizure alone. Causes may be injury to the brain, high fever (possibly due to infection), head trauma, cephalic tumor, stroke, alcohol dependence, or overintoxication. In these cases, the injury is to the neurons. Epilepsy can be diagnosed by the specific wave patterns shown in an **electroencephalogram (EEG)** recording.

electroencephalogram (EEG) a graphic record of the electrical activity of the brain.

Types and Classifications of Seizures

Seizures are classified as either partial and generalized, depending upon where the seizure begins and ends within the nervous system and the body. *Partial seizures* travel short distances on one side of the brain. *Generalized seizures* can travel anywhere throughout the brain, on both sides. Partial seizures are further classified as simple partial seizures and partial complex seizures.

Simple partial seizures affect only one side or portion of the brain and usually occur without loss of consciousness. The patient may experience an intense emotion, such as elation, sorrow, or sadness. The following characteristics are associated with simple partial seizures:

- muscle contractions of a specific body part
- abnormal sensations such as numbness and tingling, especially in the hands, feet, arms, or legs
- nausea, skin flushing, sweating, or pupil dilation
- hearing noises, seeing things, or having other hallucination-type symptoms
- loss of awareness of position for a brief time.

A patient having a *partial complex seizure* may or may not lose consciousness. All or any of the symptoms of partial simple seizures may occur, in addition to any of the following:

- being on "automatic pilot"—performance of complex behaviors (such as driving) without conscious awareness
- abnormal sensations
- changes in personality or alertness
- loss of consciousness
- olfactory or gustatory hallucinations or impairments, if the epilepsy is focused in the temporal lobe of the brain
- usually a specific body movement, such as smacking the lips or tapping the foot (often referred to as *psychomotor* manifestations)
- recalled or inappropriate emotions

Generalized seizures involve two sides of the brain and are further subclassified as tonic-clonic, myoclonic, and absence seizures.

- *Tonic-clonic,* also known as grand mal, seizures affect the whole brain. They are considered the most severe, causing the whole body to convulse with rhythmic, sustained contractions alternating with relaxation of the muscles. Infections that cause high fever may induce these seizures, called *febrile seizures,* in small children and infants. Sometimes brought on by a light or sound, the experience can last up to several minutes, with possible difficulty breathing and/or loss of bladder/bowel control.
- *Myoclonic seizures* are characterized by convulsive twitching of specific body parts or muscle groups for a brief period of time. Children with infantile spasms may present quick, "jack-knifing" muscular spasms of the head, trunk, and extremities. These seizures may become severe.
- *Absence,* also known as petit mal, seizures affect the whole brain. When a person is having an absence seizure, an onlooker may think that he is merely daydreaming or "zoning out." These patients look like most people do when bored or distracted, staring blankly into space. This type of seizure typically lasts a few seconds to two minutes. For this reason, absence seizures are difficult to diagnose. They are rare in adults and most common in girls beginning between the ages of 6 and 12. Medication usually helps, and some outgrow this type of seizure.

Status Epilepticus

Any seizures that are generalized, sustained longer than five minutes, or repeated constitute a medical emergency called *status epilepticus.* Irregular heartbeat, lack of oxygen due to difficulty breathing, and hypertension or hypotension can occur because the muscles of the heart or the diaphragm may also be convulsing. Hyperglycemia, hypoglycemia, lactic acidosis, and rise in body temperature are all due to movement. Immediate administration of IV anticonvulsant/antiepileptic medication is warranted before cerebral cortex damage or death occurs as a result of the catecholamine surge.

Treatment of status epilepticus is usually with a benzodiazepine, administered as follows:

Step 1: Uncontrolled in 2 minutes

Ativan® (lorazepam) IV—0.1 mg/kg, give 1 mg/min to a maximum of 10 mg over 10 minutes.

Versed® (midazolam)—10 mg IM (0.15–0.3 mg/kg IM).

Valium® (diazepam)—0.5–1.0 mg/kg rectally, using the IV solution per rectal tube or the diazepam gel preparation.

Step 2: Uncontrolled in 10 minutes

Cerebyx® (fosphenytoin)—20 mg/kg IV at a maximum IV rate of 150 mg/min in the average-sized adult (~3 mg/kg/min).

Step 3: an additional dose of

1. fosphenytoin—10 mg/kg IV over 5 minutes to a maximum total dose of 30 mg/kg (recommended treatment) or

2. phenobarbital—20 mg/kg IV at a maximum rate of 50–100 mg/min in the average-sized adult (~1 mg/kg/min)

Step 4: an additional dose of phenobarbital 10 mg/kg IV to a maximum total dose of 30 mg/kg or give a fourth drug loading dose IV until the seizure ceases. Pentobarbital is the "traditional" choice when using a fourth drug— 15 mg/kg (max rate of 25–50 mg/min).

Treatment of Seizures and Convulsions

Most drugs used to prevent or treat epilepsy or convulsions characteristically treat the alternate relaxation and contraction of muscles and motor centers. Antiepileptic drugs treat the CNS neuronal state of hyperactivity. As noted in the discussion on neurons, ionic concentration affects discharge or firing. Increased neuronal activity is caused by an increase of specific ions traveling into the neuron or nerve cell (*influx*).

Following are three specific MOAs to prevent and treat epilepsy and hyperexcitability of the neuron (also see Table 31-10):

- drugs that slow down an influx of sodium ions (Na^+, go outside neuron)
- drugs that slow down an influx of calcium ions (Ca^{++}, stay outside neuron)
- drugs that speed up the influx of chloride ions (Cl^-, go inside the neuron)

Parkinson's Disease

Parkinson's disease occurs as brain neurons that produce the neurotransmitter dopamine begin to malfunction and progressively die. These neurotransmitters enable the central nervous system to communicate with the somatic nervous system, to translate thought into motion. Because dopamine acts as a chemical messenger that transmits signals to other parts of the brain that control movement and coordination (the cerebral medulla and cerebellum, respectively), a change in body movement is an expected symptom of Parkinson's disease. Others include tremors, stiff or rigid muscles and joints, and/or difficulty in moving. Too much or too little dopamine can disrupt the normal balance between the dopamine system and the peripheral nervous system which uses acetylcholine; thus, the imbalance interferes with smooth and continuous movement.

Excess dopamine that does not get bound to the postsynaptic neuron is broken down by a chemical in the synapse called MAO-B. This constant transmission of dopamine to and from neurons, and its subsequent disintegration, creates a homeostasis. The balance of dopamine activity is essential to body coordination and movement.

Table 31-10   Three Major Drug Classes Used to Control Seizures

Drugs That Stimulate an Influx of Chloride Ions

BENZODIAZEPINES	BARBITURATES	MISCELLANEOUS
clonazepam (Klonopin®)	amobarbital (Amytal®)	gabapentin (Neurontin®)
clorazepate (Tranxene®)	pentobarbital (Nembutal®)	primidone (Mysoline®)
diazepam (Valium®)	phenobarbital (Luminal®)	tiagabine (Gabitril®)
lorazepam (Ativan®)	secobarbital (Seconal®)	topiramate (Topamax®)

Drugs That Delay an Influx of Sodium Ions

HYDANTOINS	MISCELLANEOUS
phenytoin (Dilantin®)	carbamazepine (Tegretol®)
fosphenytoin (Cerebyx®)	divalproex (Depakote®)
	felbamate (Felbatol®)
	lamotrigine (Lamictal®)
	valproic acid (Depakene®)
	zonisamide (Zonegran®)

Drugs That Delay an Influx of Calcium Ions

SUCCINIMIDES	MISCELLANEOUS
ethosuximide (Zarontin®)	divalproex (Depakote®)
methsuximide (Celontin®)	valproic acid (Depakene®)
phensuximide (Milontin®)	zonisamide (Zonegran®)

However, as more of the dopamine-producing cells die, less and less dopamine is produced, which causes Parkinson's disease. In addition, MAO-B continues to destroy the little remaining dopamine in the synapse. The balance of dopamine to acetylcholine is thrown off.

Factors contributing to the malfunction that causes the death of neurons that produce dopamine include:

- high fevers at a young age, such as those that accompany viral infections
- infections of the brain
- injury to the brain, specifically the basal ganglia
- antipsychotic drugs which act as dopamine antagonists and block dopamine receptors. Currently there is no way to stop the death of the cells that make dopamine. However certain drugs, such as dopamine agonists, can help the patient to "manage" the decline in motor function and activity in the early stages of the disease. By mimicking dopamine activity, dopamine agonists help to relieve symptoms such as shaking and slow movement.

Currently, there is no way to stop the death of the cells that make dopamine. However, certain drugs can help manage the decline in motor function and activity as the disease progresses.

Pharmaceutical Treatments

Levodopa is a fat-soluble substance that can cross the blood-brain barrier and then, with the help of an enzyme, be converted to dopamine in the brain. However, dopamine is a water-soluble substance and cannot cross the blood-brain barrier. One of the problems with this Parkinson's disease treatment is that the enzyme often converts levodopa before it gets a chance to cross the blood-brain barrier; the quick conversion to water-soluble dopamine keeps the dopamine away from the brain, where it is needed.

Sinemet® is the agent most commonly used in the treatment of Parkinson's (also see Table 31-11). Sinemet® is a combination of levodopa and carbidopa. The enzyme

Table 31-11   Pharmaceutical Treatment for Parkinson's Disease

DRUG TRADE/ GENERIC NAME	AVAILABILITY	DOSAGE AND ADMINISTRATION	MOA	SIDE EFFECTS AND SPECIAL NOTES
Artane® (trihexyphenidyl HCl) Cogentin® (benztropine mesylate)	Artane®: 2 mg & 5 mg tablets; 2 mg/5 mL elixir Cogentin®: 0.5 mg, 1 mg, 2 mg tablets	Artane®: Start low at 1 mg, with 2 mg/day increments. UAD: 6–10 mg. Max: 12–15 mg qd. Daily dose is given in three divided doses, usually with a meal. Cogentin®: 0.5–6 mg qd. May be given at bedtime in one dose or in divided doses.	Artane®, an antispasmodic drug, inhibits the PSNS. Cogentin® is both anticholinergic and antihistaminic. Both drugs restore the dopamine/ACh balance by reducing the activity of acetylcholine in the brain.	Used in early stages of Parkinson's, to be taken in combination with Sinemet® (adjunct therapy). Successfully reduce the tremor and muscle stiffness that result from having much more ACh than dopamine. These agents do not correct the problem of too little dopamine. Artane® side effects: dryness of the mouth, blurred vision, dizziness, mild nausea, nervousness. Artane® toxic effects: delusions, hallucinations, paranoia. Cogentin® side effects: tachycardia, constipation, dry mouth. Cogentin® toxic effects: psychosis. Contraindications: antipsychotic drugs, antidepressants.
Eldepryl® (selegiline hydrochloride)	5 mg tablets	Two 5 mg tabs; one at breakfast and one at lunch	Selective MAO Type B inhibitor. Actually blocks MAO-B, the chemical in the synapse that breaks down dopamine, thus conserving the dopamine already in the brain and keeping it in the synapse so that it can bind to postsynaptic dopamine receptors.	Side effects: nausea/ vomiting, dizziness, abdominal pain, headache. Contraindications: nonselective MAOIs, TCAs, SSRIs, meperidine. Toxic effects of these drug interactions are severe agitation, hallucinations, death.
Parlodel® (bromocriptine mesylate), Permax® (pergolide mesylate)	Parlodel®: 2.5 mg and 5 mg tablets. Permax®: 0.05 mg, 0.25 mg, 1 mg tablets	Parlodel®: Start with ½ of 2.5 mg tablet qd; increase to safe amount NTE 100 mg/day. Permax®: Start with 0.05 mg qd; increase to a max dose NTE 5 mg/day.	Dopaminergics: mimic the action of dopamine by attaching to the dopamine receptor sites on the surface of the receiving neuron (postsynaptic neuron), acting like	Dyskinesias are less common because dopamine itself is not being increased, only the dopamine-like action. Parlodel® side effects: nausea, vomiting, abnormal involuntary

Table 31-11   Pharmaceutical Treatment for Parkinson's Disease (*continued*)

DRUG TRADE/ GENERIC NAME	AVAILABILITY	DOSAGE AND ADMINISTRATION	MOA	SIDE EFFECTS AND SPECIAL NOTES
Parlodel®, Permax® (*continued*)		UAD 3 mg/day in 3 divided doses.	dopamine. This is a substitution-like action. Parlodel® is an ergot with dopamine-receptor-agonist activity. Permax® is an ergot-derivative dopamine-receptor agonist at both D_1 and D_2 receptor sites.	movements, hallucinations, confusion, dizziness, drowsiness, fainting, asthenia, abdominal discomfort, visual disturbance, ataxia, insomnia, depression, hypotension, shortness of breath, constipation, vertigo. Contraindications: decreased efficacy when taken with dopamine antagonist butyrophenones, phenothiazines, haloperidol, metoclopramide, pimozide. Permax® side effects: dyskinesia, hallucinations, somnolence, insomnia.
Sinemet®, Sinemet CR® (carbidopa and levodopa)	Tab: 10 mg/100 mg, 25 mg/100 mg, 25 mg/250 mg CR tab: 25 mg/100 mg, 50 mg/200 mg	Sinemet®: Start with one tablet qd; increase to 2 tablets qid. Sinemet CR®: UAD 200–300 mg levodopa bid or tid, NTE 1,000 mg levodopa per day in 3–4 divided doses.	Levodopa is converted to dopamine, and carbidopa slows down the conversion so that levodopa can cross the BBB.	Can be used to control symptoms for several years. As dopamine-producing cells decrease, symptoms continue to worsen, and the dose of Sinemet® has to be increased. Ultimately, the side effects of high doses of Sinemet® are unacceptable, and the drug may have to be discontinued. Dyskinesias (involuntary muscular movements) result from an overload of Sinemet® or dopamine in the brain.
Symmetrel® (amantadine hydrochloride)	100 mg gel capsules	Start with 100 mg qd UAD: 100 mg bid NTE 400 mg qd	Allows the dopamine-producing nerve cell storage sites to open more easily and wider to release dopamine from the presynaptic neuron into the synapse.	Used in milder cases of Parkinson's disease. Contraindications: decrease the dose in patients with CHF, peripheral edema, orthostatic hypotension, or impaired renal function.

carbidopa slows down the conversion of levodopa to dopamine. As Parkinson's progresses, more Sinemet® is required, which means more side effects occur. One way to prevent the need for high doses of Sinemet® is by the addition of adjunctive therapy. Two examples of adjunctive therapy are:

- Parlodel®, which mimics the action of dopamine upon attaching to the postsynaptic dopamine receptor.
- Eldepryl®, which blocks the MAO-B that destroys dopamine.

Dementia

Dementia is a progressive brain dysfunction with a loss of cognition that leads to gradually increasing restriction of daily activities. Patients with irreversible dementias, such as Alzheimer's disease, eventually become unable to care for themselves and may require around-the-clock care. According to the American Psychiatric Association (APA), Alzheimer's disease is the fourth leading cause of death in America. The changes in the brain may occur gradually or quickly, and may be caused by disease or trauma, which may determine if the dementia is permanent or temporary.

Dementia may interfere with decision making, judgment, memory, thinking, reasoning, verbal communication, and spatial orientation. Behavioral and personality changes may also result, depending on the areas of the brain affected. It is believed that the changes in the brain cause a lack of acetylcholine, which is thought to be the root of Alzheimer's disease. Treating dementia quickly may result in partial or total reversal of the disease.

Signs and Symptoms of Dementia

Early stages of dementia are characterized by loss of short-term memory. As the disease progresses, the patient has trouble with abstract thinking, which may show up as problems with counting or handling money, paying bills, understanding what was just read, or organizing daily activities. In late stages, the patient becomes disoriented about times and dates, confused, and unable to remember or describe their current residence or a recently visited place. Behavioral and personality changes may include the patient:

- being unable to dress without help
- being unable to eat, or losing the desire to eat
- having toileting problems leading to incontinence
- being unable to do self-care or grooming
- abandoning interests and hobbies
- being unable to perform routine activities, such as household tasks
- displaying personality changes, with inappropriate responses, lack of emotional control, apathy, or social withdrawal

As the disease progresses, patients with dementia may become more irritable, agitated, and quarrelsome and less neat in appearance, with diminished attention to grooming habits. In late stages of dementia, the patient stops talking, has erratic mood swings, and becomes uncooperative.

Age is the most commonly accepted contributing factor for dementia. However, according to the APA, only 15–25 percent of the elderly suffer from significant symptoms of mental illness. Untreated infections, metabolic disease, and substance abuse also can lead to dementia. The following disorders are risk factors for dementia: brain tumors, hypertension, coronary artery disease, head injury, renal failure, hepatic disease, and thyroid disease. Dietary deficiencies of vitamin B12 (cyanocobalamin), folic acid, and B1 (thiamine) have also been associated with dementia. Genetic disorders such as Huntington's, infections such as HIV/AIDS, amyotrophic lateral sclerosis (ALS, also known as Lou Gehrig's disease), and Parkinson's disease have also been associated with dementias. Substances associated with drug-induced dementias include:

- anticholinergics
- barbiturates
- benzodiazepines
- cough suppressants
- digitalis medications
- monoamine oxidase inhibitors
- tricyclic antidepressants

The most commonly used criteria for diagnosis of dementia are those in the DSM-IV. These criteria consist of two parts:

1. A deterioration of recent and remote memory.
2. An impairment of one or more of the following functions: speech, purposeful movement, comprehension/sensation, or executive function.

Treatment of Dementia

First, the underlying cause of the dementia must be treated. Infections such as HIV/AIDS are treated with antiretroviral agents. Antibiotics and antifungals are applied for neurosyphilis dementia and other infections. Antihypertensives and antihyperlipidemics are used for cardiovascular disease.

The goals of direct treatment of dementia are to improve the quality of life and maximize physical function. Some objectives include improvement of cognitive skills, mood, and behavior. Realistically, the goal of pharmacotherapy for irreversible conditions is to control symptoms and delay worsening if possible.

Tranquilizers and sedatives can modify personality changes manifested by agitation, anxiety, and aggression. Medications may be used to help manage insomnia, restlessness, and incontinence. Caretakers and family must employ safety precautions to protect the confused and disoriented patient from wandering away from home.

In 1993, the FDA approved tacrine, the first agent specifically designed for the treatment of cognitive symptoms in Alzheimer's disease. Cognex® (tacrine) is a reversible cholinesterase inhibitor and is believed to work by increasing the availability of acetylcholine in the synapses between the neurons in the brains of Alzheimer's disease patients (see Table 31-12).

Other approaches to treatment of dementias include:

- *Vitamin E*, an antioxidant, may slow nerve cell damage and death in Alzheimer's disease.
- *Eldepryl® (selegiline)*, a selective MAO-B inhibitor, is used in the United States for Parkinson's disease. It is used off-label by some doctors to slow the progression of Alzheimer's disease.
- *Ergoloid mesylates* (Hydergine), derived from rye, are used for dementias other than Alzheimer's disease and as an alternative when cholinesterase inhibitors, vitamin E, or selegiline prove ineffective in the Alzheimer's patient. UAD is 3 mg/day, NTE 9 mg/day. It is thought to enhance mental abilities by improving oxygen supply to the brain, because of its ability to act as a mild vasodilator. In addition, it is believed to possess antioxidant properties that protect the brain and heart from free-radical damage, improving the number of brain dendrites and their ability to make connections.

Table 31-12 Drugs Used to Treat Alzheimer's Disease

DRUG TRADE/ GENERIC NAME	AVAILABILITY	DOSAGE AND ADMINISTRATION	MOA	SIDE EFFECTS AND SPECIAL NOTES
Aricept® (donepezil)	Tab: 5 mg, 10 mg	1 tablet qh, NTE 10 mg/day.	Reversible acetyl-cholinesterase inhibitor; blocks the enzyme that destroys ACh.	Nausea/vomiting/diarrhea (N/V/D), insomnia, muscle cramps, fatigue, anorexia
Cognex® (tacrine)	Cap: 10 mg, 20 mg, 30 mg, 40 mg	Start with 10 mg qid. UAD: 20 mg qid. NTE 120 and 160 mg/day. Transaminase levels should be monitored every other week from at least week 4 to week 16, then decrease monitoring to every 3 months.	Parasympathomimetic reversible cholinesterase inhibitor; blocks the enzyme that destroys ACh.	N/V/D, myalgia, ataxia, anorexia; high serum ALT/SGPT or liver damage
Exelon® (rivastigmine)	Cap: 1.5 mg, 3 mg, 4.5 mg, 6 mg	Start with 1.5 mg bid, NTE 6 mg bid (12 mg/day). Take with morning and evening meals.	Reversible acetyl-cholinesterase inhibitor blocks the enzyme that destroys ACh.	Common: N/V/D, insomnia, UTI, fatigue Rare: abnormal hepatic function
Razadyne® (galantamine)	Tab: 4 g, 8 g, 12 g Oral soln: 4 mg/mL	4 mg bid, with morning and evening meals, NTE 24 mg bid.	Reversible, competitive acetylcholinesterase inhibitor.	If therapy is interrupted, patient should restart at lowest dose; lower dose for hepatically impaired patients

Migraine Headaches

A *migraine* is a very painful headache, usually on one side of the head, that tends to recur. The patient may feel nauseated, feel the urge to vomit, and be very sensitive to light and noise. Body movement can make the headache worse. Although there are many types of migraine headaches, the two major kinds are the classic and the common migraine headaches.

Classic Migraine

The major distinction of a classic migraine headache is the experience of an *aura* 10–30 minutes before the attack. The aura may manifest as flashing lights, zigzag lines in the visual field, or a temporary vision loss, and may or may not be accompanied by speech difficulty, confusion, weakness of an arm or leg, and tingling of the face or hands. The pain of a classic migraine headache is characterized by an intense throbbing or pounding in the forehead, temple, ear, jaw, or the entire area around the eyes. Beginning on one side of the head, a classic migraine may spread to the other side. It may last one to two days.

Common Migraine

The common migraine is the one most frequently observed in the general population. It is not preceded by an aura. A variety of vague symptoms may be experienced before onset of a headache, such as mental fog, mood swings, fatigue, and unusual retention of fluid. During the migraine headache phase, the patient may experience abdominal pain, polyuria, and N/V/D.

Causes and Treatment of Migraines

A classic or common migraine can occur as often as several times a week, or as rarely as once every few years. The cause of migraines may be a chemical or electrical problem in certain parts of the brain where blood flow is changed. In response to a trigger, such as stress, a food, a sound, or a smell, spasms occur at the base of the brain, which constricts some of the arteries that supply blood to the brain, thereby restricting blood flow and oxygen to the brain. Platelets clump together, releasing the chemical serotonin, a powerful constrictor of arteries; this process further reduces the blood and oxygen supply to the brain. In response to the reduced blood flow and oxygen supply, certain arteries within the brain dilate to meet the brain's energy needs. Scientists believe this vasodilation causes the pain of the migraine headache. Some migraines are influenced by hormonal changes, especially in women.

Common known migraine triggers include:

1. Medications:
   - cimetidine
   - estrogens/BCPs/HRT
   - indomethacin
   - nifedipine
   - nitroglycerin (NTG)
   - theophylline
2. Foods:
   - aged foods, including cheese, beer, wine, and hard liquor
   - yeast-containing foods, such as doughnuts and fresh breads
   - caffeine, contained in coffee, tea, colas, and some medicines
   - citrus fruits, bananas, figs, and raisins
   - dairy products
   - monosodium glutamate (MSG) and other seasonings
   - legumes, such as peas, peanuts, lima beans, and nuts
   - sulfites, aspartame, and saccharin
   - fermented foods, such as pickled herring

Nonpharmaceutical treatments of migraine headaches include:
   - stress reduction
   - biofeedback training
   - removal of certain foods from the diet
   - regular exercise to increase endorphins and reduce stress
   - reducing the inflammation of the arteries with cold packs

Table 31-13 shows some drugs used in the treatment of migraines.

Cancer Pain

The International Association for the Study of Pain defines *pain* as "an unpleasant sensory and emotional experience in association with actual or potential tissue damage, or described in terms of such damage." Approximately 30–50 percent of patients with cancer experience pain while undergoing treatment, and 70–90 percent of patients with advanced cancer experience pain.

Pain can be acute or chronic. *Acute pain* starts suddenly; it may be sharp and is often a signal of a quick onset of injury to the body. Sometimes other bodily reactions, such as sweating or elevated blood pressure, occur with pain.

Chronic pain lasts beyond the time expected for an injury to heal or an illness to be resolved. Cancer pain can be chronic, but sometimes a patient will have acute flare-ups of pain that are not completely controlled by the usual medication or therapy. This is

Table 31-13 Drugs Used in the Treatment of Migraines

DRUG TRADE/ GENERIC NAME	AVAILABILITY	DOSAGE AND ADMINISTRATION	MOA	SIDE EFFECTS AND SPECIAL NOTES
Amerge® (naratriptan)	Tab: 1 mg, 2.5 mg	2.5 mg single dose; may repeat in 4 hours, NTE 5 mg/24 hr or NTE 2.5 mg/24 hr in hepatically impaired patients	A selective 5-hydroxytryptamine$_1$ receptor subtype agonist that binds with high affinity to 5-HT$_{1D}$ and 5-HT$_{1B}$ receptors, resulting in cranial blood vessel constriction and a decrease in prostaglandin proinflammatory neuropeptide release.	Common: paresthesias, dizziness, drowsiness, malaise/fatigue Rare: fatal cardiac events, HTN crisis
Axert® (almotriptan)	Tab: 6.25 mg, 12.5 mg	NTE 12.5–25 mg/24 hr	A selective 5-HT$_{1B/1D}$ receptor subtype agonist, resulting in cranial blood vessel constriction and a decrease in prostaglandin proinflammatory neuropeptide release.	Common: paresthesias, dizziness, drowsiness, malaise/fatigue Rare: fatal cardiac events, HTN crisis
Elavil® (amitriptyline) Unlabeled use for pain associated with migraine headaches and to reduce pain perception	Tab: 10 mg, 25 mg, 50 mg, 75 mg, 100 mg, 150 mg Inj: 10 mg/mL	75–300 mg/day	TCA that blocks neuronal reuptake of NE and serotonin. Lowering serotonin lowers pain perception and causes vasodilation.	Common: skin rash, GI upset, edema, MI, hepatic failure, coma, seizures, hallucinations Drug interactions: Avoid cimetidine and MAOIs
Ergotamine + caffeine	Tab: 1 mg/100 mg	Start with 2 tablets. May take 1 additional tablet every $\frac{1}{2}$ hour, if needed for full relief NTE 6 tablets/attack, or 10 tablets/wk	Partial alpha-adrenergic agonist and antagonist, with direct stimulating effect on smooth muscle of cranial and peripheral blood vessels, causing vasoconstriction. Added caffeine is also vasoconstrictive.	Numbness and tingling of the fingers and toes, weakness in the legs, tachycardia.
Frova® (frovatriptan)	Tab: 2.5 mg	2.5 mg tab; may take a second dose in 2 hours NTE 3 tab/24 hr	A selective 5-HT$_{1B/1D}$ receptor subtype agonist, resulting in cranial blood vessel constriction and a decrease in prostaglandin proinflammatory neuropeptide release.	Common: paresthesias, dizziness, drowsiness, malaise/fatigue Rare: fatal cardiac events, HTN crisis

Table 31-13   Drugs Used in the Treatment of Migraines (*continued*)

DRUG TRADE/ GENERIC NAME	AVAILABILITY	DOSAGE AND ADMINISTRATION	MOA	SIDE EFFECTS AND SPECIAL NOTES
Imitrex® (sumatriptan)	Tab: 25 mg, 50 mg, 100 mg Nasal spray: 20 mg/spray, 5 mg/spray	po: 25–50 mg at onset. May be repeated in 2 hrs; NTE 200 mg per day Nasal: 1 spray; may repeat once in 2 hr (max 40 mg/day)	A selective 5-HT_{1D} and 5-HT_{1B} agonist, resulting in cranial blood vessel constriction and a decrease in prostaglandin pro-inflammatory neuropeptide release.	Common: diarrhea, numbness, sinusitis, tinnitus Rare: fatal cardiac events, HTN crisis.
Inderal LA® (propranolol) Used for prophylaxis of common migraine headache	Long-acting tab: 60 mg, 80 mg, 120 mg, 160 mg	Dosage varies. Start 80 mg LA UAD 160–240 mg qd	Synthetic nonselective beta-adrenergic receptor-blocking agent causing vasodilation.	Common: CHF, bradycardia, lightheadedness, insomnia, N/V/D, agranulocytosis. Contraindications: Avoid reserpine-containing drugs; may lead to bradycardia and hypotension.
Maxalt® (rizatriptan)	Tab: 5 mg, 10 mg Oral disintegrating tab: 5 mg, 10 mg	5 or 10 mg in a single dose; may be repeated in 2 hrs NTE 30 mg/24 hr	A selective $5\text{-HT}_{1B/1D}$ receptor agonist, resulting in cranial blood vessel constriction and a decrease in prostaglandin pro-inflammatory neuropeptide release.	Common: chest pain, dry mouth, GI upset, N/V, paresthesia Rare: fatal cardiac events, HTN crisis.
Relpax® (eletriptan)	Tab: 20 mg, 40 mg	UAD 20–40 mg/24 hr	A selective $5\text{-HT}_{1B/1D}$ receptor subtype agonist, resulting in cranial blood vessel constriction and a decrease in prostaglandin pro-inflammatory neuropeptide release.	Common: paresthesias, dizziness, drowsiness, malaise/fatigue Rare: fatal cardiac events, HTN crisis.
Sansert® (methysergide)	Tab: 2 mg	UAD 4–8 mg qd with meals	Ergot derivative that blocks effects of serotonin, a substance that causes vasoconstriction; also lowers pain threshold. Results in vasodilation along with ability to perceive pain differently.	Rare: May cause retroperitoneal fibrosis, pleuropulmonary fibrosis, and fibrotic thickening of cardiac valves in patients receiving long-term therapy.
Zomig® (zolmitriptan)	Tab: 2.5 mg, 5 mg Nasal spray: 5 mg/spray	1 mg, 2.5 mg, or 5 mg in a single dose; may be repeated in 2 hrs NTE 10 mg/24 hr	A selective $5\text{-HT}_{1B/1D}$ receptor agonist, resulting in cranial blood vessel constriction and a decrease in prostaglandin pro-inflammatory neuropeptide release.	Monitor hepatically impaired patients.

called *breakthrough pain*. Cancer pain is most often controlled with morphine and other opioid-like compounds.

Cancer causes pain by the mere pressure of a tumor on an organ, on bone, or on nerves. Surgical treatments and other procedures (biopsies, blood draws, lumbar punctures, and laser treatments) can also cause pain. Chemotherapy may result in the following sources of pain:

- mouth sores (*mucositis*)
- peripheral neuropathy (numb and sometimes painful sensations in the feet, legs, fingers, hands, and arms)
- GI upset—constipation, diarrhea, nausea, vomiting, abdominal cramps
- bone and joint pain

Management of cancer pain can be problematic, because some physicians do not always prescribe the right medications or permit sufficient doses of the medication. These mistakes may be due to underestimation of the degree of pain the cancer patient is experiencing and/or the doctor's concerns about the potential for addiction. The use of a pain assessment scale (for example, a scale in which "0" means "no pain at all" and "10" means "the worst pain one has ever felt before") can help the physician determine the appropriate drug and dosage.

Pain itself is both electrical and chemical in nature. When pain receptors are triggered by mechanical, chemical, or thermal stimuli, the pain signal is transmitted through the nerves to the spinal cord and then to the brain. The most common cancer pain is from tumors that metastasize to the bone. Tumors erode the bone, forming large holes that make the bone thin and weak. Nerve endings in and around the bone send pain signals to the brain.

Treatment of Cancer Pain

Analgesics do not cure the cause of the pain and provide only temporary relief. However, they may make both short-term and long-term pain tolerable.

Mild pain may be managed with nonopioid analgesics such as acetaminophen and NSAIDs. About 30 percent of cancer pain can be treated with this type of OTC medication. Severe pain is treated with opioid analgesics such as Duragesic® (fentanyl transdermal system), which provides continuous pain relief for 72 hours. Respiratory failure, hypotension, and hypoventilation may result from an overdose. Repeated administration may result in tolerance and physical and psychological dependence. Other side effects of opioid analgesics include:

- constipation, nausea, vomiting
- dry mouth, excessive sweating
- excessive sleepiness (somnolence)
- high blood pressure (hypertension) or low blood pressure (hypotension)
- confusion

Oral opioids, the most convenient and least expensive form, have a slower onset of action. Thus, they may remain in the bloodstream longer than necessary, often causing intolerable side effects such as dizziness, sedation, and vomiting.

Oral transmucosal fentanyl citrate (Actiq®) is a lozenge attached to a plastic handle, which can take 15 minutes to dissolve. There are six lozenge strengths, ranging from 200 to 1,600 mcg. The patient should not exceed 4 doses in a 24-hour period.

adjuvant helping or assisting.

Adjuvant drugs enhance the pain-relieving actions of opioid analgesics. Antidepressants used in smaller amounts than are prescribed for depression are usual choices for adjuvant drugs. Elavil® is an example.

Bone pain associated with bone fracture due to metastasis can be alleviated by bisphosphonates. These bind to the damaged areas of the bone and slow down the destruction caused by cancer cells.

Table 31-14 describes some drugs used to relieve pain.

Table 31-14 Selected Narcotics Used to Treat Pain

DRUG TRADE/ GENERIC NAME	AVAILABILITY	DOSAGE AND ADMINISTRATION	MOA	SIDE EFFECTS AND SPECIAL NOTES
Codeine Use as antitussive, prn for mild to severe pain	Tab: 15 mg, 30 mg, 60 mg Inj: 30 mL, 60 mL Oral soln: 15 mg/ 5 mL po	po, SC, IV, or IM: 15–60 mg q4–6 hr NTE 360 mg/day	Centrally active analgesic	Common side effects: constipation, dysphoria, drowsiness, N/V, respiratory depression, coma, death
Demerol® (meperidine) Postop and preop pain Obstetrical analgesia *Not* for long-term pain management	Tab: 50 mg, 100 mg Inj: 25 mg/1 mL, 50 mg/1 mL, 75 mg/1 mL, 100 mg/1 mL Syrup: 50 mg/5 mL po	50 mg–150 mg IM, SC, or po q3–4 hr prn	Opioid agonist that binds to the opioid mu receptor sites in the brain, producing analgesia and sedation and increasing tolerance to pain.	Common side effects: constipation, dysphoria, drowsiness, N/V, respiratory depression, coma, death Drug interactions: phenothiazines and many other tranquilizers increase the action of meperidine.
Dilaudid® (hydromorphone) May be used prn for pain and break-through pain	Tab: 1 mg, 2 mg, 3 mg, 4 mg Rectal supp: 3 mg Single-dose ampules for inj: 1 mg/1 mL, 2 mg/1 mL, 4 mg/1 mL Multiple-dose vials for inj: 2 mg/1 mL–20 mL	po: 2 mg q4–6 hr prn	Opioid agonist that binds to the opioid mu receptor sites in the brain, producing analgesia and sedation and increasing tolerance to pain.	Common side effects: constipation, dysphoria, drowsiness, N/V, respiratory depression, coma, death
Duragesic® (fentanyl transdermal system)	Patches: 25 mcg, 50 mcg, 75 mcg, 100 mcg	1 patch q 72 hr	Opioid agonist that binds to the opioid mu receptor sites in the brain, producing analgesia and sedation and increasing tolerance to pain.	Common side effects: constipation, dysphoria, drowsiness, N/V, respiratory depression, coma, death
Numorphan® (oxymorphone) Use prn for pain	SD ampule: 1 mg/1 mL × 1 mL Inj: 1.5 mg/1 mL × 5 mL MVD vials Rectal supp: 5 mg	1–1.5 mg q4–6 hr prn	Semisynthetic opioid agonist	Common side effects: constipation, dysphoria, drowsiness, N/V, respiratory depression, coma, death
Oramorph®, MS Contin (morphine sulfate) May be used prn for pain and break-through pain	Tab: 15 mg, 30 mg, 60 mg, 100 mg, 200 mg (immediate or slow release)	Immediate-release: 5–30 mg q4 hr prn SR: Swallow whole 15–200 mg q12 hrs NTE 400 mg/day	Opioid agonist that binds to the opioid mu receptor sites in the brain, producing analgesia and sedation and increasing tolerance to pain.	Common side effects: constipation, dysphoria, drowsiness, N/V, respiratory depression, coma, death
Oxycontin® (oxycodone) Used for continuous ATC pain, chronic/ cancer pain	CR tab: 10 mg, 20 mg, 40 mg, 80 mg, 160 mg	CR: 10–160 mg q12 hr Must be swallowed whole	Opioid agonist that binds to the opioid mu receptor sites in the brain, producing analgesia and sedation and increasing tolerance to pain.	Common side effects: constipation, dysphoria, drowsiness, N/V, respiratory depression, coma, death

Table 31-14   Selected Narcotics Used to Treat Pain (*continued*)

DRUG TRADE/ GENERIC NAME	AVAILABILITY	DOSAGE AND ADMINISTRATION	MOA	SIDE EFFECTS AND SPECIAL NOTES
Sublimaze® (fentanyl)	0.05 mg/mL	0.05–1 mg IM 30–60 minutes pre-op	Opioid agonist that binds to the opioid mu receptor sites in the brain, producing analgesia and sedation and increasing tolerance to pain.	Common side effects: constipation, dysphoria, drowsiness, N/V, respiratory depression, coma, death

Nonpharmaceutical Pain Relief

A transcutaneous electric nerve stimulation (TENS) unit produces mild electrical currents to stimulate certain nerve endings that, when activated, block pain transmission. It is a proven safe, noninvasive, and effective method for relief of many different types of pain, including neuropathic pain.

SUMMARY

The nervous system is a very complex system that interacts with every other system in the body to ensure homeostasis and to regulate the body's responses to internal and external stimuli. The nervous system communicates to all cells in the body through nerve impulses that are conducted from one part of the body to another through the transmission of chemicals called neurotransmitters.

The nervous system is divided into two parts, the central nervous system and the peripheral nervous system. The central nervous system includes the brain, the spinal column, and their nerves. The peripheral nervous system is likewise divided into two parts: the somatic nervous system, which controls voluntary movement of the body through muscles; and the autonomic nervous system, which controls involuntary motor functions such as heart rate and digestion.

Diseases and conditions affecting the nervous system include anxiety, depression, bipolar disorder, Parkinson's disease, alcohol addiction, and seizures. Pain due to injury or cancer also affects the nervous system. This chapter discusses many of these conditions and the most common treatments.

Neuropharmacology (pharmacology related to the nervous system) is one of the most diverse and complicated areas of pharmacology. A pharmacy technician must have a solid understanding of the common diseases affecting the nervous system and the pharmaceutical treatments associated with these diseases.

CHAPTER REVIEW QUESTIONS

1. The smallest functional unit of the nervous system is the:
   a. spinal cord.
   b. nerve.
   c. neuron.
   d. brain.

2. Which of the following is not part of the central nervous system?
   a. the cerebellum
   b. nerves in the hand
   c. the spinal cord
   d. the cerebrum

3. A person who is out of touch with reality is suffering from:
   a. depression.
   b. dementia.

   c. psychosis.
   d. mania.

4. Which type of molecule easily crosses the BBB?
   a. large molecules
   b. water-soluble molecule
   c. fat-soluble molecules
   d. low-fat-soluble molecules

5. Which of the following drugs is used to treat hypertension and migraine headache?
   a. Imitrex®
   b. Elavil®
   c. Sansert®
   d. Inderal® LA

6. Which of the following is responsible for the body's "fight or flight" reaction?
    a. parasympathetic nervous system
    b. somatic nervous system
    c. central nervous system
    d. sympathetic nervous system

7. The sympathetic and parasympathetic nervous systems are part of the:
    a. central nervous system.
    b. somatic nervous system.
    c. autonomic nervous system.
    d. none of the above.

8. Which of the following is responsible for the body's "rest and relaxation" response?
    a. parasympathetic nervous system
    b. somatic nervous system
    c. central nervous system
    d. sympathetic nervous system

9. Which of the following medications is not known to be a migraine trigger?
    a. cimetidine
    b. theophylline
    c. birth control pills
    d. all of the above

10. Sinemet® is indicated in the treatment of:
    a. dementia.
    b. Parkinson's disease.
    c. anxiety.
    d. seizures.

11. Phenytoin is indicated in the treatment of:
    a. dementia.
    b. Parkinson's disease.
    c. anxiety.
    d. seizures.

12. Strattera® is indicated in the treatment of:
    a. depression.
    b. anxiety.
    c. ADHD.
    d. epilepsy.

13. Celexa® is indicated in the treatment of:
    a. depression.
    b. anxiety.
    c. ADHD.
    d. epilepsy.

14. Which of the following is indicated in the treatment of bipolar disorder?
    a. nortriptyline
    b. trazodone
    c. lithium
    d. lorazepam

15. A person who has continuous and recurring obsessions that reflect exaggerated anxiety or fears is suffering from which of the following conditions?
    a. GAD
    b. SAD
    c. panic attacks
    d. OCD

CRITICAL THINKING QUESTIONS

1. How does the body react when the sympathetic nervous system is activated, as compared to when the parasympathetic nervous system is activated?

2. Why can the central nervous system be compared to a computer's CPU?

3. Why use a stimulant in the treatment of patients with ADHD when they are already hyperactive?

WEB CHALLENGE

1. Go to http://www.depression.com/understanding_depression.html to learn how depression affects the brain. What did you learn that surprised you?

2. Go to http://faculty.washington.edu/chudler/disorders.html and choose a neurological disorder you would like to find out more about. Write a one-page summary on this disorder, including an overview of the disorder, signs and symptoms, treatment(s), and prognosis.

REFERENCES AND RESOURCES

Adams, MP, Josephson, DL, & Holland, LN Jr. *Pharmacology for Nurses—A Pathophysiologic Approach*. Upper Saddle River, NJ: Pearson Education, 2008.

American Psychiatric Association: http://www.psych.org/public_info/elderly.cfm

Anxiety Disorders Association of America (ADA): http://www.adaa.org/

"Atypical antipsychotics: Mechanism of action" (accessed August 15, 2007): http://www.ncbi.nlm.nih.gov/entrez/query.fcgi?cmd=Retrieve&db=PubMed&list_uids=11873706&dopt=Abstract

"Dementia" (accessed August 15, 2007): http://penta.ufrgs.br/edu/telelab/3/dementia.htm

Drug Facts and Comparison, 2006 Ed. St. Louis: Wolters Kluwer Health, Inc.

"Effexor XR approved in the U.S. for anxiety, March 12, 1999" (accessed August 15, 2007): http://www.pslgroup.com/dg/ebe9a.htm

Family Practice Notebook. "Smoking Cessation—Tobacco Cessation" (accessed August 15, 2007): http://www.fpnotebook.com/PSY52.htm

Grieve, M. *A Modern Herbal* (1931): http://www.botanical.com/botanical/mgmh/g/guaran43.html

Holland, N, & Adams, MP. *Core Concepts in Pharmacology.* Upper Saddle River, NJ: Pearson Education, 2007.

Internet Mental Health—Monograph for Lamotrigine (accessed August 15, 2007): http://www.mentalhealth.com/drug/p30-l06.html#Head_1

Mallin, R. American Family Physician: "Smoking Cessation: Integration of Behavioral and Drug Therapies" (accessed August 15, 2007): http://www.aafp.org/afp/20020315/1107.html

"Mechanism of Action of Atypical Antipsychotic Drugs: Critical Analysis" (accessed August 15, 2007): http://www.ncbi.nlm.nih.gov/entrez/query.fcgi?cmd=Retrieve&db=PubMed&list_uids=8935797&dopt=Abstract

Merck Manual of Diagnosis and Therapy. Section 15. Psychiatric Disorders, Chapter 189. Mood Disorders—Treatment: http://www.merck.com/mrkshared/mmanual/section15/chapter189/189d.jsp

National Institute of Mental Health: http://www.nimh.nih.gov

"Schizophrenia Information" (accessed August 15, 2007): http://www.schizophrenia.com/newsletter/buckets/hypo.html

"Stimulants" (accessed August 15, 2007): http://www.drugabuse.gov/ResearchReports/Prescription/prescription4.html

Tropical Plant Database. "Guaraná *(Paullinia cupana)*" (accessed August 15, 2007): http://www.rain-tree.com/guarana.htm

Tuen, C. "Neuroland" (accessed August 15, 2007): http://neuroland.com/psy/anxiety.htm

Uchiumi, M, Isawa, S, Suzuki, M, & Murasaki, M. "The effects of zolpidem and zopiclone on daytime sleepiness and psychomotor performance" (accessed August 15, 2007): http://www.biopsychiatry.com/zolpidemvzopiclone.htm

Virtue, J. "Concerta" (accessed August 15, 2007): http://www.mental-health-matters.com/articles/article.php?artID=436

Special Topics

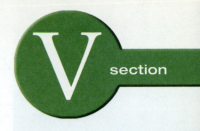

Pediatric and Neonatal Patients

neonate child from birth to 1 month of age.

infant child between the ages of 1 month and 2 years.

pharmacokinetics study of the processes of absorption, distribution, metabolism, and excretion of drugs.

LEARNING OBJECTIVES

After completing this chapter, you should be able to:

- Discuss the differences between neonatal and pediatric patients.
- Explain how the processes of pharmacokinetics in pediatric patients affect drug dosing.
- Discuss pediatric drug administration and dosage adjustment considerations.
- List two common childhood illnesses or diseases in pediatric patients.

Introduction

There are many differences between pediatric patients and adults. Pediatric patients are not just small adults, and you must consider a number of factors other than the obvious one of body weight when administering medication. **Neonates** are newborn babies from birth to one month of age; **infants** are between the ages of one month and two years. Finally, a patient is considered a *child* if he or she is between 2 and 12 years of age.

There are very significant physiological differences between pediatric patients and adults. The **pharmacokinetic** processes known as absorption, distribution, metabolism, and excretion occur quite differently in children, compared to adults, because children's organ systems are not fully developed. Providing medication therapy to pediatric patients can present a challenge if these differences are not considered (see Figure 32-1). This chapter discusses some of the pharmacological differences in neonatal, infant, and pediatric patients; special medication administration considerations; and some of the common disorders of these special patients.

Pharmacological Differences in Pediatric Patients

Compared to adults, neonates and infants weigh less and usually require a reduction in the dosage of medication. However, there are many other factors to consider when dosing these patients. Drug **absorption** is the process by which a drug enters the bloodstream, whether from the digestive system or an injection site where it is dissolved into body fluids. Neonates and infants have smaller skeletal structures, and this can affect the absorption of medication just as much as overall weight.

These youngest of patients have limited physical activity, so there is less blood flow to their muscles. Therefore, with an **intramuscular (IM)** injection medication will be absorbed more slowly, and reach the bloodstream later, than it would with an adult. The slower absorption increases the risk of muscle and nerve damage with any IM injection.

The neonate's skin is thinner than an adult's, so a topical medication, like an ointment or cream, may be absorbed more completely and rapidly into the systemic circulation. This may cause unexpected or enhanced drug effects not seen in adult patients who receive the same topical medication.

When an oral medication is given, the **pH** of the neonate's digestive system must also be considered; it is less acidic than an adult's. This can lead to decreased bioavailability and sometimes lower blood levels of the drug.

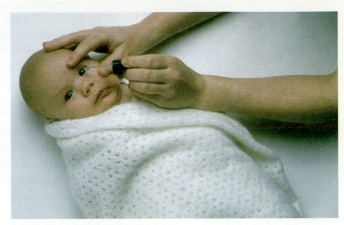

FIGURE 32-1 A baby getting eyedrops.

absorption the process by which a drug enters the bloodstream.

intramuscular (IM) within or into a muscle.

pH scale that measures the alkalinity or acidity of a substance; seven is the neutral point on this scale (less than seven is acidic and greater than 7 is alkaline).

" Workplace Wisdom Dosages for Neonates versus Infants

Remember: A dose that is appropriate for an infant or toddler may not be appropriate for a neonate. For example, digoxin dosage varies:

- For a neonate (1 month or younger), 0.03–0.04 mg/kg
- For an infant (1 month to 2 years), 0.04–0.06 mg/kg

After a medication is absorbed, it enters the bloodstream and is then distributed to the organs and tissues. Several factors, such as blood flow and plasma protein binding, influence how much of a drug reaches the target organ or area of the body. The liver and kidneys have the largest blood supply and receive a greater concentration of a drug than other organs. In addition, the adult brain has a protective barrier, called the blood-brain barrier, which protects it from **water-soluble** substances. Drugs must have a certain degree of lipid or fat solubility to penetrate this barrier and reach the brain.

In pediatric patients, liver function and the blood-brain barrier are still immature. Children usually have a higher percentage of body water and a lower percentage of body fat than adults. If a **lipid-soluble** drug is administered to a pediatric patient, there will be decreased **distribution** of the drug to the organs and body tissues because of the lower percentage of fat in the child's body. This causes more of the medication to stay in the blood, resulting in higher drug blood levels.

In comparison, water-soluble drugs administered to pediatric patients may cause lower drug concentrations in the blood because the percentage of water in the child's body is higher and thus results in more peripheral drug distribution. There are fewer plasma proteins in pediatric patients as compared to adults, which allows more of the drug to remain unbound or "free" in the body. Only unbound medications exert a drug effect, so the pediatric patient may have more effective drug in the body, enhancing the drug action and possibly even producing an overdose.

water-soluble dissolvable in water; describes drugs that are composed mostly of water and can be excreted by the kidneys.

lipid-soluble dissolvable in fats; describes drug that pass readily into cell membranes composed mostly of fatty substances, such as the brain.

distribution the process by which a drug reaches the various organs and tissues of the body.

Diarrhea and vomiting are particular concerns in the pediatric patient, as these conditions may cause them to become dehydrated very quickly. When dehydrated, children's bodies retain more of a drug in their organs, and this often leads to amplified drug effects and higher drug concentrations.

Drug Metabolism

metabolism chemical alteration of drugs, food, or foreign compounds in and by the body.

excretion elimination of a drug from the body; usually occurs through urine, feces, or the respiratory system.

Metabolism is the chemical alteration of a drug (or other substance) by the body, and **excretion** is the process by which the body eliminates a drug. The liver and the kidneys are the main organs involved in these processes, and they are not fully developed in pediatric patients. This may result in slower metabolism and excretion in children as compared to adults, so that drugs stay in their bodies for a longer period of time. This places pediatric patients at risk of drug accumulation and possible toxicity.

It should be noted that children (aged 2 to 12 years) also metabolize certain drugs more rapidly than adults. This rate usually continues to increase between 1 and 12 years. Examples of drugs that are metabolized more rapidly in children include valproic acid, which is often given for seizures; and clindamycin, often used for skin and respiratory infections. Medications containing benzyl alcohol, such as bacteriostatic sodium chloride used to dilute powder forms of injectable medications, should not be used in neonates because the alcohol can reach toxic levels. Phenobarbital and some pain medications are rapidly absorbed in some older infants, because of their liver physiology; thus, children often require larger doses or more frequent administration to reach the desired effect. Steroids can stunt pediatric growth; tetracycline can stain permanent teeth and affect bone development.

Pediatric Medication Administration

When administering medications to pediatric patients, dosage adjustments must be considered, in addition to the route and dosage forms available because of pediatric physiological differences. Compliance in pediatric patients is another important consideration; sometimes the available dosage form plays a major role in determining which medication to administer. For example, liquids are the dosage form most commonly used because color and flavors can usually be added to mask bitter or other unpleasant tastes (see Figure 32-2). Tablets and capsules are not easy for small children to swallow, and certainly are not appropriate for neonates and infants.

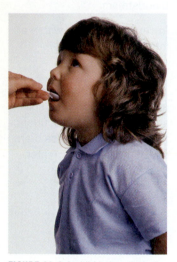

FIGURE 32-2 A child being given the liquid form of an antibiotic.

" **Workplace Wisdom** Compounding

As a pharmacy technician, you will sometimes need to compound formulations. This involves using a formula (recipe) and special equipment to create a patient-specific product. Sometimes the medication is not available commercially, or the dosage form available is not appropriate. A pharmacy technician can help ensure that a pediatric patient completes the entire course of therapy by adding flavoring to a bad-tasting medicine to make it more palatable to the child. "

Body weight is the basis of the most common method for determining the correct dose for a particular patient. Several formulas are used, including those based on weight, age, body surface area (BSA), or milligrams per body weight per day. Age is considered the least reliable of these, because a pediatric patient may be smaller or larger than the norm for his or her age.

Many over-the-counter medications are also available for pediatric patients, but often they are intended for older pediatric patients and contain no dosing instructions for very young children. Parents or caregivers with dosage questions about these OTC medicines should always be referred to a pharmacist.

─────────────────── **INFORMATION** ───────────────────

In 2007, the FDA issued a public health advisory warning about giving OTC cold and cough medicines to babies and toddlers under the age of 2, because cough and cold medicines can cause serious and potentially life-threatening side effects.

───

If the manufacturer does not suggest an exact pediatric dosage for a medication, there are several methods that may be used to calculate or estimate the proper dose (see Chapter 14 for a review). The age-based formula that is sometimes used for determining a pediatric dosage is *Young's rule*. The other formula, known as *Clark's rule*, uses only the patient's weight.

Young's rule

$$\frac{\text{Age (in years)}}{\text{Age (in years)} + 12 \text{ years}} \times \text{Adult dose} = \text{Pediatric dose}$$

Clark's rule

$$\frac{\text{Weight (in lbs.)}}{150 \text{ lbs.}} \times \text{Adult dose} = \text{Pediatric dose}$$

example 32.1

A child needs to receive a medication that has a suggested adult dose of 650 mg. The child is 5 years old and weighs 44 lbs. What would the dose be using Young's rule?

$$\frac{5 \text{ yrs old}}{5 \text{ yrs} + 12 \text{ yrs}} \times 650 \text{ mg} = 191.10 \text{ mg}$$

example 32.2

Calculate the dose for the same patient using Clark's rule.

$$\frac{44 \text{ lbs.}}{150 \text{ lbs.}} \times 650 \text{ mg} = 190.45 \text{ mg}$$

Both of these formulas use the usual adult dosage as the basis of the calculation. Clark's rule uses only the weight of the patient; Young's rule uses only the patient's age. If a pediatric patient is overweight or underweight for a particular age group, dosages could be off considerably. Also, the actual appropriate pediatric dose can vary greatly depending on the patient's condition, response, and adverse reactions to the medication. These formulas are not widely used today for this reason.

A method more commonly used to determine dosage is based on weight in kilograms and the normal adult dosage range as stated by the manufacturer. For example:

example 32.3

The manufacturer recommends a dosage of 0.5 mg/kg/day. For a child weighing 80 kg, what is the proper dose?

$$0.5 \text{ mg} \times 80 \text{ kg} = 40 \text{ mg per day}$$

Table 32-1 Recommended Acetaminophen Dosages

FORM	BRAND NAMES	CONCENTRATION	DOSAGE
Drops	Tylenol®, Liquiprin®	80 mg/0.8 mL	6–11 lbs is 0.4mL
Elixir	Tylenol®, Genapap®	160 mg/5 mL	12–17 lbs and 4–11 months is 0.5 mL
Suppositories	Uniserts®, Feverall®	80 mg, 160 mg, 325 mg, 650 mg	ages 2–3 years, 24–35 lbs =160 mg
Tablets	Tylenol®, Panadol®	325 mg, 500 mg, 650 mg	24–35 lbs, 2–3 years is 160 mg
Tablets, chewable	Tylenol®, Tempra®, Panadol®	80 mg	24–35 lbs, 2–3 years is 160 mg

Dosing tables are standard practice today and appear on many OTC packages for products such as acetaminophen and ibuprofen. Table 32-1 shows the recommended dosages for various forms of acetaminophen; these dosages are determined by the manufacturers using both the child's weight and age. For more information on calculating pediatric dosages, refer to Chapter 14.

PROFILES IN PRACTICE

Mrs. Reynolds is the mother of a 2-year-old boy. She has just filled a prescription for Augmentin® suspension for her son at your pharmacy. An hour after picking up the prescription, she calls to tell you that her son won't take the Augmentin® because it tastes bad, and asks you if there is any way to mask the taste or improve the flavor. You know that if the child does not like the way the medicine tastes, he probably will not take even another dose, let alone the entire course of the antibiotic.

• What options can you offer Mrs. Reynolds?
• Where can you find more information on safe ways to flavor Augmentin®?

Medication Errors and Pediatric Patients

Although medication errors may occur with patients of any age, pediatric patients are especially vulnerable to errors. They more often suffer from incorrect dosing, particularly dosages based on incorrect computations and wrong dosage intervals. Pediatric patients pose a unique challenge to pharmacy staff. Pre-verbal children cannot say if they have problems such as pain or nausea. The calculations often involve very small quantities, so even a slight error is potentially more serious. Calculations for drugs such as digoxin, epinephrine, theophylline, and narcotics should be checked and rechecked.

example 32.4

Digoxin is available in tablet form as 0.125 mg, 0.25 mg, and 0.5 mg. The recommended doses are as follows:

Infant: 25–35 mcg/kg

Children 1–24 months: 35–60 mcg/kg

Children 2–5 yrs: 30–40 mcg

Children 5–10 yrs: 20–35 mcg

Children over 10 yrs: 10–15 mcg

Many drugs that are used to treat pediatric illnesses are available as OTC products, but do not contain pediatric dosing indications or dosing guidelines. This greatly increases the risk of errors. As discussed previously, children vary in weight, organ maturity, and physiological differences that affect their metabolism and excretion rates. Medication improvement programs are necessary and should include every member of the healthcare team, including the family member or caregiver, the pharmacy technician, the pharmacist, and the physician. These improvement programs should also include quality performance activities and drug adverse-reaction reporting.

Pharmacy technicians play a very important role in the prevention of medication errors, and the following section discusses some preventive measures they can take. Even though pharmacy technicians work under the direct supervision of a pharmacist, they should always ensure that a medication is correct before a final check takes place. Remember, a team is only as good as its players.

Hospital-Wide Action to Prevent Medication Errors

Within the hospital setting, the following steps can help prevent medication errors:

- Provide adequate staffing.
- Establish a formulary system with therapeutic uses and evaluations for pediatric uses of certain drugs.
- Track medication errors through formal systems and report errors to families.
- Encourage a team environment.

Pharmacy Actions to Prevent Medication Errors

Within the pharmacy, the pharmacy staff can take the following steps to help prevent medication errors:

- Recheck calculations against weight-based dosage ranges.
- Reconfirm confusing orders with physician/pharmacist.
- Check for current allergies and drug compatibilities.
- Prepare drugs in a clean environment and avoid interruptions during preparation.
- Obtain the original written order before dispensing.
- If possible, use a unit-dose or ready-to-use medication form.
- Do not store sound-alike or look-alike drugs next to each other.

Pharmacy Education and Communication

Establishing best practices for ongoing education and disseminating information among the pharmacy staff can also help prevent medication errors. Steps may include the following:

- Check medication calculations with another team member, especially if unusual in dosage or amount to be given.
- Confirm patient identity and pertinent information before dispensing.
- Educate patients or caregivers about medication before dispensing.
- Implement a tracking system for errors and communicate with all staff involved, on a regular basis, to review.
- Answer all questions from caregivers and listen attentively to them.
- Double-check all orders.
- Always use proper dispensing utensils, such as droppers or medicine cups; do not use inexact utensils, such as household teaspoons, for measurement or dispensing.

Common Childhood Illnesses

Measures such as immunizations and well-baby checkups can help prevent many childhood illnesses. The FDA has a recommended schedule of vaccinations for persons from 0–6 and 7–18 years of age. These include hepatitis, whooping cough, pneumonia, measles, mumps, and rubella, as well as some other common childhood illnesses. Figure 32-3 reproduces the recommended immunization schedules approved by the FDA.

Conditions such as eye, ear, nose, and throat infections are very common in children. Before the age of 3, a child will probably have at least one ear infection. Earaches are common in the pediatric patient because the eustachian tube is narrower and shorter than in adults. This tube connects the middle ear to the back of the throat. Normally this tube allows fluid to drain from the middle ear, but if it gets infected, the tube may become inflamed, swell, and fill with mucus. Bacterial growth causes pressure on the eardrum and pain. If left untreated, this condition, known as *otitis media*, can cause temporary hearing loss and, in acute ongoing cases, even trouble with developing speech and language skills. The most common signs are pain and fever. If the child is too small to communicate pain verbally, he or she may cry or pull on the ear as an indication.

If the doctor thinks the infection is caused by bacteria, an antibiotic will be prescribed. If it is a viral infection, pain relievers and warm compresses are used. If a child has had more than three infections in six months, ear drains are often used to help balance the pressure in the ears and improve drainage. This is accomplished by surgically inserting a plastic tube into the eardrum, which allows air into the middle ear so that fluid can drain out properly. Such drains/tubes are left in for six to nine months on average.

Children who live with smokers, have a predisposing family history, attend day care, or were born prematurely are often at higher risk of infections. Viral infections such as croup, colds, and flu are often spread due to the close contact situations found in day care facilities. Bacterial infections, such as chickenpox, strep throat, and whooping cough, are also commonly transmitted in these areas. Bacterial cells can form a protective wall around themselves, and thus may persist in the environment for some time. Antibiotics can be used to destroy the wall; this kills the cells and therefore rids the body of the infection. In contrast, viruses require a host or living cell to sustain life. Because they invade the host's cells, antibiotics are ineffective against viruses.

Antibiotic medications should be used only for bacterial infections. Each time a person takes an antibiotic, some bacteria are killed. However, others "learn" to defend themselves against the antibiotic, and develop drug resistance. To prevent this, make sure the child takes the entire course of antibiotic exactly as prescribed, and use antibiotics only when the doctor says they are needed. Proper instructions regarding dosage and storage should be included in the dispensing of medication.

DEPARTMENT OF HEALTH AND HUMAN SERVICES • CENTERS FOR DISEASE CONTROL AND PREVENTION

Recommended Immunization Schedule for Persons Aged 0–6 Years—UNITED STATES • 2007

Vaccine ▼ Age ▶	Birth	1 month	2 months	4 months	6 months	12 months	15 months	18 months	19–23 months	2–3 years	4–6 years
Hepatitis B[1]	HepB	HepB		see footnote 1		HepB				HepB Series	
Rotavirus[2]			Rota	Rota	Rota						
Diphtheria, Tetanus, Pertussis[3]			DTaP	DTaP	DTaP		DTaP				DTaP
Haemophilus influenzae type b[4]			Hib	Hib	*Hib*[4]	Hib			Hib		
Pneumococcal[5]			PCV	PCV	PCV	PCV				PCV	PPV
Inactivated Poliovirus			IPV	IPV		IPV					IPV
Influenza[6]							Influenza (Yearly)				
Measles, Mumps, Rubella[7]						MMR					MMR
Varicella[8]						Varicella					Varicella
Hepatitis A[9]							HepA (2 doses)			HepA Series	
Meningococcal[10]										MPSV4	

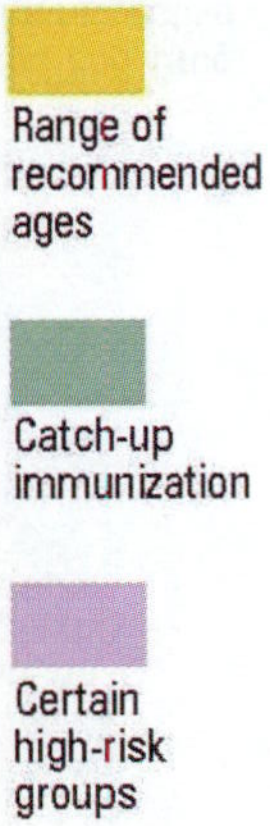

Range of recommended ages
Catch-up immunization
Certain high-risk groups

This schedule indicates the recommended ages for routine administration of currently licensed childhood vaccines, as of December 1, 2006, for children aged 0–6 years. Additional information is available at http://www.cdc.gov/nip/recs/child-schedule.htm. Any dose not administered at the recommended age should be administered at any subsequent visit, when indicated and feasible. Additional vaccines may be licensed and recommended during the year. Licensed combination vaccines may be used whenever any components of the combination are indicated and other components of the vaccine are not contraindicated and if approved by the Food and Drug Administration for that dose of the series. Providers should consult the respective Advisory Committee on Immunization Practices statement for detailed recommendations. Clinically significant adverse events that follow immunization should be reported to the Vaccine Adverse Event Reporting System (VAERS). Guidance about how to obtain and complete a VAERS form is available at http://www.vaers, hhs.gov or by telephone, 800-822-7967.

FIGURE 32-3A CDC recommended immunization schedule for persons aged 0–6 years.
(Source: Centers for Disease Control and Prevention)

Department of Health and Human Services • Centers for Disease Control and Prevention

Recommended Immunization Schedule for Persons Aged 7–18 Years—UNITED STATES • 2007

Vaccine ▼ / Age ▶	7–10 years	11–12 YEARS	13–14 years	15 years	16–18 years
Tetanus, Diphtheria, Pertussis[1]	*see footnote 1*	Tdap		Tdap	
Human Papillomavirus[2]	*see footnote 2*	HPV (3 doses)		HPV Series	
Meningococcal[3]	MPSV4	MCV4		MCV4[3] / MCV4	
Pneumococcal[4]		PPV			
Influenza[5]		Influenza (Yearly)			
Hepatitis A[6]		HepA Series			
Hepatitis B[7]		HepB Series			
Inactivated Poliovirus[8]		IPV Series			
Measles, Mumps, Rubella[9]		MMR Series			
Varicella[10]		Varicella Series			

Range of recommended ages

Catch-up immunization

Certain high-risk groups

This schedule indicates the recommended ages for routine administration of currently licensed childhood vaccines, as of December 1, 2006, for children aged 7–18 years. Additional information is available at http://www.cdc.gov/nip/recs/child-schedule.htm. Any dose not administered at the recommended age should be administered at any subsequent visit, when indicated and feasible. Additional vaccines may be licensed and recommended during the year. Licensed combination vaccines may be used whenever any components of the combination are indicated and other components of the vaccine are not contraindicated and if approved by the Food and Drug Administration for that dose of the series. Providers should consult the respective Advisory Committee on Immunization Practices statement for detailed recommendations. Clinically significant adverse events that follow immunization should be reported to the Vaccine Adverse Event Reporting System (VAERS). Guidance about how to obtain and complete a VAERS form is available at http://www.vaers.hhs.gov or by telephone, 800-822-7967.

FIGURE 32-3B CDC Recommended immunization schedule for persons aged 7–18 years.
(Source: Centers for Disease Control and Prevention)

Respiratory Diseases

Asthma is a condition that affects about 6 million children under the age of 18 each year in the United States, according to the National Institute of Allergy and Infectious Diseases (NIAID). It is the most common chronic condition among children and accounts for several million absences from school each year. Hospitalizations from asthma occur at alarming rates and treatment costs are estimated to be in the billions. Allergies are the number-one cause of asthma in pediatric patients, followed by upper respiratory infections, weather conditions, and second-hand tobacco smoke inhalation.

Early symptoms include coughing or breathing changes, reduced energy, dark circles under the eyes, and trouble sleeping. Symptoms that develop later are tightness in the chest, wheezing, and shortness of breath. Asthma can be life-threatening because it may cause respiratory failure. Children with asthma have breathing difficulties because the air passages in their lungs are narrower and do not allow correct air flow. Many triggers can bring on a full-blown asthma attack, because of the oversensitivity of lungs and airways. Diagnosis includes spirometry, with a device that measures lung function. This may be followed by chest X-rays, blood tests, and peak flow monitoring (PFM), which measures how much air a person can blow out of the lungs.

School activities such as sports and running may trigger an attack in some children. Inhalers are often prescribed to treat these attacks. Medications known as *bronchodilators* relieve the symptoms of asthma by relaxing the muscles that tighten around the airways (see Figure 32-4). Bronchodilators also help clear mucus from the lungs and open the airways. This allows more air to move in and out of the lungs, improving breathing and allowing coughing to clear mucus out of the lungs more effectively.

Another class of medications known as *anti-inflammatory agents*, is also used, often on an ongoing basis. These can actually prevent attacks because they reduce swelling and mucus production, making the airways less sensitive and less likely to react to triggers.

Treatment for pediatric patients with asthma often includes a combination of both of these drug types in the form of inhalers, nebulizers, and pills. Quick-acting medications are intended to provide prompt relief during an attack; long-term control medications can be taken to prevent attacks from occurring. In general, treatment focuses on prevention of attacks, through medication and patient or caregiver education, and long-term medications to control and prevent chronic symptoms. Added to these strategies are quick-relief medications and monitoring of daily asthma symptoms.

Other respiratory diseases include whooping cough and pneumonia. Whooping cough, also known as *pertussis*, can be fatal in young children. There is a vaccine, given during childhood along with diphtheria and tetanus (DPT) immunizations, that can prevent a child from contracting this disease. Treatment usually includes antibiotics such as erythromycin, clear liquids, and fruit juices. Pertussis can last for several weeks or even months, and is highly contagious (can be spread easily).

Croup is a viral respiratory disease in which the trachea and larynx become inflamed. It usually occurs in children between 6 months and 3 years of age, because the trachea is still very soft and pliable. The airway swells and becomes partially blocked. The child's breathing becomes difficult due to the excess mucus being produced and the partial collapse of the airway. This causes a "barking" sound when the child coughs. Once the child gets a little older, the trachea becomes more rigid, and collapse is less likely to occur. Croup usually goes away over time without treatment, and medication is not prescribed.

asthma a respiratory disease characterized by wheezing, shortness of breath, and bronchoconstriction.

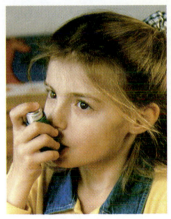

FIGURE 32-4 A child using an asthma bronchodilator.

Cardiovascular and Blood Disorders

About 50 percent of newborns will develop *jaundice* in the first 2 to 4 days post partum (after birth). This condition is caused by a buildup of excess bilirubin in the blood, and results in the skin and the whites of the eyes appearing yellow. The infant's liver cannot break down bilirubin as fast as the body makes it. It is reabsorbed in the intestines before the infant can eliminate it in the stool. If left untreated, high bilirubin levels can cause deafness, cerebral palsy, and even brain damage.

A simple test for jaundice is to press a fingertip on the tip of a child's nose: if the skin shows a yellowish color, contact a doctor. Jaundice in most infants resolves in a few days, during the first week or two of life, without intervention. If this does not occur, phototherapy can be used. In phototherapy, the infant is exposed to a special light that helps break down the bilirubin.

Kawasaki disease is a condition that causes irritation and inflammation of many body tissues, including hands, feet, mouth, lips, and throat. Lymph nodes in the neck may become swollen, and often cause heart-related complications. These may be temporary, but can turn into long-term problems, especially if related to the coronary artery. Kawasaki disease weakens the wall of the artery and causes it to balloon or bulge out. This in turn can cause an aneurysm or blood clot. Treatment includes fever reducers and increased fluid intake. Sometimes aspirin is prescribed to prevent both inflammation from the disease and clot formation.

Rheumatic fever is another pediatric disease that can cause permanent damage to the heart valves. This may occur when the underlying streptococcal infection is not treated properly, or when strep infections occur frequently. The inflammation caused by this disease may damage the heart by scarring the valves, so that the heart then has to work harder to pump blood.

Symptoms usually occur about one to five weeks after an infection by Streptococcus bacteria. The infection moves from one joint to another, causing small bumps under the skin. A pink rash follows, as do weight loss, stomach pain, and fatigue. Antibiotic therapy to kill the strep bacteria is the best way to prevent more serious damage and get rid of the infection. If heart-valve damage occurs, surgical replacement or repair may be required.

Other common pediatric diseases can also affect the heart and cardiovascular system. In addition, heart problems may be congenital (defects present at birth) or brought on by lifestyle and habits. It is estimated that about 30 percent of U.S. children aged 6 to 18 are obese. Diet and proper education of family or caregivers is important in the prevention of heart disease in the pediatric population.

SUMMARY

Pediatric patients are not just small adults. They are physiologically different, and thus present special medication considerations and challenges. Respiratory diseases such as asthma, infectious diseases such as colds, and heart diseases like rheumatic fever are just a few of the special challenges that face pediatric patients.

Dosage calculations often involve small quantities and require special formulations using manufacturers' guidelines. Lack of organ development, as well as verbal communication ability, also ensure many unique challenges when medicating this patient population. A technician should always take special precautions when calculating doses and reconfirm orders often to prevent medication errors. The healthcare team must provide education for the patient's family, as well as participating in a tracking and quality assurance system to ensure that mistakes are reviewed and learned from. These are just a few of the ways to ensure correct pediatric medication dispensing.

CHAPTER REVIEW QUESTIONS

1. Pediatric patients aged 1 month to 2 years are considered:
   a. neonates.
   b. infants.
   c. children.
   d. adolescents.

2. Neonates and infants have _____ blood flow to the muscles.
   a. rapid
   b. increased
   c. decreased
   d. slow

3. After a medication gains access to the bloodstream, it is then _____ to the organs and tissues.
   a. metabolized
   b. distributed
   c. excreted
   d. absorbed

4. Children aged 2 to 12 years metabolize certain drugs, such as pain medications, _____ adults.
   a. slower than
   b. faster than
   c. the same as
   d. none of the above

5. One way of calculating dosages for pediatric medication, based only on a child's age, is known as:
   a. Young's rule.
   b. Clark's rule.
   c. mg/kg/day.
   d. both a and c.

6. One method of preventing medication errors in the hospital is to:
   a. encourage a team environment.
   b. track errors through systems and scheduled meetings.
   c. establish a formulary.
   d. all of the above.

7. The most common physiological cause of otitis media in pediatric patients is:
   a. foreign objects placed in the ear.
   b. a middle-ear tube that is shorter than in adults.
   c. fluid buildup in the nasal cavity.
   d. bacterial drug resistance.

8. When more than 3 ear infections occur within 6 months, what is the usual treatment?
   a. Ear tubes are placed to help balance pressure.
   b. Antibiotics are given along with warm compresses.
   c. Pain relievers are used for the symptoms only.
   d. The fluid buildup is allowed to go away by itself.

9. Bronchodilators are used to treat asthma because they:
   a. reduce swelling and mucus production.
   b. kill the bacteria that cause asthma.
   c. open airways by relaxing muscles.
   d. all of the above.

10. Streptococcus bacteria can cause the following condition, which is characterized by a pink rash, if left untreated.
    a. rheumatic fever
    b. Kawasaki disease
    c. asthma
    d. otitis media

CRITICAL THINKING QUESTIONS

1. Explain why slow metabolism rates in pediatric patients can lead to toxic drug levels.

2. What pediatric dosage calculation method do you think is the best? Explain why.

3. List three ways to prevent medication errors in the pharmacy. Specify ways in which you personally can make sure that medication errors do not occur when you perform your daily tasks as a pharmacy technician.

WEB CHALLENGE

1. Look up the website for ASHP and then search for their policy position on medication misadventures. Write a one-page summary of the information you find on the website.

REFERENCES AND RESOURCES

American Academy of Allergy, Asthma, and Immunology: http://www.aaaai.org/

"Cure for the Common Cold?" (accessed April 15, 2008): http://www.quantumhealth.com/news/articlecold.html

Davidson, MR, London, ML, & Ladewig, PA (2008) *Olds' Maternal-Newborn Nursing & Women's Health Across the Lifespan*, (eighth Ed.) Upper Saddle River, NJ: Pearson Education/Prentice Hall.

"Diaphragm Development" (accessed April 15, 2008): http://www.breathing.com/articles/diaphragm-development.htm

Drug Facts and Comparisons, 2006 ed. St. Louis: Wolters Kluwer Health.

"Emphysema" (accessed April 15, 2008): http://www.wrongdiagnosis.com/e/emphysema/intro.htm

"End Allergy and Asthma Misery" (accessed April 11, 2008): http://www.acaai.org/powerpoint/online/slide1.html

"Exchange" (accessed April 15, 2008): http://www.mrothery.co.uk/exchange/exchange.htm

"Hiccup" (accessed April 15, 2008): http://www.tipsofallsorts.com/hiccup.html#facts

Holland, N, & Adams, MP. *Core Concepts in Pharmacology*. Upper Saddle River, NJ: Pearson Education, 2007.

"Into the Thorax" (accessed April 13, 2008): http://www.saburchill.com/chapters/chap0020.html

"Legal Requirement for the Sale and Purchase of Drug Products Containing Pseudoephedrine, Ephedrine, and Phenylpropanolamine" (accessed July 15, 2007): http://www.fda.gov

"Little Mystery: Why do we yawn?" (accessed April 15, 2008): http://www.msnbc.com/news/205574.asp?cp1=1

"Molecular mechanism of action of theophylline: Induction of histone deacetylase activity to decrease inflammatory gene expression" (accessed April 15, 2008): http://www.pubmedcentral.nih.gov/articlerender.fcgi?artid=124399

National Institute of Allergy and Infectious Diseases. "Common Cold" (accessed April 12, 2008): http://www.niaid.nih.gov/factsheets/cold.htm

"Pulmonary Gas Laws" (accessed March 5, 2008): http://www.mtsinai.org/pulmonary/books/scuba/sectiond.htm

"Respiratory System—Basic Function" (accessed April 15, 2008): http://www.ama-assn.org/ama/pub/category/7165.html

"Respiratory Tract" (accessed April 12, 2008): http://www.radiation-scott.org/deposition/respiratory.htm

"What allergies do you suffer from?" (accessed April 15, 2008): http://allergies.about.com/

"What Kind of Inhalers Are There?" (accessed April 15, 2008): http://www.radix.net/~mwg/inhalers.html

Geriatric Patients

33 chapter

Introduction

The number of **geriatric** patients is increasing—and this fact will affect pharmacy practice in very significant ways. There are nearly 40 million Americans who are 65 years of age or older. Advances in medical technology, and the resulting extension of life and improvements in quality of life, have increased the number of geriatric patients seeking medical treatment, as well as the number of prescriptions filled each year. Currently, geriatric prescriptions account for the greatest percentage of medication orders filled. Some experts have reported that 50 percent of all OTC products sold today, and 30 percent of prescription medications, are consumed by the elderly.

Other factors, such as physiological changes, polypharmacy, multiple diseases, and noncompliance, also affect geriatric medication therapy and should be considered when treating this population. This chapter discusses these factors and the pharmacy technician's important role in caring for the geriatric patient.

The Physiological Factors

Geriatric patients experience many changes in the body's pharmacokinetic processes as aging occurs (see Figure 33-1). These changes affect the way drugs are processed once they enter the body. Cardiac output decreases significantly with age, affecting the amount of blood that the kidneys and liver receive. By the age of 65, a person's liver and kidneys receive significantly less blood flow than they did at age 40. Because the kidneys, liver, and brain are the organs that require the most blood flow to function properly, the **metabolism** and **excretion** processes slow as people age. These changes allow certain drugs to stay in the body longer, so the drugs may cause increased **side effects**. Organs also decrease in size as patients age; this further slows the process of metabolism and may intensify any drug effects, whether intended or not.

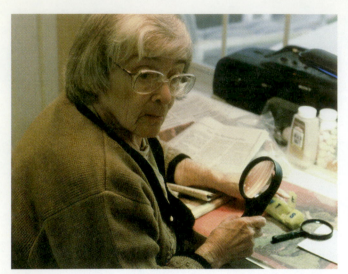

FIGURE 33-1 An elderly woman uses a magnifying glass to inspect the pills in her plastic weekly medication organizer.

metabolism chemical change of drugs or foreign compounds in and by the body.

excretion elimination of a drug from the body.

side effects drug effects other than the intended one; usually undesirable but not harmful.

absorption entrance of a drug into the bloodstream.

distribution movement of a drug from the bloodstream to organs and tissues.

half-life amount of time it takes the body to break down and excrete one-half of a drug dosage.

toxicity drug poisoning; can be life-threatening or extremely harmful.

Drug **absorption** in the geriatric patient is usually slower due to a decrease in intestinal blood flow, reduced gastric mobility, reduced stomach acid, and smaller intestinal surface area. These factors can delay the onset of action, so that it takes longer to get the desired effect. However, these same factors also mean that the drug stays in the system longer, which means the drug effect can last longer and have unwanted side effects.

Drug **distribution** is also affected in the aging adult because the percentage of lean body mass and the total percentage of body water are lower than in younger adults. Drug levels are thus lower because less water is available to distribute them throughout the body. The amount of body fat increases with age and can cause lipid-soluble drugs, such as general anesthetics, to be widely distributed to the organs that contain the most adipose tissue. This diverts such drugs away from the kidneys and liver, where the metabolism and excretion processes should occur, slowing elimination of the drug from the body and causing the drug to have a longer **half-life** and possibly greater **toxicity** because of the increased levels of medication in the bloodstream.

As mentioned previously, metabolism and excretion generally decrease during the aging process. The frequent occurrence of kidney and liver disease in the elderly can also affect these processes. Such diseases as hypertension, coronary artery disease, diabetes, and cancer reduce the blood flow and production of some important microsomal metabolizing enzymes that are necessary for the process of chemically altering a drug so that it can be distributed into the blood and tissues. Excretion is also slower, which allows drugs to stay in the body longer. Because of these changes, geriatric patients are generally more sensitive to medications than younger people, and often must take a lower dosage than the usual adult amount. In an elderly person, the dosage amount taken by a younger adult may produce a greater pharmacological effect. Therefore, drugs such as CNS depressants can actually increase mental depression and the appearance of episodes in the elderly.

Nutrition and the Presence of Disease

Nutritional status is extremely important to the geriatric patient's health (see Figure 33-2). Many elderly patients live alone and may have inadequate diets because of lack of social contact, tight finances, inability to do grocery shopping, or simple lack of appetite or interest in eating. Proper nutrition is very important to liver function and the ability to metabolize drugs. If protein intake is insufficient, the body has lower amounts of plasma protein, which is necessary for plasma protein drug binding. Many drugs bind to plasma proteins as they are distributed throughout the body, but only unbound (free) drugs cause a pharmacological effect. For example, albumin usually decreases with age. This albumin deficiency allows more unbound drug to remain in the patient's system; thus, the drug effects in the body are intensified. Nutritional deficiencies also make patients more susceptible to infections, other diseases, and drug-disease interactions.

The incidence of major chronic diseases, such as diabetes, hypertension, and mental depression, and respiratory illnesses often increases with aging, and can have a great impact on medication therapy. General good health and proper nutrition are vital to proper physiological processes.

Disease-Drug Interactions

Disease-drug interactions are medication effects that occur because of a preexisting disease or condition. Such interactions often occur because of the decrease in the number of drug receptors caused by aging. These reactions can be extreme: for example, a patient with congestive heart failure who uses drugs such as verapamil may suffer cardiac arrest; a renal disease patient who uses NSAIDs could develop complete renal failure. Patients with a chronic condition, such as anxiety or insomnia, may find that their symptoms grow worse. Drugs such as anti-anxiety agents or hypnotics may cause excessive **adverse effects** in the elderly because these patients are more sensitive to drugs that depress the central nervous system.

Certain drugs, such as antipsychotics, antidepressants, and antihistamines, can cause excessive side effects known as *anticholinergic effects,* which include urinary retention and constipation. Special consideration and attention are required when prescribing for or dispensing to an elderly patient.

Overmedication is also a growing problem for the geriatric population (see Figure 33-3). Some patients think: "If one pill is good, then two pills should be better." This philosophy can lead to increased drug interactions, increased side effects, and higher medication costs. The more medications a patient takes, the higher the chance that interactions will occur. Common side effects, such as insomnia, dizziness, and dry mouth, occur more often in older people than in younger people, and may be more intense in geriatric patients. A greatly increased risk of falls is another major negative effect of overmedication (see Figure 33-4). Falls account for 10 percent of all emergency room visits, and one out of ten results in a serious injury.

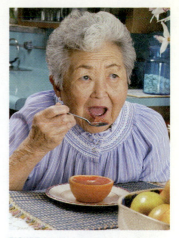

FIGURE 33-2 Maintaining proper nutrition is critical for the elderly, who often live alone.

adverse effects undesirable and potentially harmful drug effects.

INFORMATION

The following is a list of some ways a pharmacy technician can help prevent overmedication and adverse reactions in the elderly:

- Help the pharmacist create a patient profile that includes all medications.
- Make a note for the pharmacist to review the profile if you notice a duplication in medication class (for example, more than one medication in the same class being taken for high cholesterol).
- Provide nutritional information to patients to assist them in maintaining a proper diet regimen.
- Identify any over-the-counter products the patient is also taking and include them on the patient's current profile.

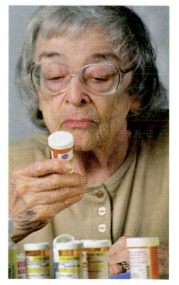

FIGURE 33-3 Overmedication is a growing problem in the elderly; patients in this population often take numerous prescription and OTC drugs at the same time.

Noncompliance

Drug *compliance*, or following a medication regimen, is another factor in geriatric medication. **Noncompliance**, which is defined as a patient's refusal or inability to follow a prescribed drug regimen, is very common in the elderly. Those who live alone, have other diseases or conditions, or have problems with memory are at greatest risk of noncompliance.

There are many reasons why a patient may not take medication as prescribed. Sometimes the dosing schedule is confusing, and the patient has difficulty understanding

noncompliance when a patient does not follow a prescribed drug regimen.

or remembering what the drug is and exactly why it was prescribed. The more complicated the drug regimen, the more likely it is that an elderly patient—or any patient, for that matter—will be noncompliant. Some other reasons for noncompliance by elderly patients include inability to afford the drug, belief that the medication is unnecessary, dislike of the drug's taste or inability to administer the dosage form, not understanding the directions, and not tolerating a drug's side effects. How can pharmacy technicians, as part of the healthcare team, help improve compliance?

Role of the Pharmacy Technician

The following are some ways in which pharmacy technicians and other healthcare team members can help ensure medication compliance.

- Greet each patient by name and mention the name often.
- Keep the directions on the prescription label as simple as possible. Make sure that directions and instructions are legible! Many patients, especially the elderly, have trouble reading small type.
- Give clear instructions on the exact treatment regimen, preferably in writing.
- Provide a card listing the medication dose, indication (reason for taking the medication), and time.
- Provide audiovisual aids, written materials, and computerized drug information.
- Ask the patient to repeat the directions on how to take the medication back to you.
- Suggest special reminder containers and calendars.
- Offer to call the patient if a refill is needed.
- Explain consequences of medication noncompliance.
- At each visit, emphasize the importance of adherence to the proper drug schedule.
- At each visit, acknowledge patients' efforts to take their medicines as ordered.
- Involve the patient's family and caregivers (see Figure 33-5).
- Avoid medical jargon when discussing the patient's medication therapy.
- Use short words and short sentences.
- Repeat instructions.
- Make advice as specific and detailed as possible.
- Find out what the patient's worries are; do not confine yourself merely to gathering objective medical information.
- Adopt a friendly demeanor rather than a strictly business-like attitude.
- Spend some time conversing about nonmedical topics.
- Suggest a behavioral contract.
- Ask patients to monitor their drug intake by keeping a log or diary.
- Help the patient link medication administration times to events in the daily routine.
- Ask the patient to recall in detail the medication(s) taken.
- Instruct patients to pay attention to adverse side effects and to inform the physician if they become concerned.
- Increase motivation by enlisting the patient in the decision-making process.
- Request that new patients bring in all medications to you to review, and create a current profile that includes them all.

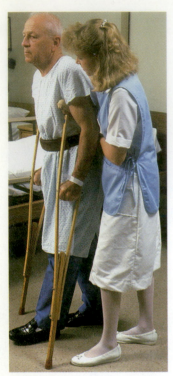

FIGURE 33-4 Elderly patients often fall because of the dizziness that some medications can cause.

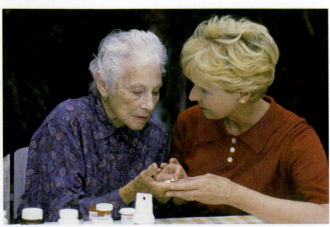

FIGURE 33-5 Involving family members in an elderly patient's drug routine can often help prevent noncompliance.

Compliance Issues Related to Dosage Forms and Timing

Another important consideration in compliance is the dosage form and administration times. Many elderly patients have difficulty swallowing, and large capsules or tablets are a problem. This requires evaluating the form to be dispensed and possibly changing to a liquid; depending on the medication, you may suggest crushing a pill into juice. Once-a-day medications are more user-friendly and easier for geriatric patients to remember.

Community-based pharmacies and nursing homes also use a packaging technique called *unit dosing*, in which each package contains a single dose of the drug(s) that should be taken at one time. This makes the drug regimen less confusing and easier for the patient to know what drugs to take and when to take them. If unit dosing is not possible, describing the different drugs as "the big green one" or the "football-shaped one" can help patients identify the correct medication and thus enhance compliance. Ideally, pharmacy instructions would be given to caregivers and family as well as to the patient.

Medication boxes and other reminders can also be very helpful in increasing medication compliance (see Figure 33-6). These devices can be used to help the patient stay on a schedule. Elderly patients may also find that associating their daily medication schedule with meals or other daily tasks, such as brushing their teeth, can act as reminders to take the medications properly.

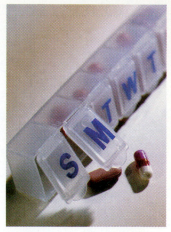

FIGURE 33-6 Encourage elderly patients to use a medication box to keep track of their daily medications.

" Workplace Wisdom Helping Patients Remember Their Medications

Many tools are available to help seniors better manage the multitude of medications they are often required to take. Pill containers, as well as some new electronic reminders, can be set up initially during a counseling session with the pharmacist. "

Another consideration is drug packaging. Lids and caps on medication bottles are sometimes hard to remove, especially if the patient has arthritis. Easy-to-open lids can be substituted. For those with impaired eyesight or who have trouble reading, large print on labels and other direction or instruction sheets is very helpful.

Polypharmacy

Polypharmacy is the administration of more medications than are clinically necessary or multiple drug prescriptions. Studies show that this occurs with 55–59 percent of the geriatric population. Due to the aging process and the incidence of multiple diseases, elderly patients often end up taking many medications (see Figure 33-7). Conditions such as diabetes, osteoporosis, Alzheimer's, dementia, and depression are very common in the elderly population, and often require complicated and multiple drug regimens, frequently prescribed by several different physicians. Good pharmacy practitioners will help patients coordinate administration of these multiple drug regimens, as well as stay alert to possible interactions and duplications in their patients' medications.

Some of these conditions affect the patient's mental abilities, but even the most alert patients can become confused about how and when to take their various medications. With each new medication, the possibility of drug-drug and drug-disease interactions increases; this includes **over-the-counter (OTC) drugs** and products. This is especially true among the elderly, who constitute only 12 to 17 percent of the population buying OTC drugs, but consume about 30 percent of all OTC medications. In fact, the elderly are projected to consume as much as 50 percent of all OTC medications by the year 2010.

polypharmacy administration of more medications than clinically indicated.

over-the-counter (OTC) drugs drugs that can be purchased without a prescription.

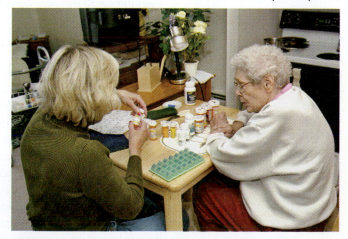

FIGURE 33-7 Keeping track of daily medications often requires the help of family members.

● ● ●

PROFILES IN PRACTICE

Mrs. Landon is an elderly patient who comes to your pharmacy with her daughter. The daughter states that her mother takes 15 medications and was recently diagnosed with and hospitalized for diabetes. The nurse in the hospital told Mrs. Landon and her daughter about certain types of infections being prominent in diabetic patients. The daughter wants to know what preventive measures she can take to help her mother, and what kind of diabetes monitoring machine she should buy.

- As a technician, what can you do to help this patient choose a diabetes monitoring system?
- What information about infection prevention can you provide for these clients?

Often patients take OTC medications without the physician's knowledge. Additionally, geriatric patients may purchase medications from more than one pharmacy and see more than one prescribing doctor. When a patient is getting prescriptions from a cardiologist, a rheumatologist, an internist, and an ophthalmologist, for example, polypharmacy is almost inevitable. Coordinating these various medications and prescriptions is critically important—and far from easy.

To help solve the problem of polypharmacy and avoid complications and adverse drug interactions, pharmacists and pharmacy technicians must record *every* medication their patients are taking and keep a current patient profile. One good way to do this is called the "brown bag method." The patient is asked to bring *all* his medications to the pharmacy, where he meets with the pharmacist so that the pharmacist can record each one. This ensures that no medication is forgotten and creates a complete profile for the pharmacy. Patients should be sure to include any herbal, diet, or vitamin supplements, topical preparations, and OTC products, as well as prescription medications. Encourage the patient to bring this "bag" in once a year for review. Emphasize the importance of notifying the pharmacy and physician of any new drugs, as soon as they are added.

Workplace Wisdom The Baby Boomers Are Aging

In the United States, there are currently 77 million "baby boomers" of middle-adult age, and the fastest-growing age group is 85 and older. By the year 2050, the population of the elderly will increase to approximately 72 million.

Medicare Part D

The Medicare Prescription Drug, Improvement, and Modernization Act of 2003 (MMA), which became effective on January 1, 2006, extends prescription coverage to all patients who are eligible for Medicare benefits. It is a voluntary insurance program to provide some drug coverage for those who experience hardships or have high-cost medications. The patient must sign up within three months of becoming eligible for Medicare (three months before reaching age 65 or three months after), or possibly face a penalty. Patients in the program are given a variety of drug coverage plans to choose from, each of which includes a yearly deductible (between $0 and $265) and a monthly premium. Each plan has its own formulary (list of drugs) and specific costs. For patients on high-cost medications, the pharmacist may provide and charge for medication management therapy (MMT). This therapy may take the form of an in-depth annual review of the patient's medications, through a program such as the "brown bag," for instance. Medication management by a pharmacist provides a safety feature and ensures a complete profile for the pharmacy record.

Pharmacy technicians can play an important role in gathering information for the pharmacist who is providing MMT, as well as participating in billing and online adjudication. A current profile that includes all of a patient's OTC medications, as well as the physicians that the patient sees, is necessary to ensure safe medication therapy. A technician is often the first person the elderly customer sees at the counter. Asking questions about these matters, finding about any allergies, and noting any changes in insurance coverage are all great ways to keep the patient's history current for the pharmacist to review.

SUMMARY

The aging process causes pharmacokinetic changes in geriatric patients, such as slower metabolism and excretion. Organ size, blood flow, and cardiac output all generally decrease with age. These factors decrease drug absorption and can delay the onset of drug action. These same factors often require a reduction in medication dosage because of the greater pharmacological effects that occur with slower metabolism and increased drug retention. Other considerations and complications, such as multiple medication therapy (polypharmacy), the presence of several diseases, and noncompliance, are significant in proper treatment of geriatric patients. Special aids, such as easy-open lids, medication organizers, complete patient profiles, and alternate dosage forms, are just a few of the ways to improve compliance and prevent drug interactions.

It is estimated that by the year 2050, geriatric persons will constitute 20.4 percent of the population. The great strides being made in the medical field increase both life expectancy and quality of life, but also increase the challenges of pharmacy, with a significantly higher number of prescriptions and demand for trained personnel to accomplish the tasks of good pharmacy practice. Education is the key to quality geriatric medication therapy. Quality therapy will take a dedicated team of healthcare workers, and the pharmacy technician will play an even greater role on this team in the future.

CHAPTER REVIEW QUESTIONS

1. Geriatric patients are those age _____ and older.
   a. 65
   b. 75
   c. 67
   d. 55

2. Geriatric patients experience a/an _____ in body fat as they age.
   a. increase
   b. delay
   c. decrease
   d. hardening

3. After a medication gains access to the blood, it is then _____ to the organs and tissues.
   a. metabolized
   b. distributed
   c. excreted
   d. absorbed

4. Geriatric patients metabolize certain drugs, such as pain medications, _____ younger adults.
   a. slower than
   b. faster than
   c. the same as
   d. none of the above

5. Geriatric patients generally require a/an _____ in medication dosages due to the _____ rate of elimination.
   a. decrease; slower
   b. increase; faster
   c. decrease; faster
   d. increase; slower

6. All of the following are methods of preventing overmedication *except*:
   a. providing the least expensive drugs available.
   b. identifying any OTC medications.
   c. making adjustments for liver impairment.
   d. weighing risks versus benefits.

7. Polypharmacy is best described as:
   a. getting prescriptions from several pharmacies.
   b. taking multiple medications.
   c. getting prescriptions from several physicians.
   d. all of the above.

8. All of the following are methods a pharmacy technician can use to aid in medication compliance, *except*:
   a. assisting in MMT information gathering for the pharmacist.
   b. counseling the patient about the "brown bag" method.
   c. aiding in Medicare online adjudication.
   d. participating in the billing process.

9. By the year 2050, geriatric persons are expected to constitute what percentage of the population?
   a. 4.1%
   b. 8.1%
   c. 12.8%
   d. 20.4%

10. As much as _____ of all over-the-counter drugs sold today are consumed by the elderly.
    a. 50%
    b. 30%
    c. 59%
    d. 55%

CRITICAL THINKING QUESTIONS

1. Explain why slow metabolism rates in geriatric patients can lead to toxic drug levels.

2. What factors contribute to noncompliance in the geriatric population and how can a pharmacy technician help prevent them?

WEB CHALLENGE

1. Look up a website for medication management and search for information about the role that pharmacy technicians will play in the future. Discuss how you as a pharmacy technician can help educate patients about better ways to manage their many medications and diseases. Give three examples of medication devices currently available for patients who may be experiencing polypharmacy situations.

2. Look up Alzheimer's disease and discuss the symptoms, treatments, and current medications being used in the treatment of this disease. Name a medication being used today and describe how it works. Are any others being researched?

REFERENCES AND RESOURCES

Alaska Mental Health Consumer Web: www.akmhcweb.org

American Society of Health System Pharmacists: www.ashp.org

Drug Facts and Comparisons, 2006 ed. St. Louis, MO: Wolters Kluwer Health.

Family Practice Notebook: www.fpnotebook.com

Hitner, N. *Pharmacology: An Introduction*. New York, NY: McGraw-Hill, 2005.

Holland, N, & Adams, MP. *Core Concepts in Pharmacology*. Upper Saddle River, NJ: Pearson Education, 2007.

Medicine Net: www.medicinenet.com

RN Web: www.rnweb.com

U.S. Department of Health and Human Services: www.medicare.gov

Biopharmaceuticals

34 chapter

LEARNING OBJECTIVES

After completing this chapter, you should be able to:

- Name at least two drugs developed by using recombinant DNA technology, and outline their uses.
- Discuss the four steps in the genetic engineering process.
- Explain briefly how a company gets approval for a biopharmaceutical drug from the FDA.
- Discuss why biopharmaceuticals, genetic engineering, and stem cell research are important in the future of pharmacy and the practice of medicine.

Introduction

Biopharmacology is a growing field of research similar to pharmacokinetics (see Chapter 19). It is the branch of pharmacology that studies the use of biologically engineered drugs. Biopharmaceuticals are substances created using biotechnology. They can be proteins like antibodies, or even consist of DNA and RNA. Research is being conducted in this area to find new therapeutic medications to treat such life-threatening diseases as AIDS, various cancers, and Parkinson's disease.

The majority of biopharmaceuticals are derived from life forms existing in nature, such as plants and animals, although the medications are produced by means other than direct extraction from a biological source. Genetic engineering is another way to create new drugs, and stem cell research offers tantalizing opportunities for new therapeutic treatments and is making significant strides in the development of new medications used today. This chapter discusses these three forms of biopharmacology, their impact on the pharmaceutical industry, and their role in the future of pharmacology.

biopharmacology branch of pharmacology that studies the use of biologically engineered drugs.

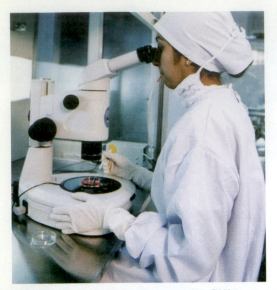

FIGURE 34-1 Scientist performing research in DNA technology.

biopharmaceuticals substances created using biotechnology.

biologics a group of varied medicinal products, such as vaccines, blood products, allergenics, and proteins.

allergenic a substance that can cause an allergic reaction.

biotechnology the use of biological substances or microorganisms to perform specific functions, such as the production of drugs, hormones, or food products.

Gaucher's disease disease in which fatty materials collect in the liver, spleen, kidneys, lungs, and brain and cause the person to be susceptible to infections.

neutropenia disease in which there is an abnormal number of the white blood cells that are responsible for fighting infections.

rheumatoid arthritis autoimmune disease that causes chronic inflammation of the joints.

What Are Biopharmaceuticals?

Biopharmaceutical drugs, also called **biopharmaceuticals** or **biologics**, are pharmaceuticals derived from life forms and used for therapeutic or diagnostic purposes. This classification includes a wide variety of medicinal products, such as vaccines, blood products, **allergenics**, and proteins (including antibodies). Biopharmaceuticals may be composed of sugars, proteins, and even living tissue or cells. Louis Pasteur's work in 1857 could be considered the first use of biotechnology, because he converted a food source into another form.

Recombinant therapeutic proteins (RTPs), which are also produced by **biotechnology**, are at the forefront of biomedical technology. RTPs are artificial forms of recombinant DNA that have been created by combining or inserting one or more DNA strands into a single molecule (see Figure 34-1). One of the first biotechnological substances to be approved by the FDA was Humulin insulin or rHI (recombinant human insulin), manufactured by the Eli Lilly Company beginning in 1982. Recombinant therapeutic proteins can also be made and used to treat a variety of medical conditions for which no other treatments are available. Some of the biopharmaceutical drugs currently being used include Cerezyme® for **Gaucher's disease**, Leukine® for **neutropenia**, and Synvisc® and Hyalgan® for **rheumatoid arthritis**.

Workplace Wisdom Storing Biological Drugs

The FDA imposes special requirements on biological drugs. These drugs are often still in the research or clinical-trial stage, and require extensive documentation for FDA review. Pharmacy technicians should always be aware of any special precautions, storage requirements, labeling instructions, or ordering and inventory information regarding these drugs. The FDA website contains all necessary information pertaining to biologicals.

Table 34-1 lists some of the biologics made with recombinant DNA technology that are currently on the market, and the diseases they are used to treat.

Process of FDA Approval

When a company develops a new biopharmaceutical drug, the company must apply for a *patent*, which gives it the sole and exclusive rights to manufacture and sell that drug. It takes approximately 12 years to move a drug from the experimental stage to the pharmacy.

During the first, "preclinical" phase, the new drug is tested against a targeted disease through laboratory and animal studies. This process also evaluates the acute toxicity of the drug, to discover if it is reasonably safe to use in humans. This entire process can take from three to five years.

Table 34-1   Biologics Made with Recombinant DNA Technology

GENERIC NAME	TRADE NAME	CONDITION USED FOR
abatacept	Orencia®	rheumatoid arthritis
adalimumab	Humira®	rheumatoid arthritis
erythropoietin	Epogen®	anemia from cancer therapy, chronic renal failure
etanercept	Enbrel®	rheumatoid arthritis, psoriasis
infliximab	Remicade®	Crohn's disease
trastuzumab	Herceptin®	breast cancer

	Preclinical Testing		Phase I	Phase II	Phase III		FDA		Phase IV
Years	3.5		1	2	3		2.5	12 Total	
Test Population	Laboratory and animal studies	File IND at FDA	20 to 80 healthy volunteers	100 to 300 patient volunteers	1000 to 3000 patient volunteers	File NDA at FDA	Review process/ Approval		Additional Post marketing testing required by FDA
Purpose	Assess safety and biological activity		Determine safety and dosage	Evaluate effectiveness, look for side effects	Verify effectiveness, monitor adverse reactions from long-term use				
Success Rate	5,000 compounds evaluated		5 enter trials				1 approved		

FIGURE 34-2 The FDA approval process for a new biopharmaceutical.
(Used with permission of the Alliance Pharmaceutical Corporation.)

After the preclinical phase, the company files an Investigational New Drug application (IND) with the Food and Drug Administration (FDA). The IND shows the results of the animal pharmacology and toxicology studies that have already been done, along with detailed information and protocols for future clinical studies that will help determine if initial-phase drug trials will be safe enough to involve human subjects. The IND must also include the chemical structure of the compound and the company's plans for its manufacture. This helps the FDA assess whether the company can produce and supply consistent batches of the drug.

The IND becomes effective if the FDA does not disapprove it within 30 days. The next three steps are clinical trials, which are conducted with volunteers in clinics and hospitals, under the care of a physician. These trials, which take several years (see Figure 34-2), use varying groups of volunteers; a study may involve as few as 20 patients or as many as 3,000.

Following the successful completion of all three IND phases, the company can then file a new drug application (NDA) with the FDA; approval of an NDA can take as long as 30 months. Once the FDA gives its approval, the drug becomes available for physicians to prescribe. However, the FDA often requires some additional annual reporting to evaluate long-term effects.

Since 1978, the number of patents on drugs has risen significantly. For example, in 1978, only 30 patents were issued for FDA-approved drugs; by 2001, more than 34,000 patents had been granted. Several countries, including Argentina, China, and Egypt, are involved in research to develop new drugs, and their respective governments are funding these endeavors with huge financial grants each year. Approval can cost a company as much as $400 million. Even after a patent is granted and the drug is released to the market, it is still monitored for several more years to ensure safety and performance.

INFORMATION

Did you know? An NDA runs 10,000 or more pages. Only about one in five drugs on which clinical testing is begun makes it through the FDA trials and approval process.

PROFILES IN PRACTICE

Mr. Jones is 67 and a regular customer at your pharmacy. He recently was diagnosed with Gaucher's disease and has a prescription for Cerezyme®, a new biopharmaceutical drug. When you call the manufacturer and try to order it, they tell you that a year's supply will cost $200,000.

- What manufacturer makes this medication?
- Is there anything you can do to help Mr. Jones get this medicine at a price he can afford?
- Are any indigency programs or patient assistance programs available for a Medicare Part D customer?

Genetic Engineering

Genetic engineering, which is the direct manipulation of an organism's genes, is another way to produce new medications. The first genetically engineered drug was approved by the FDA for therapeutic use in 1982. It was rHi, or recombinant human insulin, also known as Humulin insulin. In 1986, the FDA approved a genetically engineered vaccine for hepatitis B, and since then many new products have been approved, such as Pulmozyme® for cystic fibrosis and Alferon N® for genital warts.

The genetic engineering process has four basic steps. The first step is to isolate the desirable gene, such as resistance to a particular disease. Next, that gene is inserted into a **vector**, which is any organism that does not itself cause disease but spreads it by distributing pathogens from one host to another. Bacteria containing plasmids or extrachromosomal DNA molecules that can replicate themselves make good vectors.

During the third step, scientists use the vector to **transform**, or genetically alter, the cells of another organism. Finally, the new **genetically modified organism (GMO)** is isolated from cells that did not take up the vector. The GMO is packaged with resistant genes and then placed in a culture with penicillin to ensure that only cells that have incorporated the vector survive.

Examples of GMOs are synthetic human insulin (approved by the FDA in 1982) and a hepatitis vaccine (approved in 1987). With synthetic human insulin, the human gene that directs the production of insulin was inserted into a harmless bacterial cell. This enabled the large-scale production of insulin under controlled conditions. Genetically modified (GM) viruses have been used to treat severe immune deficiency and some genetic diseases, such as sickle cell anemia, muscular dystrophy, and cystic fibrosis. When the DNA of a virus is removed through the genetic engineering process (as described above), the virus is no longer able to inject its DNA into healthy cells. This limits the spread of disease, and enables creation of a safe vaccine. Finally, GM foods such as vegetables have been created: some resist certain bacterial infections, some were made resistant to pests, and some were modified to stay fresh longer.

vector organism that does not itself cause disease, but spreads disease by distributing or carrying pathogens from one host to another.

transform alter an organism or a cell itself in the genetic engineering process.

genetically modified organism (GMO) an organism whose genetic material has been altered using the genetic engineering techniques known as recombinant DNA technology.

INFORMATION

According to one news article, practically all genetically engineered crops contain genetic material from viruses. Some scientists think that these created viruses may cause new and more serious diseases because they could combine with other viral genes that are already present in our bodies. Even though no major health hazards from the use of GM crops have been documented since such crops were introduced (more than 13 years ago), there is still not enough data to assess the health risks from genetically engineered crops.

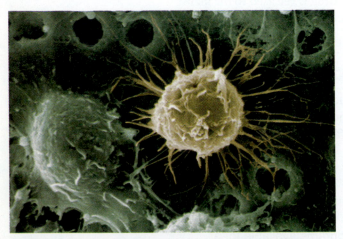

FIGURE 34-3 Color-enhanced scanning electron micrograph (SEM) of a stem cell collected from human bone marrow.

Stem Cell Research

Stem cell research also plays a significant role in the discovery of new pharmaceutical products and medical treatments (see Figure 34-3). Scientists are interested in the potential use of embryonic stem cells to treat disease for three reasons. First, stem cells have a special ability to renew themselves many times through cell division, in a process called *proliferation*. Second, unlike nerve or muscle cells, which perform specific functions in the body, stem cells are unspecialized (undifferentiated). Third, under certain conditions stem cells can transform into specialized cells, such as heart muscle, through a process called *differentiation*.

Only since 1998 have scientists been able to isolate stem cells from human embryos, so discovering the full potential of stem cells in the treatment of disease is an

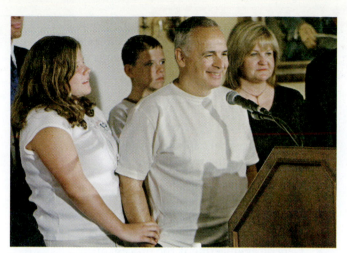

FIGURE 34-4 Nathan Klein, the first person to have gene therapy for Parkinson's disease.

ongoing process. One way they may eventually be useful is in the widespread testing of experimental medications, before the new medications are used in human clinical drug trials. Cancer research, as well as treatments for other life-threatening diseases such as Parkinson's disease, is already benefiting from the discoveries made in this area. For example, cancer cell lines are currently being used to screen for potential antitumor drugs. Stem cells could also offer a renewable source of replacement cells and tissue for treatment of diseases such as Parkinson's, diabetes, and Alzheimer's (see Figure 34-4). In Parkinson's disease, the brain cells that release dopamine die, causing a chemical imbalance in the brain. Characteristics of this chemical deficiency are tremors and a shuffling gait. Human genes that correct this imbalance were packaged in a virus and then injected into the brain cells of 59-year-old Nathan Klein, who had suffered from Parkinson's disease for more than four years. About six months after treatment, he reported feeling better.

The Political Climate

The field of biotechnology is politically charged and highly contentious. Despite the medical breakthroughs that have been accomplished through biopharmacy, genetic engineering, and stem cell research, some groups argue that biotechnology is morally wrong: first, because only God creates life, not scientists; second, because currently human embryos—potential human life—must be used as the source of stem cells. Furthermore, although some scientists argue that this research is necessary to combat both existing and future diseases, develop better medical treatments, and improve crop yields in a hungry world, others are concerned about the health consequences of consuming genetically engineered plants and animals.

Significant strides have been made in the treatment of many diseases, such as diabetes with Humulin and rheumatoid arthritis with Epogen. Companies in countries across the globe are spending millions of dollars every day on research, in a race to find new biopharmaceutical products. Imaging of the basic cellular structure has now become an integral part of clinical trials, in the hopes that one day such information will be used to develop new, better, and more effective products.

SUMMARY

Biopharmaceutical research is a growing field of pharmaceutics, and there is a growing need for the drugs that are the end products of this research. Biopharmaceuticals are used today to treat cancers, diabetes, hepatitis, multiple sclerosis (MS), and other life-threatening conditions. Genetic engineering and stem cell research play a very important role in the discovery of new products and the treatment of disease. For example, using stem cells, it may become possible to grow healthy heart muscle cells in the laboratory and then transplant those cells into patients with chronic heart disease. Genetic engineering could be used someday to repair damaged genes or replace missing genes in people who have genetic disorders such as cystic fibrosis.

Even though the FDA process for approval of a new drug is long and very expensive, the discovery of new drugs and the development of new technologies are crucial to our health. Biotechnology holds many opportunities for the future, especially as new diseases develop and old ones reemerge. The pharmaceutical industry will need to develop new vaccines and antibiotics for prevention and cure of diseases, accelerate the drug discovery process, and determine more accurate medication dosages. With today's extended life expectancy and the number of prescriptions on the rise, improved pharmacy service is even more important. As members of the pharmacy healthcare team, pharmacy technicians need to better understand diseases and find new and better ways to provide treatment, so that we can provide the best possible patient care.

CHAPTER REVIEW QUESTIONS

1. All of the following statements about biopharmaceuticals are true *except*:
   a. They are products derived from live plants and animals.
   b. They can be used for diagnostic purposes.
   c. They are not patentable.
   d. They are produced by biotechnology.

2. Artificial forms of DNA produced by biotechnology are known as:
   a. vectors.
   b. GMOs.
   c. recombinant therapeutic proteins.
   d. none of the above.

3. Enbrel® is a biologic drug made with recombinant technology and is used to treat:
   a. breast cancer.
   b. rheumatoid arthritis.
   c. tumors.
   d. Crohn's disease.

4. Infliximab is a biologic drug made with recombinant technology and is used to treat:
   a. rheumatoid arthritis.
   b. Crohn's disease.
   c. breast cancer.
   d. psoriasis.

5. In _____, 30 patents were issued for new biopharmaceutical drugs.
   a. 1970
   b. 1972
   c. 1978
   d. 2001

6. The first genetically engineered substance approved by the FDA for therapeutic use was:
   a. Enbrel®.
   b. Humira®.
   c. Humalog®.
   d. Humulin®.

7. In the process of genetic engineering, _____ is the actual alteration of the cell.
   a. isolation
   b. transformation
   c. vectoring
   d. extraction

8. Genetic engineering is the process of:
   a. direct manipulation of an organism's genes.
   b. making products using biotechnology.
   c. direct extraction from a native biological source.
   d. making cells and tissues for medical therapies.

9. It takes approximately _____ years from the time a new drug is introduced until a physician can prescribe it.
   a. 11
   b. 12
   c. 5
   d. none of the above

10. Required by the FDA, the _____ typically consists of 10,000 pages of information.
    a. IND
    b. GMO
    c. rHI
    d. NDA

CRITICAL THINKING QUESTIONS

1. Explain why some people consider stem cell research to be wrong.

2. What challenges will arise for pharmacy in the future because of the number of people living longer and requiring more medication? How can biopharmaceuticals help meet these challenges?

3. List three advantages and three disadvantages of the development of biopharmaceuticals.

WEB CHALLENGE

1. Visit the FDA's website and search for current regulations on biopharmaceutical products.

2. Using the FDA website as a source, list at least 10 biopharmaceuticals that are currently on the market, and name their therapeutic uses.

REFERENCES AND RESOURCES

Access Excellence: http://www.accessexcellence.org

American Society of Health System Pharmacists: http://www.ashp.org

Drug Facts and Comparisons, 2006 ed. St. Louis: Wolters Kluwer Health.

Food and Drug Administration: www.fda.gov

Genentech Inc.: www.genentech.com

GenWay Biotech, Inc: www.genwaybio.com

Interferon Sciences: www.Biospace.com

Medical News Today: www.medicalnewstoday.com

National Institute of Health. "Stem cell basics" (2008) (accessed February 25, 2008):
   http://stemcells.nih.gov/info/basics/basics1.asp

Appendix A:
Top 200 Drugs

BRAND NAME	GENERIC NAME	PRIMARY INDICATION/CLASSIFICATION
Lipitor	atorvastatin	Lipid/cholesterol lowering
Nexium	esomeprazole	GERD/ulcers
Prevacid	lansoprazole	GERD/ulcers
Advair Diskus	fluticasone and salmeterol	Asthma/COPD
Singulair	montelukast	Asthma
Effexor XR	venlafaxine	Antidepressant
Plavix	clopidogrel	Atherosclerosis/antiplatelet
Zocor	simvastatin	Lipid/cholesterol lowering
Norvasc	amlodipine	Hypertension/calcium channel blocker
Lexapro	escitalopram	Antidepressant
Seroquel	quetiapine	Antipsychotic
Protonix	pantoprazole	Proton pump inhibitor
Ambien	zolpidem	Insomnia/hypnotic
Actos	pioglitazone	Type 2 diabetes
Zoloft	sertraline	Antidepressant
Wellbutrin XL	bupropion	Antidepressant
Avandia	rosiglitazone	Type 2 diabetes
Risperdal	risperidone	Antipsychotic
Zyprexa	olanzapine	Antipsychotic
Topamax	topiramate	Anticonvulsant
Toprol XL	metoprolol	Hypertension/angina/beta blocker
Vytorin	ezetimibe and simvastatin	Lipid/cholesterol lowering
Fosamax	alendronate	Osteoporosis/Paget's disease
Abilify	aripiprazole	Antipsychotic
Levaquin	levofloxacin	Antibiotic
Lamictal	lamotrigine	Anticonvulsant
Celebrex	celecoxib	NSAID/arthritis
Lotrel	amlodipine and benazepril	Hypertension/ACE inhibitor/calcium channel blocker
Zyrtec	cetirizine	Antihistamine
Coreg	carvedilol	Hypertension/beta blocker
Valtrex	valacyclovir	Antiviral
Zetia	ezetimibe	Lipid/cholesterol lowering

BRAND NAME	GENERIC NAME	PRIMARY INDICATION/CLASSIFICATION
Adderall XR	amphetamine-dextroamphetamine	ADHD
Aciphex	rabeprazole	GERD/ulcers
Cymbalta	duloxetine	Antidepressant
Enbrel	etanercept	Arthritis
Crestor	rosuvastatin	Lipid/cholesterol lowering
Lantus	insulin glargine	Type 1 diabetes
Diovan	valsartan	Hypertension
Tricor	fenofibrate	Lipid/cholesterol lowering
Concerta	methylphenidate	ADD/ADHD
Diovan DCT	valsartan	Hypertension
Imitrex Oral	sumatriptan	Headache/migraine
Aricept	donepezil	Alzheimer's
Nasonex	mometasone nasal	Nasal congestions/sneezing/runny nose
Viagra	sildenafil	Erectile dysfunction
Flomax	tamsulosin	Benign prostatic hyperplasia
Actonel	risedronate	Osteoporosis
Omnicef	cefdinir	Antibiotic
Altace	ramipril	Hypertension/ACE inhibitor
OxyContin	oxycodone	Narcotic pain reliever
Lyrica	pregabalin	Anticonvulsant
Zofran	ondansetron	Antinausea/vomiting related to chemotherapy
Provigil	modafinil	Sleep apnea/narcolepsy
Lidoderm	lidocaine topical	Local anesthetic
Cozaar	losartan	Hypertension/angiotensin II receptor antagonist
Lamisil Oral	terbinafine	Antifungal
Lovenox	enoxaparin	Anticoagulant
Spiriva	tiotropium inhalation	Bronchitis/emphysema/COPD
Detrol LA	tolterodine	Bladder spasms/overactive bladder
Lunesta	eszopiclone	Sedative/hypnotic
Synthroid	levothyroxine	Hypothyroidism
Strattera	atomoxetine	ADHD
Premarin Tabs	conjugated estrogens	Female hormones/menopause
Pravachol	pravastatin	Lipid/cholesterol lowering
Truvada	emtricitabine and tenofovir	Antiviral/HIV/AIDS
Ambien CR	zolpidem	Sedative/hypnotic
Actiq	fentanyl citrate	Narcotic pain reliever
Depakote	divalproex sodium	Seizures
Combivent	albuterol and ipratropium	COPD
Humalog	insulin lispro	Diabetes

(continued)

BRAND NAME	GENERIC NAME	PRIMARY INDICATION/CLASSIFICATION
Geodon Oral	ziprasidone	Antipsychotic
Pulmicort Respules	budesonide inhalation	Asthma
Trileptal	oxcarbazepine	Anticonvulsant
Mobic	meloxicam	NSAID
Yasmin	drospirenone and ethinyl estradiol	Oral contraceptive
Evista	raloxifene	Osteoporosis
CellCept	mycophenolate mofetil	Organ transplant
Humira	adalimumab	Arthritis/Crohn's disease
Depakote ER	divalproex sodium	Seizures
Keppra	levetiracetam	Anti-epileptic
Skelaxin	metaxalone	Muscle relaxant
Flovent HFA	fluticasone inhalation	Asthma
Hyzaar	hydrochlorothiazide and losartan	Hypertension
Niaspan	niacin	Lipid/cholesterol lowering
Prograf	tacrolimus	Organ transplant
Arimidex	anastrozole	Breast cancer
Procrit	epoetin alfa	Anemia
Xalatan	latanoprost ophthalmic	Glaucoma
Asacol	mesalamine	Ulcerative colitis
Namenda	memantine	Alzheimer's
Cialis	tadalafil	Erectile dysfunction
Reyataz	atazanavir	Antiviral/HIV/AIDS
Ortho Tri-Cyclen Lo	ethinyl estradiol and norgestimate	Oral contraceptive
Avapro	irbesartan	Hypertension/angiotensin II receptor antagonist
Byetta	exenatide	Type 2 diabetes
Duragesic	fentanyl topical	Narcotic pain reliever
Combivir	lamivudine and zidovudine	Antiviral/HIV/AIDS
Kaletra	lopinavir and ritonavir	Antiviral/HIV/AIDS
Gleevec	imatinib	Leukemia
Avelox	moxifloxacin	Antibiotic
Allegra-D 12 Hour	fexofenadine and pseudoephedrine	Antihistamine/decongestant
Benicar HCT	olmesartan	Hypertension/angiotensin II receptor antagonist
Paxil CR	paroxetine	Antidepressant
Clarinex	desloratadine	Antihistamine
Xopenex	levalbuterol	Asthma/bronchitis/emphysema
Benicar	olmesartan	Hypertension/angiotensin II receptor antagonist
Copaxone	glatiramer	Multiple sclerosis
Sustiva	efavirenz	Antiviral/HIV/AIDS

BRAND NAME	GENERIC NAME	PRIMARY INDICATION/CLASSIFICATION
Avalide	hydrochlorothiazide and irbesartan	Hypertension/angiotensin II receptor antagonist
Nasacort AQ	triamcinolone	Nasal allergies
AndroGel	testosterone topical	Male hormone
Forteo	teriparatide	Osteoporosis
Patanol	olopatadine ophthalmic	Antihistamine
Avonex	interferon beta-1a	Multiple sclerosis
Flonase	fluticasone nasal	Nasal allergies
Thalomid	thalidomide	Anti-inflammatory
Boniva	ibandronate	Osteoporosis
Zofran ODT	ondansetron	Antinausea/vomiting related to chemotherapy
Caduet	amlodipine and atorvastatin	Hypertension/angina related to high cholesterol
Requip	ropinirole	Parkinson's disease
Fuzeon	enfuvirtide	Antiviral/HIV/AIDS
Rhinocort Aqua	budesonide nasal	Nasal allergies
Norvir	ritonavir	Antiviral/HIV/AIDS
Tarceva	erlotinib	Cancer
Ditropan XL	oxybutynin	Bladder spasms/overactive bladder
Aldara	imiquimod topical	Actinic keratosis/skin cancer/genital warts
NovoLog Mix 70/30	insulin aspart	Type 1 diabetes
Femara	letrozole	Breast cancer
Ortho Evra	ethinyl estradiol and norelgestromin	Oral contraceptive
Endocet	acetaminophen and oxycodone	Narcotic pain reliever
Renagel	sevelamer	End-stage renal disease
Cosopt	dorzolamide and timolol ophthalmic	Glaucoma
Viread	tenofovir	Antiviral/HIV/AIDS
Trizivir	abacavir-lamivudine-zidovudine	Antiviral/HIV/AIDS
Budeprion SR	bupropion hydrochloride	Antidepressant
Restasis	cyclosporine ophthalmic	Chronic dry eye/inflammation of the eye
Zyvox	linezolid	Antibiotic
Relpax	eletriptan	Migraine headaches
Lumigan	bimatoprost ophthalmic	Glaucoma
Benzaclin	benzoyl peroxide and clindamycin topical	Acne
Humalog Mix 75/25 Pen	insulin lispro	Diabetes
Zithromax Suspension	azithromycin	Antibiotic
Mirapex	pramipexole	Parkinson's disease/restless leg syndrome
Avodart	dutasteride	Benign prostatic hyperplasia
Casodex	bicalutamide	Prostate cancer
Astelin	azelastine nasal	Nasal allergies

(continued)

BRAND NAME	GENERIC NAME	PRIMARY INDICATION/CLASSIFICATION
Vigamox	moxifloxacin ophthalmic	Antibiotic
Epzicom	abacavir and lamivudine	Antiviral/HIV/AIDS
Lescol XL	fluvastatin	Lipid/cholesterol lowering
Xeloda	capecitabine	Cancer
Tussionex	chlorpheniramine and hydrocodone	Cough/nasal congestion
Coumadin Tablets	warfarin	Anticoagulant
Sensipar	cinacalcet	Decreases parathyroid hormone/calcium/phosphorus
Levitra	vardenafil	Erectile dysfunction
Temodar	temozolomide	Cancer
Inderal LA	propranolol	Hypertension/beta blocker
Prilosec	omeprazole	GERD/ulcers
Catapres-TTS	clonidine	Hypertension
NuvaRing	ethinyl estradiol and etonogestrel	Oral contraceptive
Biaxin XL	clarithromycin	Antibiotic
Zyrtec Syrup	cetirizine	Antihistamine
Alphagan P	brimonidine ophthalmic	Glaucoma
Differin	adapalene topical	Acne
Zyrtec-D	cetirizine	Antihistamine/decongestant
Tobradex	tobramycin and dexamethasone ophthalmic	Antibiotic
Aranesp	darbepoetin alfa	Anemia
Klor-Con	potassium chloride	Hypokalemia
Humulin N	insulin isophane	Diabetes
DuoNeb	albuterol and ipratropium	COPD
Famvir	famciclovir	Antiviral
Proscar	finasteride	Benign prostatic hyperplasia
Neupogen	filgrastim	Stimulates the growth of white blood cells
Elidel	pimecrolimus topical	Immunosuppressant
Focalin XR	dexmethylphenidate	ADHD
Levoxyl	levothyroxine	Hypothyroidism
Betaseron	interferon beta-1b	Multiple sclerosis
Ciprodex Otic	ciprofloxacin and dexamethasone otic	Antibiotic/steroid
TriNessa	ethinyl estradiol and norgestimate	Oral contraceptive
Atacand	candesartan	Hypertension/angiotensin II receptor antagonist
PEGASYS	peginterferon alfa-2a	Hepatitis B and C
Kadian	morphine	Narcotic pain reliever
Arthrotec	diclofenac and misoprostol	NSAID
Aggrenox	aspirin and dipyridamole	Antiplatelet

BRAND NAME	GENERIC NAME	PRIMARY INDICATION/CLASSIFICATION
Humulin 70/30	insulin isophane and insulin regular	Diabetes
Avinza	morphine	Narcotic pain reliever
Pulmozyme	dornase alfa	Cystic fibrosis
Travatan	travoprost ophthalmic	Glaucoma
Maxalt	rizatriptan	Headache/migraine
Dovonex	calcipotriene topical	Psoriasis
Risperdal Consta	risperidone	Antipsychotic
Tri-Sprintec	norgestimate and ethinyl estradiol	Oral contraceptive
Zomig	zolmitriptan	Headache/migraine
Maxalt MLT	rizatriptan	Headache/migraine
Prempro	conjugated estrogens and medroxyprogesterone	Female hormones/menopause
Augmentin XR	amoxicillin and clavulanate potassium	Antibiotic
Suboxone	buprenorphine and naloxone	Opiate addiction
Avandamet	metformin and rosiglitazone	Type 2 diabetes
Fosamax Plus D	alendronate and cholecalciferol	Osteoporosis

List based on gross U.S. sales for 2006.

Appendix B:
Over-the-Counter Product Guide

INDICATION (listed alphabetically)	PRODUCT NAME
Acne	Clean & Clear
	Clearasil
	Neutrogena
	Noxzema
	Oxy
	PanOxyl
	Persa Gel
	Stridex
Adult Cold—Liquid	Comtrex
	DayQuil
	Dimetapp
	NyQuil
	Robitussin
	TheraFlu
	Triaminic
	Tylenol
	Vicks 44
Adult Cold—Long Acting	Actifed
	Advil
	Chlor-Trimeton
	Claritin
	Coricidin HBP
	Delsym
	Drixoral
	Mucinex
	Robitussin
	Sudafed
	Tylenol Cold
Adult Cold—Nighttime	Benadryl
	Diabetic Tussin Nighttime
	NyQuil
	Robitussin PM
	Tylenol Nighttime
Adult Cold—Tablet/Capsule	Actifed
	Advil Cold & Sinus
	Benadryl
	Claritin
	Comtrex

INDICATION (listed alphabetically)	PRODUCT NAME
	Coricidin HBP
	Drixoral
	Motrin Cold & Sinus
	Robitussin
	Sudafed
	TheraFlu
	Tylenol Cold
Adult Cough	Benylin
	Delsym
	Mucinex
	Robitussin
Adult Expectorant	Diabetic Tussin
	Humibid
	Mucinex
	Robitussin
Allergies	Actifed
	Alavert
	Benadryl
	Chlor-Trimeton
	Claritin
	Dimetapp
	Sudafed
	Tylenol Allergy
	Zicam Allergy
Antacids/Heartburn	Gaviscon
	Maalox
	Mylanta
	Pepcid AC
	Pepcid Complete
	Pepto Bismol
	Prilosec
	Tums
	Zantac 75
Antidiarrheals	*Imodium A-D*
	Kaopectate
	Pepto-Bismol
Arthritis Pain	Advil
	Aleve
	Cosamin DS
	Motrin
	Tylenol Arthritis Pain
Athlete's Foot	*Lamisil*
	Lotrimin
	Micatin
	Tinactin

(continued)

INDICATION (listed alphabetically)	PRODUCT NAME
Blood Glucose Kits/Strips	*Accu-Chek*
	Ascensia
	FreeStyle
	Glucometer Elite
	One Touch
	True Track
Children's Analgesics	Children's Advil
	Children's Motrin
	Children's Tylenol
Children's Cold	Benadryl
	Children's Motrin
	Children's Tylenol
	Dimetapp
	Little Noses
	PediaCare
	Robitussin
	Sudafed
	Triaminic
Children's Cough	Children's Tylenol
	Delsym
	Dimetapp
	PediaCare
	Robitussin-DM
	Triaminic
Cold Sores	*Abreva*
	Campho-Phenique
	Carmex
	Herpecin
	Orajel
	Zilactin
Diaper Rash	A&D Ointment
	Aveeno
	Balmex
	Boudreaux's Butt Paste
	Desitin
	Triple Paste
Flatulence	Beano
	Gas-X
	Maalox Anti-Gas
	Mylicon
	Phazyme
Flu Relief	Advil Flu & Body Aches
	Comtrex Flu Therapy
	Coricidin D
	Oscillococcinum
	TheraFlu
	Tylenol Flu
	Vicks Cold & Flu Relief

INDICATION (listed alphabetically)	PRODUCT NAME
H2 Antagonists	Axid AR
	Pepcid AC
	Pepcid Complete
	Zantac 75
Headache	Advil
	Aleve
	Excedrin
	Motrin
	Tylenol
Hemorrhoids	Anusol
	Nupercainal
	Preparation H
	Tucks
Jock Itch	Cruex
	Lamisil
	Lotrimin
	Micatin
	Tinactin
Laxatives	Correctol
	Doxidan
	Dulcolax
	ex-lax
	Fleet
	Senokot-S
Lice	A-200
	Nix
	Rid
Migraines	Advil Migraine
	Aleve
	Excedrin Extra Strength
	Excedrin Migraine
	Motrin Migraine
	Tylenol
Motion Sickness	Bonine
	Dramamine
	Emetrol
	Seaband
Nasal Decongestants—Oral	Claritin-D
	Dimetapp
	Drixoral
	Sudafed
	Tylenol Sinus
Nasal Decongestants—Sprays	*Afrin*
	Nasalcrom
	Neo-Synephrine

(continued)

INDICATION (listed alphabetically)	PRODUCT NAME
	Vick's Sinex
	Zicam Extreme Congestion
Pregnancy Tests	Answer
	Clear Blue Easy
	e.p.t.
	Fact Plus
	First Response
Sinus Congestion	Advil Cold & Sinus
	Alavert
	Aleve Cold & Sinus
	Benadryl
	Claritin
	Motrin Sinus
	Sudafed Sinus
	Tylenol Sinus
Sleep Aids	Alluna Sleep
	Benadryl
	Hyland's Calms Forte
	Nytol
	Simply Sleep
	Sominex
	Tylenol PM
	Unisom
Sore Throat	Cepacol
	Cepastat
	Chloraseptic
	Halls Max
	Sucrets
Sore Throat—Liquids	Cepacol
	Chloraseptic
	Triaminic
	Tylenol
Stool Softener	*Colace*
	Dulcolax
	Senokot
	Surfak
Topical Analgesics	Aspercreme
	Ben-Gay
	Capsazin
	Icy Hot
	Myoflex
	Sportscreme
	Thera-gesic
	Zostrix

INDICATION (listed alphabetically)	PRODUCT NAME
Upset Stomach	Alka-Seltzer
	Emetrol
	Gaviscon
	Maalox
	Mylanta
	Pepcid AC
	Pepcid Complete
	Pepto-Bismol
	Tums
Urinary Tract Infection Pain Relief	*Azo-Standard*
	Cystex
	UriStat
Vaginal Antifungals	Gyne-Lotrimin
	Monistat
	Mycelex
	Vagistat-1
Warts	*Compound W*
	Curad Mediplast
	Dr. Scholl's Clear Away
	DuoFilm
	Wartner
Wound Care	A&D Original Ointment
	Bactine
	Betadine
	Neosporin
	Polysporin
	Triple Antibiotic Ointment

Product Names indicate the most commonly recommended by pharmacists.

Appendix C:
Advanced Career Path Options

There are numerous advanced career path opportunities for properly trained pharmacy technicians. Although the vast majority of positions available fall within standard community and health-system pharmacy settings, pharmacy technicians should consider all career opportunities available.

The following provides a brief introduction to just a few of the advanced career options for pharmacy technicians. The National Pharmacy Technician Association (NPTA) has developed a two-disc audio program, entitled *Exploring Your Career Paths in Pharmacy*, which provides insight on how to explore and evaluate 50 career path options for pharmacy technicians. For more information on this resource, go to www.pharmacytechnician.org or call 1-888-247-8700.

Clinical Pharmacy Technician

The role of *clinical pharmacy technician* is an emerging trend within certain health-system pharmacies. Rather than working within the central or satellite pharmacy, clinical pharmacy technicians are assigned to a specific unit, working with a clinical pharmacist.

Clinical pharmacy technicians have been used to manage the delivery of initial dosages, locate missing medications, review floor stock inventory levels, and assist in collecting patient-specific data for analysis by the clinical pharmacist.

Specific areas of utilization for clinical pharmacy technicians include:

- Congestive heart failure (CHF) clinics
- Coumadin therapy
- Diabetes management
- Intensive care unit (ICU) lab profiles
- Lipid clinics

Federal Pharmacy

Federal pharmacy refers to the practice of pharmacy within the federal government, such as the military, the Public Health Service, federal correctional facilities, or the Department of Veterans Affairs. Federal pharmacy is unique in that it is not regulated by a state board of pharmacy and therefore need not meet certain requirements, such as state-specified pharmacist-to-technician ratios.

Military

Military pharmacy services, which are overseen by the Department of Defense, provide pharmaceutical care for active-duty military personnel and their families. Each branch of the military (the U.S. Army, the U.S. Navy, the U.S. Air Force, the U.S. Marine Corps, and the U.S. Coast Guard) maintains its own facilities and pharmacy personnel.

Military pharmacy technicians can be either civilian or enlisted (military) personnel. Civilian pharmacy technicians are not required to complete military basic training. Enlisted pharmacy technicians, who are required to complete basic training, are classified as noncommissioned officers; they are eligible for rank advancements within the military.

Public Health Service

The *Public Health Service (PHS)*, which is part of the Department of Health and Human Services (DHHS), provides pharmaceutical care to specific populations or communities. Pharmacy technicians work in numerous divisions of PHS, including:

- Agency for Health Care Policy and Research
- Agency for Toxic Substances and Disease Registry
- Centers for Disease Control and Prevention (CDC)
- Food and Drug Administration (FDA)
- Health Resources and Services Administration
- Indian Health Service (IHS)
- National Institutes of Health (NIH)
- Substance Abuse and Mental Health Services Administration

Federal Correctional Facilities

Federal correctional facilities, also known as *federal prisons*, are responsible for providing medical and pharmaceutical care to their inmates. Pharmacists and pharmacy technicians work securely onsite at these facilities, with little to no interaction with the inmates themselves.

Department of Veterans Affairs

Through the Veterans Health Administration (VHA), the Department of Veterans Affairs (VA) provides pharmaceutical care to those who previously served in the U.S. military. There are hundreds of VA medical facilities located across the United States, including VA hospitals, and most of them employ pharmacy technicians. In addition, pharmacy technicians can work at VA mail-order facilities.

Home Infusion Pharmacy

Home infusion pharmacies prepare intravenous (IV) solutions to be administered at the patient's home. In addition to IV solutions, home infusion pharmacies prepare enteral nutrition therapy and other injectable solutions.

Home infusion pharmacies focus solely on preparation of sterile products; therefore, the pharmacists and pharmacy technicians must be properly trained in aseptic technique. After the infusion therapies have been prepared at the pharmacy, they are delivered to the patient for administration.

The most common home infusion therapies are:

- Anti-infectives, including for HIV/AIDS
- Biotechnology
- Chemotherapy
- Chronic pain management
- Hydration
- Nutrition (TPN and enteral nutrition)

Mail-Order Pharmacy

Mail-order pharmacies are facilities that dispense maintenance medications to patients via the mail (U.S. Postal Service and other carriers). Unlike community pharmacies, mail-order pharmacies are not designed to provide medications for acute needs.

Major mail-order pharmacies, such as CVS/Caremark and Medco, operate numerous facilities strategically located across the United States to provide faster deliveries to their patients. These pharmacies are considered extremely high volume, with some facilities processing and dispensing more than 30,000 prescriptions per day.

Because of the high volume of prescriptions, mail-order pharmacies employ vast numbers of pharmacists and pharmacy technicians, and generally operate 24 hours a day. Pharmacy technicians typically work in the call center or translate and input new prescription orders.

Mail-order pharmacies are completely automated, using robotics to pull, count, and label prescription orders. Each order is then verified by a staff pharmacist, who compares the prepared order with an electronic image of the original prescription and electronic images of what the medication being dispensed should look like.

Nuclear Pharmacy

Nuclear pharmacies, or *radiopharmacies*, prepare and dispense radioactive drugs, known as *radiopharmaceuticals*, which are used to diagnose and treat diseases. There are two types of nuclear pharmacies: institutional and centralized.

Institutional nuclear pharmacies operate within a large health-system's nuclear medicine department. Centralized nuclear pharmacies operate in an offsite facility and prepare radiopharmaceuticals for various facilities that outsource this service.

The two main types of radiopharmaceuticals are positron emission tomography (PET) drugs and radioactive blood elements. PET drugs are used in diagnostic imaging, and because they have a very short half-life they are prepared only in institutional nuclear pharmacies. Radioactive blood elements include red blood cells, white blood cells, and even platelets that are combined with radionuclides to be used in diagnosis.

Because they must handle advanced issues and have potential exposure to radioactive elements, pharmacy technicians must complete extensive training to work in a nuclear pharmacy. These training programs are administered by employers, such as Syncor.

Appendix D:
Professional Resources

■ = Regulatory/Governmental Agencies

■ = Associations

■ = Magazines/Conferences

■ = Certification Exams

■ Accreditation Council for Pharmacy Education (ACPE)
www.acpe-accredit.org

■ American Association of Pharmacy Technicians (AAPT)
www.pharmacytechnician.com

■ American Pharmacy Association (APhA)
www.pharmacist.com

■ American Society of Consultant Pharmacists (ASCP)
www.ascp.com

■ American Society of Health System Pharmacists (ASHP)
www.ashp.org

■ Centers for Disease Control and Prevention (CDC)
www.cdc.gov

■ Drug Enforcement Administration (DEA)
www.dea.gov

■ *Drug Topics* Magazine
www.drugtopics.com

■ Food and Drug Administration (FDA)
www.fda.gov

■ Institute for the Certification of Pharmacy Technicians (ICPT)
www.nationaltechexam.org

■ Institute for Safe Medication Practices (ISMP)
www.ismpi.org

■ Joint Commission on the Accreditation of Healthcare Organizations (JCAHO)
www.jointcommission.org

■ National Association of Boards of Pharmacy (NABP)
www.nabp.net

■ National Association of Chain Drug Stores (NACDS)
www.nacds.org

- National Community Pharmacists Association (NCPA)
  www.ncpanet.org

- National Pharmacy Technician Association (NPTA)
  www.pharmacytechnician.org

- Pharmacy Technician Certification Board (PTCB)
  www.ptcb.org

- *Pharmacy Times* Magazine
  www.pharmacytimes.com

- RxPO—Annual Pharmacy Technician Convention
  www.rxpomeeting.com

- *Today's Technician* Magazine
  www.pharmacytechnician.org

- *U.S. Pharmacist* Magazine
  www.uspharmacist.com

- *U.S. Pharmacopeia* (USP)
  www.usp.org

- World Health Organization (WHO)
  www.who.int

Appendix E:
References

Many references and resources are available to pharmacy professionals to assist in the contemporary practice of pharmacy. Pharmacy technicians should be familiar with the most common reference sources, to expedite the process of finding pertinent information when needed. Of the numerous references available, this appendix provides an overview of the 10 most commonly used.

American Hospital Formulary Service Drug Information (AHFS DI)

The American Hospital Formulary Service provides an evidence-based and peer-reviewed formulary, used primarily by hospitals. *AHFS DI*, which is derived from the American Hospital Formulary Service, contains information from medical literature that goes far beyond FDA-approved labeling and expert advice from more than 500 medical scientists, physicians, pharmacists, pharmacologists, and other professionally qualified individuals.

AHFS DI includes drug interactions, adverse reactions, cautions and toxicity, therapeutic perspective, specific dosage and administration information, preparations, chemistry, stability, pharmacology and pharmacokinetics, and contraindications for each of the formulary's approved drugs.

AHFS DI is available in an annual print edition as well as an electronic version that includes updates.

Drug Facts and Comparisons

Drug Facts and Comparisons is the most widely used reference in pharmacy. Covering 22,000 prescription drugs and 6,000 OTC products, *Drug Facts and Comparisons* is available in an annual hardbound edition, as well as looseleaf and electronic versions that are updated monthly.

Drug Facts and Comparisons is organized into five sections.

- Section 1 provides an index of trade and generic drug names.
- Section 2 lists orphan and investigational drugs.
- Section 3 contains drug monographs organized into 14 chapters based on drug classification (e.g., Cardiovascular Agents, Dermatological Agents).
- Section 4 is used in drug identification and includes full-color images of more than 250 drugs.

- Section 5 is an appendix containing various resources, such as pharmacy calculations, manufacturer abbreviation codes, and standard medical abbreviations.

Drug Topics Red Book

Drug Topics Red Book, which is referred to simply as the *Red Book*, has been published for more than 100 years. *Red Book*, which is used most commonly by community-based pharmacies, contains:

- Nationally recognized average wholesale prices (AWPs), direct prices, and federal upper-limit prices for prescription drugs
- Direct prices and federal upper-limit prices for prescription drugs
- Suggested retail prices for OTC products
- NDC numbers for all FDA-approved drugs
- Complete package information, including dosage form, route of administration, strength, and size
- "Orange Book" codes—FDA-approved drug products with therapeutic equivalent evaluations

The *Drug Topics Red Book* is available in an annual print edition.

Handbook on Injectable Drugs

The *Handbook on Injectable Drugs* provides precise stability and compatibility information for healthcare professionals involved in prescribing, preparing, or administering parenteral medications. It contains:

- More than 360 drug monographs, including 47 non-U.S. drugs.
- Index of trade and generic injectable drug names.
- AHFS classification numbers for each drug, to allow reference to therapeutic data in *AHFS Drug Information*.
- Tabulated results from primary research on the compatibility of the listed drug with infusion solutions and other drugs. Four compatibility tables are provided for each drug: solution, additive, syringe, and Y-site.
- Storage requirements and general stability information, including pH, freezing, exposure to light, sorption and filtration characteristics, and repackaging information.

- Key product data, including common sizes, strengths, volumes, and forms in which the drug is supplied. Also includes pH, osmotic value, and other important product information.

The *Handbook of Injectable Drugs* is available in an annual print edition.

Handbook of Non-Prescription Drugs

As its name implies, the *Handbook of Non-Prescription Drugs* is designed as a reference for OTC products, supplements, and therapies. The *Handbook of Non-Prescription Drugs* covers:

- Nonprescription drug pharmacotherapy
- Nutritional supplements
- Medical foods
- Nondrug and preventive measures
- Complementary and alternative therapies

It also provides FDA-approved dosing information and evidence-based research on the efficacy and safety of over-the-counter, herbal, and homeopathic medications.

The *Handbook of Non-Prescription Drugs* is available in an annual print edition as well as an electronic version.

Martindale's: The Complete Drug Reference

Martindale's: The Complete Drug Reference provides professional and comprehensive information on drugs and medicines used throughout the world. Commonly referred to as *Martindale*, it is available in annual print and electronic versions. *Martindale* includes:

- 6,300 drug monographs
- 149,000 preparations
- 14,700 manufacturers
- 660 disease reviews
- 40,700 references
- international data, including preparations used in 36 nations around the world
- drugs in clinical use
- veterinary and investigational agents
- compounds used in medicine
- pharmaceutical excipients
- herbal medicines
- toxic substances

Merck Manual

The *Merck Manual*, which is the most widely used medical reference, provides healthcare professionals with essential information on diagnosing and treating medical disorders.

Although the *Merck Manual* is more commonly used by physicians and medical students, it provides valuable information for today's pharmacy professionals to assist their patients. The *Merck Manual* is published annually in both print and electronic formats.

Physician's Desk Reference (PDR)

The *Physician's Desk Reference*, which is referred to as the *PDR*, provides extensive information on FDA-approved prescription drugs. Despite its name, the *PDR* reference is commonly used by pharmacy personnel. The *PDR* contains:

- information on more than 3,000 drugs, indexed by brand/generic name, manufacturer, and product category
- drug interactions and adverse reactions
- more than 1,800 full-color photographs cross-referenced to the drug
- phonetic spellings
- contraindications
- adult and pediatric dosages

The *PDR* is available in annual print and electronic formats.

Remington's Pharmaceutical Sciences

Remington's Pharmaceutical Sciences is a textbook and reference book on the science and practice of pharmacy. Commonly referred to as *Remington's*, this reference book is available in an annual print format.

Remington's includes information related to:

- pharmacogenomics
- application of ethical principles to practice dilemmas
- technology and automation
- professional communication
- medication errors
- reengineering of pharmacy practice
- management of special-risk medicines
- specialization in pharmacy practice
- disease state management
- emergency patient care
- wound care

United States Pharmacopeia Drug Information

The *United States Pharmacopeia Drug Information* is a three-set reference volume. Volume 1 contains drug information for healthcare professionals. Volume 2 provides information to use when advising patients on their medications. Volume 3 focuses on the federal and state requirements related to medications.

Appendix F:
Practice Certification Exams

Practice Certification Exam I

This practice test has been designed to simulate the certification exam in both the number and style of questions, as well as the content. You should complete this exam within two hours.

1. Calculate the flow rate in drops per minute if a physician orders D5W/NS 1,400 mL over 12 hr using an administration set that delivers 40 gtt/mL.

   a. 87 gtt/min

   b. 68 gtt/min

   c. 117 gtt/min

   d. 78 gtt/min

2. The drug enalapril belongs in which of the following classification groups?

   a. beta blocker

   b. ACE inhibitor

   c. NSAID

   d. antiemetic

3. The retail price of a prescription is based on AWP plus a dispensing fee. Using the following fee table, calculate the retail price of a prescription for 20 tablets if a bottle of 100 tablets has an AWP of $68.60.

AWP	DISPENSING FEE
$0–$5.00	$4.75
$5.01–$10.00	$5.75
$10.01–$20.00	$6.75
$20.00 and up	$7.75

   a. $13.72

   b. $18.47

   c. $20.47

   d. $21.47

4. A prescription for which of the following medications could not be written with refills?

   a. nifedipine

   b. lorazepam

   c. methylphenidate

   d. hydrocodone/acetaminophen

5. A technician answers the phone. The patient calling in states that after taking a medication received from the pharmacy a few hours earlier, she is not feeling well and would like to know the side effects of the medication. The technician should:

   a. tell the patient the side effects of the medication, as they are commonly known to all pharmacy personnel.

   b. put the patient on hold and notify the pharmacist of the situation.

   c. ask the patient to hold while he looks up the side effects in a reference book.

   d. tell the patient to lie down and maybe the side effects will wear off soon.

6. Diphenhydramine is the generic name for which of these drugs?

   a. Benadryl

   b. Dramamine

   c. Bentyl

   d. Soma

7. A local dermatologist has special-ordered 60 g of 1.5% hydrocortisone cream for a patient. The pharmacy has in stock a 2.5% hydrocortisone cream and a 1% hydrocortisone cream. How much of each will the technician need to correctly prepare this extemporaneous compound?

   a. 40 g of 2.5% and 20 g of 1%

   b. 40 g of 1% and 20 g of 2.5%

   c. 30 g of each strength

   d. 45 g of 1% and 15 g of 2.5%

8. Who must initiate an order for an investigational drug for patient use?

   a. a pharmacy director

   b. a pharmacist

   c. a technician

   d. a physician

9. How many 500 mg metronidazole tablets will be needed to compound the following prescription for a patient: metronidazole 3%, suspending agent 30%, simple syrup 40% qsad H_2O to 150 mL?

   a. 9

   b. 7

   c. 10

   d. 18

10. A medication given to reduce a fever is called:
    a. an analgesic.
    b. an antitussive.
    c. an anthelmintic.
    d. an antipyretic.

11. Medications that are prepackaged into unit-dose or unit-of-use containers must have the following information included on the package labeling:
    a. patient's name, dispensing date, name of medication, and directions for use.
    b. medication name and strength, lot number, and expiration date.
    c. medication name and strength, lot number, and directions for use.
    d. directions for use, medication name and strength, and expiration date.

12. A patient brings the following prescription into your pharmacy: Amoxil 400 mg po tid for 10 days. Your pharmacy has in stock an Amoxil oral suspension 250 mg/5 mL. What is the exact volume of medication you will need to correctly and completely fill the prescription for the patient?
    a. 150 mL
    b. 168 mL
    c. 240 mL
    d. 200 mL

13. When mixing cytotoxic agents for intravenous use, what type of syringe is required?
    a. glass
    b. luer-lock
    c. slip-tip
    d. reusable

14. According to the Controlled Substances Act, in what class of controlled medications is Lortab 5?
    a. V
    b. IV
    c. III
    d. II

15. *Inventory turnover rate* refers to:
    a. how often employees quit and new employees are hired to replace them.
    b. how long it takes the pharmacy to process a new prescription.
    c. how many times a year shelves are inspected for expired medications.
    d. how often medications are used and reordered.

16. The portion of the retail price of a prescription that the patient must pay is known as the:
    a. deductible.
    b. co-payment.
    c. average wholesale price.
    d. none of the above.

17. How many capsules will it take to completely fill the following prescription with the given regimen: cephalexin 500 mg, 1 po tid × 14 days?
    a. 14 capsules
    b. 21 capsules
    c. 28 capsules
    d. 42 capsules

18. Prescription medications are often referred to as _____ drugs because of the federal law that requires the packaging to display the following message: "Caution: Federal law prohibits dispensing without a prescription."
    a. controlled
    b. legend
    c. prescription
    d. none of the above

19. *Stock rotation* is the task of making sure that:
    a. the shortest expiration date is in the back.
    b. the longest expiration date is in the front.
    c. the shortest expiration date is in the front.
    d. none of the above.

20. Which of the following is classed as a beta blocker?
    a. propranolol
    b. enalapril
    c. verapamil
    d. allopurinol

21. A patient in the hospital needs KCl 8 mEq IV stat. The pharmacy stocks KCl 20 mEq/mL in a 10 mL multidose vial. What will the correct volume of the stat dose be?
    a. 2.5 mL
    b. 4 mL
    c. 0.4 mL
    d. 0.04 mL

22. What document is used as proof of receipt of a controlled substance, according to the DEA?
    a. packing slip
    b. invoice
    c. purchase order
    d. DEA Form 222c

23. The pharmacy has a 10% strength and a 2% strength of a certain ointment. A patient turns in a prescription for 4 oz. of this ointment but in a 5% strength. Which of the following would be needed to compound the ointment for the patient?
    a. 45 g of 2% ointment and 75 g of 10%
    b. 120 g of 10% ointment
    c. 75 g of 2% ointment and 45 g of 10%
    d. 75 g of 10% ointment and 45 g of 2%

24. What is the correct temperature for storing an item in the refrigerator?
    a. 2° to 8°C
    b. less than 36°F
    c. 15° to 30°C
    d. 59° to 86°F

25. In an inpatient setting, the pharmacy must receive a direct copy of a physician's order before filling an initial dose. Which of the following is not considered a direct copy?
    a. fax
    b. photocopy
    c. computer-generated transfer
    d. telephone call acknowledging the verbal order

26. 125 mL of a Cipro 5% suspension contains how many grams of active ingredient?
    a. 0.625 g
    b. 6.25 g
    c. 62.5 g
    d. 60.25 g

27. Which of the following professional concepts most specifically refers to protection of the identity and health information of patients?
    a. motility
    b. confidentiality
    c. mortality
    d. compatibility

28. According to federal law, what is the maximum number of refills permitted for a Schedule III controlled substance?
    a. six refills within one year
    b. three refills within 90 days
    c. five refills within six months
    d. no refills are allowed

29. In the NDC number 69907-3110-01, what do the numbers 3110 identify?
    a. manufacturer
    b. drug product
    c. package size
    d. number of tablets in the bottle

30. The trade name for glipizide is:
    a. Diabinese.
    b. Micronase.
    c. Glucophage.
    d. Glucotrol.

31. What is the total volume of fluid needed if D5W is to run at 50 mL/hr for 24 hr?
    a. 1,200 mL
    b. 2,083 mL
    c. 480 mL
    d. 2,000 mL

32. Gentamicin injection is normally given to a patient at 5 mg/kg/day in three divided doses. If a patient weighs 164 lb, what approximate strength per dose should the patient receive?
    a. 25 mg
    b. 75 mg
    c. 124 mg
    d. 142 mg

33. Which of the following drugs is classed as an H_2 antagonist?
    a. clonidine
    b. ranitidine
    c. loratadine
    d. clemastine

34. KCl supplements are most often used in combination with:
    a. labetalol.
    b. lisinopril.
    c. naproxen.
    d. furosemide.

35. If a patient calls in for refills on Prinivil and Diabeta, which of the following combinations of medications must be filled for the patient?
    a. lisinopril and glipizide
    b. enalapril and glyburide
    c. enalapril and glipizide
    d. lisinopril and glyburide

36. How much neomycin powder must be added to fluocinolone cream to dispense an order for 60 g of fluocinolone cream with 0.5% neomycin?
    a. 120 mg
    b. 240 mg
    c. 300 mg
    d. 600 mg

37. Which of the SIG codes given refers to the following directions: Take two tablets by mouth every 4 to 6 hours as needed?
    a. 2 tabs q4–6h prn
    b. 2 tabs po q4–6h prn
    c. 2 tabs po q4–6h
    d. none of the above

38. The pharmacy receives an order for 10% ointment. Only the 15% and 5% strengths of the particular ointment are kept in stock. In what ratio would you have to mix the two stock ointments to correctly compound the prescription order?
    a. 1:1
    b. 1:2
    c. 2:1
    d. 1:3

39. Which of the following drugs is most likely to cause photosensitivity?
    a. nifedipine
    b. naproxen
    c. tetracycline
    d. glyburide

40. How many 250 mg doses of Claforan could be withdrawn from a 2 g vial of the injection?
    a. eight doses
    b. six doses
    c. four doses
    d. two doses

41. A medication that should be protected from exposure to light is:
    a. promethazine.
    b. tetracycline.
    c. erythromycin.
    d. nitroglycerin.

42. The blower on the laminar airflow workbench should remain on at all times. If it is turned off for any reason, it should remain on for at least _____ before being used to prepare IV admixtures and other products.
    a. 15 minutes
    b. 1 hour
    c. 30 minutes
    d. 45 minutes

43. Which of the following needle sizes has the largest bore?
    a. 23 gauge
    b. 18 gauge
    c. 27 gauge
    d. 29 gauge

44. When metronidazole is dispensed for a patient, which auxiliary label should be affixed to the dispensing container?
    a. No alcohol
    b. No dairy products
    c. Take with food or milk
    d. May cause drowsiness

45. If 500 mL of a 15% solution is diluted to 1,500 mL, how would you label the final strength of the solution?
    a. 20%
    b. 5%
    c. 0.05%
    d. 0.20%

46. A prescription reading "iii gtt. as tid prn pain" should have which set of directions printed on the dispensing label?

a. Instill 3 drops in the left eye three times daily as needed for pain.
b. Instill 3 drops in the left ear three times daily as needed for pain.
c. Instill 3 drops in the right ear two times daily as needed for pain.
d. Instill 3 drops in the right eye three times daily as needed for pain.

47. A patient with a penicillin allergy is most likely to exhibit a sensitivity to:
    a. tetracycline.
    b. erythromycin.
    c. cephalexin.
    d. gentamicin.

48. A Tylenol #3 tablet contains 30 mg of codeine. The amount of codeine is also equivalent to:
    a. $\frac{1}{4}$ gr.
    b. $\frac{1}{2}$ gr.
    c. 1 gr.
    d. 2 gr.

49. An IV infusion order is written for 1 L of D5W/0.45% NS to run over 12 hours. The set that will be used delivers 15 gtt/mL. What should the flow rate be in drops per minute?
    a. 7
    b. 21
    c. 25
    d. 8

50. To ensure that it is working properly, the laminar airflow workbench should be inspected by qualified personnel at least:
    a. every six months.
    b. every year.
    c. every three years.
    d. every five years.

51. Zovirax and Epivir are both classed as _____ agents.
    a. antimalarial
    b. tuberculosis
    c. antiviral
    d. antifungal

52. A physician writes an order for a patient to receive KCl 40 mEq/1 L NS. The fluid is to be infused at 80 mL/hr. What amount of KCl will the patient receive per hour?
    a. 6.8 mEq
    b. 3.2 mEq
    c. 2.3 mEq
    d. 8.6 mEq

53. Na is the chemical symbol for which of the following elements?
    a. nitrogen
    b. nickel
    c. copper
    d. sodium

54. When withdrawing medication from an ampule, what size filter needle will be sufficient to filter out any tiny glass fragments that may have fallen into the solution?
    a. 0.2 micron
    b. 0.5 micron
    c. 2 micron
    d. 5 micron

55. Which of the following conditions is the drug rifampin used to treat?
    a. influenza
    b. tuberculosis
    c. nail fungus
    d. urinary tract infection

56. When measuring liquid in a graduated cylinder, where is the volume of liquid read?
    a. top surface of the liquid
    b. top of the meniscus
    c. center of the meniscus
    d. bottom of the meniscus

57. How many grams of 2% silver nitrate ointment will deliver 1 g of the active ingredient?
    a. 25 g
    b. 4 g
    c. 50 g
    d. 20 g

58. The federal law enacted in 1970 that requires the use of child-resistant safety caps on all dispensing containers unless otherwise desired by the patient is known as the:
    a. Controlled Substances Act.
    b. Poison Prevention Act.
    c. Bueller-Ferris Act.
    d. Harrison Narcotic Act.

59. Into what size bottle will a prescription for 180 mL of cough syrup best fit?
    a. 2 oz.
    b. 4 oz.
    c. 6 oz.
    d. 8 oz.

60. If a patient should receive a medication at 15 mg/kg/day in three equally divided doses, what will the approximate dose be if the patient weighs 142 lb?
    a. 968 mg
    b. 323 mg
    c. 2,904 mg
    d. 284 mg

61. If one of your pharmacy's patients has had an adverse drug reaction, _____ should be used to report it.
    a. the HCFA form
    b. the MedWatch form
    c. DEA Form 222c
    d. the Universal Claim Form

62. Of the following choices, which pair of drugs are H_2 antagonists?
    a. Zantac and Prevacid
    b. Prinivil and Tagamet
    c. Pepcid and Zantac
    d. Vasotec and Motrin

63. A pharmacy wants to make a 30% profit on an item that costs $4.50. What would the retail selling price have to be for the pharmacy to make such a profit?
    a. $6.23
    b. $7.10
    c. $5.85
    d. $6.40

64. Which statement is true concerning the drug tetracycline?
    a. It should be given with food or milk for best absorption.
    b. For best absorption, it should not be given with milk products or antacids.
    c. It should be given with milk because it is upsetting to the stomach.
    d. Exposure to sunlight will not affect a patient taking this medication.

65. What schedule of controlled substances does the drug Darvocet N 100 fall under?
    a. II
    b. III
    c. IV
    d. V

66. When storing an item at room temperature, the temperature of the room should be:
    a. 2° to 8°C
    b. 36° to 46°F
    c. greater than 30°C
    d. 15° to 30°C

67. A list of medications that a physician may prescribe from within a given setting is called:
    a. an MSDS.
    b. a formulary.
    c. a closed panel of drugs.
    d. an open system.

68. Which of the following SIG codes refers to these directions? Take one tablespoonful after meals as needed for indigestion.
    a. 1 Tbsp pc for indigestion
    b. 1 Tbsp pc prn for indigestion
    c. 1 tsp ac prn for indigestion
    d. 1 tsp pc prn for indigestion

69. You are preparing an IV admixture when a vial slips from your hand and breaks on the floor. A spill kit should be used to clean the area if the vial contained which of the following medications?
    a. vinblastine
    b. adenosin
    c. amphotericin b
    d. methylprednisolone

70. Which of the following statements is true about cleaning of the laminar airflow workbench in preparation to make IV admixtures?
    a. The work surface should be cleaned first using a continuous side-to-side motion.
    b. 70% isopropyl alcohol should be sprayed onto the HEPA filter to ensure its cleanliness.
    c. The sides should be cleaned from top to bottom, working outward from the filter.
    d. none of the above

71. What volume of 5% aluminum acetate solution will be needed if 120 mL of 0.05% solution is extemporaneously compounded for patient use?
    a. 12 mL
    b. 1.2 mL
    c. 8.3 mL
    d. 0.83 mL

72. Ampicillin powder for injection should be reconstituted with and diluted in _____ for best stability.
    a. D5W
    b. normal saline
    c. lactated Ringer's
    d. none of the above

73. How many 1 L bags will be needed if D5W is to run at 60 mL/hr for 16 hr?
    a. one bag
    b. two bags
    c. three bags
    d. four or more bags

74. Which of the following drugs is classified as an antidiarrheal medication?
    a. labetalol
    b. loperamide
    c. cimetidine
    d. naproxen

75. A pharmacy has 20 mL of a 1:200 solution in stock. If the pharmacist has asked the technician to dilute the solution to 500 mL, how should the final strength of the solution be labeled?
    a. 2%
    b. 2.5%
    c. 25%
    d. 0.02%

76. When an antibiotic injection is given in a small volume of solution that is connected to the main line of IV fluids the patient receives, it is commonly known as getting an:
    a. IV bag.
    b. IV injection.
    c. IV piggyback.
    d. IV push.

77. Of the drugs listed, which one could not be phoned in or filled with refills added?
    a. hydrocodone
    b. acetaminophen
    c. codeine
    d. gabapentin

78. The largest gelatin capsule used for extemporaneous compounding is:
    a. 000.
    b. 0.
    c. 10.
    d. 5.

79. All manipulations in the laminar airflow workbench should take place at least _____ within the hood.
    a. 4 in.
    b. 6 in.
    c. 8 in.
    d. 10 in.

80. Which of the following drugs is classified as a calcium channel blocker?
    a. amlodipine
    b. atenolol
    c. enalapril
    d. nitroglycerin

81. Some pharmacies operate with a manual inventory system. When using this type of system, items that must be ordered are written down. This familiar list of items to be ordered is often referred to as:
    a. a purchase order.
    b. an invoice.
    c. a want book.
    d. an MAR.

82. Which of the following DEA numbers would not be valid for Dr. Ann Cosgrove?
    a. AC6782329
    b. AC3081421
    c. AC1355672
    d. BC3421234

83. A drug subject to a _____ recall would not likely cause harm to the patient, since this recall class is the least severe.
    a. Class I
    b. Class II
    c. Class III
    d. none of the above, because any drug on recall will cause the patient harm

84. The form used for ordering Schedule II narcotics is known as:
    a. DEA Form 240.
    b. DEA Form 222c.
    c. DEA Form 121.
    d. DEA Form 200.

85. What class of drugs is used to regulate the level of fluid in the body?
    a. sedative
    b. anti-inflammatory
    c. antipyretic
    d. diuretic

86. The Orange Book is most often used to find:
    a. generic equivalents.
    b. direct prices.
    c. therapeutic equivalents.
    d. manufacturer's standards.

87. How many times a year should an ideal pharmacy's inventory be turned?
    a. 10–12
    b. 12–14
    c. 10–14
    d. 14–16

88. Which of the following pairs of medications could cause a major drug-drug interaction if taken together by a patient?
    a. hydrocodone and naproxen
    b. warfarin and aspirin
    c. penicillin and trimethoprim
    d. glyburide and metformin

89. A patient takes NPH insulin according to the following dosage regimen: 35 units sq every morning and 15 units every evening. How many vials of insulin will the patient need to last for at least 30 days?
    a. one vial
    b. two vials

90. c. three vials
    d. four or more vials

90. Which of the following medications should always be dispensed in a glass container?
    a. aminophylline
    b. dopamine
    c. potassium
    d. nitroglycerin

91. How many teaspoons are in one tablespoon?
    a. 2
    b. 3
    c. 4
    d. 5

92. When using a torsion prescription balance, the first thing you should do after placing it on a level surface is:
    a. place the weights in the left pan and the substance to be weighed in the right pan.
    b. place the weights in the right pan and the substance to be weighed in the left pan.
    c. place the substance to be weighed onto the scale.
    d. unlock the balance and level it to zero.

93. An air vent on a vented administration set should be a _____ micron filter vent to be considered a sterilizing filter.
    a. 0.2
    b. 0.5
    c. 5
    d. none of the above

94. How many tablets will a patient need if she is to take 1 tablet po bid for 10 days?
    a. 10
    b. 20
    c. 30
    d. 40

95. Of the following tasks involved in pharmacy practice, which is a pharmacy technician allowed by law to perform?
    a. giving or receiving a verbal copy
    b. counseling a patient on the use of a medication
    c. receiving a verbal order from a physician
    d. filling a unit-dose cart

96. What organization requires that oral products be stored separate from inhaled products, topical preparations be separated from injectables, and so on?
    a. ASHP
    b. PTCB
    c. APHA
    d. JCAHO

97. An automatic stop order is most likely to be issued with which of the following meds?
    a. clonidine 0.3 mg tablets
    b. acetaminophen/codeine 325 mg/60 mg tablets
    c. amlodipine 5 mg tablets
    d. furosemide 40 mg tablets

98. Which of the following is equal to $\frac{1}{2}$ pound?
    a. 454 g
    b. 1 lb
    c. 16 oz.
    d. 240 g

99. Amphotericin B should be mixed only in _____ for compatibility.
    a. 0.9% sodium chloride
    b. lactated Ringer's
    c. 0.45% sodium chloride
    d. dextrose

100. There are several different types of automated dispensing systems. Which of the following is not an automated dispensing system?
    a. Kirby-Lester
    b. Omnicell
    c. Pyxis
    d. Baker

Practice Certification Exam II

This practice test has been designed to simulate the certification exam in both the number and style of questions, as well as the content. You should complete this exam within two hours.

1. The device used to compound three-in-one total parenteral nutrition solutions is the:
    a. Readymix.
    b. Automix.
    c. Pyxis.
    d. Baker.

2. A solid dosage form containing drug substances with or without suitable diluents and prepared either by compression or molding methods is a:
    a. capsule.
    b. tablet.
    c. emulsion.
    d. paste.

3. A semisolid preparation for external application of such consistency that it may be readily applied to the skin is:
    a. a pill.
    b. a solute.
    c. an emulsifying agent.
    d. an ointment.

4. A method used to identify an employee's individual strengths and weaknesses and provide the employer with information relative to the employee's capacity for retention and promotion is the:
    a. personnel checklist.
    b. planogram.
    c. employee performance appraisal.
    d. employee handbook.

5. The _____ is used to record what the pharmacy owes its suppliers and other creditors.
    a. accounts payable ledger
    b. accounts receivable ledger
    c. purchases journal
    d. cash receipts journal

6. The failure of one or more drugs to be mixed in the same solution because of a physical or chemical interaction is:
    a. precipitation.
    b. incompatibility.
    c. intolerance.
    d. injunction.

7. A preparation of finely divided, undissolved drugs dispersed in a liquid vehicle is:
    a. an elixir.
    b. a solution.
    c. a syrup.
    d. a suspension.

8. A _____ is a system in which the item is deducted from inventory as it is sold or dispensed.
    a. turnover
    b. scantron
    c. Baker cell
    d. POS system

9. An inert substance added to the active drug ingredient to increase the bulk and make the tablet a practical size for compression is:
    a. a diluent.
    b. a binder.
    c. a facilitator.
    d. an emulsifying agent.

10. Effective communication in pharmacy practice can be hindered by:
    a. visual impairment.
    b. auditory loss.
    c. speech impairment.
    d. all of the above.

11. OBRA 90 is an acronym for the:
    a. Omnibus Budget Recommendation Act of 1990.
    b. Omnibus Budget Reconciliation Act of 1990.
    c. Omni Bus Reconciliation Act of 1990.
    d. Omni Bus Recognition Act of 1990.

12. A substance or a mixture of substances added to a tablet to facilitate its breakup or disintegration after administration is a:
    a. terminator.
    b. disintegrator.
    c. binder.
    d. diluent.

13. A solid dosage form in which the drug substance is enclosed in either a hard or soft soluble container or a shell of a suitable form of gelatin is a:
    a. capsule.
    b. pill.
    c. tablet.
    d. suppository.

14. Softening of the cornea due to vitamin A deficiency is known as:
    a. conjunctivitis.
    b. glaucoma.
    c. pellagra.
    d. keratomalacia.

15. The only drug approved to treat high blood pressure during pregnancy is:
    a. lidocaine.
    b. clonidine.
    c. metoprolol.
    d. methyldopa.

16. The only antihypertensive drug available as a transdermal delivery system is:
    a. nicotine.
    b. clonidine.
    c. nitroglycerin.
    d. lidocaine.

17. From the following formula, calculate the amount in grams of cetyl ester wax needed to make 1 lb of cold cream.

cetyl ester wax	12.5 parts
white wax	12.0 parts
mineral oil	56.0 parts
sodium borate	0.5 parts
water	19.0 parts

    a. 56.75 g
    b. 12.5 g
    c. 60 g
    d. 0.125 g

18. The drug of choice for emergency IV therapy for arrhythmias is:
    a. lidocaine.
    b. sodium bicarbonate.
    c. dopamine.
    d. adrenalin.

19. The most important drug in managing atrial flutter and fibrillation is:
    a. digitalis.
    b. amlodipine.
    c. doxazosin.
    d. quinine.

20. The antagonist to warfarin is:
    a. heparin.
    b. phytonadione.
    c. methyldopa.
    d. penicillin VK.

21. The _____ provides guidelines for the recall of devices that could cause serious adverse effects.
    a. Safe Medical Devices Act
    b. Kefauver-Harris Amendment
    c. Durham-Humphrey Amendment
    d. Medical Device Amendment

22. The functional parts of the heart include all of the following except the:
    a. blood supply.
    b. cardiac muscle.
    c. peripheral vessels.
    d. conducting system.

23. An imbalance between oxygen supply and oxygen demand in cardiac muscle may produce a condition known as:
    a. congestive heart failure.
    b. heartburn.
    c. myocardial infarction.
    d. angina pectoris.

24. From the following formula, calculate in kilograms the quantity of miconazole needed to prepare 12 kg of powder.

zinc oxide	1 part
calamine	2 parts
miconazole	1.5 parts
bismuth subgalate	3 parts
talc	8 parts

    a. 15.5 kg
    b. 0.097 kg
    c. 1.16 kg
    d. 1.5 kg

25. Frequently patients on thiazide diuretics are told to take supplements of or eat foods high in which element?
    a. calcium
    b. sodium
    c. chlorine
    d. potassium

26. Renal tubules produce urine through all of the following except:
    a. adsorption.
    b. filtration.
    c. reabsorption.
    d. secretion.

27. The structural and functional unit of the kidney is the:
    a. loop of Henle.
    b. glomerulus.
    c. nephron.
    d. cortex.

28. _____ is an antihistamine nasal spray.
    a. Nasacort
    b. Nasonex
    c. Astelin
    d. Afrin

29. _____ anesthetizes the stretch receptors in the airway, lungs, and pleura but does not affect the respiratory center.
    a. Benzonatate
    b. Guaifenesin
    c. Codeine
    d. Dextromethorphan

30. A cycle of inflammation of the nasal mucosa caused by repeated application of nasal decongestants is called:
    a. allergic rhinitis.
    b. rhinorrhea.
    c. rhinitis medicomentosa.
    d. nasal congestion.

31. In pharmacies, how may controlled substances be stored?
    a. Controlled substances may be stored in an unlocked cabinet.
    b. Controlled substances may be stored in a securely locked, substantially constructed cabinet.
    c. Controlled substances (Schedule III through V) may be stored on the pharmacy shelves among noncontrolled substances in a manner designed to deter theft.
    d. both b and c

32. _____ is a drug agent extracted from cattle lung.
    a. Proventil HFA
    b. Survanta
    c. Bonine
    d. Serevent

33. Patients taking _____ should always be warned to avoid any consumption of alcohol.
    a. metronidazole
    b. tetracycline
    c. albuterol
    d. prednisone

34. The _____ was a direct result of the thalidomide disaster and made manufacturers more accountable for their products.
    a. Comprehensive Drug Abuse Prevention and Control Act
    b. Medical Device Amendment
    c. Durham-Humphrey Amendment
    d. Kefauver-Harris Amendment

35. Patients should be advised not to drink milk or eat dairy products while taking:
    a. calcium carbonate.
    b. tetracycline.
    c. penicillin.
    d. calciferol.

36. Patients should be advised to drink plenty of water and to avoid the sun while taking:
    a. TMP-SMZ.
    b. cephalexin.
    c. propranolol.
    d. warfarin.

37. _____ are a class of pharmaceutical agents that kill or inhibit the growth of infection-causing microorganisms.
    a. Anesthetics
    b. Antilipidemics
    c. Antibiotics
    d. Antihistamines

38. A hospital-acquired infection is known as:
    a. a nosocomial infection.
    b. an institutional infection.
    c. an HA infection.
    d. a viral infection.

39. _____ means "capable of killing bacteria."
    a. Bacteriostatic
    b. Antiviral
    c. Antifungal
    d. Bactericidal

40. The agency that oversees the Controlled Substances Act is the:
    a. Central Intelligence Agency.
    b. armed forces.
    c. Food and Drug Administration.
    d. Drug Enforcement Agency.

41. _____ means "capable of inhibiting growth or multiplication of bacteria."
    a. Bacteriostatic
    b. Anti-inflammatory
    c. Antifungal
    d. Bactericidal

42. All of the following are true statements except:
    a. All controlled substances must be inventoried on the day the pharmacy first dispenses controlled substances.
    b. The inventory of Schedule II medications requires an exact count or measure, whereas other schedules may be estimated.
    c. Prescriptions are the primary records of acquisition by a pharmacy.
    d. The beginning inventory plus all acquisitions minus dispensing by prescriptions or to other practitioners should equal the current inventory count.

43. A _____ drug is active against both gram-positive and gram-negative bacteria.
    a. neg-gram
    b. bacteriostatic
    c. broad-spectrum
    d. narrow-spectrum

44. A patient weighs 165 lb. How many kilograms does the patient weigh?
    a. 165,000 kg
    b. 75 kg
    c. 363 kg
    d. 330 kg

45. _____ is a testing process to identify bacteria and to determine which drugs may effectively combat the infection.
    a. Culture and sensitivity
    b. Cross-sensitivity
    c. Cultivation
    d. A bacto-test

46. The types of ulcers include all of the following except:
    a. stress.
    b. gastric.
    c. duodenal.
    d. colon.

47. The _____ gave tax incentives to manufacturers to encourage them to develop medications for rare diseases or conditions.
    a. Orphan Drug Act
    b. Medical Device Amendment
    c. Kefauver-Harris Amendment
    d. Durham-Humphrey Amendment

48. _____ is a condition caused by increased collection of uric acid crystals in joints and soft tissue.
    a. Osteoarthritis
    b. Rheumatoid arthritis
    c. Reye's syndrome
    d. Gouty arthritis

49. Another term used to describe insulin-dependent diabetes is:
    a. non-insulin-dependent diabetes.
    b. type I diabetes.
    c. type II diabetes.
    d. diabetes insipidus.

50. Oral contraceptives interact with:
    a. antibiotics.
    b. anticonvulsants.
    c. antifungals.
    d. all of the above.

51. The _____ deals with the safety and effectiveness of life-sustaining or life-supporting devices.
    a. Prescription Drug Marketing Act
    b. Medical Device Amendment
    c. Durham-Humphrey Amendment
    d. Kefauver-Harris Amendment

52. The maximum allowable cost that an insurer will pay per tablet or dispensing unit for a given product is the:
    a. co-payment.
    b. deductible.
    c. U&C.
    d. MAC.

53. Estrogen is contraindicated with:
    a. migraines.
    b. smokers.
    c. thrombosis history.
    d. all of the above.

54. A substance with a high potential for abuse that has no currently accepted medical use in the United States and for which there is a lack of accepted safety-for-use data would be classified as:
    a. C-I.
    b. C-II.
    c. C-III.
    d. C-IV.

55. The thyroid hormones T_3 and T_4 are both stored as:
    a. serotonin.
    b. thyroglobulin.
    c. acetylcholine.
    d. norepinephrine.

56. The feedback mechanism that controls the thyroid is the:
    a. adrenocorticotropic hormone autoregulator.
    b. hypothalamic-pituitary axis.
    c. homeostasis.
    d. hirsutism.

57. The _____ requires that most prescription drugs be dispensed in childproof containers.
    a. Poison Prevention Act
    b. Safe Medical Devices Act
    c. Prescription Drug Marketing Act
    d. Medical Device Amendment

58. _____ should be taken with 8 oz. of water before the first food of the day, and the patient must avoid lying down for at least 30 minutes after taking it.
    a. Miacalcin
    b. Didronel
    c. Fosamax
    d. Hydrocortisone

59. Glial cells surrounding the capillaries in the CNS that present a barrier to many water-soluble components are referred to as:
    a. central glial cells.
    b. the blood-brain barrier.
    c. the glial barrier.
    d. the aqua barrier.

60. The _____ placed all hormones that promote muscle growth or are similar to testosterone under the Controlled Substances Act.
    a. Comprehensive Drug Abuse Prevention and Control Act
    b. Medical Device Amendment
    c. Anabolic Steroid Control Act
    d. Poison Prevention Act

61. _____ is a chemical mediator that produces intense uterine contraction, reduces blood pressure, increases heart rate and cardiac output, and inhibits gastrointestinal secretions.
    a. Epinephrine
    b. Serotonin
    c. Dopamine
    d. Prostaglandin

62. Joint action of drugs in which their combined effect is more intense or longer in duration than the sum of their individual effects is known as:
    a. opportunistic action.
    b. pharmakon.
    c. synergism.
    d. contraindication.

63. The _____ prohibits the sale of drug samples and reimportation of prescriptions and establishes fair pricing guidelines.
    a. Orphan Drug Act
    b. Prescription Drug Marketing Act
    c. Durham-Humphrey Amendment
    d. Kefauver-Harris Amendment

64. A decrease in susceptibility to a drug's effects from continued use is known as:
    a. addition.
    b. synergism.
    c. sensitivity.
    d. tolerance.

65. Which of the following DEA numbers is valid?
    a. Dr. Russ AR123456879
    b. Dr. Black AB56897
    c. Dr. Jones AJ1234563
    d. Dr. Smith CS2468217

66. The traditional agent of choice to counter accidental poisonings in the home that is commonly sold in pharmacies is:
    a. activated charcoal.
    b. demulcents.
    c. syrup of ipecac.
    d. diphenhydramine elixir.

67. _____ is a microorganism used in the production of Novo Nordisk's Novolin.
    a. Baker's yeast
    b. *Escherichia coli*
    c. Salmonella
    d. Pseudomonas

68. The rate at which inventory is used is called:
    a. sales journal.
    b. sales volume.
    c. turnover.
    d. net profit.

69. Low blood glucose is known as:
    a. glucosuria.
    b. hypoglycemia.
    c. polyuria.
    d. hyperglycemia.

70. Certain controlled substances do not bear the federal caution legend and may be sold without a prescription. These products have small quantities of controlled substances included in them and may be sold if certain requirements are met and the proper records kept. The restrictions on such sales include the following except:
    a. The sale must be made by the pharmacist or a certified pharmacy technician.

b. The purchaser must be at least 18 and must either be known to the pharmacist or have substantial identification.

c. Not more than 8 oz. or more than 48 dosage units of any substance containing opium may be furnished to the purchaser in any 48-hour period. Not more than 4 oz. or 24 dosage units of any other controlled substance may be sold in any 48-hour period.

d. Pharmacists must maintain a record in a bound book regarding the sale.

71. Sources of insulin include all of the following except:
    a. cow.
    b. horse.
    c. pig.
    d. human.

72. The human skin comprises approximately what percentage of the body weight of the average adult?
    a. 10
    b. 12.5
    c. 15
    d. 20

73. The _____ was directed toward recipients of Medicare and Medicaid. Pharmacists must offer consultation under this regulation.
    a. Durham-Humphrey Amendment
    b. Omnibus Budget Reconciliation Act
    c. Prescription Drug Marketing Act
    d. Orphan Drug Act

74. Chemicals that, in a certain concentration, redden the skin to produce a feeling of warmth but do not cause inflammation are referred to as:
    a. crepitus.
    b. thermotherapy.
    c. cryotherapy.
    d. rubefacients.

75. The National Drug Code number provides specific information about the product. Which of the following statements is true?
    a. The NDC contains ten digits.
    b. NDC numbers indicate the date the product was produced.
    c. NDC numbers are divided into two sections, with the first section indicating the manufacturer and the second section indicating the specific product.
    d. NDC numbers are divided into three sections, with the first five digits indicating the manufacturer; the next four digits indicating the product name, strength, and dosage form; and the last two digits indicating the package size.

76. A rare, acute, life-threatening condition that occurs primarily in children or teenagers in the course of or while recovering from a mild respiratory tract infection, flu, chickenpox, or other viral illness and sometimes linked to salicylate use is:
    a. Reye's syndrome.
    b. Legionnaire's disease.
    c. viral meningitis.
    d. herpes simplex.

77. A device that produces a nonheated mist to increase humidity is a:
    a. humidifier.
    b. peak flow meter.
    c. vaporizer.
    d. HEPA filter.

78. The _____ is a document that contains the goals, policies, and procedures relevant to the employee and the job the employee is performing or assuming.
    a. employee handbook
    b. corporate prospectus
    c. planogram
    d. administration handbook

79. The _____ is used to record the balances that private patients, government agencies, insurance companies, managed-care contractors, and insurers owe the pharmacy.
    a. balance sheet
    b. accounts receivable ledger
    c. cash disbursements journal
    d. sales journal

80. Control of the amount, type, and quality of health care provided to patients within a benefit program is referred to as:
    a. health insurance.
    b. managed care.
    c. benefit plans.
    d. pharmaceutical care.

81. Three systems of measurement are used in pharmacy. Which of the following is correct?
    a. metric system
       weight
       volume
       length
       apothecary system
       weight
       volume
       avoirdupois system
       weight

b. metric system
weight
volume
length
apothecary system
volume
avoirdupois system
weight

c. metric system
weight
volume
length
apothecary system
weight
volume
avoirdupois system
volume

d. metric system
weight
volume
length
height
apothecary system
weight
volume
avoirdupois system
weight

82. The principle stating that patients have the right to full disclosure of all relevant aspects of care and must give explicit consent to treatment before treatment is initiated is:
a. confidentiality.
b. fidelity.
c. informed consent.
d. moral reasoning.

83. The provision of drug therapy intended to achieve outcomes that improve the patient's quality of life as it is related to the cure or prevention of a disease, elimination or reduction of a patient's symptoms, or arresting or slowing of a disease process is:
a. pharmaceutical care.
b. managed care.
c. socialized medicine.
d. practice of pharmacy.

84. The FDA recall of a product that will cause serious or fatal consequences is classified as:
a. Class I.
b. Class II.
c. Class III.
d. Class IV.

85. Devices:
a. do not have any restrictions.
b. are defined as instruments, apparatuses, implements, machines, etc.
c. may be restricted to sale only on the written or oral order of a practitioner licensed to administer such a device.
d. both b and c.

86. _____ is a company that buys from the manufacturer and sells to hospitals, pharmacies, and other pharmaceutical dispensers.
a. The Food and Drug Administration
b. A wholesaler
c. A retailer
d. A mass merchandiser

87. Drugs that are not intended to be sold, but are intended to promote the sale of the drug, are known as:
a. legend drugs.
b. sample drugs.
c. investigational drugs.
d. over-the-counter drugs.

88. The _____ created the legend class of drugs.
a. Comprehensive Drug Abuse Prevention and Control Act
b. Medical Device Amendment
c. Durham-Humphrey Amendment
d. Kefauver-Harris Amendment

89. Mixing ingredients to provide a prescription for a specific patient or small group of patients is known as:
a. manufacturing.
b. compressing.
c. compounding.
d. adjudication.

90. A prescription is written for one pound of 3% salicylic acid in white petrolatum. How many milligrams of salicylic acid are needed?
a. 13,620 mg
b. 13.62 mg
c. 1,362 mg
d. 48 mg

91. The portion of the cost of prescriptions that patients with third-party insurance must pay is the:
a. co-payment.
b. deductible.
c. U&C.
d. MAC.

92. All of the following define the term *drugs* except:
    a. articles intended for use in the diagnosis, cure, mitigation, treatment, or prevention of disease in humans or other animals.
    b. articles recognized in the USP, the NF, and the Homeopathic Pharmacopoeia of the United States.
    c. devices that are used for life-sustaining or life-supporting functions.
    d. articles (other than food) intended to affect the structure or any function of the body.

93. All of the following methods for filing prescriptions are allowed except:
    a. a system using three prescription file drawers:
       prescriptions for C-II substances
       prescriptions for C-III, C-IV, and C-V substances
       all other prescriptions
    b. a system using two prescription file drawers:
       prescriptions for Schedule II–V substances, provided all C-III to C-V substances have a letter C no less than one inch high stamped in red ink on the lower right corner
       all other prescriptions
    c. a system using five prescription file drawers:
       Schedule II prescriptions only
       Schedule III prescriptions only
       Schedule IV prescriptions only
       Schedule V prescriptions only
       all other prescriptions
    d. a system using two prescription file drawers:
       Schedule II prescriptions only
       all other prescriptions, including C-III to C-V substances, provided the controlled prescriptions bear the red letter C as described above

94. Each of the following are characteristics desired in an intravenous solution except:
    a. pH of 6.
    b. sterility.
    c. clarity.
    d. isotonicity.

95. A prescription calls for a sliding-scale dosage of prednisone. How many 5 mg tablets would it take to fill the following?

    _____
    20 mg d × 2 d
    15 mg d × 2 d
    5 mg bid × 2 d
    2.5 mg bid × 2 d
    2.5 mg d × 2 d
    _____

    a. 20 tabs
    b. 21 tabs

    c. 22 tabs
    d. 15 tabs

96. Calculate the flow rate for an IV of 1,000 mL to run over 8 hr with a set calibrated at 20 gtt/mL.
    a. 41.6 gtt/min
    b. 17.36 gtt/min
    c. 125.1 gtt/min
    d. 50 gtt/min

97. A pharmacist may "manufacture," without registering as a manufacturer, an aqueous or oleaginous solution or solid dosage form containing a narcotic-controlled substance not exceeding _____ of the complete solution or mixture.
    a. 25%
    b. 20%
    c. 30%
    d. 50%

98. The _____ is a set amount that must be paid by the patient for each benefit period before the insurer will cover additional expenses.
    a. co-payment
    b. deductible
    c. garnishment
    d. MAC

99. An IV of 150 cc is to infuse at a rate of 80 mL/hr. What is the infusion time?
    a. 10 hr
    b. 1.8 hr
    c. 6.6 hr
    d. 47 min

100. The _____ is a device designed to reduce the risk of airborne contamination during the preparation of an IV admixture by providing an ultraclean environment.
    a. laminar airflow hood
    b. HEPA filter
    c. autoclave
    d. automix

Practice Certification Exam III

This practice test has been designed to simulate the certification exam in both the number and style of questions, as well as the content. You should complete this exam within two hours.

1. Which route of medication administration is used to inject drugs into the top skin layers?
    a. subcutaneous
    b. hypodermic
    c. intradermal
    d. intra-arterial

2. A connection between two or more computer systems that allows the transfer of data is:
   a. an interface.
   b. a terminal.
   c. a bar code.
   d. a window.

3. Certification is:
   a. the process of granting recognition or vouching for conformance with a standard.
   b. the process by which a nongovernmental agency or association grants recognition to an individual who has met certain predetermined qualifications specified by that agency or association.
   c. the general process of formally recognizing professional or technical competence.
   d. the process of making a list or being enrolled on an existing list.

4. An ongoing systematic process for monitoring, evaluating, and improving the quality of pharmacy services is:
   a. peer review.
   b. quality assurance.
   c. process validation.
   d. none of the above.

5. Sterile products should be prepared at least _____ in. inside the laminar airflow hood.
   a. 6
   b. 10
   c. 2
   d. 3

6. The main concern of pharmacy practice today is:
   a. provision of optimal drug therapy for all patients.
   b. preparation and compounding of medications for patients.
   c. bulk preparation and distribution of drug products.
   d. safe ordering, procurement, and storage of medications.

7. A policies and procedures manual may provide guidance in each of the following areas except:
   a. personnel orientation, training, and evaluation.
   b. correct aseptic (sterile) technique.
   c. activities of technicians outside the workplace.
   d. position or job descriptions.

8. All of the following are requirements for a prescription label except:
   a. name and address of the pharmacy.
   b. name of the prescriber.
   c. serial number of the prescription.
   d. telephone number of the patient.

9. A prescription can usually be refilled:
   a. only once.
   b. as many times as the pharmacist deems necessary.
   c. as many times as the prescriber indicates on the prescription within a specified time period.
   d. only at the location where it was originally filled.

10. Which of the following best describes controlled substances in Schedule I?
    a. drugs with no accepted medical use in the United States
    b. drugs with a low to moderate potential for physical dependence
    c. drugs with no potential for abuse
    d. drugs that are available without a prescription

11. A 500 mL quantity of D10W contains how many grams of dextrose?
    a. 100 g
    b. 10 g
    c. 50 g
    d. 20 g

12. What is the seventh digit of the following DEA number: AB369145_?
    a. 3
    b. 8
    c. 4
    d. 0

13. The Poison Prevention Packaging Act of 1970 mandated all of the following except:
    a. prescription drugs may be exempt if the prescriber or consumer requests noncompliant packaging.
    b. household cleaners must be packaged in childproof containers.
    c. a limited number of prescription drugs are exempt (such as sublingual nitroglycerin).
    d. the special packaging requirements are extended to nonprescription drugs.

14. Sublingual tablets are:
    a. placed under the tongue.
    b. dissolved in a liquid and release bubbles.
    c. placed inside the cheek.
    d. chewed before swallowing.

15. Which of the following terms refers to the acidic or basic nature of a solution?
    a. osmolarity
    b. osmolality
    c. isotonicity
    d. pH

16. The Omnibus Budget Reconciliation Act of 1990 (OBRA 90) requires pharmacists to perform the

following functions for patients receiving Medicaid:

a. drug therapy review.

b. counseling.

c. financial consultation.

d. both a and b.

17. A patient presents a prescription for hydrochlorothiazide (HCTZ). Other items related to his prescription that he might purchase include all of the following except:

a. home blood pressure monitoring device.

b. potassium-containing salt substitute.

c. pseudoephedrine-containing decongestant.

d. sunscreen.

18. Which statement concerning Synthroid is correct?

a. The generic name is levothyroxine.

b. The usual dose is 50–100 g/day.

c. It is usually given three times a day.

d. It is used to treat diabetes.

19. Nonprescription drugs are also known as:

a. legend drugs.

b. new drugs.

c. over-the-counter drugs.

d. investigational drugs.

20. All of the following are true concerning patient participation in an investigational drug study except:

a. the patient must sign an informed consent.

b. participation is voluntary.

c. the patient may withdraw from the study at any time.

d. the patient must be paid.

21. You receive a prescription for Ceclor suspension 125 mg/5 mL, 1.5 tsp tid × 10 days. The appropriate quantity to dispense would be:

a. 125 mL

b. 150 mL with one refill

c. 200 mL

d. 225 mL

22. When filling a prescription for Tylenol with Codeine 30 mg, a technician should do all the following except:

a. file the prescription as a Schedule III controlled substance.

b. affix an auxiliary label cautioning against performing tasks requiring alertness or driving.

c. verify that the patient is not allergic to Tylenol or codeine.

d. inform the patient that this medication is a potent anti-inflammatory agent.

23. When a prescription is received for Cortisporin drops, use as directed, the technician should:

a. have the pharmacist ascertain whether an ophthalmic or otic product is to be dispensed.

b. tell the patient to take the prescription back to the physician to be corrected.

c. affix a "For the eye" auxiliary label.

d. wash hands before dispensing so the drops will remain sterile.

24. Which of the following drug pairs is most likely to be associated with a medication error?

a. digoxin and captopril

b. prednisone and dexamethasone

c. quinidine and quinine

d. fluoxetine and fluorouracil

25. For a hospital inpatient order for ceftriaxone 1 g qd IV piggyback, the technician should do all the following except:

a. prepare the dose in the laminar airflow hood using sterile technique.

b. inform the pharmacist if the patient has a penicillin allergy recorded.

c. convert the dosage from grams to grains so the nurse will know how much to give.

d. confirm that she has the right drug—many other drugs sound similar (ceftaxime, ceftizoxime).

26. Which of the following terms may be used to describe a prepackaged unit?

a. unit dose

b. closed system

c. blister pack

d. both a and c

27. All of the following are true about cimetidine except:

a. An over-the-counter preparation is available.

b. It reduces the acidity of the stomach.

c. Using samples of this product is a good way to save money in the hospital.

d. It interacts with many other drugs.

28. The computer insurance error message "patient not found" or "invalid ID number" indicates that:

a. the customer is not a legitimate patient.

b. the patient does not appear to be enrolled in the insurance program; check for errors such as misspelling of the patient's name.

c. the patient does not have any condition that requires treatment.

d. the patient cannot find his prescription.

29. As a technician, you are asked to prepare an IV solution with insulin. Which of the following statements is true?

    a. You should use only regular insulin. The other insulins cannot be given IV.

    b. You do not need to bother making the IV in the laminar airflow hood, because insulin is an antibiotic.

    c. Because the dose is in units, you cannot measure the volume in milliliters.

    d. You must sign out the dose on the narcotic log.

30. The portion of prescription costs that the patient must pay in a given time period before a third-party insurer will begin paying is the:

    a. fee-for-service.

    b. co-payment.

    c. deductible.

    d. none of the above.

31. If a pediatric patient is to receive oral ampicillin as a suspension, which of the following is not necessary?

    a. Ensure that the patient's allergies are recorded in the computer.

    b. Affix an expiration date to the label after preparing the suspension.

    c. Affix an auxiliary label stating "Shake well before using."

    d. Prepare the medication in the laminar airflow hood.

32. A resource that may be used to determine if a parenteral medication must be filtered is:

    a. the packaging insert.

    b. the *Handbook on Injectable Drugs*.

    c. the manufacturer.

    d. all of the above.

33. The offer to counsel under OBRA 90 may be made:

    a. in writing.

    b. orally.

    c. by a technician.

    d. all of the above.

34. When filling an inpatient's medication drawer, the technician notices that the fill list contains both enalapril and lisinopril. The technician should:

    a. fill only one drug; they are both the same kind of drug.

    b. notify the pharmacist that the patient has orders for two drugs of the same class.

    c. call the doctor to see which drug to use.

    d. tell the nurse that there is a dangerous drug interaction between these drugs.

35. If you believe that someone has presented a fraudulent prescription at your pharmacy, the appropriate action would be to:

    a. call 911 immediately.

    b. call the physician whose name appears on the prescription.

    c. discreetly notify the pharmacist so that the appropriate action may be taken.

    d. ask the customer how he got the prescription.

36. You receive an order for etoposide. In preparing this drug, you should:

    a. wear gloves only if you are allergic to etoposide.

    b. flush the extra contents of the vial down the sink drain.

    c. prepare it in a biological safety cabinet (BSC).

    d. not add any extra labels—they are too confusing to the nurse.

37. While a mother is waiting for an antibiotic preparation for her 6-year-old, she asks the technician what to give the child for fever. The technician should:

    a. suggest aspirin; it is the least expensive antipyretic.

    b. inform the pharmacist that the mother would like help choosing a nonprescription product.

    c. offer to sell the mother some drug samples.

    d. suggest over-the-counter diphenhydramine.

38. You receive the following prescription: Vanceril (beclomethasone) inhaler; dispense #1; Sig: ii puffs inhaled bid. In filling the prescription, you should:

    a. inform the patient that this drug is a corticosteroid that has many serious side effects.

    b. include the following specific directions on the label: "Inhale 2 puffs into each nostril three times a day."

    c. provide the patient with the "For the patient" instructions included with the inhaler.

    d. tell the patient to use this inhaler only when she really needs it.

39. When accepting a prescription for warfarin from a patient, the technician should:

    a. notify the pharmacist if the patient is also buying aspirin; there is an interaction between these medications.

    b. give the lower dose just to be safe if the strength is unclear (10 mg versus 1.0 mg).

    c. tell the patient to take an iron supplement because this drug thins the blood.

    d. tell the patient to eat foods high in vitamin K.

40. When selling an over-the-counter nasal decongestant spray (phenylephrine), which question can the

technician answer without referring the customer to the pharmacist?

a. Can I take this drug with my blood pressure medicine?

b. I keep using this spray, but my nose seems to get stuffier. Should I use it more often?

c. Is a less expensive generic of this nose spray available?

d. I've had this cold for four weeks. Do you think I should see the doctor?

41. The pharmacist asks you to prepare the following prescription: Amoxicillin suspension 5 mL pl tid × 10 days. You notice that the prescriber did not indicate the concentration of the suspension on the prescription. You should:

a. dispense the capsules instead.

b. alert the pharmacist to the problem.

c. ask the patient which concentration he prefers.

d. prepare the prescription with a 250 mg/mL concentration, because it is most frequently ordered.

42. Which of the following could contribute to a medication error?

a. failure to rotate stock appropriately

b. preparing one prescription at a time

c. reading the drug product label carefully

d. none of the above

43. The risk of a decimal point error is reduced by writing "seven milligrams" as:

a. 0.7 g

b. 7 mg

c. 7.0 mg

d. 0.70 g

44. Pharmaceutical compounding may involve which of the following ingredients?

a. Aquaphor

b. simple syrup

c. coal tar

d. all of the above

45. A patient calls the pharmacy asking why his heart medication is white instead of the usual yellow color. Upon investigation, you learn that the prescription was filled with 0.25 mg digoxin instead of the 0.125 mg strength. Which of the following is the most appropriate action to take?

a. Tell the patient to cut the tablets in half and take one-half tablet daily.

b. Ask the patient to bring the prescription back to the pharmacy so that you can secretly exchange it for the correct dose.

c. Explain the situation to the pharmacist, correct the error, and document the error per procedures.

d. Prepare a new prescription with the 0.125 mg strength and inform the patient that pharmacists are solely responsible for the accuracy of prescriptions.

46. Position or job descriptions:

a. are the same for technicians from hospital to hospital.

b. are written descriptions outlining employee responsibilities.

c. are the same for pharmacists and technicians.

d. apply only to upper-level hospital managers.

47. Which of the following reasons corresponds to why it is important to follow established policies and procedures at your institution or company to prevent medication errors?

a. Policies and procedures formally establish a system to prevent the occurrence of medication errors.

b. It is important to follow policies and procedures for good performance in your position.

c. Policies and procedures are a good resource when you are confronted with an unusual request by a patient.

d. Patients usually ask the technicians if policies and procedures are followed in the institution or company.

48. A technician reading a medication order for a patient notices an abbreviation with which she is not familiar. Which of the following are acceptable ways to clarify the meaning of the abbreviation?

a. Call the prescriber and ask the meaning of the abbreviation.

b. Ask the pharmacist the meaning of the abbreviation.

c. Refer to the lists of approved abbreviations in the policy and procedure manual.

d. Both b and c.

49. A physician calls the pharmacy asking about the maximum dose of a new medication. The technician answering the phone remembers hearing the pharmacist answer this question earlier that same day. How should the technician handle this call?

a. Inform the physician that the maximum dose is 500 mg twice daily, because that was the dose the pharmacist described earlier that day.

b. Ask another technician and relay the information to the physician.

c. Look up the answer to the question in *Drug Facts and Comparisons* and inform the physician.

d. Refer the question to the pharmacist.

50. A prescription with directions to be given a.d. should be administered to:
    a. both eyes.
    b. the left eye.
    c. the right ear.
    d. the left ear.

51. The usual dose of milk of magnesia is 30 cc. This is equivalent to:
    a. 3 Tbsp.
    b. 3 tsp.
    c. 1 tsp.
    d. 2 Tbsp.

52. Which vaccine has to be stored frozen before use?
    a. oral polio
    b. injectable polio
    c. influenza
    d. pneumococcal

53. If a product is labeled to expire 8/05, what is the last date it should be used by?
    a. 8/01/05
    b. 9/01/05
    c. 7/31/05
    d. 8/31/05

54. The only type of insulin that may be added to an IV solution is:
    a. isophane insulin.
    b. regular insulin.
    c. NPH insulin.
    d. extended insulin zinc.

55. Which agent is not used for the treatment of tuberculosis?
    a. pyrazinamide
    b. rifampin
    c. ethambutol
    d. vinblastine

56. Refill limitations for a Schedule III controlled substance prescription are:
    a. maximum of five refills and not more than six months after date of issuance.
    b. maximum of five refills and not more than one year after date of issuance.
    c. maximum of ten refills and not more than six months after date of issuance.
    d. maximum of ten refills and not more than one year after date of issuance.

57. Which cytotoxic drug does not require refrigeration?
    a. vinblastine
    b. cyclophosphamide
    c. asparaginase
    d. carmustine

58. The set of procedures for preparation of sterile products that is designed to prevent contamination is called:
    a. eutectic mixing.
    b. filtration.
    c. trituration.
    d. aseptic technique.

59. An example of a drug used as an anticonvulsant is:
    a. aspirin.
    b. levothyroxine.
    c. phenobarbital.
    d. lithium.

60. Which of the following statements is true regarding quality?
    a. Quality control is a process of checks and balances.
    b. Quality is defined by what our customers perceive.
    c. Quality improvement is an important part of meeting regulatory agency (such as JCAHO) requirements.
    d. All of the above.

61. Triazolam would most likely be ordered as:
    a. tid prn.
    b. bid.
    c. qAM.
    d. qHS prn.

62. Cortisporin is ordered "a.u." Which of the following medications should be dispensed?
    a. otic suspension
    b. ophthalmic solution
    c. topical ointment
    d. ophthalmic ointment

63. The reasons why a technician should always refer patients with medication or health-related questions to a pharmacist include:
    a. the possibility of drug-drug interaction.
    b. the possibility of drug-disease state interaction.
    c. the need for physician referral.
    d. all of the above.

64. A type of reimbursement whereby a pharmacy receives a predetermined amount of money for a defined group of patients regardless of the number of prescriptions filled is:
    a. fee-for-service.
    b. co-payment.
    c. capitation.
    d. no payment.

65. Typical data collected from the patient at the prescription take-in window include:

    a. weight for children and infants.

    b. allergies.

    c. emergency phone numbers.

    d. all of the above.

66. If a patient is noted to have experienced an allergic reaction to a medication, the technician should:

    a. tell the patient that the doctor made a mistake, and refuse to fill the prescription.

    b. tell the patient to take the medication anyway, because the doctor ordered it.

    c. ask the patient the type of allergic reaction experienced, note the patient's response, and alert the pharmacist.

    d. none of the above.

67. If a prescription is written generically and is marked "may not substitute":

    a. a generic drug can usually be dispensed (state law may vary).

    b. the specific brand-name drug must be dispensed because the prescription is marked "may not substitute."

    c. send the patient back to the physician's office for clarification.

    d. none of the above.

68. Endocarditis is an infection involving which part of the body?

    a. bone

    b. heart

    c. joint

    d. skin

69. Three fluid ounces is equal to _____ mL.

    a. 120

    b. 90

    c. 100

    d. 150

70. Fentanyl has a concentration of 0.05 mg/mL. How many milliliters do you need for a 950 μg dose?

    a. 190 mL

    b. 0.19 mL

    c. 19 mL

    d. 1.9 mL

71. According to most insurance coverage, if a prescription is written for a brand-name product and "may substitute" is marked on it:

    a. the brand-name drug must be dispensed.

    b. the generic drug must be dispensed.

    c. the generic drug can be dispensed if the patient and the pharmacist agree.

    d. the prescription is written incorrectly.

72. The last step in the prescription-processing function is:

    a. computer data entry.

    b. prescription filling.

    c. dispensing.

    d. compounding.

73. During prescription computer entry, the technician is responsible for all of the following except:

    a. entering accurate patient demographic information.

    b. entering any allergies the patient reports.

    c. handling insurance claims messaging.

    d. handling drug interaction messaging.

74. The computer error message "refill too soon" indicates that:

    a. the patient is attempting to get the prescription earlier than the "days supply" indicated.

    b. the pharmacy should not refill the prescription under any circumstances.

    c. both a and b.

    d. none of the above.

75. You receive an order for amoxicillin suspension (125 mg/5 mL) with a dose of 250 mg tid for 10 days. How many milliliters do you need to dispense?

    a. 300 mL

    b. 150 mL

    c. 100 mL

    d. 120 mL

76. When receiving a drug-drug, drug-disease state, or drug-allergy interaction computer message, the technician should:

    a. inform the patient that the prescription cannot be filled.

    b. alert the doctor to the mistake.

    c. ignore the message if the technician has seen the interaction before.

    d. alert the pharmacist to the problem.

77. All of the following drugs are antidotes except:

    a. activated charcoal.

    b. Digibind.

    c. cefazolin.

    d. naloxone.

78. Which of the following is not required on a prescription label?

    a. the prescription number

    b. directions on how to take the medication

c. the prescribing physician's name

d. the physician's DEA number

79. The sterile parts of a syringe that may never be touched are the:

a. plunger and barrel.

b. tip and plunger.

c. barrel and hub.

d. tip and hub.

80. The advantage of using a vertical laminar airflow hood in preparing chemotherapy medication is:

a. there is no advantage.

b. contaminated air is not blown at the operator.

c. the vertical airflow hood provides a better sterile environment than horizontal airflow hoods.

d. horizontal airflow hoods are to be used in preparing chemotherapy medications.

81. Which of the following medications must be protected from light?

a. amphotericin B

b. heparin

c. tobramycin

d. lanoxin

82. All of the following medications must be stored in the refrigerator, but not frozen, except:

a. tetanus toxoid.

b. insulin.

c. tobramycin.

d. nitroglycerin.

83. Which of the following is not commonly treated in the home care environment?

a. sepsis

b. osteomyelitis

c. chronic pain

d. malnutrition

84. All of the following medications must be prepared in a vertical laminar airflow hood except:

a. cisplatin.

b. cyclophosphamide.

c. cefotaxime.

d. etoposide.

85. All of the following drugs are laxatives except:

a. bisacodyl tablets.

b. Citrucel powder.

c. FiberCon tablets.

d. Pancrease capsules.

86. Examples of quality control measures utilized when preparing an IVPB include:

a. pulling the drug from the shelf and double-checking to ensure that the vial is correct.

b. calculating the correct dose and volume to withdraw from the vial to ensure that the vial is correct.

c. checking the IVPB for particulate matter after injecting the medication.

d. all of the above.

87. All of the following drugs are scheduled narcotics except:

a. Vicodin tablets.

b. Seconal capsules.

c. Duragesic patches.

d. Toradol tablets.

88. The concentration of tobramycin is 80 mg/2 mL. An order is written for 130 mg of tobramycin in 100 mL NS. How many milliliters of tobramycin do you inject into the IVPB bag?

a. 0.325 mL

b. 3.25 mL

c. 1.625 mL

d. 16.25 mL

89. A 1,000 mL bag of Ringer's lactate is to infuse over 8 hr. What is the flow rate of the infusion?

a. 62.5 mL/hr

b. 12.5 mL/hr

c. 6.25 mL/hr

d. 125 mL/hr

90. Schedule II narcotic prescriptions may be refilled how many times?

a. 6

b. 1

c. 0

d. 12

91. A bulk vial of cefazolin indicates an expiration date of May 2005. Which of the following statements is true regarding the use of this cefazolin vial?

a. The vial may be used for up to one year after the printed expiration date.

b. The vial must be used by May 1, 2005.

c. The vial can be used through the last day of May 2005.

d. The vial may be used for up to six months after the printed expiration date.

92. A patient is receiving Timentin 3.1 g q6 hr via a CADD Plus pump at home. Which of the following information is mandatory on a label in the home care setting?

a. patient name

b. prescription serial number

c. drug name

d. all of the above

93. Routine practice for clean rooms includes washing the walls at least how often?

    a. weekly

    b. daily

    c. monthly

    d. semiannually

94. You receive an order to prepare 250 mg of dobutamine in a 100 mL CADD cassette with NS as the diluent. Dobutamine is available as a 12.5 mg/mL solution. How many milliliters of dobutamine do you need to prepare this prescription?

    a. 20 mL

    b. 40 mL

    c. 200 mL

    d. 400 mL

95. Because of incompatibility concerns, which of the following additives should be added first to a total-nutrient admixture that will contain calcium gluconate?

    a. sodium chloride

    b. magnesium sulfate

    c. potassium acetate

    d. potassium phosphate

96. You are asked to make fluorouracil 4,000 mg in 1,000 mL of sodium chloride 0.9%. What auxiliary label should be placed on the prepared admixture?

    a. Protect from light

    b. Caution: Federal law prohibits the transfer of this drug to any person other than the patient for whom it was prescribed

    c. Chemotherapy/biohazard

    d. Administer with food or milk

97. A pharmacy technician is preparing heparin 25,000 units in 500 mL of dextrose 5% in water. The appropriate concentration on the label should read:

    a. 100 units/mL

    b. 125 units/mL

    c. 75 units/mL

    d. 50 units/mL

98. The pharmacist asks you to check the compatibility of parenteral phenytoin with sodium chloride 0.9%. Which reference would you select to find this information?

    a. *Handbook of Injectable Drugs*

    b. *Remington's Pharmaceutical Sciences*

    c. *Medication Teaching Manual: The Guide to Patient Drug Information*

    d. none of the above

99. In which of the following functions may a well-trained technician participate?

    a. documenting investigational drug use

    b. preparing chemotherapeutic agents

    c. purchasing and inventory control

    d. all of the above

100. Checking the temperature of a refrigerator that stores medications on a daily basis is all of the following except:

    a. an example of a quality-control mechanism used to meet JCAHO requirements.

    b. a method to assure proper storage of medications and avoid waste.

    c. a mechanism to satisfy a paperwork quota set by the pharmacy director.

    d. all of the above.

Glossary

absorption the process by which a drug is moved from the site of administration into the bloodstream.

Acceptable Macronutrient Distribution Range (AMDR) the range of intake levels that provide adequate amount of a nutrient and are associated with a reduced risk of disease.

acidosis excessive acid in the body fluids.

acne a bacterial infection accompanied by an overproduction of sebum.

addiction a pattern of compulsive substance abuse characterized by a continued psychological and physiological craving or need for the substance and its effects.

adipose fat.

adjudication the process of transmitting a prescription electronically to the proper insurance company or third-party biller for approval and billing.

adjuvant helping or assisting.

adulterated altered and causing an undesirable effect.

adverse effects undesirable and potentially harmful drug effects.

aerobic requires oxygen for life.

afferent sending an impulse toward the CNS.

agonist a type of drug that activates the receptor to produce a predicted action.

allegation a principle relating to the solution of questions concerning the compounding or mixing of different ingredients.

allergen a substance capable of causing a hypersensitivity reaction.

allergy the result of the immune system's reaction to a foreign substance.

ambulatory pharmacy community-based pharmacy; includes chain retail drugstores, grocery store pharmacies, home health care, mail-order facilities, and other pharmacies from which patients can obtain medications without living onsite.

anaerobic does not require oxygen for life.

anhydrous without water.

antagonist a type of drug that prevents receptor activation.

antibodies proteins that specifically seek and bind to the surface of pathogens or antigens.

antigens specific molecules that trigger an immune response.

antineoplastics agents, such as medications, that prevent the growth of malignant cells.

antioxidant molecule that slows or prevents the oxidation of other molecules.

anxiety a mental state characterized by apprehension and uneasiness stemming from the anticipation of danger.

anxiolytic a drug used in the treatment of anxiety.

apothecary Latin term for pharmacist; also used as a general term to refer to the early practice of pharmacy.

apothecary system an old English system of measurement of weight, based on the grain.

applications software programs designed to perform specific functions, such as creating databases, spreadsheets, e-mail, or graphics, or performing word processing.

aqueous containing water; water-soluble.

aromatic having a strong or fragrant smell (aroma).

arterioles the smallest arteries.

aseptic technique the process of performing a procedure under controlled conditions in a manner that minimizes the chance of contamination of the preparation.

association a group of individuals who voluntarily form an organization to accomplish a common purpose.

asthma a respiratory disease characterized by wheezing, shortness of breath, and bronchoconstriction.

asymptomatic showing no evidence of disease or disordered condition.

atrioventricular valves include the tricuspid and mitral valves of the heart.

attire clothing.

attitude a way of acting, thinking, or believing.

autonomy the condition or quality of being independent.

avoirdupois system the current American system of measurement of weight, based on a pound being equivalent to 16 ounces.

bactericidal kills microorganisms.

bacteriostatic inhibits the growth and/or reproduction of microorganisms.

bench (countertop) model a horizontal laminar flow hood that sits on top of a counter; the space underneath it can be used for storage.

beneficence the quality of being kind or charitable.

bevel the sharp, pointed, diagonally cut end of a needle.

bilirubin substance produced by the breakdown of hemoglobin.

bioavailability the degree to which a drug becomes available to body tissue(s) after administration.

biological safety cabinet a vertical laminar flow hood used to provide protection for the worker, the work environment, and the drug.

biologics a group of varied medicinal products, such as vaccines, blood products, allergenics, and proteins.

biometrics technology that measures and analyzes human body characteristics, such as fingerprints, for authentication purposes.

biopharmaceuticals substances created using biotechnology.

biopharmacology branch of pharmacology that studies the use of biologically engineered drugs.

biotechnology the use of biological substances or microorganisms to perform specific functions, such as the production or modification of drugs, hormones, or food products.

blepharitis inflammation of the eyelid margins accompanied by redness.

blister packs unit-dose packages.

bone marrow the spongy type of tissue found inside most bones; responsible for the manufacture of red blood cells, some white blood cells, and platelets. Also acts as storage area for fat.

bones specialized form of dense connective tissue consisting of calcified intercellular substance that provides the shape and support for the body. Bones are made of calcium and phosphate. Injuries can result in fractures.

buffer capacity the ability of a solution to resist a change in pH when either an acidic or an alkaline substance is added to the solution.

capsule a solid dosage form in which the active ingredient and any excipients are enclosed in a soluble gelatin shell that will dissolve in the stomach.

carcinoma malignant tumor.

carrier/insurer/provider the insurance company.

cartilage soft tissues that line every joint and give shape to the ears and nose. Injuries can result in tears or degeneration of the cartilage and arthritis.

cassette systems drug containers that can hold hundreds or thousands of tablets and are affixed to a counting machine.

cataract an ocular opacity or obscurity in the lens of the eye.

cellulitis   inflammation of the connective tissue of the skin.

Celsius (centigrade)   international unit of measurement for temperature.

central nervous system (CNS)   the part of the nervous system made up of the brain and spinal cord.

central processing unit (CPU)   the brain of a computer system; it interprets commands, connects the various hardware components, runs software applications, and controls speed and use of memory space.

centralized pharmacy system   system in which all pharmacy-related activities are performed from one location and medications are delivered to various patient care units throughout the facility.

cerebrospinal fluid (CSF)   the fluid surrounding the brain and spinal cord.

certification   recognition granted by a nongovernmental agency attesting that an individual has met the required levels of competency.

certified nursing assistant (CNA)   an individual who is certified to assist RNs and LPNs in providing patient care, but is not permitted to administer medication.

certified pharmacy technician (CPhT)   an individual who is certified to assist pharmacists in providing pharmaceutical care, but is not permitted to dispense medication or counsel patients; certification is achieved by passing a national certification exam.

chain pharmacy   a retail, or ambulatory, pharmacy that is owned by a corporation operating multiple pharmacy facilities at various locations.

channel   a gesture, action, sound, written or spoken word, or visual image used in transmitting information.

chemotherapy   drug therapy used to treat cancer and other diseases.

chronic obstructive pulmonary disease (COPD)   a condition resulting from continual blockage of oxygen exchange in the lungs; an umbrella term for emphysema and chronic bronchitis.

chyme   the liquid that food turns into before it passes into the small intestine.

cilia   the tiny hair-like organelles found in the nose and bronchial passageways.

civil law   Any law dealing with the rights of private citizens.

claim   a request for reimbursement, for products or services rendered, from a healthcare provider to an insurance provider.

Clark's Rule   formula for solving pediatric dosage calculations based on the patient's weight in pounds.

class 100 environment   the classification of an airflow unit capable of producing an environment containing no more than 100 airborne particles of a size 0.5 micron or larger, per cubic foot of air.

clearance   the time it takes a drug to be eliminated from the body.

combining form   a root word with an added vowel.

comminuting   the process of reducing the particle size of a substance by grinding; also known as trituration.

common fractions   fractions written with a numerator that is separated by a fraction line and positioned above a denominator.

community pharmacy   name commonly used for an ambulatory or retail pharmacy.

compassion   a deep awareness of and sympathy for another's suffering.

complement   a large group of proteins that are activated in sequence when cells are exposed to a foreign substance; activation eventually results in the death or destruction of the substance. In general, complements amplify or enhance the effects of antibodies and inflammation.

complex fraction   a fraction in which both the numerator and the denominator are themselves common fractions.

compounding   the practice of extemporaneously preparing medications to meet the unique need of an individual patient according to the specific order of a prescriber; producing, mixing, or preparing a drug by combining two or more ingredients.

concentration   term for the strength of active pharmaceutical ingredient in a medication.

conjunctivitis   acute or chronic inflammation of the eye conjunctiva.

consequentialism   the theory that the value of an action derives solely from the value of its consequences.

console model   a horizontal laminar flow hood that sits on the floor.

context   the setting, or circumstances, in which communication occurs.

contraception   birth control.

contractility   the ability to contract; also, the degree of contraction.

contracts   written agreements.

co-pay   a portion of the cost of a service or product that a patient pays out of pocket each time it is provided.

correctional facilities   more commonly referred to as prisons; places in which individuals are physically confined and usually deprived of a range of personal freedoms.

corticosteroid   steroidal hormones produced in the adrenal cortex.

counseling   the process of providing patients and customers with pharmaceutical and general health-related advice; provided only by registered pharmacists or doctors of pharmacy.

counting machines   electronic devices that automatically and precisely count capsules and tablets, based on weight.

criminal law   any law dealing with crime or punishment.

cross-multiplication   a principle used in solving pharmacy calculations; you set up two ratios or fractions in relationship to each other as a proportion and solve for the unknown variable.

cycloplegic   causing relaxation and paralysis of the intraocular muscles.

cytotoxic   poisonous or destructive to cells.

databases   lists of information, ordered in specific ways.

DAW   instructions from the prescriber to "dispense as written," without generic substitution.

days supply   the expected duration for a prescription being dispensed; how long the amount of medication dispensed will last if taken as directed.

decentralized pharmacy system   pharmacy service system consisting of a central, or inpatient, pharmacy and multiple satellite pharmacies, as well as an outpatient pharmacy.

decimal fractions   fractions written as a whole number with a zero and a decimal point in front of the value.

deductible   a set amount that a client pays up front before insurance coverage applies.

deep venous thrombosis (DVT)   a blood clot in one of the veins of the legs or other deep veins.

defendant   the party against which a legal action is brought.

defense mechanisms   unconscious mental processes used to protect one's ego.

denial   a defense mechanism characterized by refusal to acknowledge painful realities, thoughts, or feelings.

denominator   the bottom value of a fraction; placed beneath the fraction line.

dependency   the state of being dependent.

depression   a mental state characterized by lack of energy, feelings of despair, guilt, and misery, and changes in sleep pattern and eating habits.

dialysis   a medical procedure that removes waste from the blood of patients with renal failure.

diction   clarity and distinctness of pronunciation in speech.

Dietary Reference Intakes (DRI)   nutritional guidelines that include both recommended intakes and tolerable upper intake levels.

diluent   a substance used to dilute another substance.

"dispense as written" (DAW)   notation by the prescriber instructing the pharmacy to use the exact drug written (usually brand).

dispensing quantity   the total amount of medication to be dispensed.

displacement   a defense mechanism in which there is an unconscious shift of emotions, affect, or desires from the original object to a more acceptable or immediate substitute.

distribution   the process by which an absorbed drug is moved from the bloodstream to body tissues or receptors.

DNA   deoxyribonucleic acid; a nucleic acid that carries genetic information and is capable of self-replication and synthesis of RNA.

doctor of medicine (MD)   a licensed individual, trained to examine patients, diagnose illnesses, and prescribe and administer medication.

doctor of osteopathy (DO)   a licensed individual, trained to examine patients, diagnose illnesses, and prescribe and administer treatments using manipulative techniques on the musculoskeletal system in conjunction with conventional treatments.

doctor of pharmacy (PharmD)   an individual who has completed a doctoral degree in pharmacy and is licensed to practice pharmacy in a specific state.

dosage calculations   pharmacy calculations pertaining to the number of doses, dispensing quantities, and/or ingredient quantities.

dosage form   the actual form of the drug (tablet, capsule, suppository, solution, etc.); also called dosage formulation.

dose   the amount of medication prescribed to be taken at one time.

drop factor   an abbreviated form referring to a specific drip rate.

drops per minute (gtts/min)   the volume of medication to be administered each minute.

drug-drug interaction   an interaction between two or more drugs administered to a patient, resulting in either an increase or a decrease in the therapeutic effects of one or more of the drugs, or an adverse effect.

drug of choice (DOC)   the drug preferred for treatment of a particular condition or disease.

drug per hour (mg/hr)   the dosage, or amount of medication in milligrams, that will be administered per hour of infusion.

dyscrasia   an abnormal condition of the body, especially a blood imbalance.

eczema   an inflammatory skin condition characterized by itching, redness, blistering, and oozing.

edema   swelling.

efferent   sending impulses away from the CNS.

electroencephalogram (EEG)   a graphic record of the electrical activity of the brain.

emergency medication order   a specific type of STAT order for a medication that is required for a physician to be able to respond to a medical emergency.

empathy   a feeling of concern and understanding for another's situation or feelings.

emollient   softening and soothing to the skin.

emulsion   a suspension that consists of two immiscible liquids and an emulsifying agent to hold them together; liquid mixture of water and oil.

endometrium   the lining of the uterus.

epiglottis   the small, leaf-shaped cartilage attached to the tongue that prevents substances other than air from entering the trachea.

epitope   a region on the surface of an antigen that is capable of producing an immune response.

ethics   a system of principles and duties; often associated with a profession.

excipient   any substance added to a prescription to confer a suitable consistency or form to the drug.

excretion   the process by which drugs are eliminated from the body; usually occurs through urine, feces, or the respiratory system.

exogenous   from outside the organism.

expired drugs   drugs that have not been dispensed as of the manufacturer's printed expiration date.

Fahrenheit   American unit of measurement for temperature.

feedback   the return of information, or a message, in the communication process.

felony   a serious crime, such as rape or murder.

fidelity   faithfulness to obligations and duties.

floor stock   distribution system in which medications are kept on each floor for distribution to patients.

flow rate duration   length of time for which an IV will be administered, or how long an IV bag will last before it must be changed.

flow rates   a term used to describe a number of common pharmacy calculations used in the preparation of IV infusions.

formulary   a listing of drugs approved for specific uses or for reimbursement.

fortified   with an added nutrient for enrichment.

fraction line   symbol representing the division of two values; placed between the numerator and the denominator of a fraction.

franchise pharmacy   a retail, or ambulatory, pharmacy that consists of facilities at multiple locations, although each pharmacy may be separately owned.

Fried's Rule   formula for solving pediatric dosage calculations based on the patient's age in months.

front end   the over-the-counter (OTC) section of a retail pharmacy.

Gaucher's disease   disease in which fatty materials collect in the liver, spleen, kidneys, lungs, and brain and cause the person to be susceptible to infections.

genetically modified organism (GMO)   an organism whose genetic material has been altered using the genetic engineering techniques known as recombinant DNA technology.

geometric dilution   technique of starting with the ingredient of the smallest amount and doubling the portion by adding the other ingredients, in order of quantity, until fully mixed.

geriatric   refers to persons over the age of 65.

glaucoma   a group of eye diseases characterized by an increase in intraocular pressure.

gonads   testes and ovaries.

grain   the primary unit of weight in the apothecary system.

gram   metric system's primary unit of weight.

gray matter   a major component of the nervous system, composed of nonmyelinated nerve tissue with a gray-brown color.

group purchasing system   a purchasing system in which a pharmacy joins a group purchasing organization (GPO), which contracts with pharmaceutical manufacturers collectively for all members of that GPO.

half-life   the time required for serum concentration levels of an absorbed and distributed drug to decrease by one-half.

hard drive   the main storage device of a computer; can be either external or internal.

hardware   the mechanical and electrical components that make up a computer system.

health maintenance organization (HMO)   a type of health care/insurance plan.

health-system pharmacy   classification of pharmacy setting in which patients reside onsite at the facility where the pharmacy is located (such as hospitals, nursing homes, and long-term care facilities).

hematopoiesis   the formation and development of blood cells.

hematopoietic   blood-forming.

hematuria   blood in the urine.

HEPA   a high-efficiency particulate air filter; used in flow hoods.

high-density lipoprotein (HDL)   good cholesterol.

homeostasis   a stable and constant environment.

homogenous   having all the same qualities within a group.

hordeolum   an infection of one (or more) of the sebaceous glands of the eye.

hormone   a chemical substance, produced by an organ or gland, that travels through the bloodstream to regulate certain bodily functions and/or the activity of other organs and glands.

hospice   provides palliative care (care designed to help ease suffering) and supportive services to individuals at the end of their lives.

hospital pharmacy the most common type of health-system pharmacy; a pharmacy located within a hospital facility serving patients who have been admitted or are being discharged.

household system the measurement system commonly used by Americans for general measuring and cooking.

humor a body fluid.

hydrophobic repels water.

hyperlipidemia high concentrations of lipids in the blood.

hypermetabolic metabolizing at an increased rate.

hyperplasia the reproduction of cells within an organ at an increased rate.

hypersensitivity allergy.

hypertension high blood pressure.

hypertonic solutions solutions that have greater osmotic pressure than cell contents. Hypertonic solutions cause cells to dehydrate and shrink.

hypotension abnormally low blood pressure.

hypotonic solutions solutions that have a lower osmotic pressure than cell contents. Hypotonic solutions cause cells to take on water and expand.

improper fraction a fraction in which the value of the numerator is larger than the value of the denominator.

independent purchasing system a purchasing system in which the pharmacy establishes contracts directly with each pharmaceutical manufacturer.

infant child between the ages of 1 month and 2 years.

infection invasion of pathogens into the body; an infection occurs when a pathogenic microbe is able to multiply in the tissues (colonize).

inflection alteration in pitch or tone of the voice.

infusion a relatively large volume of solution given at a constant rate.

inpatient pharmacy (IP) portion of a facility that is responsible for medication packaging, centralized inventory, sterile product preparation, and the preparation and delivery of medication carts. It provides pharmaceutical services to patients admitted to a facility.

input devices hardware that allows information, or data, to be entered into a computer system.

institutional pharmacy a pharmacy found in places such as hospitals, long-term-care facilities, extended-living facilities, and retirement homes, which require patients to reside onsite.

intellectualization a defense mechanism used to protect oneself from the emotional stress and anxiety associated with confronting painful personal fears or problems; characterized by excessive reasoning.

International Units (IU) measurement of a drug in terms of its action, not its physical weight.

intradermal parenteral injection in the dermis of the skin.

intramuscular (IM) within or into a muscle; parenteral injection in the muscle.

intraocular within the eye.

intrathecal parenteral injection in the spine.

intravenous parenteral injection in the vein.

investigational medication order an order for medication used in facilities that participate in research programs.

iridotomy an incision made in the iris of the eye to enlarge the pupil.

isotonic containing the same tonicity concentration as red blood cells.

isotonic solutions solutions that have an osmotic pressure equal to that of cell contents.

IV admixture a mixture of a solution and drug(s) prepared aseptically to be administered via a vein.

IV infusion a compounded solution that provides fluids, specific medications, nutrients, electrolytes, and minerals to a patient.

joint the location or position where bones are connected to each other. A joint contains synovial fluid and cartilage.

justice the principle of moral rightness and equity.

Kegel exercises pelvic muscle training and toning exercises.

ketone a by-product of fat metabolism.

keyboard the primary input device of a computer system, used to enter information (both alphabetic and numeric) into the computer.

kilocalories (kcal) unit of measurement for food energy.

laminar flow hood a device containing a HEPA filter; used for preparing sterile products.

larynx the voicebox.

leukocyte white blood cell.

licensed nursing assistant (LNA) an individual who is licensed to assist RNs and LPNs in providing patient care, but is not permitted to administer medication.

licensed practical nurse (LPN) an individual who is licensed to provide basic care, such as administering medication, under the supervision of a registered nurse.

licensing permission granted by a government entity for an individual to perform an activity.

ligaments strong fibrous bands of connective tissue that hold bones together. Injuries can result in sprains.

lipid fat.

lipid-soluble dissolvable in fats; describes drugs that pass readily into cell membranes composed mostly of fatty substances, such as the brain.

liter metric system's primary unit of volume.

long-term care (LTC) facility facility that provides rehabilitative, restorative, or ongoing skilled nursing care to individuals who need assistance with activities of daily living.

low-density lipoprotein (LDL) bad cholesterol.

lozenge a solid dosage form administered orally to be dissolved in the mouth.

lumen the hollow space inside a needle.

lymphocyte type of white blood cell.

lysis the destruction of cells.

macrophage white blood cell, found primarily in connective tissue and the bloodstream.

malabsorption an abnormality in digestion that causes nutrients to be absorbed poorly or not at all.

mastication chewing.

Medicaid the health insurance program for individuals and families with low incomes or disabilities.

medical device any instrument or apparatus used in the diagnosis, prevention, monitoring, treatment, or alleviation of disease.

medical ethics principles and moral values of proper medical care.

medical malpractice the negligent treatment of a patient by a health-care professional.

Medicare the health insurance program for individuals aged 65 or older, younger people with disabilities, and people with end-stage renal disease.

medication order term for a patient prescription in a health system.

message the substance, or information, being transferred in communication.

metabolism chemical alteration of drugs, food, or foreign compounds in and by the body; the process of transforming drugs in the body; also known as biotransformation.

metabolite any substance produced by the metabolic process.

meter metric system's primary unit of length.

metric system the international and scientific standard system of measurement; based on the meter, the gram, and the liter.

mg/kg/day formula for solving dosage calculations based on the patient's weight in kilograms.

microdrip the most commonly used drip rate; 60 gtts/mL.

µg   microgram.

milliequivalent (mEq)   unit of measurement based on the number of grams of a drug in 1 mL of a normal solution.

misbranded drug   a drug that has been misleadingly or fraudulently labeled.

misdemeanor   an offense or infraction less serious than a felony.

mitigate   to lessen or decrease severity.

modem   hardware device used for connecting computer systems that are remotely located, via a telephone line or cable; can be installed either internally or externally.

monitor   the visual display screen of the computer system.

monocyte   type of white blood cell.

monograph   a detailed document pertaining to a specific drug.

monosaccharide   simplest form of carbohydrate (e.g., glucose, fructose).

mouse   a device that rolls on a hard, flat surface and controls the movement of the cursor, or pointer, on the screen.

mucopurulent   containing or composed of mucus and pus.

multiple sclerosis (MS)   a chronic, inflammatory disease of the white-matter areas of the brain and spinal cord in the central nervous system. In later stages of the disease, some level of permanent disability affects the patient.

muscle   specialized tissue that contracts when stimulated.

mydriatic   causing dilation of the pupil of the eye.

myocyte   a muscle cell.

narcolepsy   a condition characterized by frequent and uncontrolled periods of deep sleep.

National Drug Code (NDC) number   a unique identifying number assigned to each drug by the manufacturer.

negative feedback   the process by which the body is able to return to homeostasis.

neighborhood pharmacy   an independent pharmacy that is privately owned, small in size, and usually fills an average of 100 to 300 prescriptions per day.

neonate   child from birth to 1 month of age.

neutropenia   disease in which there is an abnormal number of the white blood cells that are responsible for fighting infections.

nomenclature   set of names; way of naming.

noncompliance   when a patient does not follow a prescribed drug regimen.

nonconsequentialism   the theory that certain actions, in and of themselves, are wrong.

nonverbal communication   the imparting or interchanging of thoughts, opinions, or information without the use of spoken words.

numerator   the top value of a fraction; placed above the fraction line.

nurse practitioner (NP)   an individual who is licensed to work closely with a physician in providing patient care, and typically may prescribe medications under the supervision of a physician.

nursing home   facility that provides skilled and custodial care to older Americans who do not need the intensive, acute care of a hospital but who can no longer manage independent living.

occlusive   closing or blocking; refers to a substance that closes or covers a wound and keeps the air from reaching the wound.

ointment   a semisolid topical preparation that is applied to the skin or mucous membranes.

oleaginous   containing oil; having oil-like properties.

oocyte   an immature egg.

operating system   the primary software program used to connect the various hardware components of a computer and allow them to perform their essential functions.

ophthalmic   pertaining to the eye.

otic   for or of the ear.

otitis media   infection and inflammation of the middle ear.

outpatient pharmacy   a pharmacy that is available to patients who are being discharged from the hospital, or who are being treated by a physician without requiring overnight admission.

output devices   hardware devices that produce and release data in a visual or tangible, printed form.

ovaries   the female reproductive organs that produce eggs.

over-the-counter (OTC) products   medications and devices that do not require a prescription for purchase and use.

ovulation   the process in which the ovarian follicle ruptures and releases the egg.

ovum   a mature egg.

palliative   reducing the severity of symptoms.

parasite   an organism that lives on or inside another organism.

parenteral nutrition   complex admixtures used to provide nutritional support to patients who are unable to take in adequate nutrients through the gastrointestinal tract.

pathogen   disease-causing microorganism.

patient prescription stock system   a system in which medication orders are reviewed, prepared, and verified, and then the medications are taken to the floor and dispensed to the patient.

patient profile   an electronic record, stored in the pharmacy computer system, that details the patient's personal and billing information, prescription records, and medical conditions.

pepsin   digestive enzyme needed to break down food proteins.

pepsinogen   precursor to pepsin.

percent strength   representation of the number of grams of active ingredient contained in 100 mL.

% Volume/Volume (%v/v)   percent strength concentration of a liquid active ingredient contained within a liquid base.

% Weight/Volume (%w/v)   percent strength concentration of a solid active ingredient contained within a liquid base.

% Weight/Weight (%w/w)   percent strength concentration of a solid active ingredient contained within a solid base.

peripheral nervous system (PNS)   all parts of the nervous system excluding the brain and spinal cord.

personal digital assistant (PDA)   handheld electronic device that is battery powered and operates like a computer.

pH   the measure of acidity or alkalinity of a solution or substance; seven is the neutral point on this scale (less than seven is acidic and greater than seven is alkaline).

phagocyte   specialized cell that engulfs and ingests other cells.

pharmacist   educated, skilled individual licensed to practice pharmacy and dispense medication.

pharmacist in charge (PIC)   an individual designated on the records of the State Board of Pharmacy as the primary, onsite pharmacist.

pharmacodynamics   the study of the biochemical and physiologic effects of drugs and their mechanisms of action.

pharmacogenomics   the study of individual genetic differences in response to drug therapy.

pharmacokinetics   study of the processes of absorption, distribution, metabolism, and excretion of drugs; study of the time course of a drug and its metabolites in the body following drug administration.

pharmacology   the study of drugs.

pharmacopoeia   a compilation or listing of pharmaceutical products that also contains their formulas and methods of preparation.

pharmacy   the profession of preparing and dispensing medications, as well as supplying drug-related information to patients and consumers.

pharmacy clerk/cashier   a noncertified/unlicensed individual who is authorized to do only nonpharmacy-related tasks, such as operating the cash register.

pharmacy manager   an individual, almost always a pharmacist, who is appointed to supervise all aspects of the daily pharmacy operations.

pharmacy technician educated, skilled individual trained to work in a pharmacy, under the supervision of a pharmacist.

pharynx the part of the throat from the back of the nasal cavity to the larynx.

physician assistant (PA) a licensed individual who is trained to coordinate patient care under the supervision of a medical or osteopathic doctor.

piggyback bags minibags that hold 50 mL or 100 mL of solution and are used to administer drugs intermittently.

pigmentation color.

pitch the property of sound that is determined by the frequency of sound-wave vibrations reaching the ear.

plaintiff the party that initiates a legal action.

plaque fatty deposit that is high in cholesterol.

POE system a point-of-entry computer system, networked within the health system to allow prescribers and nurses to enter medication orders directly for the pharmacy; sometimes referred to as a computerized physician order entry (CPOE) system.

polydipsia ingestion of abnormally large amounts of fluids.

polyphagia excessive hunger or eating.

polypharmacy administration of more medications than clinically indicated.

polyuria excessive urination.

powder a solid dosage form made from blended active ingredients and excipients.

precipitate a solid that forms within a solution.

prefix a part of a word attached to the beginning of the root word that gives a specific meaning to the root.

prescription an order, by an authorized individual, for the preparation or dispensing of a medication.

priapism painful, extended-duration erection.

printer the primary output device of a computer system, used to produce paper documents.

PRN order a medication order used when a patient is to receive a medication only as necessary, as with pain medication.

processing components hardware devices used to organize, manage, and store data.

processor a company hired by the insurer to process claims.

profession an occupation that requires advanced education and training.

projection a defense mechanism whereby one's own attitudes, feelings, or suppositions are attributed to others.

pronunciation the manner in which someone utters a word.

proper fraction a fraction in which the value of the numerator is smaller than the value of the denominator.

proportion two, or more, equivalent ratios or fractions that both represent the same value.

protease enzyme that begins protein breakdown.

psoriasis a noncontagious, chronic skin disease characterized by rapid skin cell turnover resulting in thick, red, scaly skin.

psychotic refers to a mental state characterized by a loss of orientation to reality.

pulmonary edema fluid collection in the pulmonary vessels or lungs.

purchasing system an organization's strategy or procedure for obtaining medications, devices, and products.

quality assurance (QA) a program of activities used to ensure that the procedures used in the preparation of compounded products meet specific standards.

random-access memory (RAM) temporary memory used while information is being input into the computer.

rash a skin condition characterized by redness and inflammation.

ratio the expression of a relationship of two numbers, separated by a colon (:).

rationalization a defense mechanism whereby one's true motivation is concealed by explaining one's actions and feelings in a way that is not threatening.

reaction formation a defense mechanism characterized by action at the opposite extreme of one's true feelings, as overcompensation for unacceptable impulses.

read-only memory (ROM) permanent memory used for essential operating instructions for the computer system.

recall the process in which a drug manufacturer or the FDA requires that specific drugs or devices be returned to the manufacturer, because of a specific concern about the recalled product.

receiver the person to whom a communication message is sent.

receptor molecular structure located on the surface of the cell that binds with a particular chemical or chemicals. When a chemical binds with a receptor, the receptor is stimulated to either produce or inhibit a specific action.

registered nurse (RN) an individual who is registered to assist physicians with specific procedures, administer medications, and provide patient care.

registered pharmacist (RPh) an individual who has completed a bachelor's degree in pharmacy and is licensed to practice pharmacy in a specific state.

registration the process of listing, or being named to a list.

regression a defense mechanism characterized by reverting to an earlier or less mature pattern of feeling or behavior.

repression a defense mechanism characterized by the exclusion of painful impulses, desires, or fears from the conscious mind.

retinopathy a noninflammatory disease in which the retina of the eye is damaged.

rheumatoid arthritis autoimmune disease that causes chronic inflammation of the joints.

rhinitis inflammation of the nasal passages.

rhinorrhea runny nose.

RNA ribonucleic acid; a nucleic acid needed for the metabolic processes of protein synthesis. In viruses, RNA may carry the genetic information of the virus.

Roman numerals letters and symbols used to represent numbers.

root words words or parts of a word that identify the major meaning of a term.

rosacea a facial skin disorder accompanied by chronic redness and inflammation, and/or acne.

route of administration how a drug is introduced into or on the body.

Rx abbreviation for prescription.

sarcomere one of the segments into which a fibril of striated muscle is divided.

satellite pharmacies subunits of a central pharmacy, located near specific patient care areas in a facility, such as cardiology, operating rooms, and chemotherapy treatment centers.

scanner a hardware device used to input a photographic image into the computer system.

sebum oily substance produced by the sebaceous glands in the skin.

seizure a disturbance of brain activity characterized by changes in consciousness, activity, and sensation.

semilunar valves include the aortic and pulmonary valves of the heart.

semi-synthetic a naturally occurring compound that has been chemically altered.

sender the person who originates or imparts a communication message.

sexually transmitted disease (STD) a disease caused by a pathogen (virus, bacterium, parasite, or fungus) that is spread from person to person through sexual contact.

sexually transmitted infection (STI) a sexually transmitted disease.

side effects drug effects other than the intended one; usually undesirable but not harmful.

SIG   specific directions provided on a prescription for the patient to follow, such as dosages, schedule and frequency of administration, and additional instructions.

simple fraction   a proper fraction, with both the numerator and denominator reduced to lowest terms.

site of action   the location where a drug will exert its effect.

social contract   an understood agreement between individual members of a society.

software   the programs and applications that control the functioning of computer hardware and direct the operation of the computer.

specific gravity   a measure of the density of a substance as compared to water; the specific gravity of water is 1.

standing order   a medication order used when a patient is to receive a specific medication at specific intervals throughout the day; also called a scheduled order.

STAT order   a medication order used when a patient requires a medication immediately; this is an urgent order and thus takes priority over other orders and requests.

statute   a law, decree, or edict.

sterile   free from bacteria and other microorganisms.

store manager   an individual appointed to supervise all aspects of the daily store operations, including the pharmacy department.

stye   an infection of one (or more) of the sebaceous glands of the eye.

subcutaneous   parenteral injection in the skin.

sublimation   a defense mechanism in which unacceptable instinctual drives and wishes are modified to take more personally and socially acceptable forms.

sublingually   under the tongue; preparations may be administered by placing them under the tongue and allowing them to dissolve.

suffix   a part of a word attached to the end of the root word that gives a specific meaning to the root.

suppository   a solid dosage form used to administer medication by way of the rectum, vagina, or urethral tract.

suspension   liquid containing ingredients that are not soluble in the vehicle.

synovial fluid   liquid that fills the space between the cartilage of each bone; provides smooth movement by lubricating the cartilage.

synthesized   produced in a laboratory to imitate a naturally occurring compound.

synthetic   drugs that are not naturally occurring; produced in a laboratory.

tablet   a solid dosage form that may be administered orally, sublingually, vaginally, or under the skin.

target cell   general term referring to a large number of cells, all of which are similar, on which a particular drug is intended to act.

telepharmacy   the practice of using advanced telecommunications technology to provide pharmaceutical care to patients in rural and medically underserved areas from a distance.

tendons   cords of connective tissue that attach muscle to bone. Injuries can result in strains, ruptures, or inflammation.

teratogenic   causing congenital malformations (birth defects).

testes   The male reproductive organs that produce sperm.

thrombi   blood clots (singular, thrombus).

thrombophlebitis   inflammation of a vein with a thrombus.

tinnitus   ringing or buzzing in the ear that is not caused by an external source; may be caused by infection or a reaction to a drug.

tolerance   when a person requires (psychologically or physiologically) larger doses of a drug to achieve the same effect.

tonicity   a state of normal tension of the tissues by virtue of which the parts are kept in shape, alert, and able to function properly.

total parenteral nutrition (TPN)   a solution made to supply many of the body's basic nutritional needs via parenteral administration.

toxicity   drug poisoning; can be life-threatening or extremely harmful.

trachea   the windpipe.

transdermal gel   a gel that penetrates the skin and allows the active ingredient to be easily absorbed into the body; also known as a PLO gel.

transfer   situation in which the patient would like to have the prescription refilled at a pharmacy other than where it was originally delivered or filled.

transform   alter an organism or a cell itself in the genetic engineering process.

trituration   the process of reducing the particle size of a substance by grinding; also known as comminuting.

troche   interchangeable term for lozenge, but sometimes prepared in soft form.

type 1 diabetes mellitus   a metabolic disorder formerly called insulin-dependent diabetes mellitus (IDDM).

type 2 diabetes mellitus   a metabolic disorder formerly called noninsulin-dependent diabetes mellitus (NIDDM).

unit-dose   a distribution system in which each medication order is filled in the pharmacy in a way that provides each dose in a package ready to administer to the patient. Usually, not more than a 24-hour supply is dispensed at one time.

urobilinogen   substance produced by the breakdown of bilirubin.

vector   organism that does not itself cause disease, but spreads disease by distributing or carrying pathogens from one host to another.

venules   the smallest veins.

veracity   truthfulness; the quality of conforming with the truth.

verbal communication   the imparting or interchanging of thoughts, opinions, or information through the use of spoken words.

viscous   thick; almost jelly-like.

void   empty the bladder.

volatile   evaporates rapidly.

volume   the loudness of a communication.

volume per hour (mL/hr)   the amount of fluid, or solution, that will be administered to the patient intravenously per hour.

water-soluble   dissolvable in water; describes drugs that are composed mostly of water and can be excreted by the kidneys.

white matter   a major component of the CNS, composed of myelinated nerve tissue that is white in color.

written communication   the imparting or interchanging of thoughts, opinions, or information through the use of written words.

Young's Rule   formula for solving pediatric dosage calculations based on the patient's age in years.

Index